HEALTH CARE STATE RANKINGS
1995

Health Care in the 50 United States

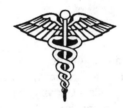

Kathleen O'Leary Morgan, Scott Morgan and Neal Quitno, Editors

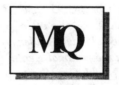

Morgan Quitno Press
© Copyright 1995, All Rights Reserved

P.O. Box 1656, Lawrence, KS 66044
800-457-0742 or 913-841-3534

3246432 (handwritten)

ISBN:
0-56692-302-6 (paper)
0-56692-306-9 (cloth)
ISSN: 1065-1403

Health Care State Rankings 1995 sells for $43.95 paper, $67.95 cloth. For those who prefer ranking information tailored to a particular state, we also offer Health Care State Perspectives, state-specific reports for each of the 50 states. These individual guides provide information on a state's data and rank for each of the categories featured in the national Health Care State Rankings volume. Perspectives sell for $18.00, $9.00 if ordered with Health Care State Rankings. If crime statistics are your interest, please ask about our annual Crime State Rankings ($43.95 paper, $67.95 cloth). If you are interested in city and metropolitan crime data, we offer City Crime Rankings for $19.95. If you are interested in a general view of the states, please ask about our annual State Rankings ($43.95 paper, $67.95 cloth). We also offer the data in our books on diskette (.dbf format).

Third Edition
Printed in the United States of America
May 1995

PREFACE

Concerns over the health care system in the United States have not gone away. While Congress and the President seem to have reached an impasse over how to better regulate the health care industry, problems with rising health care costs and delivery remain. Given this uncertainty, it is essential to have access to sound statistical information that provides nothing but straightforward health care facts.

This third edition of *Health Care State Rankings* provides a huge collection of objective, up-to-date statistics for numerous health care areas: insurance and finance, health care facilities, health care providers, incidence of disease, physical fitness, deaths, births and reproductive health. Data from a number of government and private sources are pulled together into one comprehensive health care reference guide.

Important Notes About *Health Care State Rankings*

This newest edition of *Health Care State Rankings* features some significant improvements from previous versions. Most notably, the format is quite different, with all categories now reported in both alphabetical and rank order. This way readers can quickly find data for their state and just as quickly discover which states rank above and below that state for a particular category. While the format has changed, many of the features that have made *Health Care State Rankings* so popular with readers and reviewers have not. Sources and other pertinent footnotes are shown at the bottom of each page. National totals, rates and percentages are prominently displayed at the top of each table. Every other line is shaded in gray for easier reading. In addition, numerous information finding tools are retained: a thorough table of contents, table listings at the beginning of each chapter, a roster of sources with addresses and phone numbers, a detailed index and a chapter thumb index all help to ease the search for data.

As in all of our reference books, the numbers shown in *Health Care State Rankings* are "complete," meaning that no additional calculations are required to convert them from millions, thousands, etc. All states are ranked on a high to low basis, with any ties among the states listed alphabetically for a given ranking. Negative numbers are shown in parentheses "( )." For tables with national totals (as opposed to rates, per capitas, etc.) a separate column is included showing what percent of the national total each individual state's total represents. This column is headed by "% of USA." This percentage figure is particularly interesting when compared with a state's share of the nation's population for a particular year.

For those interested in information for a particular state, we once again are offering our *Health Care State Perspective* series of publications. These 23-page comb bound reports feature data and ranking information for an individual state, pulled from the national *Health Care State Rankings* book. (For example *California Health Care in Perspective* features information about the state of California only.) They serve as handy, quick reference guides for those who do not want to page through the entire *Health Care State Rankings* volume searching for information for their particular state. When purchased by themselves, *Health Care State Perspectives* sell for $18. When purchased with a copy of *Health Care State Rankings*, these handy quick reference guides are just $9.

Other Books From Morgan Quitno Press

In addition to *Health Care State Rankings*, our company offers three other rankings reference books. The first of these, *State Rankings*, provides a general view of the states. Statistics are featured in a wide variety of categories including agriculture, transportation, government finance, health, crime, education, social welfare, energy and environment. In its sixth edition for 1995, this book has received great acclaim for its ease of use and simple presentation of state data.

Another popular state reference book is *Crime State Rankings*, an annual compilation of state crime data. Statistics on law enforcement personnel and expenditures, corrections, arrests and offenses are presented in an easy to use, instantly-understandable format. The second edition of this book, *Crime State Rankings 1995*, is now available. *Crime State Rankings* proved to be so popular in its first year that we have since launched a companion volume of crime data, *City Crime Rankings*. Making its debut in February of 1995, this newest reference book ranks U.S. metropolitan areas and 100 largest cities in all major crime categories. Numbers of crimes, crime rates, changes in crime rates over one and five years are presented for all major crime categories reported by the FBI.

The *City Crime Rankings* book sells for $19.95. The *State Rankings* and *Crime State Rankings* books each are available for $43.95 paper, $67.95 cloth. All of the data in our books is also available on diskette (.dbf format). If you would like a brochure or further information, please give us a call at 1-800-457-0742.

Finally, we want to thank the many librarians, government and health care industry officials who helped us in developing, designing and producing this book. Their suggestions and contributions of data are much appreciated. Thanks also to the many users of *Health Care State Rankings* who have made suggestions about how to improve the collection of data in the book. We appreciate those comments and encourage your input -- so please call or write us.

THE EDITORS

WHICH STATE IS HEALTHIEST?

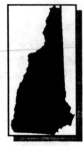 Each year we take a step back from our objective reporting of health statistics, throw some basic figures in to our computer and determine the Healthiest State. This year New Hampshire grabs the title as winner of the 1995 Healthiest State Award.

Based on the 23 categories listed below, the Granite State beat out its neighbor Vermont as well as Utah, Connecticut and Hawaii as the top of the top five healthiest states. Last year's winner, Minnesota, fell to a still healthy sixth. Ranking last for the second year in a row (with apologies to the Clintons) is Arkansas, preceded by Louisiana, Florida, Delaware and West Virginia.

Of course, the categories selected have a lot to do with the outcome of the award. A few factors used last year were replaced with what we believe to be more telling statistics. Overall, the factors chosen reflect affordability of health care, access to health care and a generally healthy population. All factors were given equal weight.

1995 HEALTHIEST STATE AWARD

RANK	STATE	AVG	'94	RANK	STATE	AVG	'94
1	New Hampshire	36.45	3	26	Colorado	24.30	13
2	Vermont	36.26	2	27	Illinois	24.13	32
3	Utah	34.48	6	28	Arizona	24.09	33
4	Connecticut	33.17	8	29	New Mexico	24.04	27
5	Hawaii	32.00	5	30	Ohio	23.87	29
6	Minnesota	31.91	1	31	Pennsylvania	23.70	28
7	Maine	31.45	17	32	Alabama	23.17	42
8	Iowa	30.39	21	33	Michigan	22.87	30
9	Idaho	30.18	13	33	New York	22.87	34
10	Virginia	30.17	22	35	North Carolina	22.61	36
11	Washington	30.04	7	35	Texas	22.61	37
12	Kansas	29.96	18	37	Georgia	22.26	39
13	Alaska	29.04	26	38	Nevada	21.91	45
13	Nebraska	29.04	4	39	Indiana	21.57	31
15	Massachusetts	28.91	9	40	Tennessee	21.17	41
16	Wisconsin	28.74	20	41	Kentucky	20.83	44
17	Oregon	28.04	15	42	Missouri	19.61	47
18	Maryland	27.70	19	43	South Carolina	19.57	35
19	California	27.61	23	44	Oklahoma	19.22	43
20	Wyoming	26.58	16	45	Mississippi	18.43	38
21	New Jersey	26.48	24	46	West Virginia	18.22	39
22	Rhode Island	26.30	11	47	Delaware	17.78	46
23	South Dakota	26.13	25	48	Florida	17.52	48
24	Montana	25.30	12	49	Louisiana	16.78	48
25	North Dakota	25.27	10	50	Arkansas	15.43	50

Once the factors were determined, we averaged each state's rankings for the 23 categories. Based on these averages, states were then ranked from "healthiest" (highest average ranking) to "least healthy" (lowest average ranking). States with no data available for a given category were assigned a zero for that category and ranked on the remaining factors. In our book, data are listed from highest to lowest. However, for purposes of this award, we inverted rankings for those factors we determined to be "positive." Thus the state with the highest rate of physicians in the book (ranking 1st) would be given a "50" for purposes of this award.

The table above shows how each state fared in the 1995 Healthiest State Award as well as its placement in 1994. We were pleased last year with the level of discussion generated by this award in many state capitals. We hope that such useful discussion will again result. Congratulations to the fine (and healthy) people of New Hampshire!

The Editors

POSITIVE (+) AND NEGATIVE (-) FACTORS CONSIDERED:
1. Births of Low Birthweight as a Percent of All Births (Table 15) -
2. Births to Teenage Mothers as a Percent of Live Births (Table 28) -
3. Percent of Receiving Late or No Prenatal Care (Table 50) -
4. Death Rate (Table 76) -
5. Infant Mortality Rate (Table 85) -
6. Death Rate by AIDS (Table 106) -
7. Estimated Death Rate by Cancer (Table 108) -
8. Death Rate by Suicide (Table 161) -
9. Percent of Population Not Covered by Health Insurance (Table 229) -
10. Change in Percent of Population Uninsured: 1991 to 1993 (Table 236) -
11. Per Capita Health Payments (Table 250) -
12. Percent of Average Family Income Spent on Health Care (Table 255) -
13. Estimated Rate of New Cancer Cases (Table 316) -
14. Combined Notifiable Disease Rate (Tables 341-380) -
15. Adult Apparent Per Capita Alcohol Consumption (Table 451) -
16. Percent of Adults Who Smoke (Table 460) -
17. Percent of Adults Overweight (Table 462) -
18. Number of Days in Past Month When Physical Health was "Not Good" (Table 463) -
19. Beds in Community Hospitals per 100,000 Population (Table 175) +
20. Community Hospitals per 1,000 Square Miles (Table 176) +
21. Percent of Kindergarteners Entering School in 1993 Who Were Fully Immunized at Age Two (Table 381) +
22. Rate of Nonfederal Physicians (Table 396) +
23. Safety Belt Usage Rate (Table 471) +

TABLE OF CONTENTS

I. Births and Reproductive Health

TABLE OF CONTENTS (continued)

Abortions

II. Deaths

TABLE OF CONTENTS (continued)

TABLE OF CONTENTS (continued)

III. Facilities

TABLE OF CONTENTS (continued)

IV. Finance

TABLE OF CONTENTS (continued)

V. Incidence of Disease

TABLE OF CONTENTS (continued)

VI. Personnel

TABLE OF CONTENTS (continued)

VII. Physical Fitness

TABLE OF CONTENTS (continued)

VIII. Appendix

IX. Sources

X. Index

I. BIRTHS AND REPRODUCTIVE HEALTH

1   Births in 1993
2   Birth Rate in 1993
3   Births in 1992
4   Birth Rate in 1992
5   Births in 1990
6   Birth Rate in 1990
7   Births in 1980
8   Birth Rate in 1980
9   Fertility Rate in 1992
10   Births to White Women in 1992
11   White Births as a Percent of All Births in 1992
12   Births to Black Women in 1992
13   Black Births as a Percent of All Births in 1992
14   Births of Low Birthweight in 1992
15   Births of Low Birthweight as a Percent of All Births in 1992
16   Births of Low Birthweight to White Women in 1992
17   Births of Low Birthweight to White Women as a Percent of All Births to White Women in 1992
18   Births of Low Birthweight to Black Women in 1992
19   Births of Low Birthweight to Black Women as a Percent of All Births to Black Women in 1992
20   Births to Unmarried Women in 1992
21   Births to Unmarried Women as a Percent of All Births in 1992
22   Births to Unmarried White Women in 1992
23   Births to Unmarried White Women as a Percent of All Births to White Women in 1992
24   Births to Unmarried Black Women in 1992
25   Births to Unmarried Black Women as a Percent of All Births to Black Women in 1992
26   Births to Teenage Mothers in 1992
27   Teenage Birth Rate in 1992
28   Births to Teenage Mothers as a Percent of Live Births in 1992
29   Pregnancy Rate for 15 to 19 Year Old Women in 1990
30   Births to Teenage Mothers in 1990
31   Teenage Birth Rate in 1990
32   Births to Teenage Mothers in 1980
33   Teenage Birth Rate in 1980
34   Percent Change in Teenage Birth Rate: 1980 to 1990
35   Births to White Teenage Mothers in 1992
36   Births to White Teenage Mothers as a Percent of White Births in 1992
37   Births to Black Teenage Mothers in 1992
38   Births to Black Teenage Mothers as a Percent of Black Births in 1992
39   Births to Women 35 to 49 Years Old in 1992
40   Births to Women 35 to 49 Years Old as a Percent of All Births in 1992
41   Births by Vaginal Delivery in 1992
42   Percent of Births by Vaginal Delivery in 1992
43   Births by Cesarean Delivery in 1992
44   Percent of Births by Cesarean Delivery in 1992
45   Births by Vaginal Delivery after a Previous Cesarean Delivery (VBAC) in 1992
46   Rate of Vaginal Births after a Previous Cesarean (VBAC) in 1992
47   Percent of Mothers Beginning Prenatal Care in First Trimester in 1992
48   Percent of White Mothers Beginning Prenatal Care in First Trimester in 1992
49   Percent of Black Mothers Beginning Prenatal Care in First Trimester in 1992
50   Percent of Mothers Receiving Late or No Prenatal Care in 1992
51   Percent of White Mothers Receiving Late or No Prenatal Care in 1992
52   Percent of Black Mothers Receiving Late or No Prenatal Care in 1992
53   Median Weight Gain During Pregnancy in 1992
54   Percent of Births to Women Considered Alcoholic Drinkers During Pregnancy in 1992
55   Percent of Births to Women Who Smoked During Pregnancy in 1992
56   Percent of Births Not in a Hospital in 1992
57   Percent of Births Attended by Midwives in 1992

I. BIRTHS AND REPRODUCTIVE HEALTH (CONTINUED)

Abortions

Births in 1993

National Total = 4,039,000 Live Births*

ALPHA ORDER

RANK	STATE	BIRTHS	% of USA
23	Alabama	63,332	1.57%
46	Alaska	10,555	0.26%
19	Arizona	70,770	1.75%
34	Arkansas	34,248	0.85%
1	California	589,685	14.60%
24	Colorado	54,817	1.36%
28	Connecticut	45,821	1.13%
46	Delaware	10,555	0.26%
4	Florida	193,087	4.78%
10	Georgia	112,400	2.78%
39	Hawaii	19,589	0.48%
40	Idaho	17,162	0.42%
5	Illinois	191,042	4.73%
14	Indiana	84,644	2.10%
32	Iowa	37,044	0.92%
31	Kansas	38,040	0.94%
26	Kentucky	52,256	1.29%
20	Louisiana	69,819	1.73%
41	Maine	15,027	0.37%
16	Maryland	75,526	1.87%
13	Massachusetts	86,317	2.14%
8	Michigan	143,576	3.55%
22	Minnesota	63,761	1.58%
30	Mississippi	42,160	1.04%
15	Missouri	77,424	1.92%
44	Montana	11,450	0.28%
36	Nebraska	22,847	0.57%
38	Nevada	21,129	0.52%
42	New Hampshire	14,952	0.37%
9	New Jersey	123,020	3.05%
35	New Mexico	27,658	0.68%
3	New York	278,307	6.89%
11	North Carolina	100,597	2.49%
48	North Dakota	8,746	0.22%
7	Ohio	156,748	3.88%
27	Oklahoma	46,711	1.16%
29	Oregon	42,195	1.04%
6	Pennsylvania	159,189	3.94%
43	Rhode Island	14,275	0.35%
25	South Carolina	53,997	1.34%
45	South Dakota	10,830	0.27%
17	Tennessee	73,613	1.82%
2	Texas	330,596	8.19%
33	Utah	36,462	0.90%
49	Vermont	7,286	0.18%
12	Virginia	95,161	2.36%
18	Washington	71,437	1.77%
37	West Virginia	22,044	0.55%
21	Wisconsin	69,289	1.72%
50	Wyoming	6,662	0.16%

RANK ORDER

RANK	STATE	BIRTHS	% of USA
1	California	589,685	14.60%
2	Texas	330,596	8.19%
3	New York	278,307	6.89%
4	Florida	193,087	4.78%
5	Illinois	191,042	4.73%
6	Pennsylvania	159,189	3.94%
7	Ohio	156,748	3.88%
8	Michigan	143,576	3.55%
9	New Jersey	123,020	3.05%
10	Georgia	112,400	2.78%
11	North Carolina	100,597	2.49%
12	Virginia	95,161	2.36%
13	Massachusetts	86,317	2.14%
14	Indiana	84,644	2.10%
15	Missouri	77,424	1.92%
16	Maryland	75,526	1.87%
17	Tennessee	73,613	1.82%
18	Washington	71,437	1.77%
19	Arizona	70,770	1.75%
20	Louisiana	69,819	1.73%
21	Wisconsin	69,289	1.72%
22	Minnesota	63,761	1.58%
23	Alabama	63,332	1.57%
24	Colorado	54,817	1.36%
25	South Carolina	53,997	1.34%
26	Kentucky	52,256	1.29%
27	Oklahoma	46,711	1.16%
28	Connecticut	45,821	1.13%
29	Oregon	42,195	1.04%
30	Mississippi	42,160	1.04%
31	Kansas	38,040	0.94%
32	Iowa	37,044	0.92%
33	Utah	36,462	0.90%
34	Arkansas	34,248	0.85%
35	New Mexico	27,658	0.68%
36	Nebraska	22,847	0.57%
37	West Virginia	22,044	0.55%
38	Nevada	21,129	0.52%
39	Hawaii	19,589	0.48%
40	Idaho	17,162	0.42%
41	Maine	15,027	0.37%
42	New Hampshire	14,952	0.37%
43	Rhode Island	14,275	0.35%
44	Montana	11,450	0.28%
45	South Dakota	10,830	0.27%
46	Alaska	10,555	0.26%
46	Delaware	10,555	0.26%
48	North Dakota	8,746	0.22%
49	Vermont	7,286	0.18%
50	Wyoming	6,662	0.16%
	District of Columbia	9,780	0.24%

Source: U.S. Department of Health and Human Services, National Center for Health Statistics
"Monthly Vital Statistics Report" (Vol. 42, No. 13, October 11, 1994)
*Data are provisional estimates by state of residence.

Birth Rate in 1993

National Rate = 15.7 Live Births per 1,000 Population*

ALPHA ORDER				RANK ORDER		
RANK	**STATE**	**RATE**		**RANK**	**STATE**	**RATE**
18	Alabama	15.1		1	Utah	19.6
5	Alaska	17.6		2	California	18.9
4	Arizona	18.0		3	Texas	18.3
34	Arkansas	14.1		4	Arizona	18.0
2	California	18.9		5	Alaska	17.6
14	Colorado	15.4		6	New Mexico	17.1
38	Connecticut	14.0		7	Hawaii	16.7
18	Delaware	15.1		8	Illinois	16.3
34	Florida	14.1		8	Louisiana	16.3
10	Georgia	16.2		10	Georgia	16.2
7	Hawaii	16.7		11	Mississippi	16.0
12	Idaho	15.6		12	Idaho	15.6
8	Illinois	16.3		12	New Jersey	15.6
23	Indiana	14.8		14	Colorado	15.4
46	Iowa	13.2		15	New York	15.3
22	Kansas	15.0		16	Maryland	15.2
40	Kentucky	13.8		16	Nevada	15.2
8	Louisiana	16.3		18	Alabama	15.1
49	Maine	12.1		18	Delaware	15.1
16	Maryland	15.2		18	Michigan	15.1
29	Massachusetts	14.4		18	South Dakota	15.1
18	Michigan	15.1		22	Kansas	15.0
34	Minnesota	14.1		23	Indiana	14.8
11	Mississippi	16.0		23	Missouri	14.8
23	Missouri	14.8		23	South Carolina	14.8
43	Montana	13.6		26	Virginia	14.7
32	Nebraska	14.2		27	North Carolina	14.5
16	Nevada	15.2		27	Oklahoma	14.5
45	New Hampshire	13.3		29	Massachusetts	14.4
12	New Jersey	15.6		29	Tennessee	14.4
6	New Mexico	17.1		31	Rhode Island	14.3
15	New York	15.3		32	Nebraska	14.2
27	North Carolina	14.5		32	Wyoming	14.2
40	North Dakota	13.8		34	Arkansas	14.1
34	Ohio	14.1		34	Florida	14.1
27	Oklahoma	14.5		34	Minnesota	14.1
39	Oregon	13.9		34	Ohio	14.1
46	Pennsylvania	13.2		38	Connecticut	14.0
31	Rhode Island	14.3		39	Oregon	13.9
23	South Carolina	14.8		40	Kentucky	13.8
18	South Dakota	15.1		40	North Dakota	13.8
29	Tennessee	14.4		40	Wisconsin	13.8
3	Texas	18.3		43	Montana	13.6
1	Utah	19.6		43	Washington	13.6
48	Vermont	12.6		45	New Hampshire	13.3
26	Virginia	14.7		46	Iowa	13.2
43	Washington	13.6		46	Pennsylvania	13.2
49	West Virginia	12.1		48	Vermont	12.6
40	Wisconsin	13.8		49	Maine	12.1
32	Wyoming	14.2		49	West Virginia	12.1
					District of Columbia	16.9

Source: U.S. Department of Health and Human Services, National Center for Health Statistics
"Monthly Vital Statistics Report" (Vol. 42, No. 13, October 11, 1994)
Data are provisional estimates by state of residence.

Births in 1992

National Total = 4,065,014 Live Births*

ALPHA ORDER

RANK ORDER

RANK	STATE	BIRTHS	% of USA		RANK	STATE	BIRTHS	% of USA
23	Alabama	62,260	1.53%		1	California	601,730	14.80%
44	Alaska	11,726	0.29%		2	Texas	320,845	7.89%
21	Arizona	68,829	1.69%		3	New York	287,887	7.08%
34	Arkansas	34,820	0.86%		4	Florida	191,713	4.72%
1	California	601,730	14.80%		5	Illinois	191,396	4.71%
25	Colorado	54,535	1.34%		6	Pennsylvania	164,625	4.05%
27	Connecticut	47,573	1.17%		7	Ohio	162,247	3.99%
47	Delaware	10,656	0.26%		8	Michigan	144,089	3.54%
4	Florida	191,713	4.72%		9	New Jersey	119,909	2.95%
10	Georgia	111,116	2.73%		10	Georgia	111,116	2.73%
39	Hawaii	19,864	0.49%		11	North Carolina	103,967	2.56%
40	Idaho	17,362	0.43%		12	Virginia	97,198	2.39%
5	Illinois	191,396	4.71%		13	Massachusetts	87,231	2.15%
14	Indiana	84,140	2.07%		14	Indiana	84,140	2.07%
31	Iowa	38,469	0.95%		15	Washington	79,450	1.95%
32	Kansas	38,027	0.94%		16	Maryland	77,815	1.91%
26	Kentucky	53,840	1.32%		17	Missouri	76,301	1.88%
19	Louisiana	70,707	1.74%		18	Tennessee	73,614	1.81%
41	Maine	16,057	0.40%		19	Louisiana	70,707	1.74%
16	Maryland	77,815	1.91%		20	Wisconsin	70,670	1.74%
13	Massachusetts	87,231	2.15%		21	Arizona	68,829	1.69%
8	Michigan	144,089	3.54%		22	Minnesota	65,607	1.61%
22	Minnesota	65,607	1.61%		23	Alabama	62,260	1.53%
29	Mississippi	42,681	1.05%		24	South Carolina	56,192	1.38%
17	Missouri	76,301	1.88%		25	Colorado	54,535	1.34%
45	Montana	11,472	0.28%		26	Kentucky	53,840	1.32%
36	Nebraska	23,397	0.58%		27	Connecticut	47,573	1.17%
37	Nevada	22,374	0.55%		28	Oklahoma	47,557	1.17%
42	New Hampshire	15,990	0.39%		29	Mississippi	42,681	1.05%
9	New Jersey	119,909	2.95%		30	Oregon	42,035	1.03%
35	New Mexico	27,922	0.69%		31	Iowa	38,469	0.95%
3	New York	287,887	7.08%		32	Kansas	38,027	0.94%
11	North Carolina	103,967	2.56%		33	Utah	37,200	0.92%
48	North Dakota	8,811	0.22%		34	Arkansas	34,820	0.86%
7	Ohio	162,247	3.99%		35	New Mexico	27,922	0.69%
28	Oklahoma	47,557	1.17%		36	Nebraska	23,397	0.58%
30	Oregon	42,035	1.03%		37	Nevada	22,374	0.55%
6	Pennsylvania	164,625	4.05%		38	West Virginia	22,170	0.55%
43	Rhode Island	14,500	0.36%		39	Hawaii	19,864	0.49%
24	South Carolina	56,192	1.38%		40	Idaho	17,362	0.43%
46	South Dakota	11,018	0.27%		41	Maine	16,057	0.40%
18	Tennessee	73,614	1.81%		42	New Hampshire	15,990	0.39%
2	Texas	320,845	7.89%		43	Rhode Island	14,500	0.36%
33	Utah	37,200	0.92%		44	Alaska	11,726	0.29%
49	Vermont	7,737	0.19%		45	Montana	11,472	0.28%
12	Virginia	97,198	2.39%		46	South Dakota	11,018	0.27%
15	Washington	79,450	1.95%		47	Delaware	10,656	0.26%
38	West Virginia	22,170	0.55%		48	North Dakota	8,811	0.22%
20	Wisconsin	70,670	1.74%		49	Vermont	7,737	0.19%
50	Wyoming	6,723	0.17%		50	Wyoming	6,723	0.17%
						District of Columbia	10,960	0.27%

Source: U.S. Department of Health and Human Services, National Center for Health Statistics
"Monthly Vital Statistics Report" (Vol. 43, No. 5, Supplement, October 25, 1994)
*Final data by state of residence.

Birth Rate in 1992

National Rate = 15.9 Live Births per 1,000 Population*

ALPHA ORDER			RANK ORDER		
RANK	STATE	RATE	RANK	STATE	RATE
26	Alabama	15.0	1	Utah	20.5
2	Alaska	20.0	2	Alaska	20.0
5	Arizona	18.0	3	California	19.5
35	Arkansas	14.5	4	Texas	18.1
3	California	19.5	5	Arizona	18.0
16	Colorado	15.7	6	New Mexico	17.7
35	Connecticut	14.5	7	Hawaii	17.2
19	Delaware	15.4	8	Nevada	16.7
41	Florida	14.2	9	Illinois	16.5
11	Georgia	16.4	9	Louisiana	16.5
7	Hawaii	17.2	11	Georgia	16.4
12	Idaho	16.3	12	Idaho	16.3
9	Illinois	16.5	12	Mississippi	16.3
27	Indiana	14.9	14	New York	15.9
46	Iowa	13.7	15	Maryland	15.8
25	Kansas	15.1	16	Colorado	15.7
39	Kentucky	14.3	17	South Carolina	15.6
9	Louisiana	16.5	17	South Dakota	15.6
49	Maine	13.0	19	Delaware	15.4
15	Maryland	15.8	19	Washington	15.4
32	Massachusetts	14.6	21	Michigan	15.3
21	Michigan	15.3	21	New Jersey	15.3
29	Minnesota	14.7	23	North Carolina	15.2
12	Mississippi	16.3	23	Virginia	15.2
29	Missouri	14.7	25	Kansas	15.1
44	Montana	14.0	26	Alabama	15.0
32	Nebraska	14.6	27	Indiana	14.9
8	Nevada	16.7	28	Oklahoma	14.8
39	New Hampshire	14.3	29	Minnesota	14.7
21	New Jersey	15.3	29	Missouri	14.7
6	New Mexico	17.7	29	Ohio	14.7
14	New York	15.9	32	Massachusetts	14.6
23	North Carolina	15.2	32	Nebraska	14.6
45	North Dakota	13.9	32	Tennessee	14.6
29	Ohio	14.7	35	Arkansas	14.5
28	Oklahoma	14.8	35	Connecticut	14.5
43	Oregon	14.1	35	Rhode Island	14.5
46	Pennsylvania	13.7	35	Wyoming	14.5
35	Rhode Island	14.5	39	Kentucky	14.3
17	South Carolina	15.6	39	New Hampshire	14.3
17	South Dakota	15.6	41	Florida	14.2
32	Tennessee	14.6	41	Wisconsin	14.2
4	Texas	18.1	43	Oregon	14.1
1	Utah	20.5	44	Montana	14.0
48	Vermont	13.5	45	North Dakota	13.9
23	Virginia	15.2	46	Iowa	13.7
19	Washington	15.4	46	Pennsylvania	13.7
50	West Virginia	12.3	48	Vermont	13.5
41	Wisconsin	14.2	49	Maine	13.0
35	Wyoming	14.5	50	West Virginia	12.3
				District of Columbia	18.7

Source: U.S. Department of Health and Human Services, National Center for Health Statistics
  "Monthly Vital Statistics Report" (Vol. 43, No. 5, Supplement, October 25, 1994)
Final data by state of residence.

Births in 1990

National Total = 4,158,212 Live Births*

ALPHA ORDER

RANK ORDER

RANK	STATE	BIRTHS	% of USA	RANK	STATE	BIRTHS	% of USA
23	Alabama	63,487	1.53%	1	California	612,628	14.73%
44	Alaska	11,902	0.29%	2	Texas	316,423	7.61%
21	Arizona	68,995	1.66%	3	New York	297,576	7.16%
33	Arkansas	36,457	0.88%	4	Florida	199,339	4.79%
1	California	612,628	14.73%	5	Illinois	195,790	4.71%
26	Colorado	53,525	1.29%	6	Pennsylvania	171,961	4.14%
27	Connecticut	50,123	1.21%	7	Ohio	166,913	4.01%
46	Delaware	11,113	0.27%	8	Michigan	153,700	3.70%
4	Florida	199,339	4.79%	9	New Jersey	122,289	2.94%
10	Georgia	112,666	2.71%	10	Georgia	112,666	2.71%
39	Hawaii	20,489	0.49%	11	North Carolina	104,525	2.51%
42	Idaho	16,433	0.40%	12	Virginia	99,352	2.39%
5	Illinois	195,790	4.71%	13	Massachusetts	92,654	2.23%
14	Indiana	86,214	2.07%	14	Indiana	86,214	2.07%
31	Iowa	39,409	0.95%	15	Maryland	80,245	1.93%
32	Kansas	39,020	0.94%	16	Missouri	79,260	1.91%
25	Kentucky	54,362	1.31%	17	Washington	79,251	1.91%
20	Louisiana	72,192	1.74%	18	Tennessee	74,962	1.80%
41	Maine	17,359	0.42%	19	Wisconsin	72,895	1.75%
15	Maryland	80,245	1.93%	20	Louisiana	72,192	1.74%
13	Massachusetts	92,654	2.23%	21	Arizona	68,995	1.66%
8	Michigan	153,700	3.70%	22	Minnesota	68,013	1.64%
22	Minnesota	68,013	1.64%	23	Alabama	63,487	1.53%
29	Mississippi	43,563	1.05%	24	South Carolina	58,610	1.41%
16	Missouri	79,260	1.91%	25	Kentucky	54,362	1.31%
45	Montana	11,613	0.28%	26	Colorado	53,525	1.29%
36	Nebraska	24,380	0.59%	27	Connecticut	50,123	1.21%
38	Nevada	21,599	0.52%	28	Oklahoma	47,649	1.15%
40	New Hampshire	17,569	0.42%	29	Mississippi	43,563	1.05%
9	New Jersey	122,289	2.94%	30	Oregon	42,891	1.03%
35	New Mexico	27,402	0.66%	31	Iowa	39,409	0.95%
3	New York	297,576	7.16%	32	Kansas	39,020	0.94%
11	North Carolina	104,525	2.51%	33	Arkansas	36,457	0.88%
48	North Dakota	9,250	0.22%	34	Utah	36,277	0.87%
7	Ohio	166,913	4.01%	35	New Mexico	27,402	0.66%
28	Oklahoma	47,649	1.15%	36	Nebraska	24,380	0.59%
30	Oregon	42,891	1.03%	37	West Virginia	22,585	0.54%
6	Pennsylvania	171,961	4.14%	38	Nevada	21,599	0.52%
43	Rhode Island	15,195	0.37%	39	Hawaii	20,489	0.49%
24	South Carolina	58,610	1.41%	40	New Hampshire	17,569	0.42%
47	South Dakota	10,999	0.26%	41	Maine	17,359	0.42%
18	Tennessee	74,962	1.80%	42	Idaho	16,433	0.40%
2	Texas	316,423	7.61%	43	Rhode Island	15,195	0.37%
34	Utah	36,277	0.87%	44	Alaska	11,902	0.29%
49	Vermont	8,273	0.20%	45	Montana	11,613	0.28%
12	Virginia	99,352	2.39%	46	Delaware	11,113	0.27%
17	Washington	79,251	1.91%	47	South Dakota	10,999	0.26%
37	West Virginia	22,585	0.54%	48	North Dakota	9,250	0.22%
19	Wisconsin	72,895	1.75%	49	Vermont	8,273	0.20%
50	Wyoming	6,985	0.17%	50	Wyoming	6,985	0.17%
					District of Columbia	11,850	0.28%

Source: U.S. Department of Health and Human Services, National Center for Health Statistics
"Monthly Vital Statistics Report" (Vol. 41, No. 9, Supplement, February 25, 1993)
Final data by state of residence.

Birth Rate in 1990

National Rate = 16.7 Births per 1,000 Population*

ALPHA ORDER			RANK ORDER		
RANK	STATE	RATE	RANK	STATE	RATE
26	Alabama	15.7	1	Alaska	21.6
1	Alaska	21.6	2	Utah	21.1
4	Arizona	18.8	3	California	20.6
29	Arkansas	15.5	4	Arizona	18.8
3	California	20.6	5	Texas	18.6
20	Colorado	16.2	6	Hawaii	18.5
38	Connecticut	15.2	7	New Mexico	18.1
15	Delaware	16.7	8	Nevada	18.0
32	Florida	15.4	9	Georgia	17.4
9	Georgia	17.4	10	Illinois	17.1
6	Hawaii	18.5	10	Louisiana	17.1
18	Idaho	16.3	12	Mississippi	16.9
10	Illinois	17.1	13	Maryland	16.8
28	Indiana	15.6	13	South Carolina	16.8
48	Iowa	14.2	15	Delaware	16.7
26	Kansas	15.7	16	Michigan	16.5
43	Kentucky	14.8	16	New York	16.5
10	Louisiana	17.1	18	Idaho	16.3
49	Maine	14.1	18	Washington	16.3
13	Maryland	16.8	20	Colorado	16.2
32	Massachusetts	15.4	21	Virginia	16.1
16	Michigan	16.5	22	New Hampshire	15.8
29	Minnesota	15.5	22	New Jersey	15.8
12	Mississippi	16.9	22	North Carolina	15.8
29	Missouri	15.5	22	South Dakota	15.8
45	Montana	14.5	26	Alabama	15.7
32	Nebraska	15.4	26	Kansas	15.7
8	Nevada	18.0	28	Indiana	15.6
22	New Hampshire	15.8	29	Arkansas	15.5
22	New Jersey	15.8	29	Minnesota	15.5
7	New Mexico	18.1	29	Missouri	15.5
16	New York	16.5	32	Florida	15.4
22	North Carolina	15.8	32	Massachusetts	15.4
45	North Dakota	14.5	32	Nebraska	15.4
32	Ohio	15.4	32	Ohio	15.4
39	Oklahoma	15.1	32	Tennessee	15.4
39	Oregon	15.1	32	Wyoming	15.4
45	Pennsylvania	14.5	38	Connecticut	15.2
39	Rhode Island	15.1	39	Oklahoma	15.1
13	South Carolina	16.8	39	Oregon	15.1
22	South Dakota	15.8	39	Rhode Island	15.1
32	Tennessee	15.4	42	Wisconsin	14.9
5	Texas	18.6	43	Kentucky	14.8
2	Utah	21.1	44	Vermont	14.7
44	Vermont	14.7	45	Montana	14.5
21	Virginia	16.1	45	North Dakota	14.5
18	Washington	16.3	45	Pennsylvania	14.5
50	West Virginia	12.6	48	Iowa	14.2
42	Wisconsin	14.9	49	Maine	14.1
32	Wyoming	15.4	50	West Virginia	12.6
				District of Columbia	19.5

Source: U.S. Department of Health and Human Services, National Center for Health Statistics
  "Monthly Vital Statistics Report" (Vol. 41, No. 9, Supplement, February 25, 1993)
*Final data by state of residence.

Births in 1980

National Total = 3,612,000 Births*

ALPHA ORDER					RANK ORDER			
RANK	STATE	BIRTHS	% of USA		RANK	STATE	BIRTHS	% of USA
21	Alabama	64,000	1.77%		1	California	403,000	11.16%
48	Alaska	10,000	0.28%		2	Texas	274,000	7.59%
26	Arizona	50,000	1.38%		3	New York	239,000	6.62%
34	Arkansas	37,000	1.02%		4	Illinois	190,000	5.26%
1	California	403,000	11.16%		5	Ohio	169,000	4.68%
26	Colorado	50,000	1.38%		6	Pennsylvania	159,000	4.40%
33	Connecticut	39,000	1.08%		7	Michigan	146,000	4.04%
49	Delaware	9,000	0.25%		8	Florida	132,000	3.65%
8	Florida	132,000	3.65%		9	New Jersey	97,000	2.69%
10	Georgia	92,000	2.55%		10	Georgia	92,000	2.55%
39	Hawaii	18,000	0.50%		11	Indiana	88,000	2.44%
38	Idaho	20,000	0.55%		12	North Carolina	84,000	2.33%
4	Illinois	190,000	5.26%		13	Louisiana	82,000	2.27%
11	Indiana	88,000	2.44%		14	Missouri	79,000	2.19%
28	Iowa	48,000	1.33%		15	Virginia	78,000	2.16%
32	Kansas	41,000	1.14%		16	Wisconsin	75,000	2.08%
22	Kentucky	60,000	1.66%		17	Massachusetts	73,000	2.02%
13	Louisiana	82,000	2.27%		18	Tennessee	69,000	1.91%
40	Maine	16,000	0.44%		19	Minnesota	68,000	1.88%
22	Maryland	60,000	1.66%		19	Washington	68,000	1.88%
17	Massachusetts	73,000	2.02%		21	Alabama	64,000	1.77%
7	Michigan	146,000	4.04%		22	Kentucky	60,000	1.66%
19	Minnesota	68,000	1.88%		22	Maryland	60,000	1.66%
28	Mississippi	48,000	1.33%		24	Oklahoma	52,000	1.44%
14	Missouri	79,000	2.19%		24	South Carolina	52,000	1.44%
41	Montana	14,000	0.39%		26	Arizona	50,000	1.38%
36	Nebraska	27,000	0.75%		26	Colorado	50,000	1.38%
43	Nevada	13,000	0.36%		28	Iowa	48,000	1.33%
41	New Hampshire	14,000	0.39%		28	Mississippi	48,000	1.33%
9	New Jersey	97,000	2.69%		30	Oregon	43,000	1.19%
37	New Mexico	26,000	0.72%		31	Utah	42,000	1.16%
3	New York	239,000	6.62%		32	Kansas	41,000	1.14%
12	North Carolina	84,000	2.33%		33	Connecticut	39,000	1.08%
45	North Dakota	12,000	0.33%		34	Arkansas	37,000	1.02%
5	Ohio	169,000	4.68%		35	West Virginia	29,000	0.80%
24	Oklahoma	52,000	1.44%		36	Nebraska	27,000	0.75%
30	Oregon	43,000	1.19%		37	New Mexico	26,000	0.72%
6	Pennsylvania	159,000	4.40%		38	Idaho	20,000	0.55%
45	Rhode Island	12,000	0.33%		39	Hawaii	18,000	0.50%
24	South Carolina	52,000	1.44%		40	Maine	16,000	0.44%
43	South Dakota	13,000	0.36%		41	Montana	14,000	0.39%
18	Tennessee	69,000	1.91%		41	New Hampshire	14,000	0.39%
2	Texas	274,000	7.59%		43	Nevada	13,000	0.36%
31	Utah	42,000	1.16%		43	South Dakota	13,000	0.36%
50	Vermont	8,000	0.22%		45	North Dakota	12,000	0.33%
15	Virginia	78,000	2.16%		45	Rhode Island	12,000	0.33%
19	Washington	68,000	1.88%		47	Wyoming	11,000	0.30%
35	West Virginia	29,000	0.80%		48	Alaska	10,000	0.28%
16	Wisconsin	75,000	2.08%		49	Delaware	9,000	0.25%
47	Wyoming	11,000	0.30%		50	Vermont	8,000	0.22%
						District of Columbia	9,000	0.25%

Source: U.S. Department of Health and Human Services, National Center for Health Statistics
"Vital Statistics of the United States, 1980" and "Monthly Vital Statistics Report"
*Live births by state of residence.

Birth Rate in 1980

National Rate = 15.9 Births per 1,000 Population*

ALPHA ORDER			RANK ORDER		
RANK	STATE	RATE	RANK	STATE	RATE
27	Alabama	16.3	1	Utah	28.6
2	Alaska	23.7	2	Alaska	23.7
11	Arizona	18.4	3	Wyoming	22.5
27	Arkansas	16.3	4	Idaho	21.4
18	California	17.0	5	New Mexico	20.0
15	Colorado	17.2	6	Louisiana	19.5
50	Connecticut	12.5	7	South Dakota	19.2
33	Delaware	15.8	7	Texas	19.2
45	Florida	13.5	9	Mississippi	19.0
19	Georgia	16.9	10	Hawaii	18.8
10	Hawaii	18.8	11	Arizona	18.4
4	Idaho	21.4	11	North Dakota	18.4
20	Illinois	16.6	13	Montana	18.1
30	Indiana	16.1	14	Nebraska	17.4
24	Iowa	16.4	15	Colorado	17.2
15	Kansas	17.2	15	Kansas	17.2
27	Kentucky	16.3	15	Oklahoma	17.2
6	Louisiana	19.5	18	California	17.0
41	Maine	14.6	19	Georgia	16.9
43	Maryland	14.2	20	Illinois	16.6
49	Massachusetts	12.7	20	Minnesota	16.6
34	Michigan	15.7	20	Nevada	16.6
20	Minnesota	16.6	20	South Carolina	16.6
9	Mississippi	19.0	24	Iowa	16.4
30	Missouri	16.1	24	Oregon	16.4
13	Montana	18.1	24	Washington	16.4
14	Nebraska	17.4	27	Alabama	16.3
20	Nevada	16.6	27	Arkansas	16.3
39	New Hampshire	14.9	27	Kentucky	16.3
47	New Jersey	13.2	30	Indiana	16.1
5	New Mexico	20.0	30	Missouri	16.1
44	New York	13.6	32	Wisconsin	15.9
42	North Carolina	14.4	33	Delaware	15.8
11	North Dakota	18.4	34	Michigan	15.7
34	Ohio	15.7	34	Ohio	15.7
15	Oklahoma	17.2	36	Vermont	15.4
24	Oregon	16.4	37	Tennessee	15.1
46	Pennsylvania	13.4	37	West Virginia	15.1
48	Rhode Island	12.9	39	New Hampshire	14.9
20	South Carolina	16.6	40	Virginia	14.7
7	South Dakota	19.2	41	Maine	14.6
37	Tennessee	15.1	42	North Carolina	14.4
7	Texas	19.2	43	Maryland	14.2
1	Utah	28.6	44	New York	13.6
36	Vermont	15.4	45	Florida	13.5
40	Virginia	14.7	46	Pennsylvania	13.4
24	Washington	16.4	47	New Jersey	13.2
37	West Virginia	15.1	48	Rhode Island	12.9
32	Wisconsin	15.9	49	Massachusetts	12.7
3	Wyoming	22.5	50	Connecticut	12.5
				District of Columbia	14.7

Source: U.S. Department of Health and Human Services, National Center for Health Statistics
"Vital Statistics of the United States, 1980" and "Monthly Vital Statistics Report"
*Live births by state of residence.

Fertility Rate in 1992

National Rate = 68.9 Live Births per 1,000 Women 15 to 44 Years Old*

ALPHA ORDER

RANK	STATE	RATE
29	Alabama	64.8
3	Alaska	82.0
4	Arizona	80.4
20	Arkansas	66.2
2	California	83.1
28	Colorado	65.0
36	Connecticut	63.2
26	Delaware	65.2
16	Florida	68.0
17	Georgia	66.9
7	Hawaii	75.2
9	Idaho	73.5
11	Illinois	71.4
31	Indiana	64.0
36	Iowa	63.2
14	Kansas	68.2
45	Kentucky	61.5
13	Louisiana	69.8
49	Maine	56.3
25	Maryland	65.3
46	Massachusetts	60.8
26	Michigan	65.2
33	Minnesota	63.7
12	Mississippi	70.2
23	Missouri	65.5
34	Montana	63.6
22	Nebraska	66.0
8	Nevada	73.6
47	New Hampshire	59.5
18	New Jersey	66.8
5	New Mexico	77.0
15	New York	68.1
30	North Carolina	64.7
34	North Dakota	63.6
32	Ohio	63.9
19	Oklahoma	66.5
39	Oregon	62.7
44	Pennsylvania	61.6
41	Rhode Island	62.5
23	South Carolina	65.5
10	South Dakota	73.0
41	Tennessee	62.5
6	Texas	76.1
1	Utah	88.5
48	Vermont	58.6
40	Virginia	62.6
21	Washington	66.1
50	West Virginia	54.6
43	Wisconsin	62.4
38	Wyoming	62.9

RANK ORDER

RANK	STATE	RATE
1	Utah	88.5
2	California	83.1
3	Alaska	82.0
4	Arizona	80.4
5	New Mexico	77.0
6	Texas	76.1
7	Hawaii	75.2
8	Nevada	73.6
9	Idaho	73.5
10	South Dakota	73.0
11	Illinois	71.4
12	Mississippi	70.2
13	Louisiana	69.8
14	Kansas	68.2
15	New York	68.1
16	Florida	68.0
17	Georgia	66.9
18	New Jersey	66.8
19	Oklahoma	66.5
20	Arkansas	66.2
21	Washington	66.1
22	Nebraska	66.0
23	Missouri	65.5
23	South Carolina	65.5
25	Maryland	65.3
26	Delaware	65.2
26	Michigan	65.2
28	Colorado	65.0
29	Alabama	64.8
30	North Carolina	64.7
31	Indiana	64.0
32	Ohio	63.9
33	Minnesota	63.7
34	Montana	63.6
34	North Dakota	63.6
36	Connecticut	63.2
36	Iowa	63.2
38	Wyoming	62.9
39	Oregon	62.7
40	Virginia	62.6
41	Rhode Island	62.5
41	Tennessee	62.5
43	Wisconsin	62.4
44	Pennsylvania	61.6
45	Kentucky	61.5
46	Massachusetts	60.8
47	New Hampshire	59.5
48	Vermont	58.6
49	Maine	56.3
50	West Virginia	54.6
	District of Columbia	71.2

Source: U.S. Department of Health and Human Services, National Center for Health Statistics
"Monthly Vital Statistics Report" (Vol. 43, No. 5, Supplement, October 25, 1994)
*Final data by state of residence.

Births to White Women in 1992

National Total = 3,201,678 Live Births to White Women*

ALPHA ORDER				RANK ORDER			
RANK	STATE	BIRTHS	% of USA	RANK	STATE	BIRTHS	% of USA
25	Alabama	40,180	1.25%	1	California	492,487	15.38%
45	Alaska	7,934	0.25%	2	Texas	270,198	8.44%
18	Arizona	59,432	1.86%	3	New York	212,579	6.64%
33	Arkansas	26,289	0.82%	4	Florida	143,463	4.48%
1	California	492,487	15.38%	5	Illinois	142,842	4.46%
21	Colorado	49,644	1.55%	6	Pennsylvania	135,996	4.25%
24	Connecticut	40,278	1.26%	7	Ohio	134,344	4.20%
46	Delaware	7,901	0.25%	8	Michigan	112,169	3.50%
4	Florida	143,463	4.48%	9	New Jersey	90,823	2.84%
15	Georgia	68,819	2.15%	10	Massachusetts	75,141	2.35%
50	Hawaii	5,738	0.18%	11	Indiana	73,914	2.31%
39	Idaho	16,834	0.53%	12	North Carolina	70,772	2.21%
5	Illinois	142,842	4.46%	13	Virginia	70,137	2.19%
11	Indiana	73,914	2.31%	14	Washington	70,081	2.19%
29	Iowa	36,567	1.14%	15	Georgia	68,819	2.15%
32	Kansas	33,674	1.05%	16	Missouri	61,908	1.93%
23	Kentucky	48,227	1.51%	17	Wisconsin	60,689	1.90%
26	Louisiana	39,757	1.24%	18	Arizona	59,432	1.86%
40	Maine	15,762	0.49%	19	Minnesota	59,187	1.85%
22	Maryland	49,619	1.55%	20	Tennessee	55,279	1.73%
10	Massachusetts	75,141	2.35%	21	Colorado	49,644	1.55%
8	Michigan	112,169	3.50%	22	Maryland	49,619	1.55%
19	Minnesota	59,187	1.85%	23	Kentucky	48,227	1.51%
35	Mississippi	21,704	0.68%	24	Connecticut	40,278	1.26%
16	Missouri	61,908	1.93%	25	Alabama	40,180	1.25%
43	Montana	9,981	0.31%	26	Louisiana	39,757	1.24%
36	Nebraska	21,403	0.67%	27	Oregon	39,068	1.22%
38	Nevada	18,962	0.59%	28	Oklahoma	37,305	1.17%
41	New Hampshire	15,714	0.49%	29	Iowa	36,567	1.14%
9	New Jersey	90,823	2.84%	30	Utah	35,317	1.10%
34	New Mexico	23,159	0.72%	31	South Carolina	33,977	1.06%
3	New York	212,579	6.64%	32	Kansas	33,674	1.05%
12	North Carolina	70,772	2.21%	33	Arkansas	26,289	0.82%
47	North Dakota	7,831	0.24%	34	New Mexico	23,159	0.72%
7	Ohio	134,344	4.20%	35	Mississippi	21,704	0.68%
28	Oklahoma	37,305	1.17%	36	Nebraska	21,403	0.67%
27	Oregon	39,068	1.22%	37	West Virginia	21,248	0.66%
6	Pennsylvania	135,996	4.25%	38	Nevada	18,962	0.59%
42	Rhode Island	12,673	0.40%	39	Idaho	16,834	0.53%
31	South Carolina	33,977	1.06%	40	Maine	15,762	0.49%
44	South Dakota	9,110	0.28%	41	New Hampshire	15,714	0.49%
20	Tennessee	55,279	1.73%	42	Rhode Island	12,673	0.40%
2	Texas	270,198	8.44%	43	Montana	9,981	0.31%
30	Utah	35,317	1.10%	44	South Dakota	9,110	0.28%
48	Vermont	7,629	0.24%	45	Alaska	7,934	0.25%
13	Virginia	70,137	2.19%	46	Delaware	7,901	0.25%
14	Washington	70,081	2.19%	47	North Dakota	7,831	0.24%
37	West Virginia	21,248	0.66%	48	Vermont	7,629	0.24%
17	Wisconsin	60,689	1.90%	49	Wyoming	6,326	0.20%
49	Wyoming	6,326	0.20%	50	Hawaii	5,738	0.18%
					District of Columbia	1,607	0.05%

Source: U.S. Department of Health and Human Services, National Center for Health Statistics
   "Monthly Vital Statistics Report" (Vol. 43, No. 5, Supplement, October 25, 1994)
*Final data by state of residence. By race of mother.

White Births as a Percent of All Births in 1992

National Percent = 78.76% of Live Births*

ALPHA ORDER

RANK ORDER

RANK	STATE	PERCENT	RANK	STATE	PERCENT
44	Alabama	64.54	1	Vermont	98.60
43	Alaska	67.66	2	New Hampshire	98.27
20	Arizona	86.35	3	Maine	98.16
35	Arkansas	75.50	4	Idaho	96.96
30	California	81.85	5	West Virginia	95.84
11	Colorado	91.03	6	Iowa	95.06
24	Connecticut	84.67	7	Utah	94.94
39	Delaware	74.15	8	Wyoming	94.09
37	Florida	74.83	9	Oregon	92.94
46	Georgia	61.93	10	Nebraska	91.48
50	Hawaii	28.89	11	Colorado	91.03
4	Idaho	96.96	12	Minnesota	90.21
38	Illinois	74.63	13	Kentucky	89.57
17	Indiana	87.85	14	North Dakota	88.88
6	Iowa	95.06	15	Kansas	88.55
15	Kansas	88.55	16	Washington	88.21
13	Kentucky	89.57	17	Indiana	87.85
48	Louisiana	56.23	18	Rhode Island	87.40
3	Maine	98.16	19	Montana	87.00
45	Maryland	63.77	20	Arizona	86.35
21	Massachusetts	86.14	21	Massachusetts	86.14
33	Michigan	77.85	22	Wisconsin	85.88
12	Minnesota	90.21	23	Nevada	84.75
49	Mississippi	50.85	24	Connecticut	84.67
31	Missouri	81.14	25	Texas	84.21
19	Montana	87.00	26	New Mexico	82.94
10	Nebraska	91.48	27	Ohio	82.80
23	Nevada	84.75	28	South Dakota	82.68
2	New Hampshire	98.27	29	Pennsylvania	82.61
34	New Jersey	75.74	30	California	81.85
26	New Mexico	82.94	31	Missouri	81.14
40	New York	73.84	32	Oklahoma	78.44
42	North Carolina	68.07	33	Michigan	77.85
14	North Dakota	88.88	34	New Jersey	75.74
27	Ohio	82.80	35	Arkansas	75.50
32	Oklahoma	78.44	36	Tennessee	75.09
9	Oregon	92.94	37	Florida	74.83
29	Pennsylvania	82.61	38	Illinois	74.63
18	Rhode Island	87.40	39	Delaware	74.15
47	South Carolina	60.47	40	New York	73.84
28	South Dakota	82.68	41	Virginia	72.16
36	Tennessee	75.09	42	North Carolina	68.07
25	Texas	84.21	43	Alaska	67.66
7	Utah	94.94	44	Alabama	64.54
1	Vermont	98.60	45	Maryland	63.77
41	Virginia	72.16	46	Georgia	61.93
16	Washington	88.21	47	South Carolina	60.47
5	West Virginia	95.84	48	Louisiana	56.23
22	Wisconsin	85.88	49	Mississippi	50.85
8	Wyoming	94.09	50	Hawaii	28.89

| | | | | District of Columbia | 14.66 |

Source: Morgan Quitno Press using data from U.S. Department of Health and Human Services, National Center for Health "Monthly Vital Statistics Report" (Vol. 43, No. 5, Supplement, October 25, 1994)
*Final data by state of residence. By race of mother.

Births to Black Women in 1992

National Total = 673,633 Live Births to Black Women*

<u>ALPHA ORDER</u>

RANK	STATE	BIRTHS	% of USA
16	Alabama	21,522	3.19%
40	Alaska	542	0.08%
32	Arizona	2,448	0.36%
22	Arkansas	8,152	1.21%
2	California	46,509	6.90%
29	Colorado	3,008	0.45%
24	Connecticut	6,145	0.91%
31	Delaware	2,553	0.38%
3	Florida	44,970	6.68%
6	Georgia	40,382	5.99%
39	Hawaii	685	0.10%
48	Idaho	58	0.01%
5	Illinois	42,923	6.37%
20	Indiana	9,426	1.40%
36	Iowa	1,184	0.18%
27	Kansas	3,314	0.49%
25	Kentucky	5,188	0.77%
8	Louisiana	29,841	4.43%
44	Maine	82	0.01%
11	Maryland	25,426	3.77%
21	Massachusetts	8,647	1.28%
9	Michigan	29,742	4.42%
30	Minnesota	2,916	0.43%
17	Mississippi	20,524	3.05%
19	Missouri	13,315	1.98%
49	Montana	49	0.01%
34	Nebraska	1,312	0.19%
33	Nevada	2,163	0.32%
43	New Hampshire	109	0.02%
14	New Jersey	23,406	3.47%
41	New Mexico	513	0.08%
1	New York	60,990	9.05%
7	North Carolina	30,333	4.50%
46	North Dakota	75	0.01%
10	Ohio	25,994	3.86%
26	Oklahoma	5,164	0.77%
37	Oregon	955	0.14%
12	Pennsylvania	25,405	3.77%
35	Rhode Island	1,186	0.18%
15	South Carolina	21,604	3.21%
45	South Dakota	79	0.01%
18	Tennessee	17,510	2.60%
4	Texas	43,016	6.39%
42	Utah	245	0.04%
50	Vermont	34	0.01%
13	Virginia	23,854	3.54%
28	Washington	3,145	0.47%
38	West Virginia	815	0.12%
23	Wisconsin	7,307	1.08%
47	Wyoming	65	0.01%

<u>RANK ORDER</u>

RANK	STATE	BIRTHS	% of USA
1	New York	60,990	9.05%
2	California	46,509	6.90%
3	Florida	44,970	6.68%
4	Texas	43,016	6.39%
5	Illinois	42,923	6.37%
6	Georgia	40,382	5.99%
7	North Carolina	30,333	4.50%
8	Louisiana	29,841	4.43%
9	Michigan	29,742	4.42%
10	Ohio	25,994	3.86%
11	Maryland	25,426	3.77%
12	Pennsylvania	25,405	3.77%
13	Virginia	23,854	3.54%
14	New Jersey	23,406	3.47%
15	South Carolina	21,604	3.21%
16	Alabama	21,522	3.19%
17	Mississippi	20,524	3.05%
18	Tennessee	17,510	2.60%
19	Missouri	13,315	1.98%
20	Indiana	9,426	1.40%
21	Massachusetts	8,647	1.28%
22	Arkansas	8,152	1.21%
23	Wisconsin	7,307	1.08%
24	Connecticut	6,145	0.91%
25	Kentucky	5,188	0.77%
26	Oklahoma	5,164	0.77%
27	Kansas	3,314	0.49%
28	Washington	3,145	0.47%
29	Colorado	3,008	0.45%
30	Minnesota	2,916	0.43%
31	Delaware	2,553	0.38%
32	Arizona	2,448	0.36%
33	Nevada	2,163	0.32%
34	Nebraska	1,312	0.19%
35	Rhode Island	1,186	0.18%
36	Iowa	1,184	0.18%
37	Oregon	955	0.14%
38	West Virginia	815	0.12%
39	Hawaii	685	0.10%
40	Alaska	542	0.08%
41	New Mexico	513	0.08%
42	Utah	245	0.04%
43	New Hampshire	109	0.02%
44	Maine	82	0.01%
45	South Dakota	79	0.01%
46	North Dakota	75	0.01%
47	Wyoming	65	0.01%
48	Idaho	58	0.01%
49	Montana	49	0.01%
50	Vermont	34	0.01%
	District of Columbia	8,803	1.31%

Source: U.S. Department of Health and Human Services, National Center for Health Statistics
"Monthly Vital Statistics Report" (Vol. 43, No. 5, Supplement, October 25, 1994)
*Final data by state of residence. By race of mother.

Black Births as a Percent of All Births in 1992

National Percent = 16.57% of Live Births*

<table>
<tr><td colspan="3">ALPHA ORDER</td><td colspan="3">RANK ORDER</td></tr>
<tr><td>RANK</td><td>STATE</td><td>PERCENT</td><td>RANK</td><td>STATE</td><td>PERCENT</td></tr>
<tr><td>5</td><td>Alabama</td><td>34.57</td><td>1</td><td>Mississippi</td><td>48.09</td></tr>
<tr><td>33</td><td>Alaska</td><td>4.62</td><td>2</td><td>Louisiana</td><td>42.20</td></tr>
<tr><td>37</td><td>Arizona</td><td>3.56</td><td>3</td><td>South Carolina</td><td>38.45</td></tr>
<tr><td>12</td><td>Arkansas</td><td>23.41</td><td>4</td><td>Georgia</td><td>36.34</td></tr>
<tr><td>30</td><td>California</td><td>7.73</td><td>5</td><td>Alabama</td><td>34.57</td></tr>
<tr><td>32</td><td>Colorado</td><td>5.52</td><td>6</td><td>Maryland</td><td>32.67</td></tr>
<tr><td>21</td><td>Connecticut</td><td>12.92</td><td>7</td><td>North Carolina</td><td>29.18</td></tr>
<tr><td>9</td><td>Delaware</td><td>23.96</td><td>8</td><td>Virginia</td><td>24.54</td></tr>
<tr><td>11</td><td>Florida</td><td>23.46</td><td>9</td><td>Delaware</td><td>23.96</td></tr>
<tr><td>4</td><td>Georgia</td><td>36.34</td><td>10</td><td>Tennessee</td><td>23.79</td></tr>
<tr><td>38</td><td>Hawaii</td><td>3.45</td><td>11</td><td>Florida</td><td>23.46</td></tr>
<tr><td>50</td><td>Idaho</td><td>0.33</td><td>12</td><td>Arkansas</td><td>23.41</td></tr>
<tr><td>13</td><td>Illinois</td><td>22.43</td><td>13</td><td>Illinois</td><td>22.43</td></tr>
<tr><td>22</td><td>Indiana</td><td>11.20</td><td>14</td><td>New York</td><td>21.19</td></tr>
<tr><td>39</td><td>Iowa</td><td>3.08</td><td>15</td><td>Michigan</td><td>20.64</td></tr>
<tr><td>28</td><td>Kansas</td><td>8.71</td><td>16</td><td>New Jersey</td><td>19.52</td></tr>
<tr><td>27</td><td>Kentucky</td><td>9.64</td><td>17</td><td>Missouri</td><td>17.45</td></tr>
<tr><td>2</td><td>Louisiana</td><td>42.20</td><td>18</td><td>Ohio</td><td>16.02</td></tr>
<tr><td>47</td><td>Maine</td><td>0.51</td><td>19</td><td>Pennsylvania</td><td>15.43</td></tr>
<tr><td>6</td><td>Maryland</td><td>32.67</td><td>20</td><td>Texas</td><td>13.41</td></tr>
<tr><td>25</td><td>Massachusetts</td><td>9.91</td><td>21</td><td>Connecticut</td><td>12.92</td></tr>
<tr><td>15</td><td>Michigan</td><td>20.64</td><td>22</td><td>Indiana</td><td>11.20</td></tr>
<tr><td>34</td><td>Minnesota</td><td>4.44</td><td>23</td><td>Oklahoma</td><td>10.86</td></tr>
<tr><td>1</td><td>Mississippi</td><td>48.09</td><td>24</td><td>Wisconsin</td><td>10.34</td></tr>
<tr><td>17</td><td>Missouri</td><td>17.45</td><td>25</td><td>Massachusetts</td><td>9.91</td></tr>
<tr><td>49</td><td>Montana</td><td>0.43</td><td>26</td><td>Nevada</td><td>9.67</td></tr>
<tr><td>31</td><td>Nebraska</td><td>5.61</td><td>27</td><td>Kentucky</td><td>9.64</td></tr>
<tr><td>26</td><td>Nevada</td><td>9.67</td><td>28</td><td>Kansas</td><td>8.71</td></tr>
<tr><td>45</td><td>New Hampshire</td><td>0.68</td><td>29</td><td>Rhode Island</td><td>8.18</td></tr>
<tr><td>16</td><td>New Jersey</td><td>19.52</td><td>30</td><td>California</td><td>7.73</td></tr>
<tr><td>41</td><td>New Mexico</td><td>1.84</td><td>31</td><td>Nebraska</td><td>5.61</td></tr>
<tr><td>14</td><td>New York</td><td>21.19</td><td>32</td><td>Colorado</td><td>5.52</td></tr>
<tr><td>7</td><td>North Carolina</td><td>29.18</td><td>33</td><td>Alaska</td><td>4.62</td></tr>
<tr><td>43</td><td>North Dakota</td><td>0.85</td><td>34</td><td>Minnesota</td><td>4.44</td></tr>
<tr><td>18</td><td>Ohio</td><td>16.02</td><td>35</td><td>Washington</td><td>3.96</td></tr>
<tr><td>23</td><td>Oklahoma</td><td>10.86</td><td>36</td><td>West Virginia</td><td>3.68</td></tr>
<tr><td>40</td><td>Oregon</td><td>2.27</td><td>37</td><td>Arizona</td><td>3.56</td></tr>
<tr><td>19</td><td>Pennsylvania</td><td>15.43</td><td>38</td><td>Hawaii</td><td>3.45</td></tr>
<tr><td>29</td><td>Rhode Island</td><td>8.18</td><td>39</td><td>Iowa</td><td>3.08</td></tr>
<tr><td>3</td><td>South Carolina</td><td>38.45</td><td>40</td><td>Oregon</td><td>2.27</td></tr>
<tr><td>44</td><td>South Dakota</td><td>0.72</td><td>41</td><td>New Mexico</td><td>1.84</td></tr>
<tr><td>10</td><td>Tennessee</td><td>23.79</td><td>42</td><td>Wyoming</td><td>0.97</td></tr>
<tr><td>20</td><td>Texas</td><td>13.41</td><td>43</td><td>North Dakota</td><td>0.85</td></tr>
<tr><td>46</td><td>Utah</td><td>0.66</td><td>44</td><td>South Dakota</td><td>0.72</td></tr>
<tr><td>48</td><td>Vermont</td><td>0.44</td><td>45</td><td>New Hampshire</td><td>0.68</td></tr>
<tr><td>8</td><td>Virginia</td><td>24.54</td><td>46</td><td>Utah</td><td>0.66</td></tr>
<tr><td>35</td><td>Washington</td><td>3.96</td><td>47</td><td>Maine</td><td>0.51</td></tr>
<tr><td>36</td><td>West Virginia</td><td>3.68</td><td>48</td><td>Vermont</td><td>0.44</td></tr>
<tr><td>24</td><td>Wisconsin</td><td>10.34</td><td>49</td><td>Montana</td><td>0.43</td></tr>
<tr><td>42</td><td>Wyoming</td><td>0.97</td><td>50</td><td>Idaho</td><td>0.33</td></tr>
<tr><td></td><td></td><td></td><td></td><td>District of Columbia</td><td>80.32</td></tr>
</table>

Source: Morgan Quitno Press using data from U.S. Department of Health and Human Services, National Center for Health "Monthly Vital Statistics Report" (Vol. 43, No. 5, Supplement, October 25, 1994)
*Final data by state of residence. By race of mother.

Births of Low Birthweight in 1992

National Total = 287,493 Live Births*

ALPHA ORDER					RANK ORDER			
RANK	**STATE**		**BIRTHS**	**% of USA**	**RANK**	**STATE**	**BIRTHS**	**% of USA**
18	Alabama		5,264	1.83%	1	California	35,704	12.42%
46	Alaska		577	0.20%	2	Texas	22,388	7.79%
22	Arizona		4,419	1.54%	3	New York	21,841	7.60%
30	Arkansas		2,835	0.99%	4	Illinois	14,772	5.14%
1	California		35,704	12.42%	5	Florida	14,239	4.95%
21	Colorado		4,632	1.61%	6	Ohio	11,920	4.15%
28	Connecticut		3,264	1.14%	7	Pennsylvania	11,799	4.10%
44	Delaware		806	0.28%	8	Michigan	10,780	3.75%
5	Florida		14,239	4.95%	9	Georgia	9,490	3.30%
9	Georgia		9,490	3.30%	10	North Carolina	8,737	3.04%
38	Hawaii		1,430	0.50%	11	New Jersey	8,664	3.01%
40	Idaho		955	0.33%	12	Virginia	7,158	2.49%
4	Illinois		14,772	5.14%	13	Louisiana	6,620	2.30%
16	Indiana		5,635	1.96%	14	Maryland	6,432	2.24%
32	Iowa		2,200	0.77%	15	Tennessee	6,241	2.17%
31	Kansas		2,451	0.85%	16	Indiana	5,635	1.96%
26	Kentucky		3,681	1.28%	17	Missouri	5,587	1.94%
13	Louisiana		6,620	2.30%	18	Alabama	5,264	1.83%
43	Maine		808	0.28%	19	Massachusetts	5,185	1.80%
14	Maryland		6,432	2.24%	20	South Carolina	5,066	1.76%
19	Massachusetts		5,185	1.80%	21	Colorado	4,632	1.61%
8	Michigan		10,780	3.75%	22	Arizona	4,419	1.54%
27	Minnesota		3,408	1.19%	23	Mississippi	4,221	1.47%
23	Mississippi		4,221	1.47%	24	Washington	4,205	1.46%
17	Missouri		5,587	1.94%	25	Wisconsin	4,193	1.46%
45	Montana		688	0.24%	26	Kentucky	3,681	1.28%
39	Nebraska		1,315	0.46%	27	Minnesota	3,408	1.19%
36	Nevada		1,599	0.56%	28	Connecticut	3,264	1.14%
42	New Hampshire		841	0.29%	29	Oklahoma	3,175	1.10%
11	New Jersey		8,664	3.01%	30	Arkansas	2,835	0.99%
35	New Mexico		2,013	0.70%	31	Kansas	2,451	0.85%
3	New York		21,841	7.60%	32	Iowa	2,200	0.77%
10	North Carolina		8,737	3.04%	33	Oregon	2,175	0.76%
49	North Dakota		448	0.16%	34	Utah	2,085	0.73%
6	Ohio		11,920	4.15%	35	New Mexico	2,013	0.70%
29	Oklahoma		3,175	1.10%	36	Nevada	1,599	0.56%
33	Oregon		2,175	0.76%	36	West Virginia	1,599	0.56%
7	Pennsylvania		11,799	4.10%	38	Hawaii	1,430	0.50%
41	Rhode Island		897	0.31%	39	Nebraska	1,315	0.46%
20	South Carolina		5,066	1.76%	40	Idaho	955	0.33%
47	South Dakota		573	0.20%	41	Rhode Island	897	0.31%
15	Tennessee		6,241	2.17%	42	New Hampshire	841	0.29%
2	Texas		22,388	7.79%	43	Maine	808	0.28%
34	Utah		2,085	0.73%	44	Delaware	806	0.28%
50	Vermont		431	0.15%	45	Montana	688	0.24%
12	Virginia		7,158	2.49%	46	Alaska	577	0.20%
24	Washington		4,205	1.46%	47	South Dakota	573	0.20%
36	West Virginia		1,599	0.56%	48	Wyoming	491	0.17%
25	Wisconsin		4,193	1.46%	49	North Dakota	448	0.16%
48	Wyoming		491	0.17%	50	Vermont	431	0.15%
						District of Columbia	1,556	0.54%

Source: U.S. Department of Health and Human Services, National Center for Health Statistics
"Monthly Vital Statistics Report" (Vol. 43, No. 5, Supplement, October 25, 1994)
*Final data by state of residence. Births of less than 2,500 grams (5 pounds 8 ounces).

Births of Low Birthweight as a Percent of All Births in 1992

National Percent = 7.1% of Live Births*

ALPHA ORDER			RANK ORDER		
RANK	STATE	PERCENT	RANK	STATE	PERCENT
4	Alabama	8.5	1	Mississippi	9.9
50	Alaska	4.9	2	Louisiana	9.4
31	Arizona	6.4	3	South Carolina	9.0
10	Arkansas	8.2	4	Alabama	8.5
36	California	5.9	4	Colorado	8.5
4	Colorado	8.5	4	Georgia	8.5
27	Connecticut	6.9	4	Tennessee	8.5
12	Delaware	7.6	8	North Carolina	8.4
15	Florida	7.4	9	Maryland	8.3
4	Georgia	8.5	10	Arkansas	8.2
20	Hawaii	7.2	11	Illinois	7.7
42	Idaho	5.5	12	Delaware	7.6
11	Illinois	7.7	12	New York	7.6
29	Indiana	6.7	14	Michigan	7.5
38	Iowa	5.7	15	Florida	7.4
31	Kansas	6.4	15	Ohio	7.4
28	Kentucky	6.8	15	Virginia	7.4
2	Louisiana	9.4	18	Missouri	7.3
49	Maine	5.0	18	Wyoming	7.3
9	Maryland	8.3	20	Hawaii	7.2
34	Massachusetts	6.0	20	New Jersey	7.2
14	Michigan	7.5	20	New Mexico	7.2
45	Minnesota	5.2	20	Pennsylvania	7.2
1	Mississippi	9.9	20	West Virginia	7.2
18	Missouri	7.3	25	Nevada	7.1
34	Montana	6.0	26	Texas	7.0
39	Nebraska	5.6	27	Connecticut	6.9
25	Nevada	7.1	28	Kentucky	6.8
43	New Hampshire	5.3	29	Indiana	6.7
20	New Jersey	7.2	29	Oklahoma	6.7
20	New Mexico	7.2	31	Arizona	6.4
12	New York	7.6	31	Kansas	6.4
8	North Carolina	8.4	33	Rhode Island	6.3
48	North Dakota	5.1	34	Massachusetts	6.0
15	Ohio	7.4	34	Montana	6.0
29	Oklahoma	6.7	36	California	5.9
45	Oregon	5.2	36	Wisconsin	5.9
20	Pennsylvania	7.2	38	Iowa	5.7
33	Rhode Island	6.3	39	Nebraska	5.6
3	South Carolina	9.0	39	Utah	5.6
45	South Dakota	5.2	39	Vermont	5.6
4	Tennessee	8.5	42	Idaho	5.5
26	Texas	7.0	43	New Hampshire	5.3
39	Utah	5.6	43	Washington	5.3
39	Vermont	5.6	45	Minnesota	5.2
15	Virginia	7.4	45	Oregon	5.2
43	Washington	5.3	45	South Dakota	5.2
20	West Virginia	7.2	48	North Dakota	5.1
36	Wisconsin	5.9	49	Maine	5.0
18	Wyoming	7.3	50	Alaska	4.9

District of Columbia	14.3

Source: U.S. Department of Health and Human Services, National Center for Health Statistics
"Monthly Vital Statistics Report" (Vol. 43, No. 5, Supplement, October 25, 1994)
*Final data by state of residence. Births of less than 2,500 grams (5 pounds 8 ounces).

Births of Low Birthweight to White Women in 1992

National Total = 185,662 Live Births*

ALPHA ORDER

RANK	STATE	BIRTHS	% of USA
25	Alabama	2,470	1.33%
49	Alaska	344	0.19%
18	Arizona	3,684	1.98%
33	Arkansas	1,720	0.93%
1	California	25,890	13.94%
15	Colorado	3,964	2.14%
26	Connecticut	2,324	1.25%
45	Delaware	459	0.25%
4	Florida	8,596	4.63%
12	Georgia	4,105	2.21%
50	Hawaii	309	0.17%
39	Idaho	922	0.50%
6	Illinois	8,114	4.37%
11	Indiana	4,422	2.38%
30	Iowa	1,989	1.07%
29	Kansas	2,007	1.08%
20	Kentucky	3,050	1.64%
24	Louisiana	2,477	1.33%
41	Maine	793	0.43%
23	Maryland	2,799	1.51%
13	Massachusetts	4,019	2.16%
8	Michigan	6,257	3.37%
22	Minnesota	2,867	1.54%
36	Mississippi	1,473	0.79%
17	Missouri	3,701	1.99%
43	Montana	600	0.32%
38	Nebraska	1,124	0.61%
37	Nevada	1,218	0.66%
40	New Hampshire	821	0.44%
9	New Jersey	5,136	2.77%
34	New Mexico	1,696	0.91%
3	New York	12,924	6.96%
10	North Carolina	4,499	2.42%
48	North Dakota	390	0.21%
5	Ohio	8,190	4.41%
27	Oklahoma	2,252	1.21%
32	Oregon	1,938	1.04%
7	Pennsylvania	7,897	4.25%
42	Rhode Island	738	0.40%
28	South Carolina	2,146	1.16%
44	South Dakota	462	0.25%
16	Tennessee	3,722	2.00%
2	Texas	16,277	8.77%
31	Utah	1,964	1.06%
47	Vermont	422	0.23%
14	Virginia	3,968	2.14%
19	Washington	3,458	1.86%
35	West Virginia	1,489	0.80%
21	Wisconsin	3,046	1.64%
46	Wyoming	457	0.25%

RANK ORDER

RANK	STATE	BIRTHS	% of USA
1	California	25,890	13.94%
2	Texas	16,277	8.77%
3	New York	12,924	6.96%
4	Florida	8,596	4.63%
5	Ohio	8,190	4.41%
6	Illinois	8,114	4.37%
7	Pennsylvania	7,897	4.25%
8	Michigan	6,257	3.37%
9	New Jersey	5,136	2.77%
10	North Carolina	4,499	2.42%
11	Indiana	4,422	2.38%
12	Georgia	4,105	2.21%
13	Massachusetts	4,019	2.16%
14	Virginia	3,968	2.14%
15	Colorado	3,964	2.14%
16	Tennessee	3,722	2.00%
17	Missouri	3,701	1.99%
18	Arizona	3,684	1.98%
19	Washington	3,458	1.86%
20	Kentucky	3,050	1.64%
21	Wisconsin	3,046	1.64%
22	Minnesota	2,867	1.54%
23	Maryland	2,799	1.51%
24	Louisiana	2,477	1.33%
25	Alabama	2,470	1.33%
26	Connecticut	2,324	1.25%
27	Oklahoma	2,252	1.21%
28	South Carolina	2,146	1.16%
29	Kansas	2,007	1.08%
30	Iowa	1,989	1.07%
31	Utah	1,964	1.06%
32	Oregon	1,938	1.04%
33	Arkansas	1,720	0.93%
34	New Mexico	1,696	0.91%
35	West Virginia	1,489	0.80%
36	Mississippi	1,473	0.79%
37	Nevada	1,218	0.66%
38	Nebraska	1,124	0.61%
39	Idaho	922	0.50%
40	New Hampshire	821	0.44%
41	Maine	793	0.43%
42	Rhode Island	738	0.40%
43	Montana	600	0.32%
44	South Dakota	462	0.25%
45	Delaware	459	0.25%
46	Wyoming	457	0.25%
47	Vermont	422	0.23%
48	North Dakota	390	0.21%
49	Alaska	344	0.19%
50	Hawaii	309	0.17%
	District of Columbia	73	0.04%

Source: U.S. Department of Health and Human Services, National Center for Health Statistics
"Monthly Vital Statistics Report" (Vol. 43, No. 5, Supplement, October 25, 1994)
*Final data by state of residence. Births of less than 2,500 grams (5 pounds 8 ounces).

Births of Low Birthweight to White Women
As a Percent of All Births to White Women in 1992
National Percent = 5.8% of Live Births to White Women*

ALPHA ORDER

RANK	STATE	PERCENT
12	Alabama	6.2
50	Alaska	4.3
12	Arizona	6.2
7	Arkansas	6.5
40	California	5.3
1	Colorado	8.0
26	Connecticut	5.8
26	Delaware	5.8
18	Florida	6.0
18	Georgia	6.0
37	Hawaii	5.4
35	Idaho	5.5
29	Illinois	5.7
18	Indiana	6.0
37	Iowa	5.4
18	Kansas	6.0
10	Kentucky	6.3
12	Louisiana	6.2
44	Maine	5.0
29	Maryland	5.7
37	Massachusetts	5.4
33	Michigan	5.6
49	Minnesota	4.8
5	Mississippi	6.8
18	Missouri	6.0
18	Montana	6.0
40	Nebraska	5.3
8	Nevada	6.4
42	New Hampshire	5.2
29	New Jersey	5.7
2	New Mexico	7.3
15	New York	6.1
8	North Carolina	6.4
44	North Dakota	5.0
15	Ohio	6.1
15	Oklahoma	6.1
44	Oregon	5.0
26	Pennsylvania	5.8
25	Rhode Island	5.9
10	South Carolina	6.3
43	South Dakota	5.1
6	Tennessee	6.7
18	Texas	6.0
33	Utah	5.6
35	Vermont	5.5
29	Virginia	5.7
48	Washington	4.9
4	West Virginia	7.0
44	Wisconsin	5.0
3	Wyoming	7.2

RANK ORDER

RANK	STATE	PERCENT
1	Colorado	8.0
2	New Mexico	7.3
3	Wyoming	7.2
4	West Virginia	7.0
5	Mississippi	6.8
6	Tennessee	6.7
7	Arkansas	6.5
8	Nevada	6.4
8	North Carolina	6.4
10	Kentucky	6.3
10	South Carolina	6.3
12	Alabama	6.2
12	Arizona	6.2
12	Louisiana	6.2
15	New York	6.1
15	Ohio	6.1
15	Oklahoma	6.1
18	Florida	6.0
18	Georgia	6.0
18	Indiana	6.0
18	Kansas	6.0
18	Missouri	6.0
18	Montana	6.0
18	Texas	6.0
25	Rhode Island	5.9
26	Connecticut	5.8
26	Delaware	5.8
26	Pennsylvania	5.8
29	Illinois	5.7
29	Maryland	5.7
29	New Jersey	5.7
29	Virginia	5.7
33	Michigan	5.6
33	Utah	5.6
35	Idaho	5.5
35	Vermont	5.5
37	Hawaii	5.4
37	Iowa	5.4
37	Massachusetts	5.4
40	California	5.3
40	Nebraska	5.3
42	New Hampshire	5.2
43	South Dakota	5.1
44	Maine	5.0
44	North Dakota	5.0
44	Oregon	5.0
44	Wisconsin	5.0
48	Washington	4.9
49	Minnesota	4.8
50	Alaska	4.3

District of Columbia   4.6

Source: U.S. Department of Health and Human Services, National Center for Health Statistics
"Monthly Vital Statistics Report" (Vol. 43, No. 5, Supplement, October 25, 1994)
*Final data by state of residence. Births of less than 2,500 grams (5 pounds 8 ounces).

Births of Low Birthweight to Black Women in 1992

National Total = 89,517 Live Births*

ALPHA ORDER

RANK ORDER

RANK	STATE	BIRTHS	% of USA	RANK	STATE	BIRTHS	% of USA
16	Alabama	2,763	3.09%	1	New York	7,973	8.91%
41	Alaska	58	0.06%	2	Illinois	6,258	6.99%
32	Arizona	306	0.34%	3	California	5,880	6.57%
21	Arkansas	1,095	1.22%	4	Texas	5,583	6.24%
3	California	5,880	6.57%	5	Florida	5,408	6.04%
27	Colorado	509	0.57%	6	Georgia	5,267	5.88%
24	Connecticut	857	0.96%	7	Michigan	4,393	4.91%
30	Delaware	333	0.37%	8	Louisiana	4,080	4.56%
5	Florida	5,408	6.04%	9	North Carolina	4,015	4.49%
6	Georgia	5,267	5.88%	10	Pennsylvania	3,689	4.12%
39	Hawaii	73	0.08%	11	Ohio	3,600	4.02%
48	Idaho	5	0.01%	12	Maryland	3,464	3.87%
2	Illinois	6,258	6.99%	13	New Jersey	3,143	3.51%
20	Indiana	1,165	1.30%	14	Virginia	3,000	3.35%
35	Iowa	152	0.17%	15	South Carolina	2,879	3.22%
28	Kansas	383	0.43%	16	Alabama	2,763	3.09%
26	Kentucky	611	0.68%	17	Mississippi	2,705	3.02%
8	Louisiana	4,080	4.56%	18	Tennessee	2,451	2.74%
48	Maine	5	0.01%	19	Missouri	1,811	2.02%
12	Maryland	3,464	3.87%	20	Indiana	1,165	1.30%
23	Massachusetts	940	1.05%	21	Arkansas	1,095	1.22%
7	Michigan	4,393	4.91%	22	Wisconsin	982	1.10%
30	Minnesota	333	0.37%	23	Massachusetts	940	1.05%
17	Mississippi	2,705	3.02%	24	Connecticut	857	0.96%
19	Missouri	1,811	2.02%	25	Oklahoma	634	0.71%
48	Montana	5	0.01%	26	Kentucky	611	0.68%
34	Nebraska	155	0.17%	27	Colorado	509	0.57%
33	Nevada	298	0.33%	28	Kansas	383	0.43%
44	New Hampshire	9	0.01%	29	Washington	373	0.42%
13	New Jersey	3,143	3.51%	30	Delaware	333	0.37%
40	New Mexico	68	0.08%	30	Minnesota	333	0.37%
1	New York	7,973	8.91%	32	Arizona	306	0.34%
9	North Carolina	4,015	4.49%	33	Nevada	298	0.33%
43	North Dakota	10	0.01%	34	Nebraska	155	0.17%
11	Ohio	3,600	4.02%	35	Iowa	152	0.17%
25	Oklahoma	634	0.71%	36	Rhode Island	109	0.12%
37	Oregon	104	0.12%	37	Oregon	104	0.12%
10	Pennsylvania	3,689	4.12%	38	West Virginia	101	0.11%
36	Rhode Island	109	0.12%	39	Hawaii	73	0.08%
15	South Carolina	2,879	3.22%	40	New Mexico	68	0.08%
46	South Dakota	7	0.01%	41	Alaska	58	0.06%
18	Tennessee	2,451	2.74%	42	Utah	22	0.02%
4	Texas	5,583	6.24%	43	North Dakota	10	0.01%
42	Utah	22	0.02%	44	New Hampshire	9	0.01%
47	Vermont	6	0.01%	44	Wyoming	9	0.01%
14	Virginia	3,000	3.35%	46	South Dakota	7	0.01%
29	Washington	373	0.42%	47	Vermont	6	0.01%
38	West Virginia	101	0.11%	48	Idaho	5	0.01%
22	Wisconsin	982	1.10%	48	Maine	5	0.01%
44	Wyoming	9	0.01%	48	Montana	5	0.01%
					District of Columbia	1,438	1.61%

Source: U.S. Department of Health and Human Services, National Center for Health Statistics
"Monthly Vital Statistics Report" (Vol. 43, No. 5, Supplement, October 25, 1994)
*Final data by state of residence. Births of less than 2,500 grams (5 pounds 8 ounces).

Births of Low Birthweight to Black Women
As a Percent of All Births to Black Women in 1992
National Percent = 13.3% of Live Births to Black Women*

ALPHA ORDER

RANK	STATE	PERCENT
24	Alabama	12.8
39	Alaska	10.7
27	Arizona	12.5
12	Arkansas	13.5
25	California	12.6
1	Colorado	16.9
5	Connecticut	14.0
19	Delaware	13.1
31	Florida	12.0
19	Georgia	13.1
39	Hawaii	10.7
NA	Idaho**	NA
3	Illinois	14.6
28	Indiana	12.4
23	Iowa	12.9
35	Kansas	11.6
33	Kentucky	11.8
9	Louisiana	13.7
NA	Maine**	NA
9	Maryland	13.7
37	Massachusetts	10.9
2	Michigan	14.8
36	Minnesota	11.4
17	Mississippi	13.2
11	Missouri	13.6
NA	Montana**	NA
33	Nebraska	11.8
8	Nevada	13.8
NA	New Hampshire**	NA
12	New Jersey	13.5
15	New Mexico	13.3
19	New York	13.1
17	North Carolina	13.2
NA	North Dakota**	NA
7	Ohio	13.9
28	Oklahoma	12.4
37	Oregon	10.9
4	Pennsylvania	14.5
41	Rhode Island	9.3
15	South Carolina	13.3
NA	South Dakota**	NA
5	Tennessee	14.0
22	Texas	13.0
42	Utah	9.0
NA	Vermont**	NA
25	Virginia	12.6
32	Washington	11.9
28	West Virginia	12.4
14	Wisconsin	13.4
NA	Wyoming**	NA

RANK ORDER

RANK	STATE	PERCENT
1	Colorado	16.9
2	Michigan	14.8
3	Illinois	14.6
4	Pennsylvania	14.5
5	Connecticut	14.0
5	Tennessee	14.0
7	Ohio	13.9
8	Nevada	13.8
9	Louisiana	13.7
9	Maryland	13.7
11	Missouri	13.6
12	Arkansas	13.5
12	New Jersey	13.5
14	Wisconsin	13.4
15	New Mexico	13.3
15	South Carolina	13.3
17	Mississippi	13.2
17	North Carolina	13.2
19	Delaware	13.1
19	Georgia	13.1
19	New York	13.1
22	Texas	13.0
23	Iowa	12.9
24	Alabama	12.8
25	California	12.6
25	Virginia	12.6
27	Arizona	12.5
28	Indiana	12.4
28	Oklahoma	12.4
28	West Virginia	12.4
31	Florida	12.0
32	Washington	11.9
33	Kentucky	11.8
33	Nebraska	11.8
35	Kansas	11.6
36	Minnesota	11.4
37	Massachusetts	10.9
37	Oregon	10.9
39	Alaska	10.7
39	Hawaii	10.7
41	Rhode Island	9.3
42	Utah	9.0
NA	Idaho**	NA
NA	Maine**	NA
NA	Montana**	NA
NA	New Hampshire**	NA
NA	North Dakota**	NA
NA	South Dakota**	NA
NA	Vermont**	NA
NA	Wyoming**	NA

	District of Columbia	16.4

*Source: U.S. Department of Health and Human Services, National Center for Health Statistics
"Monthly Vital Statistics Report" (Vol. 43, No. 5, Supplement, October 25, 1994)*
Final data by state of residence. Births of less than 2,500 grams (5 pounds 8 ounces).
***Insufficient data.*

Births to Unmarried Women in 1992

National Total = 1,224,876 Live Births*

<table>
<tr><td colspan="4"><u>ALPHA ORDER</u></td><td colspan="4"><u>RANK ORDER</u></td></tr>
<tr><td>RANK</td><td>STATE</td><td>BIRTHS</td><td>% of USA</td><td>RANK</td><td>STATE</td><td>BIRTHS</td><td>% of USA</td></tr>
<tr><td>20</td><td>Alabama</td><td>20,272</td><td>1.66%</td><td>1</td><td>California</td><td>206,396</td><td>16.85%</td></tr>
<tr><td>43</td><td>Alaska</td><td>3,215</td><td>0.26%</td><td>2</td><td>New York</td><td>100,260</td><td>8.19%</td></tr>
<tr><td>14</td><td>Arizona</td><td>24,939</td><td>2.04%</td><td>3</td><td>Florida</td><td>65,491</td><td>5.35%</td></tr>
<tr><td>32</td><td>Arkansas</td><td>10,781</td><td>0.88%</td><td>4</td><td>Illinois</td><td>63,979</td><td>5.22%</td></tr>
<tr><td>1</td><td>California</td><td>206,396</td><td>16.85%</td><td>5</td><td>Texas</td><td>55,994</td><td>4.57%</td></tr>
<tr><td>29</td><td>Colorado</td><td>12,971</td><td>1.06%</td><td>6</td><td>Pennsylvania</td><td>51,959</td><td>4.24%</td></tr>
<tr><td>27</td><td>Connecticut</td><td>13,657</td><td>1.11%</td><td>7</td><td>Ohio</td><td>51,317</td><td>4.19%</td></tr>
<tr><td>42</td><td>Delaware</td><td>3,470</td><td>0.28%</td><td>8</td><td>Georgia</td><td>38,925</td><td>3.18%</td></tr>
<tr><td>3</td><td>Florida</td><td>65,491</td><td>5.35%</td><td>9</td><td>Michigan</td><td>38,620</td><td>3.15%</td></tr>
<tr><td>8</td><td>Georgia</td><td>38,925</td><td>3.18%</td><td>10</td><td>North Carolina</td><td>32,547</td><td>2.66%</td></tr>
<tr><td>39</td><td>Hawaii</td><td>5,204</td><td>0.42%</td><td>11</td><td>New Jersey</td><td>31,631</td><td>2.58%</td></tr>
<tr><td>44</td><td>Idaho</td><td>3,179</td><td>0.26%</td><td>12</td><td>Louisiana</td><td>28,452</td><td>2.32%</td></tr>
<tr><td>4</td><td>Illinois</td><td>63,979</td><td>5.22%</td><td>13</td><td>Virginia</td><td>27,538</td><td>2.25%</td></tr>
<tr><td>15</td><td>Indiana</td><td>24,786</td><td>2.02%</td><td>14</td><td>Arizona</td><td>24,939</td><td>2.04%</td></tr>
<tr><td>34</td><td>Iowa</td><td>9,058</td><td>0.74%</td><td>15</td><td>Indiana</td><td>24,786</td><td>2.02%</td></tr>
<tr><td>33</td><td>Kansas</td><td>9,224</td><td>0.75%</td><td>16</td><td>Tennessee</td><td>24,061</td><td>1.96%</td></tr>
<tr><td>26</td><td>Kentucky</td><td>14,181</td><td>1.16%</td><td>17</td><td>Missouri</td><td>24,049</td><td>1.96%</td></tr>
<tr><td>12</td><td>Louisiana</td><td>28,452</td><td>2.32%</td><td>18</td><td>Maryland</td><td>23,717</td><td>1.94%</td></tr>
<tr><td>41</td><td>Maine</td><td>4,063</td><td>0.33%</td><td>19</td><td>Massachusetts</td><td>22,618</td><td>1.85%</td></tr>
<tr><td>18</td><td>Maryland</td><td>23,717</td><td>1.94%</td><td>20</td><td>Alabama</td><td>20,272</td><td>1.66%</td></tr>
<tr><td>19</td><td>Massachusetts</td><td>22,618</td><td>1.85%</td><td>21</td><td>Washington</td><td>20,116</td><td>1.64%</td></tr>
<tr><td>9</td><td>Michigan</td><td>38,620</td><td>3.15%</td><td>22</td><td>South Carolina</td><td>19,934</td><td>1.63%</td></tr>
<tr><td>25</td><td>Minnesota</td><td>15,058</td><td>1.23%</td><td>23</td><td>Wisconsin</td><td>18,444</td><td>1.51%</td></tr>
<tr><td>24</td><td>Mississippi</td><td>18,312</td><td>1.50%</td><td>24</td><td>Mississippi</td><td>18,312</td><td>1.50%</td></tr>
<tr><td>17</td><td>Missouri</td><td>24,049</td><td>1.96%</td><td>25</td><td>Minnesota</td><td>15,058</td><td>1.23%</td></tr>
<tr><td>46</td><td>Montana</td><td>3,032</td><td>0.25%</td><td>26</td><td>Kentucky</td><td>14,181</td><td>1.16%</td></tr>
<tr><td>38</td><td>Nebraska</td><td>5,290</td><td>0.43%</td><td>27</td><td>Connecticut</td><td>13,657</td><td>1.11%</td></tr>
<tr><td>35</td><td>Nevada</td><td>7,449</td><td>0.61%</td><td>28</td><td>Oklahoma</td><td>13,486</td><td>1.10%</td></tr>
<tr><td>45</td><td>New Hampshire</td><td>3,068</td><td>0.25%</td><td>29</td><td>Colorado</td><td>12,971</td><td>1.06%</td></tr>
<tr><td>11</td><td>New Jersey</td><td>31,631</td><td>2.58%</td><td>30</td><td>Oregon</td><td>11,343</td><td>0.93%</td></tr>
<tr><td>31</td><td>New Mexico</td><td>11,023</td><td>0.90%</td><td>31</td><td>New Mexico</td><td>11,023</td><td>0.90%</td></tr>
<tr><td>2</td><td>New York</td><td>100,260</td><td>8.19%</td><td>32</td><td>Arkansas</td><td>10,781</td><td>0.88%</td></tr>
<tr><td>10</td><td>North Carolina</td><td>32,547</td><td>2.66%</td><td>33</td><td>Kansas</td><td>9,224</td><td>0.75%</td></tr>
<tr><td>48</td><td>North Dakota</td><td>1,995</td><td>0.16%</td><td>34</td><td>Iowa</td><td>9,058</td><td>0.74%</td></tr>
<tr><td>7</td><td>Ohio</td><td>51,317</td><td>4.19%</td><td>35</td><td>Nevada</td><td>7,449</td><td>0.61%</td></tr>
<tr><td>28</td><td>Oklahoma</td><td>13,486</td><td>1.10%</td><td>36</td><td>West Virginia</td><td>6,149</td><td>0.50%</td></tr>
<tr><td>30</td><td>Oregon</td><td>11,343</td><td>0.93%</td><td>37</td><td>Utah</td><td>5,634</td><td>0.46%</td></tr>
<tr><td>6</td><td>Pennsylvania</td><td>51,959</td><td>4.24%</td><td>38</td><td>Nebraska</td><td>5,290</td><td>0.43%</td></tr>
<tr><td>40</td><td>Rhode Island</td><td>4,298</td><td>0.35%</td><td>39</td><td>Hawaii</td><td>5,204</td><td>0.42%</td></tr>
<tr><td>22</td><td>South Carolina</td><td>19,934</td><td>1.63%</td><td>40</td><td>Rhode Island</td><td>4,298</td><td>0.35%</td></tr>
<tr><td>47</td><td>South Dakota</td><td>2,933</td><td>0.24%</td><td>41</td><td>Maine</td><td>4,063</td><td>0.33%</td></tr>
<tr><td>16</td><td>Tennessee</td><td>24,061</td><td>1.96%</td><td>42</td><td>Delaware</td><td>3,470</td><td>0.28%</td></tr>
<tr><td>5</td><td>Texas</td><td>55,994</td><td>4.57%</td><td>43</td><td>Alaska</td><td>3,215</td><td>0.26%</td></tr>
<tr><td>37</td><td>Utah</td><td>5,634</td><td>0.46%</td><td>44</td><td>Idaho</td><td>3,179</td><td>0.26%</td></tr>
<tr><td>49</td><td>Vermont</td><td>1,811</td><td>0.15%</td><td>45</td><td>New Hampshire</td><td>3,068</td><td>0.25%</td></tr>
<tr><td>13</td><td>Virginia</td><td>27,538</td><td>2.25%</td><td>46</td><td>Montana</td><td>3,032</td><td>0.25%</td></tr>
<tr><td>21</td><td>Washington</td><td>20,116</td><td>1.64%</td><td>47</td><td>South Dakota</td><td>2,933</td><td>0.24%</td></tr>
<tr><td>36</td><td>West Virginia</td><td>6,149</td><td>0.50%</td><td>48</td><td>North Dakota</td><td>1,995</td><td>0.16%</td></tr>
<tr><td>23</td><td>Wisconsin</td><td>18,444</td><td>1.51%</td><td>49</td><td>Vermont</td><td>1,811</td><td>0.15%</td></tr>
<tr><td>50</td><td>Wyoming</td><td>1,613</td><td>0.13%</td><td>50</td><td>Wyoming</td><td>1,613</td><td>0.13%</td></tr>
<tr><td></td><td></td><td></td><td></td><td></td><td>District of Columbia</td><td>7,334</td><td>0.60%</td></tr>
</table>

Source: U.S. Department of Health and Human Services, National Center for Health Statistics
"Monthly Vital Statistics Report" (Vol. 43, No. 5, Supplement, October 25, 1994)
*Final data by state of residence.

Births to Unmarried Women as a Percent of All Births in 1992

National Percent = 30.1% of Live Births to Unmarried Women*

ALPHA ORDER

RANK	STATE	PERCENT
13	Alabama	32.6
27	Alaska	27.4
4	Arizona	36.2
19	Arkansas	31.0
8	California	34.3
41	Colorado	23.8
23	Connecticut	28.7
13	Delaware	32.6
9	Florida	34.2
6	Georgia	35.0
34	Hawaii	26.2
48	Idaho	18.3
10	Illinois	33.4
22	Indiana	29.5
42	Iowa	23.5
39	Kansas	24.3
33	Kentucky	26.3
2	Louisiana	40.2
37	Maine	25.3
20	Maryland	30.5
36	Massachusetts	25.9
29	Michigan	26.8
44	Minnesota	23.0
1	Mississippi	42.9
17	Missouri	31.5
31	Montana	26.4
45	Nebraska	22.6
11	Nevada	33.3
47	New Hampshire	19.2
31	New Jersey	26.4
3	New Mexico	39.5
7	New York	34.8
18	North Carolina	31.3
45	North Dakota	22.6
15	Ohio	31.6
24	Oklahoma	28.4
28	Oregon	27.0
15	Pennsylvania	31.6
21	Rhode Island	29.6
5	South Carolina	35.5
30	South Dakota	26.6
12	Tennessee	32.7
49	Texas	17.5
50	Utah	15.1
43	Vermont	23.4
25	Virginia	28.3
37	Washington	25.3
26	West Virginia	27.7
35	Wisconsin	26.1
40	Wyoming	24.0

RANK ORDER

RANK	STATE	PERCENT
1	Mississippi	42.9
2	Louisiana	40.2
3	New Mexico	39.5
4	Arizona	36.2
5	South Carolina	35.5
6	Georgia	35.0
7	New York	34.8
8	California	34.3
9	Florida	34.2
10	Illinois	33.4
11	Nevada	33.3
12	Tennessee	32.7
13	Alabama	32.6
13	Delaware	32.6
15	Ohio	31.6
15	Pennsylvania	31.6
17	Missouri	31.5
18	North Carolina	31.3
19	Arkansas	31.0
20	Maryland	30.5
21	Rhode Island	29.6
22	Indiana	29.5
23	Connecticut	28.7
24	Oklahoma	28.4
25	Virginia	28.3
26	West Virginia	27.7
27	Alaska	27.4
28	Oregon	27.0
29	Michigan	26.8
30	South Dakota	26.6
31	Montana	26.4
31	New Jersey	26.4
33	Kentucky	26.3
34	Hawaii	26.2
35	Wisconsin	26.1
36	Massachusetts	25.9
37	Maine	25.3
37	Washington	25.3
39	Kansas	24.3
40	Wyoming	24.0
41	Colorado	23.8
42	Iowa	23.5
43	Vermont	23.4
44	Minnesota	23.0
45	Nebraska	22.6
45	North Dakota	22.6
47	New Hampshire	19.2
48	Idaho	18.3
49	Texas	17.5
50	Utah	15.1

| | District of Columbia | 66.9 |

Source: U.S. Department of Health and Human Services, National Center for Health Statistics
"Monthly Vital Statistics Report" (Vol. 43, No. 5, Supplement, October 25, 1994)
*Final data by state of residence.

Births to Unmarried White Women in 1992

National Total = 721,986 Live Births*

<table>
<tr><td colspan="4">ALPHA ORDER</td><td colspan="4">RANK ORDER</td></tr>
<tr><td>RANK</td><td>STATE</td><td>BIRTHS</td><td>% of USA</td><td>RANK</td><td>STATE</td><td>BIRTHS</td><td>% of USA</td></tr>
<tr><td>33</td><td>Alabama</td><td>5,517</td><td>0.76%</td><td>1</td><td>California</td><td>167,651</td><td>23.22%</td></tr>
<tr><td>47</td><td>Alaska</td><td>1,505</td><td>0.21%</td><td>2</td><td>New York</td><td>56,641</td><td>7.85%</td></tr>
<tr><td>8</td><td>Arizona</td><td>19,443</td><td>2.69%</td><td>3</td><td>Texas</td><td>35,324</td><td>4.89%</td></tr>
<tr><td>36</td><td>Arkansas</td><td>4,886</td><td>0.68%</td><td>4</td><td>Florida</td><td>33,993</td><td>4.71%</td></tr>
<tr><td>1</td><td>California</td><td>167,651</td><td>23.22%</td><td>5</td><td>Pennsylvania</td><td>31,183</td><td>4.32%</td></tr>
<tr><td>21</td><td>Colorado</td><td>10,801</td><td>1.50%</td><td>6</td><td>Ohio</td><td>31,024</td><td>4.30%</td></tr>
<tr><td>24</td><td>Connecticut</td><td>8,934</td><td>1.24%</td><td>7</td><td>Illinois</td><td>29,544</td><td>4.09%</td></tr>
<tr><td>46</td><td>Delaware</td><td>1,593</td><td>0.22%</td><td>8</td><td>Arizona</td><td>19,443</td><td>2.69%</td></tr>
<tr><td>4</td><td>Florida</td><td>33,993</td><td>4.71%</td><td>9</td><td>Indiana</td><td>17,461</td><td>2.42%</td></tr>
<tr><td>17</td><td>Georgia</td><td>11,607</td><td>1.61%</td><td>10</td><td>Michigan</td><td>16,838</td><td>2.33%</td></tr>
<tr><td>50</td><td>Hawaii</td><td>888</td><td>0.12%</td><td>11</td><td>Washington</td><td>16,448</td><td>2.28%</td></tr>
<tr><td>41</td><td>Idaho</td><td>3,016</td><td>0.42%</td><td>12</td><td>Massachusetts</td><td>16,368</td><td>2.27%</td></tr>
<tr><td>7</td><td>Illinois</td><td>29,544</td><td>4.09%</td><td>13</td><td>New Jersey</td><td>15,821</td><td>2.19%</td></tr>
<tr><td>9</td><td>Indiana</td><td>17,461</td><td>2.42%</td><td>14</td><td>Missouri</td><td>13,340</td><td>1.85%</td></tr>
<tr><td>28</td><td>Iowa</td><td>7,990</td><td>1.11%</td><td>15</td><td>Virginia</td><td>11,924</td><td>1.65%</td></tr>
<tr><td>30</td><td>Kansas</td><td>6,789</td><td>0.94%</td><td>16</td><td>Wisconsin</td><td>11,685</td><td>1.62%</td></tr>
<tr><td>22</td><td>Kentucky</td><td>10,455</td><td>1.45%</td><td>17</td><td>Georgia</td><td>11,607</td><td>1.61%</td></tr>
<tr><td>29</td><td>Louisiana</td><td>7,350</td><td>1.02%</td><td>18</td><td>Minnesota</td><td>11,451</td><td>1.59%</td></tr>
<tr><td>38</td><td>Maine</td><td>3,980</td><td>0.55%</td><td>19</td><td>North Carolina</td><td>11,394</td><td>1.58%</td></tr>
<tr><td>25</td><td>Maryland</td><td>8,089</td><td>1.12%</td><td>20</td><td>Tennessee</td><td>11,088</td><td>1.54%</td></tr>
<tr><td>12</td><td>Massachusetts</td><td>16,368</td><td>2.27%</td><td>21</td><td>Colorado</td><td>10,801</td><td>1.50%</td></tr>
<tr><td>10</td><td>Michigan</td><td>16,838</td><td>2.33%</td><td>22</td><td>Kentucky</td><td>10,455</td><td>1.45%</td></tr>
<tr><td>18</td><td>Minnesota</td><td>11,451</td><td>1.59%</td><td>23</td><td>Oregon</td><td>10,059</td><td>1.39%</td></tr>
<tr><td>39</td><td>Mississippi</td><td>3,291</td><td>0.46%</td><td>24</td><td>Connecticut</td><td>8,934</td><td>1.24%</td></tr>
<tr><td>14</td><td>Missouri</td><td>13,340</td><td>1.85%</td><td>25</td><td>Maryland</td><td>8,089</td><td>1.12%</td></tr>
<tr><td>43</td><td>Montana</td><td>2,076</td><td>0.29%</td><td>26</td><td>Oklahoma</td><td>8,025</td><td>1.11%</td></tr>
<tr><td>37</td><td>Nebraska</td><td>4,019</td><td>0.56%</td><td>27</td><td>New Mexico</td><td>8,003</td><td>1.11%</td></tr>
<tr><td>34</td><td>Nevada</td><td>5,462</td><td>0.76%</td><td>28</td><td>Iowa</td><td>7,990</td><td>1.11%</td></tr>
<tr><td>42</td><td>New Hampshire</td><td>3,000</td><td>0.42%</td><td>29</td><td>Louisiana</td><td>7,350</td><td>1.02%</td></tr>
<tr><td>13</td><td>New Jersey</td><td>15,821</td><td>2.19%</td><td>30</td><td>Kansas</td><td>6,789</td><td>0.94%</td></tr>
<tr><td>27</td><td>New Mexico</td><td>8,003</td><td>1.11%</td><td>31</td><td>South Carolina</td><td>5,693</td><td>0.79%</td></tr>
<tr><td>2</td><td>New York</td><td>56,641</td><td>7.85%</td><td>32</td><td>West Virginia</td><td>5,559</td><td>0.77%</td></tr>
<tr><td>19</td><td>North Carolina</td><td>11,394</td><td>1.58%</td><td>33</td><td>Alabama</td><td>5,517</td><td>0.76%</td></tr>
<tr><td>48</td><td>North Dakota</td><td>1,425</td><td>0.20%</td><td>34</td><td>Nevada</td><td>5,462</td><td>0.76%</td></tr>
<tr><td>6</td><td>Ohio</td><td>31,024</td><td>4.30%</td><td>35</td><td>Utah</td><td>5,004</td><td>0.69%</td></tr>
<tr><td>26</td><td>Oklahoma</td><td>8,025</td><td>1.11%</td><td>36</td><td>Arkansas</td><td>4,886</td><td>0.68%</td></tr>
<tr><td>23</td><td>Oregon</td><td>10,059</td><td>1.39%</td><td>37</td><td>Nebraska</td><td>4,019</td><td>0.56%</td></tr>
<tr><td>5</td><td>Pennsylvania</td><td>31,183</td><td>4.32%</td><td>38</td><td>Maine</td><td>3,980</td><td>0.55%</td></tr>
<tr><td>40</td><td>Rhode Island</td><td>3,256</td><td>0.45%</td><td>39</td><td>Mississippi</td><td>3,291</td><td>0.46%</td></tr>
<tr><td>31</td><td>South Carolina</td><td>5,693</td><td>0.79%</td><td>40</td><td>Rhode Island</td><td>3,256</td><td>0.45%</td></tr>
<tr><td>45</td><td>South Dakota</td><td>1,652</td><td>0.23%</td><td>41</td><td>Idaho</td><td>3,016</td><td>0.42%</td></tr>
<tr><td>20</td><td>Tennessee</td><td>11,088</td><td>1.54%</td><td>42</td><td>New Hampshire</td><td>3,000</td><td>0.42%</td></tr>
<tr><td>3</td><td>Texas</td><td>35,324</td><td>4.89%</td><td>43</td><td>Montana</td><td>2,076</td><td>0.29%</td></tr>
<tr><td>35</td><td>Utah</td><td>5,004</td><td>0.69%</td><td>44</td><td>Vermont</td><td>1,774</td><td>0.25%</td></tr>
<tr><td>44</td><td>Vermont</td><td>1,774</td><td>0.25%</td><td>45</td><td>South Dakota</td><td>1,652</td><td>0.23%</td></tr>
<tr><td>15</td><td>Virginia</td><td>11,924</td><td>1.65%</td><td>46</td><td>Delaware</td><td>1,593</td><td>0.22%</td></tr>
<tr><td>11</td><td>Washington</td><td>16,448</td><td>2.28%</td><td>47</td><td>Alaska</td><td>1,505</td><td>0.21%</td></tr>
<tr><td>32</td><td>West Virginia</td><td>5,559</td><td>0.77%</td><td>48</td><td>North Dakota</td><td>1,425</td><td>0.20%</td></tr>
<tr><td>16</td><td>Wisconsin</td><td>11,685</td><td>1.62%</td><td>49</td><td>Wyoming</td><td>1,423</td><td>0.20%</td></tr>
<tr><td>49</td><td>Wyoming</td><td>1,423</td><td>0.20%</td><td>50</td><td>Hawaii</td><td>888</td><td>0.12%</td></tr>
<tr><td></td><td></td><td></td><td></td><td></td><td>District of Columbia</td><td>244</td><td>0.03%</td></tr>
</table>

Source: U.S. Department of Health and Human Services, National Center for Health Statistics
"Monthly Vital Statistics Report" (Vol. 43, No. 5, Supplement, October 25, 1994)
*Final data by state of residence.

Births to Unmarried White Women as a Percent of All Births to White Women in 1992

National Percent = 22.6% of Live Births*

ALPHA ORDER

RANK ORDER

RANK	STATE	PERCENT		RANK	STATE	PERCENT
49	Alabama	13.7		1	New Mexico	34.6
32	Alaska	19.0		2	California	34.0
3	Arizona	32.7		3	Arizona	32.7
34	Arkansas	18.6		4	Nevada	28.8
2	California	34.0		5	New York	26.6
19	Colorado	21.8		6	West Virginia	26.2
17	Connecticut	22.2		7	Oregon	25.7
26	Delaware	20.2		7	Rhode Island	25.7
10	Florida	23.7		9	Maine	25.3
41	Georgia	16.9		10	Florida	23.7
45	Hawaii	15.5		11	Indiana	23.6
38	Idaho	17.9		12	Washington	23.5
25	Illinois	20.7		13	Vermont	23.3
11	Indiana	23.6		14	Ohio	23.1
18	Iowa	21.9		15	Pennsylvania	22.9
26	Kansas	20.2		16	Wyoming	22.5
21	Kentucky	21.7		17	Connecticut	22.2
35	Louisiana	18.5		18	Iowa	21.9
9	Maine	25.3		19	Colorado	21.8
43	Maryland	16.3		19	Massachusetts	21.8
19	Massachusetts	21.8		21	Kentucky	21.7
47	Michigan	15.0		22	Missouri	21.5
29	Minnesota	19.3		22	Oklahoma	21.5
46	Mississippi	15.2		24	Montana	20.8
22	Missouri	21.5		25	Illinois	20.7
24	Montana	20.8		26	Delaware	20.2
33	Nebraska	18.8		26	Kansas	20.2
4	Nevada	28.8		28	Tennessee	20.1
31	New Hampshire	19.1		29	Minnesota	19.3
39	New Jersey	17.4		29	Wisconsin	19.3
1	New Mexico	34.6		31	New Hampshire	19.1
5	New York	26.6		32	Alaska	19.0
44	North Carolina	16.1		33	Nebraska	18.8
36	North Dakota	18.2		34	Arkansas	18.6
14	Ohio	23.1		35	Louisiana	18.5
22	Oklahoma	21.5		36	North Dakota	18.2
7	Oregon	25.7		37	South Dakota	18.1
15	Pennsylvania	22.9		38	Idaho	17.9
7	Rhode Island	25.7		39	New Jersey	17.4
42	South Carolina	16.8		40	Virginia	17.0
37	South Dakota	18.1		41	Georgia	16.9
28	Tennessee	20.1		42	South Carolina	16.8
50	Texas	13.1		43	Maryland	16.3
48	Utah	14.2		44	North Carolina	16.1
13	Vermont	23.3		45	Hawaii	15.5
40	Virginia	17.0		46	Mississippi	15.2
12	Washington	23.5		47	Michigan	15.0
6	West Virginia	26.2		48	Utah	14.2
29	Wisconsin	19.3		49	Alabama	13.7
16	Wyoming	22.5		50	Texas	13.1
					District of Columbia	15.2

Source: U.S. Department of Health and Human Services, National Center for Health Statistics
"Monthly Vital Statistics Report" (Vol. 43, No. 5, Supplement, October 25, 1994)
*Final data by state of residence.

Births to Unmarried Black Women in 1992

National Total = 458,969 Live Births*

ALPHA ORDER

RANK	STATE	BIRTHS	% of USA
16	Alabama	14,680	3.20%
40	Alaska	191	0.04%
32	Arizona	1,598	0.35%
22	Arkansas	5,822	1.27%
4	California	29,226	6.37%
31	Colorado	1,686	0.37%
24	Connecticut	4,347	0.95%
29	Delaware	1,853	0.40%
3	Florida	30,963	6.75%
5	Georgia	27,103	5.91%
41	Hawaii	133	0.03%
47	Idaho	21	0.00%
2	Illinois	33,993	7.41%
20	Indiana	7,237	1.58%
35	Iowa	889	0.19%
27	Kansas	2,180	0.47%
25	Kentucky	3,659	0.80%
7	Louisiana	20,899	4.55%
45	Maine	30	0.01%
13	Maryland	15,303	3.33%
23	Massachusetts	5,446	1.19%
6	Michigan	21,431	4.67%
28	Minnesota	2,170	0.47%
15	Mississippi	14,872	3.24%
19	Missouri	10,474	2.28%
48	Montana	17	0.00%
34	Nebraska	954	0.21%
33	Nevada	1,555	0.34%
43	New Hampshire	54	0.01%
12	New Jersey	15,385	3.35%
39	New Mexico	298	0.06%
1	New York	41,360	9.01%
8	North Carolina	20,262	4.41%
49	North Dakota	15	0.00%
10	Ohio	20,051	4.37%
26	Oklahoma	3,532	0.77%
37	Oregon	676	0.15%
9	Pennsylvania	20,181	4.40%
36	Rhode Island	797	0.17%
17	South Carolina	14,173	3.09%
46	South Dakota	26	0.01%
18	Tennessee	12,829	2.80%
11	Texas	20,032	4.36%
42	Utah	127	0.03%
50	Vermont	13	0.00%
14	Virginia	15,237	3.32%
30	Washington	1,740	0.38%
38	West Virginia	581	0.13%
21	Wisconsin	6,007	1.31%
44	Wyoming	33	0.01%

RANK ORDER

RANK	STATE	BIRTHS	% of USA
1	New York	41,360	9.01%
2	Illinois	33,993	7.41%
3	Florida	30,963	6.75%
4	California	29,226	6.37%
5	Georgia	27,103	5.91%
6	Michigan	21,431	4.67%
7	Louisiana	20,899	4.55%
8	North Carolina	20,262	4.41%
9	Pennsylvania	20,181	4.40%
10	Ohio	20,051	4.37%
11	Texas	20,032	4.36%
12	New Jersey	15,385	3.35%
13	Maryland	15,303	3.33%
14	Virginia	15,237	3.32%
15	Mississippi	14,872	3.24%
16	Alabama	14,680	3.20%
17	South Carolina	14,173	3.09%
18	Tennessee	12,829	2.80%
19	Missouri	10,474	2.28%
20	Indiana	7,237	1.58%
21	Wisconsin	6,007	1.31%
22	Arkansas	5,822	1.27%
23	Massachusetts	5,446	1.19%
24	Connecticut	4,347	0.95%
25	Kentucky	3,659	0.80%
26	Oklahoma	3,532	0.77%
27	Kansas	2,180	0.47%
28	Minnesota	2,170	0.47%
29	Delaware	1,853	0.40%
30	Washington	1,740	0.38%
31	Colorado	1,686	0.37%
32	Arizona	1,598	0.35%
33	Nevada	1,555	0.34%
34	Nebraska	954	0.21%
35	Iowa	889	0.19%
36	Rhode Island	797	0.17%
37	Oregon	676	0.15%
38	West Virginia	581	0.13%
39	New Mexico	298	0.06%
40	Alaska	191	0.04%
41	Hawaii	133	0.03%
42	Utah	127	0.03%
43	New Hampshire	54	0.01%
44	Wyoming	33	0.01%
45	Maine	30	0.01%
46	South Dakota	26	0.01%
47	Idaho	21	0.00%
48	Montana	17	0.00%
49	North Dakota	15	0.00%
50	Vermont	13	0.00%
	District of Columbia	6,828	1.49%

Source: U.S. Department of Health and Human Services, National Center for Health Statistics
"Monthly Vital Statistics Report" (Vol. 43, No. 5, Supplement, October 25, 1994)
*Final data by state of residence.

Births to Unmarried Black Women as a Percent of All Births to Black Women in 1992

National Percent = 68.1% of Live Births*

ALPHA ORDER			RANK ORDER		
RANK	STATE	PERCENT	RANK	STATE	PERCENT
23	Alabama	68.2	1	Wisconsin	82.2
45	Alaska	35.2	2	Pennsylvania	79.4
31	Arizona	65.3	3	Illinois	79.2
15	Arkansas	71.4	4	Missouri	78.7
34	California	62.8	5	Ohio	77.1
37	Colorado	56.1	6	Indiana	76.8
18	Connecticut	70.7	7	Iowa	75.1
11	Delaware	72.6	8	Minnesota	74.4
21	Florida	68.9	9	Tennessee	73.3
26	Georgia	67.1	10	Nebraska	72.7
47	Hawaii	19.4	11	Delaware	72.6
44	Idaho	36.2	12	Mississippi	72.5
3	Illinois	79.2	13	Michigan	72.1
6	Indiana	76.8	14	Nevada	71.9
7	Iowa	75.1	15	Arkansas	71.4
28	Kansas	65.8	16	West Virginia	71.3
19	Kentucky	70.5	17	Oregon	70.8
20	Louisiana	70.0	18	Connecticut	70.7
43	Maine	36.6	19	Kentucky	70.5
35	Maryland	60.2	20	Louisiana	70.0
33	Massachusetts	63.0	21	Florida	68.9
13	Michigan	72.1	22	Oklahoma	68.4
8	Minnesota	74.4	23	Alabama	68.2
12	Mississippi	72.5	24	New York	67.8
4	Missouri	78.7	25	Rhode Island	67.2
NA	Montana**	NA	26	Georgia	67.1
10	Nebraska	72.7	27	North Carolina	66.8
14	Nevada	71.9	28	Kansas	65.8
41	New Hampshire	49.5	29	New Jersey	65.7
29	New Jersey	65.7	30	South Carolina	65.6
36	New Mexico	58.1	31	Arizona	65.3
24	New York	67.8	32	Virginia	63.9
27	North Carolina	66.8	33	Massachusetts	63.0
NA	North Dakota**	NA	34	California	62.8
5	Ohio	77.1	35	Maryland	60.2
22	Oklahoma	68.4	36	New Mexico	58.1
17	Oregon	70.8	37	Colorado	56.1
2	Pennsylvania	79.4	38	Washington	55.3
25	Rhode Island	67.2	39	Utah	51.8
30	South Carolina	65.6	40	Wyoming	50.8
46	South Dakota	32.9	41	New Hampshire	49.5
9	Tennessee	73.3	42	Texas	46.6
42	Texas	46.6	43	Maine	36.6
39	Utah	51.8	44	Idaho	36.2
NA	Vermont**	NA	45	Alaska	35.2
32	Virginia	63.9	46	South Dakota	32.9
38	Washington	55.3	47	Hawaii	19.4
16	West Virginia	71.3	NA	Montana**	NA
1	Wisconsin	82.2	NA	North Dakota**	NA
40	Wyoming	50.8	NA	Vermont**	NA
				District of Columbia	77.6

Source: U.S. Department of Health and Human Services, National Center for Health Statistics
 "Monthly Vital Statistics Report" (Vol. 43, No. 5, Supplement, October 25, 1994)
*Final data by state of residence.
**Insufficient data.

Births to Teenage Mothers in 1992

National Total = 505,415 Live Births*

ALPHA ORDER

RANK ORDER

RANK	STATE	BIRTHS	% of USA		RANK	STATE	BIRTHS	% of USA
14	Alabama	10,960	2.17%		1	California	69,401	13.73%
45	Alaska	1,260	0.25%		2	Texas	49,805	9.85%
17	Arizona	10,147	2.01%		3	New York	25,363	5.02%
27	Arkansas	6,554	1.30%		4	Florida	25,213	4.99%
1	California	69,401	13.73%		5	Illinois	23,981	4.74%
28	Colorado	6,401	1.27%		6	Ohio	21,539	4.26%
36	Connecticut	3,701	0.73%		7	Michigan	18,374	3.64%
44	Delaware	1,265	0.25%		8	Georgia	17,462	3.45%
4	Florida	25,213	4.99%		9	Pennsylvania	16,835	3.33%
8	Georgia	17,462	3.45%		10	North Carolina	15,653	3.10%
40	Hawaii	1,956	0.39%		11	Louisiana	12,392	2.45%
39	Idaho	2,229	0.44%		12	Tennessee	12,127	2.40%
5	Illinois	23,981	4.74%		13	Indiana	11,668	2.31%
13	Indiana	11,668	2.31%		14	Alabama	10,960	2.17%
33	Iowa	3,872	0.77%		15	Missouri	10,857	2.15%
32	Kansas	4,640	0.92%		16	Virginia	10,465	2.07%
21	Kentucky	8,710	1.72%		17	Arizona	10,147	2.01%
11	Louisiana	12,392	2.45%		18	New Jersey	9,262	1.83%
41	Maine	1,625	0.32%		19	South Carolina	9,052	1.79%
24	Maryland	7,356	1.46%		20	Mississippi	8,810	1.74%
26	Massachusetts	6,558	1.30%		21	Kentucky	8,710	1.72%
7	Michigan	18,374	3.64%		22	Washington	8,303	1.64%
29	Minnesota	5,210	1.03%		23	Oklahoma	7,858	1.55%
20	Mississippi	8,810	1.74%		24	Maryland	7,356	1.46%
15	Missouri	10,857	2.15%		25	Wisconsin	7,050	1.39%
43	Montana	1,345	0.27%		26	Massachusetts	6,558	1.30%
38	Nebraska	2,285	0.45%		27	Arkansas	6,554	1.30%
37	Nevada	2,719	0.54%		28	Colorado	6,401	1.27%
47	New Hampshire	1,062	0.21%		29	Minnesota	5,210	1.03%
18	New Jersey	9,262	1.83%		30	Oregon	5,125	1.01%
31	New Mexico	4,670	0.92%		31	New Mexico	4,670	0.92%
3	New York	25,363	5.02%		32	Kansas	4,640	0.92%
10	North Carolina	15,653	3.10%		33	Iowa	3,872	0.77%
49	North Dakota	811	0.16%		34	Utah	3,869	0.77%
6	Ohio	21,539	4.26%		35	West Virginia	3,758	0.74%
23	Oklahoma	7,858	1.55%		36	Connecticut	3,701	0.73%
30	Oregon	5,125	1.01%		37	Nevada	2,719	0.54%
9	Pennsylvania	16,835	3.33%		38	Nebraska	2,285	0.45%
42	Rhode Island	1,381	0.27%		39	Idaho	2,229	0.44%
19	South Carolina	9,052	1.79%		40	Hawaii	1,956	0.39%
46	South Dakota	1,245	0.25%		41	Maine	1,625	0.32%
12	Tennessee	12,127	2.40%		42	Rhode Island	1,381	0.27%
2	Texas	49,805	9.85%		43	Montana	1,345	0.27%
34	Utah	3,869	0.77%		44	Delaware	1,265	0.25%
50	Vermont	649	0.13%		45	Alaska	1,260	0.25%
16	Virginia	10,465	2.07%		46	South Dakota	1,245	0.25%
22	Washington	8,303	1.64%		47	New Hampshire	1,062	0.21%
35	West Virginia	3,758	0.74%		48	Wyoming	878	0.17%
25	Wisconsin	7,050	1.39%		49	North Dakota	811	0.16%
48	Wyoming	878	0.17%		50	Vermont	649	0.13%
						District of Columbia	1,704	0.34%

Source: Morgan Quitno Press using data from U.S. Dept of Health & Human Services, National Center for Health Statistics (unpublished data, Table 1-60)

*Live births to women age 15 to 19 years old.

Teenage Birth Rate in 1992

National Rate = 61 Births per 1,000 Teenage Women*

ALPHA ORDER			RANK ORDER		
RANK	**STATE**	**RATE**	**RANK**	**STATE**	**RATE**
9	Alabama	73	1	Mississippi	84
18	Alaska	64	2	Arizona	82
2	Arizona	82	3	New Mexico	80
6	Arkansas	75	4	Texas	79
8	California	74	5	Louisiana	76
15	Colorado	68	6	Arkansas	75
44	Connecticut	39	6	Georgia	75
21	Delaware	60	8	California	74
16	Florida	66	9	Alabama	73
6	Georgia	75	10	Nevada	71
28	Hawaii	54	10	Tennessee	71
30	Idaho	52	12	North Carolina	70
18	Illinois	64	12	Oklahoma	70
22	Indiana	59	12	South Carolina	70
42	Iowa	41	15	Colorado	68
25	Kansas	56	16	Florida	66
16	Kentucky	66	16	Kentucky	66
5	Louisiana	76	18	Alaska	64
40	Maine	43	18	Illinois	64
32	Maryland	51	20	Missouri	63
46	Massachusetts	38	21	Delaware	60
24	Michigan	57	22	Indiana	59
48	Minnesota	36	23	Ohio	58
1	Mississippi	84	24	Michigan	57
20	Missouri	63	25	Kansas	56
36	Montana	46	25	West Virginia	56
42	Nebraska	41	25	Wyoming	56
10	Nevada	71	28	Hawaii	54
50	New Hampshire	31	29	Oregon	53
44	New Jersey	39	30	Idaho	52
3	New Mexico	80	30	Virginia	52
38	New York	45	32	Maryland	51
12	North Carolina	70	32	Washington	51
47	North Dakota	37	34	Rhode Island	48
23	Ohio	58	34	South Dakota	48
12	Oklahoma	70	36	Montana	46
29	Oregon	53	36	Utah	46
38	Pennsylvania	45	38	New York	45
34	Rhode Island	48	38	Pennsylvania	45
12	South Carolina	70	40	Maine	43
34	South Dakota	48	41	Wisconsin	42
10	Tennessee	71	42	Iowa	41
4	Texas	79	42	Nebraska	41
36	Utah	46	44	Connecticut	39
48	Vermont	36	44	New Jersey	39
30	Virginia	52	46	Massachusetts	38
32	Washington	51	47	North Dakota	37
25	West Virginia	56	48	Minnesota	36
41	Wisconsin	42	48	Vermont	36
25	Wyoming	56	50	New Hampshire	31
				District of Columbia	116

Source: U.S. Department of Health and Human Services, Centers for Disease Control and Prevention
   Forthcoming in "Vital Statistics of the United States, 1992" (Vol. 1, Natality)
*Women aged 15 to 19 years old.

Births to Teenage Mothers as a Percent of Live Births in 1992

National Percent = 12.43% of Live Births*

ALPHA ORDER			RANK ORDER		
RANK	STATE	PERCENT	RANK	STATE	PERCENT
3	Alabama	17.60	1	Mississippi	20.64
32	Alaska	10.75	2	Arkansas	18.82
14	Arizona	14.74	3	Alabama	17.60
2	Arkansas	18.82	4	Louisiana	17.53
29	California	11.53	5	West Virginia	16.95
27	Colorado	11.74	6	New Mexico	16.73
47	Connecticut	7.78	7	Oklahoma	16.52
26	Delaware	11.87	8	Tennessee	16.47
18	Florida	13.15	9	Kentucky	16.18
11	Georgia	15.72	10	South Carolina	16.11
39	Hawaii	9.85	11	Georgia	15.72
20	Idaho	12.84	12	Texas	15.52
22	Illinois	12.53	13	North Carolina	15.06
16	Indiana	13.87	14	Arizona	14.74
37	Iowa	10.07	15	Missouri	14.23
23	Kansas	12.20	16	Indiana	13.87
9	Kentucky	16.18	17	Ohio	13.28
4	Louisiana	17.53	18	Florida	13.15
36	Maine	10.12	19	Wyoming	13.06
42	Maryland	9.45	20	Idaho	12.84
49	Massachusetts	7.52	21	Michigan	12.75
21	Michigan	12.75	22	Illinois	12.53
46	Minnesota	7.94	23	Kansas	12.20
1	Mississippi	20.64	24	Oregon	12.19
15	Missouri	14.23	25	Nevada	12.15
28	Montana	11.72	26	Delaware	11.87
40	Nebraska	9.77	27	Colorado	11.74
25	Nevada	12.15	28	Montana	11.72
50	New Hampshire	6.64	29	California	11.53
48	New Jersey	7.72	30	South Dakota	11.30
6	New Mexico	16.73	31	Virginia	10.77
44	New York	8.81	32	Alaska	10.75
13	North Carolina	15.06	33	Washington	10.45
43	North Dakota	9.20	34	Utah	10.40
17	Ohio	13.28	35	Pennsylvania	10.23
7	Oklahoma	16.52	36	Maine	10.12
24	Oregon	12.19	37	Iowa	10.07
35	Pennsylvania	10.23	38	Wisconsin	9.98
41	Rhode Island	9.52	39	Hawaii	9.85
10	South Carolina	16.11	40	Nebraska	9.77
30	South Dakota	11.30	41	Rhode Island	9.52
8	Tennessee	16.47	42	Maryland	9.45
12	Texas	15.52	43	North Dakota	9.20
34	Utah	10.40	44	New York	8.81
45	Vermont	8.39	45	Vermont	8.39
31	Virginia	10.77	46	Minnesota	7.94
33	Washington	10.45	47	Connecticut	7.78
5	West Virginia	16.95	48	New Jersey	7.72
38	Wisconsin	9.98	49	Massachusetts	7.52
19	Wyoming	13.06	50	New Hampshire	6.64
				District of Columbia	15.55

Source: Morgan Quitno Press using data from U.S. Dept of Health & Human Services, National Center for Health Statistics
(unpublished data, Table 1-60)
*Women age 15 to 19 years old.

Pregnancy Rate for 15 to 19 Year Old Women in 1990

National Average = 83.0 Births and Abortions per 1,000 Women 15 to 19 Years Old*

ALPHA ORDER

RANK	STATE	RATE
NA	Alabama**	NA
NA	Alaska**	NA
5	Arizona	101.8
8	Arkansas	98.4
NA	California**	NA
22	Colorado	82.3
NA	Connecticut**	NA
NA	Delaware**	NA
NA	Florida**	NA
1	Georgia	110.8
16	Hawaii	88.2
38	Idaho	58.8
NA	Illinois**	NA
28	Indiana	74.3
NA	Iowa**	NA
24	Kansas	81.1
14	Kentucky	91.0
13	Louisiana	92.1
32	Maine	68.4
20	Maryland	84.7
31	Massachusetts	71.1
19	Michigan	85.2
37	Minnesota	62.0
9	Mississippi	97.8
21	Missouri	82.6
23	Montana	81.7
29	Nebraska	74.2
2	Nevada	107.5
NA	New Hampshire**	NA
25	New Jersey	75.3
7	New Mexico	100.4
12	New York	92.9
3	North Carolina	106.4
40	North Dakota	56.4
27	Ohio	74.5
NA	Oklahoma**	NA
15	Oregon	89.2
26	Pennsylvania	74.6
17	Rhode Island	87.7
11	South Carolina	95.0
39	South Dakota	56.9
5	Tennessee	101.8
4	Texas	102.7
35	Utah	63.0
30	Vermont	72.1
18	Virginia	86.4
10	Washington	95.4
33	West Virginia	67.4
34	Wisconsin	66.6
36	Wyoming	62.2

RANK ORDER

RANK	STATE	RATE
1	Georgia	110.8
2	Nevada	107.5
3	North Carolina	106.4
4	Texas	102.7
5	Arizona	101.8
5	Tennessee	101.8
7	New Mexico	100.4
8	Arkansas	98.4
9	Mississippi	97.8
10	Washington	95.4
11	South Carolina	95.0
12	New York	92.9
13	Louisiana	92.1
14	Kentucky	91.0
15	Oregon	89.2
16	Hawaii	88.2
17	Rhode Island	87.7
18	Virginia	86.4
19	Michigan	85.2
20	Maryland	84.7
21	Missouri	82.6
22	Colorado	82.3
23	Montana	81.7
24	Kansas	81.1
25	New Jersey	75.3
26	Pennsylvania	74.6
27	Ohio	74.5
28	Indiana	74.3
29	Nebraska	74.2
30	Vermont	72.1
31	Massachusetts	71.1
32	Maine	68.4
33	West Virginia	67.4
34	Wisconsin	66.6
35	Utah	63.0
36	Wyoming	62.2
37	Minnesota	62.0
38	Idaho	58.8
39	South Dakota	56.9
40	North Dakota	56.4
NA	Alabama**	NA
NA	Alaska**	NA
NA	California**	NA
NA	Connecticut**	NA
NA	Delaware**	NA
NA	Florida**	NA
NA	Illinois**	NA
NA	Iowa**	NA
NA	New Hampshire**	NA
NA	Oklahoma**	NA

District of Columbia	255.2

Source: U.S. Department of Health and Human Services, Centers for Disease Control and Prevention
"Surveillance for Pregnancy and Birth Rates Among Teenagers" (MMWR, Vol. 42, No. SS-6, 12/17/93)
*The sum of live births and legal induced abortions per 1,000 women aged 15–19 years old. Births by state of residence, abortions by state of occurrence. National average is simply the average of the rates of reporting states (excluding Washington, DC).

**Not available.

Births to Teenage Mothers in 1990

National Total = 521,826 Live Births*

<table>
<tr><td colspan="4">ALPHA ORDER</td><td colspan="4">RANK ORDER</td></tr>
<tr><th>RANK</th><th>STATE</th><th>BIRTHS</th><th>% of USA</th><th>RANK</th><th>STATE</th><th>BIRTHS</th><th>% of USA</th></tr>
<tr><td>15</td><td>Alabama</td><td>11,252</td><td>2.16%</td><td>1</td><td>California</td><td>69,712</td><td>13.36%</td></tr>
<tr><td>47</td><td>Alaska</td><td>1,142</td><td>0.22%</td><td>2</td><td>Texas</td><td>48,302</td><td>9.26%</td></tr>
<tr><td>19</td><td>Arizona</td><td>9,612</td><td>1.84%</td><td>3</td><td>Florida</td><td>27,017</td><td>5.18%</td></tr>
<tr><td>27</td><td>Arkansas</td><td>7,011</td><td>1.34%</td><td>4</td><td>New York</td><td>26,608</td><td>5.10%</td></tr>
<tr><td>1</td><td>California</td><td>69,712</td><td>13.36%</td><td>5</td><td>Illinois</td><td>24,967</td><td>4.78%</td></tr>
<tr><td>28</td><td>Colorado</td><td>5,975</td><td>1.15%</td><td>6</td><td>Ohio</td><td>22,690</td><td>4.35%</td></tr>
<tr><td>33</td><td>Connecticut</td><td>4,038</td><td>0.77%</td><td>7</td><td>Michigan</td><td>20,312</td><td>3.89%</td></tr>
<tr><td>44</td><td>Delaware</td><td>1,277</td><td>0.24%</td><td>8</td><td>Georgia</td><td>18,369</td><td>3.52%</td></tr>
<tr><td>3</td><td>Florida</td><td>27,017</td><td>5.18%</td><td>9</td><td>Pennsylvania</td><td>18,216</td><td>3.49%</td></tr>
<tr><td>8</td><td>Georgia</td><td>18,369</td><td>3.52%</td><td>10</td><td>North Carolina</td><td>16,506</td><td>3.16%</td></tr>
<tr><td>39</td><td>Hawaii</td><td>2,122</td><td>0.41%</td><td>11</td><td>Tennessee</td><td>12,928</td><td>2.48%</td></tr>
<tr><td>40</td><td>Idaho</td><td>2,009</td><td>0.38%</td><td>12</td><td>Indiana</td><td>12,335</td><td>2.36%</td></tr>
<tr><td>5</td><td>Illinois</td><td>24,967</td><td>4.78%</td><td>13</td><td>Louisiana</td><td>12,270</td><td>2.35%</td></tr>
<tr><td>12</td><td>Indiana</td><td>12,335</td><td>2.36%</td><td>14</td><td>Virginia</td><td>11,353</td><td>2.18%</td></tr>
<tr><td>34</td><td>Iowa</td><td>3,989</td><td>0.76%</td><td>15</td><td>Alabama</td><td>11,252</td><td>2.16%</td></tr>
<tr><td>31</td><td>Kansas</td><td>4,722</td><td>0.90%</td><td>16</td><td>Missouri</td><td>11,227</td><td>2.15%</td></tr>
<tr><td>20</td><td>Kentucky</td><td>9,349</td><td>1.79%</td><td>17</td><td>New Jersey</td><td>10,068</td><td>1.93%</td></tr>
<tr><td>13</td><td>Louisiana</td><td>12,270</td><td>2.35%</td><td>18</td><td>South Carolina</td><td>9,721</td><td>1.86%</td></tr>
<tr><td>41</td><td>Maine</td><td>1,857</td><td>0.36%</td><td>19</td><td>Arizona</td><td>9,612</td><td>1.84%</td></tr>
<tr><td>23</td><td>Maryland</td><td>8,143</td><td>1.56%</td><td>20</td><td>Kentucky</td><td>9,349</td><td>1.79%</td></tr>
<tr><td>26</td><td>Massachusetts</td><td>7,266</td><td>1.39%</td><td>21</td><td>Mississippi</td><td>8,909</td><td>1.71%</td></tr>
<tr><td>7</td><td>Michigan</td><td>20,312</td><td>3.89%</td><td>22</td><td>Washington</td><td>8,397</td><td>1.61%</td></tr>
<tr><td>29</td><td>Minnesota</td><td>5,342</td><td>1.02%</td><td>23</td><td>Maryland</td><td>8,143</td><td>1.56%</td></tr>
<tr><td>21</td><td>Mississippi</td><td>8,909</td><td>1.71%</td><td>24</td><td>Oklahoma</td><td>7,590</td><td>1.45%</td></tr>
<tr><td>16</td><td>Missouri</td><td>11,227</td><td>2.15%</td><td>25</td><td>Wisconsin</td><td>7,281</td><td>1.40%</td></tr>
<tr><td>43</td><td>Montana</td><td>1,331</td><td>0.26%</td><td>26</td><td>Massachusetts</td><td>7,266</td><td>1.39%</td></tr>
<tr><td>38</td><td>Nebraska</td><td>2,352</td><td>0.45%</td><td>27</td><td>Arkansas</td><td>7,011</td><td>1.34%</td></tr>
<tr><td>37</td><td>Nevada</td><td>2,663</td><td>0.51%</td><td>28</td><td>Colorado</td><td>5,975</td><td>1.15%</td></tr>
<tr><td>45</td><td>New Hampshire</td><td>1,258</td><td>0.24%</td><td>29</td><td>Minnesota</td><td>5,342</td><td>1.02%</td></tr>
<tr><td>17</td><td>New Jersey</td><td>10,068</td><td>1.93%</td><td>30</td><td>Oregon</td><td>5,084</td><td>0.97%</td></tr>
<tr><td>32</td><td>New Mexico</td><td>4,367</td><td>0.84%</td><td>31</td><td>Kansas</td><td>4,722</td><td>0.90%</td></tr>
<tr><td>4</td><td>New York</td><td>26,608</td><td>5.10%</td><td>32</td><td>New Mexico</td><td>4,367</td><td>0.84%</td></tr>
<tr><td>10</td><td>North Carolina</td><td>16,506</td><td>3.16%</td><td>33</td><td>Connecticut</td><td>4,038</td><td>0.77%</td></tr>
<tr><td>49</td><td>North Dakota</td><td>793</td><td>0.15%</td><td>34</td><td>Iowa</td><td>3,989</td><td>0.76%</td></tr>
<tr><td>6</td><td>Ohio</td><td>22,690</td><td>4.35%</td><td>35</td><td>West Virginia</td><td>3,976</td><td>0.76%</td></tr>
<tr><td>24</td><td>Oklahoma</td><td>7,590</td><td>1.45%</td><td>36</td><td>Utah</td><td>3,707</td><td>0.71%</td></tr>
<tr><td>30</td><td>Oregon</td><td>5,084</td><td>0.97%</td><td>37</td><td>Nevada</td><td>2,663</td><td>0.51%</td></tr>
<tr><td>9</td><td>Pennsylvania</td><td>18,216</td><td>3.49%</td><td>38</td><td>Nebraska</td><td>2,352</td><td>0.45%</td></tr>
<tr><td>42</td><td>Rhode Island</td><td>1,564</td><td>0.30%</td><td>39</td><td>Hawaii</td><td>2,122</td><td>0.41%</td></tr>
<tr><td>18</td><td>South Carolina</td><td>9,721</td><td>1.86%</td><td>40</td><td>Idaho</td><td>2,009</td><td>0.38%</td></tr>
<tr><td>46</td><td>South Dakota</td><td>1,172</td><td>0.22%</td><td>41</td><td>Maine</td><td>1,857</td><td>0.36%</td></tr>
<tr><td>11</td><td>Tennessee</td><td>12,928</td><td>2.48%</td><td>42</td><td>Rhode Island</td><td>1,564</td><td>0.30%</td></tr>
<tr><td>2</td><td>Texas</td><td>48,302</td><td>9.26%</td><td>43</td><td>Montana</td><td>1,331</td><td>0.26%</td></tr>
<tr><td>36</td><td>Utah</td><td>3,707</td><td>0.71%</td><td>44</td><td>Delaware</td><td>1,277</td><td>0.24%</td></tr>
<tr><td>50</td><td>Vermont</td><td>702</td><td>0.13%</td><td>45</td><td>New Hampshire</td><td>1,258</td><td>0.24%</td></tr>
<tr><td>14</td><td>Virginia</td><td>11,353</td><td>2.18%</td><td>46</td><td>South Dakota</td><td>1,172</td><td>0.22%</td></tr>
<tr><td>22</td><td>Washington</td><td>8,397</td><td>1.61%</td><td>47</td><td>Alaska</td><td>1,142</td><td>0.22%</td></tr>
<tr><td>35</td><td>West Virginia</td><td>3,976</td><td>0.76%</td><td>48</td><td>Wyoming</td><td>943</td><td>0.18%</td></tr>
<tr><td>25</td><td>Wisconsin</td><td>7,281</td><td>1.40%</td><td>49</td><td>North Dakota</td><td>793</td><td>0.15%</td></tr>
<tr><td>48</td><td>Wyoming</td><td>943</td><td>0.18%</td><td>50</td><td>Vermont</td><td>702</td><td>0.13%</td></tr>
<tr><td></td><td></td><td></td><td></td><td></td><td>District of Columbia</td><td>2,030</td><td>0.39%</td></tr>
</table>

Source: U.S. Department of Health and Human Services, Centers for Disease Control and Prevention
"Surveillance for Pregnancy and Birth Rates Among Teenagers" (MMWR, Vol. 42, No. SS-6, 12/17/93)
*Women aged 15 to 19 years old.

Teenage Birth Rate in 1990

National Rate = 59.9 Live Births per 1,000 Teenage Women*

ALPHA ORDER			RANK ORDER		
RANK	STATE	RATE	RANK	STATE	RATE
11	Alabama	71.0	1	Mississippi	81.0
17	Alaska	65.3	2	Arkansas	80.1
4	Arizona	75.5	3	New Mexico	78.2
2	Arkansas	80.1	4	Arizona	75.5
12	California	70.6	4	Georgia	75.5
28	Colorado	54.5	6	Texas	75.3
45	Connecticut	38.8	7	Louisiana	74.2
28	Delaware	54.5	8	Nevada	73.3
13	Florida	69.1	9	Tennessee	72.3
4	Georgia	75.5	10	South Carolina	71.3
20	Hawaii	61.2	11	Alabama	71.0
33	Idaho	50.6	12	California	70.6
18	Illinois	62.9	13	Florida	69.1
22	Indiana	58.6	14	Kentucky	67.6
43	Iowa	40.5	14	North Carolina	67.6
26	Kansas	56.1	16	Oklahoma	66.8
14	Kentucky	67.6	17	Alaska	65.3
7	Louisiana	74.2	18	Illinois	62.9
40	Maine	43.0	19	Missouri	62.8
30	Maryland	53.2	20	Hawaii	61.2
48	Massachusetts	35.1	21	Michigan	59.0
21	Michigan	59.0	22	Indiana	58.6
46	Minnesota	36.3	23	Ohio	57.9
1	Mississippi	81.0	24	West Virginia	57.3
19	Missouri	62.8	25	Wyoming	56.3
35	Montana	48.4	26	Kansas	56.1
42	Nebraska	42.3	27	Oregon	54.6
8	Nevada	73.3	28	Colorado	54.5
50	New Hampshire	33.0	28	Delaware	54.5
43	New Jersey	40.5	30	Maryland	53.2
3	New Mexico	78.2	31	Washington	53.1
39	New York	43.6	32	Virginia	52.9
14	North Carolina	67.6	33	Idaho	50.6
47	North Dakota	35.4	34	Utah	48.5
23	Ohio	57.9	35	Montana	48.4
16	Oklahoma	66.8	36	South Dakota	46.8
27	Oregon	54.6	37	Pennsylvania	44.9
37	Pennsylvania	44.9	38	Rhode Island	43.9
38	Rhode Island	43.9	39	New York	43.6
10	South Carolina	71.3	40	Maine	43.0
36	South Dakota	46.8	41	Wisconsin	42.6
9	Tennessee	72.3	42	Nebraska	42.3
6	Texas	75.3	43	Iowa	40.5
34	Utah	48.5	43	New Jersey	40.5
49	Vermont	34.0	45	Connecticut	38.8
32	Virginia	52.9	46	Minnesota	36.3
31	Washington	53.1	47	North Dakota	35.4
24	West Virginia	57.3	48	Massachusetts	35.1
41	Wisconsin	42.6	49	Vermont	34.0
25	Wyoming	56.3	50	New Hampshire	33.0
				District of Columbia	93.1

Source: U.S. Department of Health and Human Services, Centers for Disease Control and Prevention
"Surveillance for Pregnancy and Birth Rates Among Teenagers" (MMWR, Vol. 42, No. SS-6, 12/17/93)
Women aged 15 to 19 years old.

Births to Teenage Mothers in 1980

National Total = 562,330 Live Births*

ALPHA ORDER					RANK ORDER			
RANK	STATE		BIRTHS	% of USA	RANK	STATE	BIRTHS	% of USA
15	Alabama		13,096	2.33%	1	California	56,138	9.98%
49	Alaska		1,123	0.20%	2	Texas	50,125	8.91%
25	Arizona		8,235	1.46%	3	Illinois	29,798	5.30%
26	Arkansas		8,060	1.43%	4	New York	28,206	5.02%
1	California		56,138	9.98%	5	Ohio	26,567	4.72%
29	Colorado		6,592	1.17%	6	Florida	24,042	4.28%
36	Connecticut		4,408	0.78%	7	Pennsylvania	22,029	3.92%
45	Delaware		1,572	0.28%	8	Michigan	20,401	3.63%
6	Florida		24,042	4.28%	9	Georgia	19,137	3.40%
9	Georgia		19,137	3.40%	10	Louisiana	16,504	2.93%
40	Hawaii		2,085	0.37%	11	North Carolina	16,192	2.88%
38	Idaho		2,645	0.47%	12	Indiana	15,331	2.73%
3	Illinois		29,798	5.30%	13	Tennessee	13,792	2.45%
12	Indiana		15,331	2.73%	14	Missouri	13,312	2.37%
31	Iowa		5,962	1.06%	15	Alabama	13,096	2.33%
30	Kansas		6,090	1.08%	16	Kentucky	12,559	2.23%
16	Kentucky		12,559	2.23%	17	Virginia	12,138	2.16%
10	Louisiana		16,504	2.93%	18	New Jersey	11,904	2.12%
39	Maine		2,522	0.45%	19	Mississippi	11,079	1.97%
23	Maryland		8,885	1.58%	20	South Carolina	10,282	1.83%
27	Massachusetts		7,765	1.38%	21	Oklahoma	10,206	1.81%
8	Michigan		20,401	3.63%	22	Wisconsin	9,220	1.64%
28	Minnesota		7,048	1.25%	23	Maryland	8,885	1.58%
19	Mississippi		11,079	1.97%	24	Washington	8,495	1.51%
14	Missouri		13,312	2.37%	25	Arizona	8,235	1.46%
43	Montana		1,761	0.31%	26	Arkansas	8,060	1.43%
37	Nebraska		3,313	0.59%	27	Massachusetts	7,765	1.38%
41	Nevada		2,048	0.36%	28	Minnesota	7,048	1.25%
47	New Hampshire		1,475	0.26%	29	Colorado	6,592	1.17%
18	New Jersey		11,904	2.12%	30	Kansas	6,090	1.08%
34	New Mexico		4,758	0.85%	31	Iowa	5,962	1.06%
4	New York		28,206	5.02%	32	West Virginia	5,911	1.05%
11	North Carolina		16,192	2.88%	33	Oregon	5,731	1.02%
48	North Dakota		1,304	0.23%	34	New Mexico	4,758	0.85%
5	Ohio		26,567	4.72%	35	Utah	4,594	0.82%
21	Oklahoma		10,206	1.81%	36	Connecticut	4,408	0.78%
33	Oregon		5,731	1.02%	37	Nebraska	3,313	0.59%
7	Pennsylvania		22,029	3.92%	38	Idaho	2,645	0.47%
46	Rhode Island		1,502	0.27%	39	Maine	2,522	0.45%
20	South Carolina		10,282	1.83%	40	Hawaii	2,085	0.37%
42	South Dakota		1,797	0.32%	41	Nevada	2,048	0.36%
13	Tennessee		13,792	2.45%	42	South Dakota	1,797	0.32%
2	Texas		50,125	8.91%	43	Montana	1,761	0.31%
35	Utah		4,594	0.82%	44	Wyoming	1,634	0.29%
50	Vermont		1,024	0.18%	45	Delaware	1,572	0.28%
17	Virginia		12,138	2.16%	46	Rhode Island	1,502	0.27%
24	Washington		8,495	1.51%	47	New Hampshire	1,475	0.26%
32	West Virginia		5,911	1.05%	48	North Dakota	1,304	0.23%
22	Wisconsin		9,220	1.64%	49	Alaska	1,123	0.20%
44	Wyoming		1,634	0.29%	50	Vermont	1,024	0.18%
						District of Columbia	1,933	0.34%

Source: U.S. Department of Health and Human Services, National Center for Health Statistics
"Vital Statistics of the United States, 1980" (Vol. I-Natality, issued 1984)
*Births to women age 15 to 19 years old.

Teenage Birth Rate in 1980

National Rate = 53.0 Live Births per 1,000 Teenage Women*

ALPHA ORDER				RANK ORDER		
RANK	**STATE**	**RATE**		**RANK**	**STATE**	**RATE**
10	Alabama	68.3		1	Mississippi	83.7
15	Alaska	64.4		2	Wyoming	78.7
12	Arizona	65.5		3	Louisiana	76.0
5	Arkansas	74.5		4	Oklahoma	74.6
25	California	53.3		5	Arkansas	74.5
31	Colorado	49.9		6	Texas	74.3
49	Connecticut	30.5		7	Kentucky	72.3
28	Delaware	51.2		8	Georgia	71.9
18	Florida	58.5		9	New Mexico	71.8
8	Georgia	71.9		10	Alabama	68.3
30	Hawaii	50.7		11	West Virginia	67.8
17	Idaho	59.5		12	Arizona	65.5
24	Illinois	55.8		13	Utah	65.2
21	Indiana	57.5		14	South Carolina	64.8
39	Iowa	43.0		15	Alaska	64.4
23	Kansas	56.8		16	Tennessee	64.1
7	Kentucky	72.3		17	Idaho	59.5
3	Louisiana	76.0		18	Florida	58.5
34	Maine	47.4		18	Nevada	58.5
38	Maryland	43.4		20	Missouri	57.8
50	Massachusetts	28.1		21	Indiana	57.5
37	Michigan	45.0		21	North Carolina	57.5
44	Minnesota	35.4		23	Kansas	56.8
1	Mississippi	83.7		24	Illinois	55.8
20	Missouri	57.8		25	California	53.3
32	Montana	48.5		26	South Dakota	52.6
36	Nebraska	45.1		27	Ohio	52.5
18	Nevada	58.5		28	Delaware	51.2
47	New Hampshire	33.6		29	Oregon	50.9
45	New Jersey	35.2		30	Hawaii	50.7
9	New Mexico	71.8		31	Colorado	49.9
46	New York	34.8		32	Montana	48.5
21	North Carolina	57.5		33	Virginia	48.3
40	North Dakota	41.7		34	Maine	47.4
27	Ohio	52.5		35	Washington	46.7
4	Oklahoma	74.6		36	Nebraska	45.1
29	Oregon	50.9		37	Michigan	45.0
41	Pennsylvania	40.5		38	Maryland	43.4
48	Rhode Island	33.0		39	Iowa	43.0
14	South Carolina	64.8		40	North Dakota	41.7
26	South Dakota	52.6		41	Pennsylvania	40.5
16	Tennessee	64.1		42	Vermont	39.5
6	Texas	74.3		42	Wisconsin	39.5
13	Utah	65.2		44	Minnesota	35.4
42	Vermont	39.5		45	New Jersey	35.2
33	Virginia	48.3		46	New York	34.8
35	Washington	46.7		47	New Hampshire	33.6
11	West Virginia	67.8		48	Rhode Island	33.0
42	Wisconsin	39.5		49	Connecticut	30.5
2	Wyoming	78.7		50	Massachusetts	28.1

District of Columbia   62.4

Source: U.S. Department of Health and Human Services, Centers for Disease Control and Prevention
"Surveillance for Pregnancy and Birth Rates Among Teenagers" (MMWR, Vol. 42, No. SS-6, 12/17/93)
Women aged 15 to 19 years old.

Percent Change in Teenage Birth Rate: 1980 to 1990

National Percent Change = 13% Increase*

<table>
<tr><td colspan="3">ALPHA ORDER</td><td colspan="3">RANK ORDER</td></tr>
<tr><td>RANK</td><td>STATE</td><td>PERCENT CHANGE</td><td>RANK</td><td>STATE</td><td>PERCENT CHANGE</td></tr>
<tr><td>29</td><td>Alabama</td><td>4</td><td>1</td><td>Rhode Island</td><td>33</td></tr>
<tr><td>32</td><td>Alaska</td><td>1</td><td>2</td><td>California</td><td>32</td></tr>
<tr><td>12</td><td>Arizona</td><td>15</td><td>3</td><td>Michigan</td><td>31</td></tr>
<tr><td>25</td><td>Arkansas</td><td>7</td><td>4</td><td>Connecticut</td><td>27</td></tr>
<tr><td>2</td><td>California</td><td>32</td><td>5</td><td>Massachusetts</td><td>25</td></tr>
<tr><td>20</td><td>Colorado</td><td>9</td><td>5</td><td>Nevada</td><td>25</td></tr>
<tr><td>4</td><td>Connecticut</td><td>27</td><td>5</td><td>New York</td><td>25</td></tr>
<tr><td>27</td><td>Delaware</td><td>6</td><td>8</td><td>Maryland</td><td>23</td></tr>
<tr><td>10</td><td>Florida</td><td>18</td><td>9</td><td>Hawaii</td><td>21</td></tr>
<tr><td>28</td><td>Georgia</td><td>5</td><td>10</td><td>Florida</td><td>18</td></tr>
<tr><td>9</td><td>Hawaii</td><td>21</td><td>10</td><td>North Carolina</td><td>18</td></tr>
<tr><td>46</td><td>Idaho</td><td>(15)</td><td>12</td><td>Arizona</td><td>15</td></tr>
<tr><td>15</td><td>Illinois</td><td>13</td><td>12</td><td>New Jersey</td><td>15</td></tr>
<tr><td>30</td><td>Indiana</td><td>2</td><td>14</td><td>Washington</td><td>14</td></tr>
<tr><td>39</td><td>Iowa</td><td>(6)</td><td>15</td><td>Illinois</td><td>13</td></tr>
<tr><td>35</td><td>Kansas</td><td>(1)</td><td>15</td><td>Tennessee</td><td>13</td></tr>
<tr><td>41</td><td>Kentucky</td><td>(7)</td><td>17</td><td>Pennsylvania</td><td>11</td></tr>
<tr><td>36</td><td>Louisiana</td><td>(2)</td><td>18</td><td>Ohio</td><td>10</td></tr>
<tr><td>42</td><td>Maine</td><td>(9)</td><td>18</td><td>South Carolina</td><td>10</td></tr>
<tr><td>8</td><td>Maryland</td><td>23</td><td>20</td><td>Colorado</td><td>9</td></tr>
<tr><td>5</td><td>Massachusetts</td><td>25</td><td>20</td><td>Missouri</td><td>9</td></tr>
<tr><td>3</td><td>Michigan</td><td>31</td><td>20</td><td>New Mexico</td><td>9</td></tr>
<tr><td>30</td><td>Minnesota</td><td>2</td><td>20</td><td>Virginia</td><td>9</td></tr>
<tr><td>38</td><td>Mississippi</td><td>(3)</td><td>24</td><td>Wisconsin</td><td>8</td></tr>
<tr><td>20</td><td>Missouri</td><td>9</td><td>25</td><td>Arkansas</td><td>7</td></tr>
<tr><td>34</td><td>Montana</td><td>0</td><td>25</td><td>Oregon</td><td>7</td></tr>
<tr><td>39</td><td>Nebraska</td><td>(6)</td><td>27</td><td>Delaware</td><td>6</td></tr>
<tr><td>5</td><td>Nevada</td><td>25</td><td>28</td><td>Georgia</td><td>5</td></tr>
<tr><td>36</td><td>New Hampshire</td><td>(2)</td><td>29</td><td>Alabama</td><td>4</td></tr>
<tr><td>12</td><td>New Jersey</td><td>15</td><td>30</td><td>Indiana</td><td>2</td></tr>
<tr><td>20</td><td>New Mexico</td><td>9</td><td>30</td><td>Minnesota</td><td>2</td></tr>
<tr><td>5</td><td>New York</td><td>25</td><td>32</td><td>Alaska</td><td>1</td></tr>
<tr><td>10</td><td>North Carolina</td><td>18</td><td>32</td><td>Texas</td><td>1</td></tr>
<tr><td>46</td><td>North Dakota</td><td>(15)</td><td>34</td><td>Montana</td><td>0</td></tr>
<tr><td>18</td><td>Ohio</td><td>10</td><td>35</td><td>Kansas</td><td>(1)</td></tr>
<tr><td>43</td><td>Oklahoma</td><td>(10)</td><td>36</td><td>Louisiana</td><td>(2)</td></tr>
<tr><td>25</td><td>Oregon</td><td>7</td><td>36</td><td>New Hampshire</td><td>(2)</td></tr>
<tr><td>17</td><td>Pennsylvania</td><td>11</td><td>38</td><td>Mississippi</td><td>(3)</td></tr>
<tr><td>1</td><td>Rhode Island</td><td>33</td><td>39</td><td>Iowa</td><td>(6)</td></tr>
<tr><td>18</td><td>South Carolina</td><td>10</td><td>39</td><td>Nebraska</td><td>(6)</td></tr>
<tr><td>44</td><td>South Dakota</td><td>(11)</td><td>41</td><td>Kentucky</td><td>(7)</td></tr>
<tr><td>15</td><td>Tennessee</td><td>13</td><td>42</td><td>Maine</td><td>(9)</td></tr>
<tr><td>32</td><td>Texas</td><td>1</td><td>43</td><td>Oklahoma</td><td>(10)</td></tr>
<tr><td>49</td><td>Utah</td><td>(26)</td><td>44</td><td>South Dakota</td><td>(11)</td></tr>
<tr><td>45</td><td>Vermont</td><td>(14)</td><td>45</td><td>Vermont</td><td>(14)</td></tr>
<tr><td>20</td><td>Virginia</td><td>9</td><td>46</td><td>Idaho</td><td>(15)</td></tr>
<tr><td>14</td><td>Washington</td><td>14</td><td>46</td><td>North Dakota</td><td>(15)</td></tr>
<tr><td>46</td><td>West Virginia</td><td>(15)</td><td>46</td><td>West Virginia</td><td>(15)</td></tr>
<tr><td>24</td><td>Wisconsin</td><td>8</td><td>49</td><td>Utah</td><td>(26)</td></tr>
<tr><td>50</td><td>Wyoming</td><td>(29)</td><td>50</td><td>Wyoming</td><td>(29)</td></tr>
<tr><td></td><td></td><td></td><td></td><td>District of Columbia</td><td>49</td></tr>
</table>

Source: U.S. Department of Health and Human Services, Centers for Disease Control and Prevention
"Surveillance for Pregnancy and Birth Rates Among Teenagers" (MMWR, Vol. 42, No. SS-6, 12/17/93)
Women aged 15 to 19 years old.

Births to White Teenage Mothers in 1992

National Total = 342,739 Live Births*

ALPHA ORDER					RANK ORDER			
RANK	STATE	BIRTHS	% of USA		RANK	STATE	BIRTHS	% of USA
20	Alabama	5,494	1.60%		1	California	57,690	16.83%
46	Alaska	719	0.21%		2	Texas	39,502	11.53%
10	Arizona	8,478	2.47%		3	New York	15,879	4.63%
26	Arkansas	4,187	1.22%		4	Ohio	15,012	4.38%
1	California	57,690	16.83%		5	Florida	14,720	4.29%
18	Colorado	5,588	1.63%		6	Illinois	13,103	3.82%
36	Connecticut	2,606	0.76%		7	Pennsylvania	11,172	3.26%
47	Delaware	659	0.19%		8	Michigan	10,748	3.14%
5	Florida	14,720	4.29%		9	Indiana	9,063	2.64%
11	Georgia	8,335	2.43%		10	Arizona	8,478	2.47%
50	Hawaii	326	0.10%		11	Georgia	8,335	2.43%
37	Idaho	2,144	0.63%		12	North Carolina	8,237	2.40%
6	Illinois	13,103	3.82%		13	Tennessee	7,839	2.29%
9	Indiana	9,063	2.64%		14	Kentucky	7,428	2.17%
33	Iowa	3,495	1.02%		15	Missouri	7,343	2.14%
30	Kansas	3,713	1.08%		16	Washington	7,040	2.05%
14	Kentucky	7,428	2.17%		17	Virginia	5,852	1.71%
22	Louisiana	4,989	1.46%		18	Colorado	5,588	1.63%
40	Maine	1,596	0.47%		19	Oklahoma	5,574	1.63%
35	Maryland	3,013	0.88%		20	Alabama	5,494	1.60%
21	Massachusetts	5,085	1.48%		21	Massachusetts	5,085	1.48%
8	Michigan	10,748	3.14%		22	Louisiana	4,989	1.46%
28	Minnesota	3,928	1.15%		23	New Jersey	4,733	1.38%
34	Mississippi	3,190	0.93%		24	Oregon	4,643	1.35%
15	Missouri	7,343	2.14%		25	Wisconsin	4,490	1.31%
43	Montana	1,012	0.30%		26	Arkansas	4,187	1.22%
39	Nebraska	1,852	0.54%		27	South Carolina	4,062	1.19%
38	Nevada	2,097	0.61%		28	Minnesota	3,928	1.15%
42	New Hampshire	1,037	0.30%		29	New Mexico	3,897	1.14%
23	New Jersey	4,733	1.38%		30	Kansas	3,713	1.08%
29	New Mexico	3,897	1.14%		31	Utah	3,633	1.06%
3	New York	15,879	4.63%		32	West Virginia	3,571	1.04%
12	North Carolina	8,237	2.40%		33	Iowa	3,495	1.02%
49	North Dakota	617	0.18%		34	Mississippi	3,190	0.93%
4	Ohio	15,012	4.38%		35	Maryland	3,013	0.88%
19	Oklahoma	5,574	1.63%		36	Connecticut	2,606	0.76%
24	Oregon	4,643	1.35%		37	Idaho	2,144	0.63%
7	Pennsylvania	11,172	3.26%		38	Nevada	2,097	0.61%
41	Rhode Island	1,055	0.31%		39	Nebraska	1,852	0.54%
27	South Carolina	4,062	1.19%		40	Maine	1,596	0.47%
45	South Dakota	793	0.23%		41	Rhode Island	1,055	0.31%
13	Tennessee	7,839	2.29%		42	New Hampshire	1,037	0.30%
2	Texas	39,502	11.53%		43	Montana	1,012	0.30%
31	Utah	3,633	1.06%		44	Wyoming	807	0.24%
48	Vermont	636	0.19%		45	South Dakota	793	0.23%
17	Virginia	5,852	1.71%		46	Alaska	719	0.21%
16	Washington	7,040	2.05%		47	Delaware	659	0.19%
32	West Virginia	3,571	1.04%		48	Vermont	636	0.19%
25	Wisconsin	4,490	1.31%		49	North Dakota	617	0.18%
44	Wyoming	807	0.24%		50	Hawaii	326	0.10%
						District of Columbia	57	0.02%

Source: U.S. Department of Health and Human Services, National Center for Health Statistics
(unpublished data, Table 1-60)
*Births to women age 15 to 19 years old.

Births to White Teenage Mothers as a Percent of White Births in 1992

National Percent = 10.70% of White Live Births*

ALPHA ORDER

RANK	STATE	PERCENT
10	Alabama	13.67
33	Alaska	9.06
8	Arizona	14.27
3	Arkansas	15.93
19	California	11.71
21	Colorado	11.26
47	Connecticut	6.47
36	Delaware	8.34
26	Florida	10.26
15	Georgia	12.11
49	Hawaii	5.68
12	Idaho	12.74
32	Illinois	9.17
14	Indiana	12.26
31	Iowa	9.56
24	Kansas	11.03
4	Kentucky	15.40
13	Louisiana	12.55
28	Maine	10.13
48	Maryland	6.07
44	Massachusetts	6.77
30	Michigan	9.58
45	Minnesota	6.64
6	Mississippi	14.70
18	Missouri	11.86
27	Montana	10.14
35	Nebraska	8.65
23	Nevada	11.06
46	New Hampshire	6.60
50	New Jersey	5.21
1	New Mexico	16.83
42	New York	7.47
20	North Carolina	11.64
41	North Dakota	7.88
22	Ohio	11.17
5	Oklahoma	14.94
17	Oregon	11.88
40	Pennsylvania	8.21
39	Rhode Island	8.32
16	South Carolina	11.96
34	South Dakota	8.70
9	Tennessee	14.18
7	Texas	14.62
25	Utah	10.29
36	Vermont	8.34
36	Virginia	8.34
29	Washington	10.05
2	West Virginia	16.81
43	Wisconsin	7.40
11	Wyoming	12.76

RANK ORDER

RANK	STATE	PERCENT
1	New Mexico	16.83
2	West Virginia	16.81
3	Arkansas	15.93
4	Kentucky	15.40
5	Oklahoma	14.94
6	Mississippi	14.70
7	Texas	14.62
8	Arizona	14.27
9	Tennessee	14.18
10	Alabama	13.67
11	Wyoming	12.76
12	Idaho	12.74
13	Louisiana	12.55
14	Indiana	12.26
15	Georgia	12.11
16	South Carolina	11.96
17	Oregon	11.88
18	Missouri	11.86
19	California	11.71
20	North Carolina	11.64
21	Colorado	11.26
22	Ohio	11.17
23	Nevada	11.06
24	Kansas	11.03
25	Utah	10.29
26	Florida	10.26
27	Montana	10.14
28	Maine	10.13
29	Washington	10.05
30	Michigan	9.58
31	Iowa	9.56
32	Illinois	9.17
33	Alaska	9.06
34	South Dakota	8.70
35	Nebraska	8.65
36	Delaware	8.34
36	Vermont	8.34
36	Virginia	8.34
39	Rhode Island	8.32
40	Pennsylvania	8.21
41	North Dakota	7.88
42	New York	7.47
43	Wisconsin	7.40
44	Massachusetts	6.77
45	Minnesota	6.64
46	New Hampshire	6.60
47	Connecticut	6.47
48	Maryland	6.07
49	Hawaii	5.68
50	New Jersey	5.21

	District of Columbia	3.55

Source: Morgan Quitno Press using data from US Dept of Health & Human Services, National Center for Health Statistics (unpublished data, Table 1-60)

*Births to women age 15 to 19 years old.

Births to Black Teenage Mothers in 1992

National Total = 146,800 Live Births*

RANK	STATE	BIRTHS	% of USA
13	Alabama	5,428	3.70%
40	Alaska	76	0.05%
32	Arizona	559	0.38%
21	Arkansas	2,324	1.58%
6	California	7,920	5.40%
29	Colorado	603	0.41%
26	Connecticut	1,041	0.71%
30	Delaware	590	0.40%
2	Florida	10,283	7.00%
5	Georgia	9,031	6.15%
41	Hawaii	59	0.04%
45	Idaho	9	0.01%
1	Illinois	10,732	7.31%
20	Indiana	2,553	1.74%
35	Iowa	316	0.22%
27	Kansas	825	0.56%
24	Kentucky	1,257	0.86%
8	Louisiana	7,304	4.98%
47	Maine	8	0.01%
17	Maryland	4,275	2.91%
23	Massachusetts	1,283	0.87%
7	Michigan	7,395	5.04%
28	Minnesota	716	0.49%
11	Mississippi	5,552	3.78%
19	Missouri	3,429	2.34%
49	Montana	5	0.00%
34	Nebraska	321	0.22%
33	Nevada	489	0.33%
43	New Hampshire	18	0.01%
16	New Jersey	4,421	3.01%
39	New Mexico	111	0.08%
4	New York	9,139	6.23%
9	North Carolina	6,972	4.75%
45	North Dakota	9	0.01%
10	Ohio	6,418	4.37%
25	Oklahoma	1,237	0.84%
36	Oregon	254	0.17%
12	Pennsylvania	5,484	3.74%
37	Rhode Island	244	0.17%
14	South Carolina	4,950	3.37%
48	South Dakota	7	0.00%
18	Tennessee	4,227	2.88%
3	Texas	9,929	6.76%
42	Utah	45	0.03%
49	Vermont	5	0.00%
15	Virginia	4,499	3.06%
31	Washington	570	0.39%
38	West Virginia	181	0.12%
22	Wisconsin	2,092	1.43%
44	Wyoming	14	0.01%

RANK	STATE	BIRTHS	% of USA
1	Illinois	10,732	7.31%
2	Florida	10,283	7.00%
3	Texas	9,929	6.76%
4	New York	9,139	6.23%
5	Georgia	9,031	6.15%
6	California	7,920	5.40%
7	Michigan	7,395	5.04%
8	Louisiana	7,304	4.98%
9	North Carolina	6,972	4.75%
10	Ohio	6,418	4.37%
11	Mississippi	5,552	3.78%
12	Pennsylvania	5,484	3.74%
13	Alabama	5,428	3.70%
14	South Carolina	4,950	3.37%
15	Virginia	4,499	3.06%
16	New Jersey	4,421	3.01%
17	Maryland	4,275	2.91%
18	Tennessee	4,227	2.88%
19	Missouri	3,429	2.34%
20	Indiana	2,553	1.74%
21	Arkansas	2,324	1.58%
22	Wisconsin	2,092	1.43%
23	Massachusetts	1,283	0.87%
24	Kentucky	1,257	0.86%
25	Oklahoma	1,237	0.84%
26	Connecticut	1,041	0.71%
27	Kansas	825	0.56%
28	Minnesota	716	0.49%
29	Colorado	603	0.41%
30	Delaware	590	0.40%
31	Washington	570	0.39%
32	Arizona	559	0.38%
33	Nevada	489	0.33%
34	Nebraska	321	0.22%
35	Iowa	316	0.22%
36	Oregon	254	0.17%
37	Rhode Island	244	0.17%
38	West Virginia	181	0.12%
39	New Mexico	111	0.08%
40	Alaska	76	0.05%
41	Hawaii	59	0.04%
42	Utah	45	0.03%
43	New Hampshire	18	0.01%
44	Wyoming	14	0.01%
45	Idaho	9	0.01%
45	North Dakota	9	0.01%
47	Maine	8	0.01%
48	South Dakota	7	0.00%
49	Montana	5	0.00%
49	Vermont	5	0.00%
	District of Columbia	1,591	1.08%

Source: U.S. Department of Health and Human Services, National Center for Health Statistics
    unpublished data
    (unpublished data, Table 1-60)
*Births to women age 15 to 19 years old.

Births to Black Teenage Mothers as a Percent of Black Births in 1992

National Percent = 21.79% of Black Live Births*

ALPHA ORDER				RANK ORDER		
RANK	STATE	BIRTHS		RANK	STATE	BIRTHS
8	Alabama	25.22		1	Wisconsin	28.63
45	Alaska	14.02		2	Arkansas	28.51
24	Arizona	22.83		3	Indiana	27.08
2	Arkansas	28.51		4	Mississippi	27.05
37	California	17.03		5	Iowa	26.69
32	Colorado	20.05		6	Oregon	26.60
38	Connecticut	16.94		7	Missouri	25.75
19	Delaware	23.11		8	Alabama	25.22
23	Florida	22.87		9	Illinois	25.00
26	Georgia	22.36		10	Kansas	24.89
50	Hawaii	8.61		11	Michigan	24.86
41	Idaho	15.52		12	Ohio	24.69
9	Illinois	25.00		13	Minnesota	24.55
3	Indiana	27.08		14	Louisiana	24.48
5	Iowa	26.69		15	Nebraska	24.47
10	Kansas	24.89		16	Kentucky	24.23
16	Kentucky	24.23		17	Tennessee	24.14
14	Louisiana	24.48		18	Oklahoma	23.95
48	Maine	9.76		19	Delaware	23.11
39	Maryland	16.81		20	Texas	23.08
43	Massachusetts	14.84		21	North Carolina	22.98
11	Michigan	24.86		22	South Carolina	22.91
13	Minnesota	24.55		23	Florida	22.87
4	Mississippi	27.05		24	Arizona	22.83
7	Missouri	25.75		25	Nevada	22.61
47	Montana	10.20		26	Georgia	22.36
15	Nebraska	24.47		27	West Virginia	22.21
25	Nevada	22.61		28	New Mexico	21.64
40	New Hampshire	16.51		29	Pennsylvania	21.59
33	New Jersey	18.89		30	Wyoming	21.54
28	New Mexico	21.64		31	Rhode Island	20.57
42	New York	14.98		32	Colorado	20.05
21	North Carolina	22.98		33	New Jersey	18.89
46	North Dakota	12.00		34	Virginia	18.86
12	Ohio	24.69		35	Utah	18.37
18	Oklahoma	23.95		36	Washington	18.12
6	Oregon	26.60		37	California	17.03
29	Pennsylvania	21.59		38	Connecticut	16.94
31	Rhode Island	20.57		39	Maryland	16.81
22	South Carolina	22.91		40	New Hampshire	16.51
49	South Dakota	8.86		41	Idaho	15.52
17	Tennessee	24.14		42	New York	14.98
20	Texas	23.08		43	Massachusetts	14.84
35	Utah	18.37		44	Vermont	14.71
44	Vermont	14.71		45	Alaska	14.02
34	Virginia	18.86		46	North Dakota	12.00
36	Washington	18.12		47	Montana	10.20
27	West Virginia	22.21		48	Maine	9.76
1	Wisconsin	28.63		49	South Dakota	8.86
30	Wyoming	21.54		50	Hawaii	8.61
					District of Columbia	18.07

Source: Morgan Quitno Press using data from US Dept of Health & Human Services, National Center for Health Statistics
(unpublished data, Table 1-60)
*Births to women age 15 to 19 years old.

Births to Women 35 to 49 Years Old in 1992

National Total = 402,354 Live Births

ALPHA ORDER					RANK ORDER			
RANK	STATE	BIRTHS	% of USA		RANK	STATE	BIRTHS	% of USA
27	Alabama	3,962	0.98%		1	California	70,383	17.49%
44	Alaska	1,334	0.33%		2	New York	37,357	9.28%
20	Arizona	6,140	1.53%		3	Texas	26,237	6.52%
38	Arkansas	1,965	0.49%		4	Illinois	19,213	4.78%
1	California	70,383	17.49%		5	Florida	18,714	4.65%
19	Colorado	6,286	1.56%		6	Pennsylvania	17,305	4.30%
18	Connecticut	6,346	1.58%		7	New Jersey	16,495	4.10%
46	Delaware	924	0.23%		8	Ohio	13,833	3.44%
5	Florida	18,714	4.65%		9	Michigan	12,897	3.21%
14	Georgia	8,622	2.14%		10	Massachusetts	12,143	3.02%
33	Hawaii	2,479	0.62%		11	Virginia	10,265	2.55%
41	Idaho	1,478	0.37%		12	Maryland	9,242	2.30%
4	Illinois	19,213	4.78%		13	Washington	9,100	2.26%
22	Indiana	6,012	1.49%		14	Georgia	8,622	2.14%
32	Iowa	3,068	0.76%		15	North Carolina	7,736	1.92%
30	Kansas	3,261	0.81%		16	Minnesota	7,086	1.76%
28	Kentucky	3,479	0.86%		17	Wisconsin	6,659	1.66%
24	Louisiana	5,030	1.25%		18	Connecticut	6,346	1.58%
43	Maine	1,431	0.36%		19	Colorado	6,286	1.56%
12	Maryland	9,242	2.30%		20	Arizona	6,140	1.53%
10	Massachusetts	12,143	3.02%		21	Missouri	6,107	1.52%
9	Michigan	12,897	3.21%		22	Indiana	6,012	1.49%
16	Minnesota	7,086	1.76%		23	Tennessee	5,166	1.28%
35	Mississippi	2,430	0.60%		24	Louisiana	5,030	1.25%
21	Missouri	6,107	1.52%		25	Oregon	4,526	1.12%
45	Montana	1,153	0.29%		26	South Carolina	4,002	0.99%
36	Nebraska	2,224	0.55%		27	Alabama	3,962	0.98%
37	Nevada	1,984	0.49%		28	Kentucky	3,479	0.86%
39	New Hampshire	1,808	0.45%		29	Utah	3,395	0.84%
7	New Jersey	16,495	4.10%		30	Kansas	3,261	0.81%
34	New Mexico	2,469	0.61%		31	Oklahoma	3,118	0.77%
2	New York	37,357	9.28%		32	Iowa	3,068	0.76%
15	North Carolina	7,736	1.92%		33	Hawaii	2,479	0.62%
49	North Dakota	785	0.20%		34	New Mexico	2,469	0.61%
8	Ohio	13,833	3.44%		35	Mississippi	2,430	0.60%
31	Oklahoma	3,118	0.77%		36	Nebraska	2,224	0.55%
25	Oregon	4,526	1.12%		37	Nevada	1,984	0.49%
6	Pennsylvania	17,305	4.30%		38	Arkansas	1,965	0.49%
40	Rhode Island	1,585	0.39%		39	New Hampshire	1,808	0.45%
26	South Carolina	4,002	0.99%		40	Rhode Island	1,585	0.39%
47	South Dakota	914	0.23%		41	Idaho	1,478	0.37%
23	Tennessee	5,166	1.28%		42	West Virginia	1,438	0.36%
3	Texas	26,237	6.52%		43	Maine	1,431	0.36%
29	Utah	3,395	0.84%		44	Alaska	1,334	0.33%
48	Vermont	908	0.23%		45	Montana	1,153	0.29%
11	Virginia	10,265	2.55%		46	Delaware	924	0.23%
13	Washington	9,100	2.26%		47	South Dakota	914	0.23%
42	West Virginia	1,438	0.36%		48	Vermont	908	0.23%
17	Wisconsin	6,659	1.66%		49	North Dakota	785	0.20%
50	Wyoming	573	0.14%		50	Wyoming	573	0.14%
						District of Columbia	1,287	0.32%

Source: Morgan Quitno Press using data from U.S. Dept of Health & Human Services, National Center for Health Statistics
(unpublished data, Table 1-60)

Births to Women 35 to 49 Years Old as a Percent of All Births in 1992

National Percent = 9.90% of Live Births

<table>
<tr><td colspan="3"><u>ALPHA ORDER</u></td><td colspan="3"><u>RANK ORDER</u></td></tr>
<tr><td>RANK</td><td>STATE</td><td>PERCENT</td><td>RANK</td><td>STATE</td><td>PERCENT</td></tr>
<tr><td>48</td><td>Alabama</td><td>6.36</td><td>1</td><td>Massachusetts</td><td>13.92</td></tr>
<tr><td>11</td><td>Alaska</td><td>11.38</td><td>2</td><td>New Jersey</td><td>13.76</td></tr>
<tr><td>25</td><td>Arizona</td><td>8.92</td><td>3</td><td>Connecticut</td><td>13.34</td></tr>
<tr><td>50</td><td>Arkansas</td><td>5.64</td><td>4</td><td>New York</td><td>12.98</td></tr>
<tr><td>8</td><td>California</td><td>11.70</td><td>5</td><td>Hawaii</td><td>12.48</td></tr>
<tr><td>9</td><td>Colorado</td><td>11.53</td><td>6</td><td>Maryland</td><td>11.88</td></tr>
<tr><td>3</td><td>Connecticut</td><td>13.34</td><td>7</td><td>Vermont</td><td>11.74</td></tr>
<tr><td>30</td><td>Delaware</td><td>8.67</td><td>8</td><td>California</td><td>11.70</td></tr>
<tr><td>20</td><td>Florida</td><td>9.76</td><td>9</td><td>Colorado</td><td>11.53</td></tr>
<tr><td>39</td><td>Georgia</td><td>7.76</td><td>10</td><td>Washington</td><td>11.45</td></tr>
<tr><td>5</td><td>Hawaii</td><td>12.48</td><td>11</td><td>Alaska</td><td>11.38</td></tr>
<tr><td>34</td><td>Idaho</td><td>8.51</td><td>12</td><td>New Hampshire</td><td>11.31</td></tr>
<tr><td>19</td><td>Illinois</td><td>10.04</td><td>13</td><td>Rhode Island</td><td>10.93</td></tr>
<tr><td>41</td><td>Indiana</td><td>7.15</td><td>14</td><td>Minnesota</td><td>10.80</td></tr>
<tr><td>38</td><td>Iowa</td><td>7.98</td><td>15</td><td>Oregon</td><td>10.77</td></tr>
<tr><td>31</td><td>Kansas</td><td>8.58</td><td>16</td><td>Virginia</td><td>10.56</td></tr>
<tr><td>47</td><td>Kentucky</td><td>6.46</td><td>17</td><td>Pennsylvania</td><td>10.51</td></tr>
<tr><td>43</td><td>Louisiana</td><td>7.11</td><td>18</td><td>Montana</td><td>10.05</td></tr>
<tr><td>26</td><td>Maine</td><td>8.91</td><td>19</td><td>Illinois</td><td>10.04</td></tr>
<tr><td>6</td><td>Maryland</td><td>11.88</td><td>20</td><td>Florida</td><td>9.76</td></tr>
<tr><td>1</td><td>Massachusetts</td><td>13.92</td><td>21</td><td>Nebraska</td><td>9.51</td></tr>
<tr><td>24</td><td>Michigan</td><td>8.95</td><td>22</td><td>Wisconsin</td><td>9.42</td></tr>
<tr><td>14</td><td>Minnesota</td><td>10.80</td><td>23</td><td>Utah</td><td>9.13</td></tr>
<tr><td>49</td><td>Mississippi</td><td>5.69</td><td>24</td><td>Michigan</td><td>8.95</td></tr>
<tr><td>37</td><td>Missouri</td><td>8.00</td><td>25</td><td>Arizona</td><td>8.92</td></tr>
<tr><td>18</td><td>Montana</td><td>10.05</td><td>26</td><td>Maine</td><td>8.91</td></tr>
<tr><td>21</td><td>Nebraska</td><td>9.51</td><td>26</td><td>North Dakota</td><td>8.91</td></tr>
<tr><td>28</td><td>Nevada</td><td>8.87</td><td>28</td><td>Nevada</td><td>8.87</td></tr>
<tr><td>12</td><td>New Hampshire</td><td>11.31</td><td>29</td><td>New Mexico</td><td>8.84</td></tr>
<tr><td>2</td><td>New Jersey</td><td>13.76</td><td>30</td><td>Delaware</td><td>8.67</td></tr>
<tr><td>29</td><td>New Mexico</td><td>8.84</td><td>31</td><td>Kansas</td><td>8.58</td></tr>
<tr><td>4</td><td>New York</td><td>12.98</td><td>32</td><td>Ohio</td><td>8.53</td></tr>
<tr><td>40</td><td>North Carolina</td><td>7.44</td><td>33</td><td>Wyoming</td><td>8.52</td></tr>
<tr><td>26</td><td>North Dakota</td><td>8.91</td><td>34</td><td>Idaho</td><td>8.51</td></tr>
<tr><td>32</td><td>Ohio</td><td>8.53</td><td>35</td><td>South Dakota</td><td>8.30</td></tr>
<tr><td>45</td><td>Oklahoma</td><td>6.56</td><td>36</td><td>Texas</td><td>8.18</td></tr>
<tr><td>15</td><td>Oregon</td><td>10.77</td><td>37</td><td>Missouri</td><td>8.00</td></tr>
<tr><td>17</td><td>Pennsylvania</td><td>10.51</td><td>38</td><td>Iowa</td><td>7.98</td></tr>
<tr><td>13</td><td>Rhode Island</td><td>10.93</td><td>39</td><td>Georgia</td><td>7.76</td></tr>
<tr><td>42</td><td>South Carolina</td><td>7.12</td><td>40</td><td>North Carolina</td><td>7.44</td></tr>
<tr><td>35</td><td>South Dakota</td><td>8.30</td><td>41</td><td>Indiana</td><td>7.15</td></tr>
<tr><td>44</td><td>Tennessee</td><td>7.02</td><td>42</td><td>South Carolina</td><td>7.12</td></tr>
<tr><td>36</td><td>Texas</td><td>8.18</td><td>43</td><td>Louisiana</td><td>7.11</td></tr>
<tr><td>23</td><td>Utah</td><td>9.13</td><td>44</td><td>Tennessee</td><td>7.02</td></tr>
<tr><td>7</td><td>Vermont</td><td>11.74</td><td>45</td><td>Oklahoma</td><td>6.56</td></tr>
<tr><td>16</td><td>Virginia</td><td>10.56</td><td>46</td><td>West Virginia</td><td>6.49</td></tr>
<tr><td>10</td><td>Washington</td><td>11.45</td><td>47</td><td>Kentucky</td><td>6.46</td></tr>
<tr><td>46</td><td>West Virginia</td><td>6.49</td><td>48</td><td>Alabama</td><td>6.36</td></tr>
<tr><td>22</td><td>Wisconsin</td><td>9.42</td><td>49</td><td>Mississippi</td><td>5.69</td></tr>
<tr><td>33</td><td>Wyoming</td><td>8.52</td><td>50</td><td>Arkansas</td><td>5.64</td></tr>
<tr><td></td><td></td><td></td><td></td><td>District of Columbia</td><td>11.74</td></tr>
</table>

Source: Morgan Quitno Press using data from U.S. Dept of Health & Human Services, National Center for Health Statistics
(unpublished data, Table 1-60)

Births by Vaginal Delivery in 1992

National Total = 3,100,710 Live Births

RANK	STATE	BIRTHS	% of USA
23	Alabama	46,696	1.51%
44	Alaska	9,800	0.32%
18	Arizona	56,424	1.82%
34	Arkansas	24,871	0.80%
1	California	471,726	15.21%
24	Colorado	45,675	1.47%
28	Connecticut	33,019	1.06%
47	Delaware	8,242	0.27%
5	Florida	145,185	4.68%
10	Georgia	86,112	2.78%
39	Hawaii	16,002	0.52%
40	Idaho	14,458	0.47%
4	Illinois	149,062	4.81%
14	Indiana	65,828	2.12%
31	Iowa	30,683	0.99%
33	Kansas	29,234	0.94%
26	Kentucky	39,237	1.27%
22	Louisiana	50,466	1.63%
42	Maine	12,522	0.40%
21	Maryland	52,195	1.68%
13	Massachusetts	67,722	2.18%
8	Michigan	112,248	3.62%
20	Minnesota	52,952	1.71%
29	Mississippi	30,981	1.00%
16	Missouri	58,932	1.90%
45	Montana	9,128	0.29%
36	Nebraska	18,853	0.61%
37	Nevada	17,704	0.57%
41	New Hampshire	12,601	0.41%
9	New Jersey	90,318	2.91%
35	New Mexico	22,564	0.73%
2	New York	216,665	6.99%
11	North Carolina	80,452	2.59%
48	North Dakota	7,125	0.23%
7	Ohio	124,133	4.00%
32	Oklahoma	30,454	0.98%
27	Oregon	34,300	1.11%
6	Pennsylvania	128,394	4.14%
43	Rhode Island	10,840	0.35%
25	South Carolina	43,179	1.39%
46	South Dakota	8,648	0.28%
19	Tennessee	56,271	1.81%
3	Texas	213,452	6.88%
30	Utah	30,718	0.99%
49	Vermont	6,309	0.20%
12	Virginia	74,507	2.40%
15	Washington	64,827	2.09%
38	West Virginia	16,409	0.53%
17	Wisconsin	58,773	1.90%
50	Wyoming	5,368	0.17%

RANK	STATE	BIRTHS	% of USA
1	California	471,726	15.21%
2	New York	216,665	6.99%
3	Texas	213,452	6.88%
4	Illinois	149,062	4.81%
5	Florida	145,185	4.68%
6	Pennsylvania	128,394	4.14%
7	Ohio	124,133	4.00%
8	Michigan	112,248	3.62%
9	New Jersey	90,318	2.91%
10	Georgia	86,112	2.78%
11	North Carolina	80,452	2.59%
12	Virginia	74,507	2.40%
13	Massachusetts	67,722	2.18%
14	Indiana	65,828	2.12%
15	Washington	64,827	2.09%
16	Missouri	58,932	1.90%
17	Wisconsin	58,773	1.90%
18	Arizona	56,424	1.82%
19	Tennessee	56,271	1.81%
20	Minnesota	52,952	1.71%
21	Maryland	52,195	1.68%
22	Louisiana	50,466	1.63%
23	Alabama	46,696	1.51%
24	Colorado	45,675	1.47%
25	South Carolina	43,179	1.39%
26	Kentucky	39,237	1.27%
27	Oregon	34,300	1.11%
28	Connecticut	33,019	1.06%
29	Mississippi	30,981	1.00%
30	Utah	30,718	0.99%
31	Iowa	30,683	0.99%
32	Oklahoma	30,454	0.98%
33	Kansas	29,234	0.94%
34	Arkansas	24,871	0.80%
35	New Mexico	22,564	0.73%
36	Nebraska	18,853	0.61%
37	Nevada	17,704	0.57%
38	West Virginia	16,409	0.53%
39	Hawaii	16,002	0.52%
40	Idaho	14,458	0.47%
41	New Hampshire	12,601	0.41%
42	Maine	12,522	0.40%
43	Rhode Island	10,840	0.35%
44	Alaska	9,800	0.32%
45	Montana	9,128	0.29%
46	South Dakota	8,648	0.28%
47	Delaware	8,242	0.27%
48	North Dakota	7,125	0.23%
49	Vermont	6,309	0.20%
50	Wyoming	5,368	0.17%
	District of Columbia	8,446	0.27%

Source: U.S. Department of Health and Human Services, National Center for Health Statistics
(unpublished data, table 1–168, May 24, 1994)

Percent of Births by Vaginal Delivery in 1992

National Percent = 76.28% of Live Births

ALPHA ORDER			RANK ORDER		
RANK	STATE	PERCENT	RANK	STATE	PERCENT
40	Alabama	75.00	1	Colorado	83.75
2	Alaska	83.57	2	Alaska	83.57
6	Arizona	81.98	3	Idaho	83.27
45	Arkansas	71.43	4	Wisconsin	83.17
21	California	78.39	5	Utah	82.58
1	Colorado	83.75	6	Arizona	81.98
47	Connecticut	69.41	7	Oregon	81.60
30	Delaware	77.35	8	Washington	81.59
37	Florida	75.73	9	Vermont	81.54
28	Georgia	77.50	10	North Dakota	80.86
14	Hawaii	80.56	11	New Mexico	80.81
3	Idaho	83.27	12	Minnesota	80.71
26	Illinois	77.88	13	Nebraska	80.58
22	Indiana	78.24	14	Hawaii	80.56
16	Iowa	79.76	15	Wyoming	79.85
32	Kansas	76.88	16	Iowa	79.76
43	Kentucky	72.88	17	Montana	79.57
46	Louisiana	71.37	18	Nevada	79.13
24	Maine	77.98	19	New Hampshire	78.81
48	Maryland	67.08	20	South Dakota	78.49
27	Massachusetts	77.64	21	California	78.39
25	Michigan	77.90	22	Indiana	78.24
12	Minnesota	80.71	23	Pennsylvania	77.99
44	Mississippi	72.59	24	Maine	77.98
31	Missouri	77.24	25	Michigan	77.90
17	Montana	79.57	26	Illinois	77.88
13	Nebraska	80.58	27	Massachusetts	77.64
18	Nevada	79.13	28	Georgia	77.50
19	New Hampshire	78.81	29	North Carolina	77.38
38	New Jersey	75.32	30	Delaware	77.35
11	New Mexico	80.81	31	Missouri	77.24
39	New York	75.26	32	Kansas	76.88
29	North Carolina	77.38	33	South Carolina	76.84
10	North Dakota	80.86	34	Virginia	76.65
35	Ohio	76.51	35	Ohio	76.51
50	Oklahoma	64.04	36	Tennessee	76.44
7	Oregon	81.60	37	Florida	75.73
23	Pennsylvania	77.99	38	New Jersey	75.32
41	Rhode Island	74.76	39	New York	75.26
33	South Carolina	76.84	40	Alabama	75.00
20	South Dakota	78.49	41	Rhode Island	74.76
36	Tennessee	76.44	42	West Virginia	74.01
49	Texas	66.53	43	Kentucky	72.88
5	Utah	82.58	44	Mississippi	72.59
9	Vermont	81.54	45	Arkansas	71.43
34	Virginia	76.65	46	Louisiana	71.37
8	Washington	81.59	47	Connecticut	69.41
42	West Virginia	74.01	48	Maryland	67.08
4	Wisconsin	83.17	49	Texas	66.53
15	Wyoming	79.85	50	Oklahoma	64.04
				District of Columbia	77.06

Source: Morgan Quitno Press using data from US Dept of Health & Human Services, National Center for Health Statistics
(unpublished data, table 1-168, May 24, 1994)

Births by Cesarean Delivery in 1992

National Total = 888,622 Live Cesarean Births

RANK	STATE	BIRTHS	% of USA
19	Alabama	15,458	1.74%
47	Alaska	1,865	0.21%
23	Arizona	12,206	1.37%
27	Arkansas	9,800	1.10%
1	California	129,726	14.60%
29	Colorado	8,700	0.98%
30	Connecticut	8,683	0.98%
44	Delaware	2,382	0.27%
4	Florida	45,692	5.14%
10	Georgia	23,839	2.68%
39	Hawaii	3,853	0.43%
42	Idaho	2,882	0.32%
5	Illinois	41,453	4.66%
15	Indiana	18,102	2.04%
32	Iowa	7,656	0.86%
31	Kansas	8,145	0.92%
21	Kentucky	12,893	1.45%
13	Louisiana	20,164	2.27%
40	Maine	3,424	0.39%
18	Maryland	16,489	1.86%
14	Massachusetts	19,310	2.17%
8	Michigan	30,653	3.45%
26	Minnesota	10,512	1.18%
25	Mississippi	11,593	1.30%
16	Missouri	17,025	1.92%
45	Montana	2,290	0.26%
37	Nebraska	4,507	0.51%
38	Nevada	4,502	0.51%
41	New Hampshire	3,336	0.38%
9	New Jersey	28,922	3.25%
36	New Mexico	5,250	0.59%
3	New York	66,002	7.43%
11	North Carolina	23,125	2.60%
48	North Dakota	1,666	0.19%
6	Ohio	37,421	4.21%
28	Oklahoma	9,577	1.08%
33	Oregon	7,648	0.86%
7	Pennsylvania	35,859	4.04%
43	Rhode Island	2,555	0.29%
22	South Carolina	12,888	1.45%
46	South Dakota	2,227	0.25%
17	Tennessee	16,863	1.90%
2	Texas	76,573	8.62%
34	Utah	6,373	0.72%
49	Vermont	1,426	0.16%
12	Virginia	22,282	2.51%
20	Washington	13,530	1.52%
35	West Virginia	5,698	0.64%
24	Wisconsin	11,825	1.33%
50	Wyoming	1,345	0.15%

RANK	STATE	BIRTHS	% of USA
1	California	129,726	14.60%
2	Texas	76,573	8.62%
3	New York	66,002	7.43%
4	Florida	45,692	5.14%
5	Illinois	41,453	4.66%
6	Ohio	37,421	4.21%
7	Pennsylvania	35,859	4.04%
8	Michigan	30,653	3.45%
9	New Jersey	28,922	3.25%
10	Georgia	23,839	2.68%
11	North Carolina	23,125	2.60%
12	Virginia	22,282	2.51%
13	Louisiana	20,164	2.27%
14	Massachusetts	19,310	2.17%
15	Indiana	18,102	2.04%
16	Missouri	17,025	1.92%
17	Tennessee	16,863	1.90%
18	Maryland	16,489	1.86%
19	Alabama	15,458	1.74%
20	Washington	13,530	1.52%
21	Kentucky	12,893	1.45%
22	South Carolina	12,888	1.45%
23	Arizona	12,206	1.37%
24	Wisconsin	11,825	1.33%
25	Mississippi	11,593	1.30%
26	Minnesota	10,512	1.18%
27	Arkansas	9,800	1.10%
28	Oklahoma	9,577	1.08%
29	Colorado	8,700	0.98%
30	Connecticut	8,683	0.98%
31	Kansas	8,145	0.92%
32	Iowa	7,656	0.86%
33	Oregon	7,648	0.86%
34	Utah	6,373	0.72%
35	West Virginia	5,698	0.64%
36	New Mexico	5,250	0.59%
37	Nebraska	4,507	0.51%
38	Nevada	4,502	0.51%
39	Hawaii	3,853	0.43%
40	Maine	3,424	0.39%
41	New Hampshire	3,336	0.38%
42	Idaho	2,882	0.32%
43	Rhode Island	2,555	0.29%
44	Delaware	2,382	0.27%
45	Montana	2,290	0.26%
46	South Dakota	2,227	0.25%
47	Alaska	1,865	0.21%
48	North Dakota	1,666	0.19%
49	Vermont	1,426	0.16%
50	Wyoming	1,345	0.15%
	District of Columbia	2,427	0.27%

Source: U.S. Department of Health and Human Services, National Center for Health Statistics (unpublished data, table 1–168, May 24, 1994)

Percent of Births by Cesarean Delivery in 1992

National Percent = 22.3% of Live Births

ALPHA ORDER			RANK ORDER		
RANK	STATE	PERCENT	RANK	STATE	PERCENT
6	Alabama	24.9	1	Louisiana	28.5
49	Alaska	16.0	2	Arkansas	28.3
43	Arizona	17.8	3	Mississippi	27.2
2	Arkansas	28.3	4	Texas	26.4
25	California	21.6	5	West Virginia	25.8
49	Colorado	16.0	6	Alabama	24.9
30	Connecticut	20.8	7	Kentucky	24.7
17	Delaware	22.4	8	New Jersey	24.3
10	Florida	23.9	9	Maryland	24.0
24	Georgia	21.7	10	Florida	23.9
36	Hawaii	19.4	10	Oklahoma	23.9
47	Idaho	16.6	12	New York	23.3
21	Illinois	21.8	13	Ohio	23.2
25	Indiana	21.6	14	Tennessee	23.1
34	Iowa	20.0	15	South Carolina	23.0
21	Kansas	21.8	15	Virginia	23.0
7	Kentucky	24.7	17	Delaware	22.4
1	Louisiana	28.5	17	Missouri	22.4
27	Maine	21.5	19	North Carolina	22.3
9	Maryland	24.0	20	Massachusetts	22.2
20	Massachusetts	22.2	21	Illinois	21.8
27	Michigan	21.5	21	Kansas	21.8
47	Minnesota	16.6	21	Pennsylvania	21.8
3	Mississippi	27.2	24	Georgia	21.7
17	Missouri	22.4	25	California	21.6
33	Montana	20.1	25	Indiana	21.6
37	Nebraska	19.3	27	Maine	21.5
32	Nevada	20.3	27	Michigan	21.5
29	New Hampshire	20.9	29	New Hampshire	20.9
8	New Jersey	24.3	30	Connecticut	20.8
40	New Mexico	18.9	31	South Dakota	20.5
12	New York	23.3	32	Nevada	20.3
19	North Carolina	22.3	33	Montana	20.1
39	North Dakota	19.0	34	Iowa	20.0
13	Ohio	23.2	34	Wyoming	20.0
10	Oklahoma	23.9	36	Hawaii	19.4
42	Oregon	18.2	37	Nebraska	19.3
21	Pennsylvania	21.8	38	Rhode Island	19.1
38	Rhode Island	19.1	39	North Dakota	19.0
15	South Carolina	23.0	40	New Mexico	18.9
31	South Dakota	20.5	41	Vermont	18.4
14	Tennessee	23.1	42	Oregon	18.2
4	Texas	26.4	43	Arizona	17.8
45	Utah	17.2	44	Washington	17.3
41	Vermont	18.4	45	Utah	17.2
15	Virginia	23.0	46	Wisconsin	16.7
44	Washington	17.3	47	Idaho	16.6
5	West Virginia	25.8	47	Minnesota	16.6
46	Wisconsin	16.7	49	Alaska	16.0
34	Wyoming	20.0	49	Colorado	16.0
				District of Columbia	22.3

Source: U.S. Department of Health and Human Services, National Center for Health Statistics
(unpublished data, table 1-168, May 24, 1994)

Births by Vaginal Delivery after a Previous Cesarean Delivery (VBAC) in 1992

National Total = 97,549 Live VBAC Births

ALPHA ORDER

RANK	STATE	BIRTHS	% of USA
26	Alabama	1,185	1.21%
41	Alaska	431	0.44%
19	Arizona	1,716	1.76%
37	Arkansas	628	0.64%
1	California	11,767	12.06%
22	Colorado	1,554	1.59%
24	Connecticut	1,324	1.36%
46	Delaware	346	0.35%
6	Florida	4,543	4.66%
14	Georgia	2,336	2.39%
40	Hawaii	507	0.52%
38	Idaho	545	0.56%
5	Illinois	4,588	4.70%
20	Indiana	1,710	1.75%
25	Iowa	1,193	1.22%
29	Kansas	948	0.97%
27	Kentucky	1,034	1.06%
31	Louisiana	859	0.88%
43	Maine	408	0.42%
18	Maryland	1,924	1.97%
11	Massachusetts	2,448	2.51%
8	Michigan	3,632	3.72%
12	Minnesota	2,359	2.42%
34	Mississippi	713	0.73%
17	Missouri	2,212	2.27%
45	Montana	371	0.38%
35	Nebraska	690	0.71%
36	Nevada	655	0.67%
39	New Hampshire	523	0.54%
9	New Jersey	2,847	2.92%
33	New Mexico	748	0.77%
2	New York	9,689	9.93%
13	North Carolina	2,351	2.41%
49	North Dakota	258	0.26%
7	Ohio	4,212	4.32%
32	Oklahoma	816	0.84%
21	Oregon	1,592	1.63%
3	Pennsylvania	4,862	4.98%
42	Rhode Island	414	0.42%
28	South Carolina	1,027	1.05%
48	South Dakota	260	0.27%
23	Tennessee	1,459	1.50%
4	Texas	4,789	4.91%
30	Utah	901	0.92%
47	Vermont	271	0.28%
16	Virginia	2,253	2.31%
10	Washington	2,472	2.53%
44	West Virginia	397	0.41%
15	Wisconsin	2,256	2.31%
50	Wyoming	206	0.21%

RANK ORDER

RANK	STATE	BIRTHS	% of USA
1	California	11,767	12.06%
2	New York	9,689	9.93%
3	Pennsylvania	4,862	4.98%
4	Texas	4,789	4.91%
5	Illinois	4,588	4.70%
6	Florida	4,543	4.66%
7	Ohio	4,212	4.32%
8	Michigan	3,632	3.72%
9	New Jersey	2,847	2.92%
10	Washington	2,472	2.53%
11	Massachusetts	2,448	2.51%
12	Minnesota	2,359	2.42%
13	North Carolina	2,351	2.41%
14	Georgia	2,336	2.39%
15	Wisconsin	2,256	2.31%
16	Virginia	2,253	2.31%
17	Missouri	2,212	2.27%
18	Maryland	1,924	1.97%
19	Arizona	1,716	1.76%
20	Indiana	1,710	1.75%
21	Oregon	1,592	1.63%
22	Colorado	1,554	1.59%
23	Tennessee	1,459	1.50%
24	Connecticut	1,324	1.36%
25	Iowa	1,193	1.22%
26	Alabama	1,185	1.21%
27	Kentucky	1,034	1.06%
28	South Carolina	1,027	1.05%
29	Kansas	948	0.97%
30	Utah	901	0.92%
31	Louisiana	859	0.88%
32	Oklahoma	816	0.84%
33	New Mexico	748	0.77%
34	Mississippi	713	0.73%
35	Nebraska	690	0.71%
36	Nevada	655	0.67%
37	Arkansas	628	0.64%
38	Idaho	545	0.56%
39	New Hampshire	523	0.54%
40	Hawaii	507	0.52%
41	Alaska	431	0.44%
42	Rhode Island	414	0.42%
43	Maine	408	0.42%
44	West Virginia	397	0.41%
45	Montana	371	0.38%
46	Delaware	346	0.35%
47	Vermont	271	0.28%
48	South Dakota	260	0.27%
49	North Dakota	258	0.26%
50	Wyoming	206	0.21%
	District of Columbia	320	0.33%

Source: U.S. Department of Health and Human Services, National Center for Health Statistics
(unpublished data, table 1–168, May 24, 1994)

Rate of Vaginal Births after a Previous Cesarean (VBAC) in 1992

National Percent = 22.6% of Live Births to Women Who Had Had a Cesarean*

ALPHA ORDER				RANK ORDER		
RANK	STATE	PERCENT		RANK	STATE	PERCENT
44	Alabama	17.6		1	Alaska	39.3
1	Alaska	39.3		2	Minnesota	36.9
19	Arizona	28.2		3	Oregon	36.1
47	Arkansas	14.5		4	Colorado	35.5
40	California	19.4		5	Vermont	33.9
4	Colorado	35.5		6	Washington	32.7
11	Connecticut	29.5		6	Wisconsin	32.7
14	Delaware	28.6		8	Idaho	31.1
36	Florida	21.4		9	Rhode Island	30.8
37	Georgia	21.0		10	Montana	29.8
21	Hawaii	27.4		11	Connecticut	29.5
8	Idaho	31.1		12	Wyoming	29.3
33	Illinois	22.2		13	New Hampshire	29.2
41	Indiana	19.3		14	Delaware	28.6
18	Iowa	28.3		14	New Mexico	28.6
34	Kansas	22.1		16	Nevada	28.5
45	Kentucky	17.5		17	New York	28.4
50	Louisiana	10.4		18	Iowa	28.3
28	Maine	24.4		19	Arizona	28.2
24	Maryland	25.9		20	Nebraska	28.0
27	Massachusetts	25.0		21	Hawaii	27.4
30	Michigan	23.5		21	North Dakota	27.4
2	Minnesota	36.9		23	Missouri	26.0
49	Mississippi	13.5		24	Maryland	25.9
23	Missouri	26.0		25	Pennsylvania	25.6
10	Montana	29.8		26	Utah	25.2
20	Nebraska	28.0		27	Massachusetts	25.0
16	Nevada	28.5		28	Maine	24.4
13	New Hampshire	29.2		29	North Carolina	23.9
38	New Jersey	20.7		30	Michigan	23.5
14	New Mexico	28.6		31	South Dakota	22.9
17	New York	28.4		31	Virginia	22.9
29	North Carolina	23.9		33	Illinois	22.2
21	North Dakota	27.4		34	Kansas	22.1
35	Ohio	21.9		35	Ohio	21.9
42	Oklahoma	17.8		36	Florida	21.4
3	Oregon	36.1		37	Georgia	21.0
25	Pennsylvania	25.6		38	New Jersey	20.7
9	Rhode Island	30.8		39	Tennessee	19.5
42	South Carolina	17.8		40	California	19.4
31	South Dakota	22.9		41	Indiana	19.3
39	Tennessee	19.5		42	Oklahoma	17.8
48	Texas	13.7		42	South Carolina	17.8
26	Utah	25.2		44	Alabama	17.6
5	Vermont	33.9		45	Kentucky	17.5
31	Virginia	22.9		46	West Virginia	16.0
6	Washington	32.7		47	Arkansas	14.5
46	West Virginia	16.0		48	Texas	13.7
6	Wisconsin	32.7		49	Mississippi	13.5
12	Wyoming	29.3		50	Louisiana	10.4
					District of Columbia	25.5

Source: U.S. Department of Health and Human Services, National Center for Health Statistics
(unpublished data, table 1-168, May 24, 1994)

*Vaginal births after a cesarean delivery as a percent of all births to women with a previous cesarean delivery giving birth in 1992.

Percent of Mothers Beginning Prenatal Care in First Trimester in 1992

National Percent = 77.7% of Mothers*

ALPHA ORDER RANK ORDER

RANK	STATE	PERCENT	RANK	STATE	PERCENT
35	Alabama	77.1	1	Rhode Island	88.5
11	Alaska	83.1	2	Connecticut	87.5
47	Arizona	71.3	3	Maine	87.3
45	Arkansas	72.3	3	New Hampshire	87.3
40	California	75.1	5	Massachusetts	87.2
27	Colorado	79.0	6	Iowa	86.2
2	Connecticut	87.5	7	Maryland	85.0
20	Delaware	80.5	7	Utah	85.0
34	Florida	77.9	9	Vermont	84.5
39	Georgia	75.8	10	Kansas	83.6
44	Hawaii	73.6	11	Alaska	83.1
37	Idaho	76.6	12	Nebraska	82.3
32	Illinois	78.2	12	Ohio	82.3
31	Indiana	78.3	14	North Dakota	82.2
6	Iowa	86.2	15	Wisconsin	82.0
10	Kansas	83.6	16	Minnesota	81.8
22	Kentucky	80.1	16	Virginia	81.8
38	Louisiana	76.3	18	New Jersey	81.5
3	Maine	87.3	19	Michigan	80.8
7	Maryland	85.0	20	Delaware	80.5
5	Massachusetts	87.2	20	Missouri	80.5
19	Michigan	80.8	22	Kentucky	80.1
16	Minnesota	81.8	23	Washington	79.8
41	Mississippi	74.9	24	Pennsylvania	79.6
20	Missouri	80.5	24	Tennessee	79.6
32	Montana	78.2	26	North Carolina	79.4
12	Nebraska	82.3	27	Colorado	79.0
46	Nevada	71.5	27	South Dakota	79.0
3	New Hampshire	87.3	27	Wyoming	79.0
18	New Jersey	81.5	30	Oregon	78.7
50	New Mexico	61.7	31	Indiana	78.3
42	New York	74.7	32	Illinois	78.2
26	North Carolina	79.4	32	Montana	78.2
14	North Dakota	82.2	34	Florida	77.9
12	Ohio	82.3	35	Alabama	77.1
43	Oklahoma	74.6	36	West Virginia	76.7
30	Oregon	78.7	37	Idaho	76.6
24	Pennsylvania	79.6	38	Louisiana	76.3
1	Rhode Island	88.5	39	Georgia	75.8
47	South Carolina	71.3	40	California	75.1
27	South Dakota	79.0	41	Mississippi	74.9
24	Tennessee	79.6	42	New York	74.7
49	Texas	70.3	43	Oklahoma	74.6
7	Utah	85.0	44	Hawaii	73.6
9	Vermont	84.5	45	Arkansas	72.3
16	Virginia	81.8	46	Nevada	71.5
23	Washington	79.8	47	Arizona	71.3
36	West Virginia	76.7	47	South Carolina	71.3
15	Wisconsin	82.0	49	Texas	70.3
27	Wyoming	79.0	50	New Mexico	61.7
				District of Columbia	56.9

Source: U.S. Department of Health and Human Services, National Center for Health Statistics
"Monthly Vital Statistics Report" (Vol. 43, No. 5, Supplement, October 25, 1994)
*Final data by state of residence.

Percent of White Mothers Beginning Prenatal Care in First Trimester in 1992

National Percent = 80.8% of White Mothers*

ALPHA ORDER				RANK ORDER		
RANK	STATE	PERCENT		RANK	STATE	PERCENT
24	Alabama	84.2		1	Maryland	90.7
12	Alaska	85.8		2	Rhode Island	90.4
48	Arizona	73.0		3	Connecticut	89.8
43	Arkansas	77.0		4	Massachusetts	89.1
46	California	74.9		5	New Hampshire	87.5
37	Colorado	80.1		6	Maine	87.4
3	Connecticut	89.8		7	Iowa	86.9
8	Delaware	86.7		8	Delaware	86.7
31	Florida	82.2		9	Virginia	86.6
28	Georgia	82.6		10	New Jersey	86.1
44	Hawaii	76.8		11	Utah	86.0
44	Idaho	76.8		12	Alaska	85.8
28	Illinois	82.6		12	North Carolina	85.8
36	Indiana	80.4		12	Wisconsin	85.8
7	Iowa	86.9		15	Louisiana	85.5
17	Kansas	85.0		16	Ohio	85.3
32	Kentucky	81.6		17	Kansas	85.0
15	Louisiana	85.5		18	Michigan	84.9
6	Maine	87.4		18	Minnesota	84.9
1	Maryland	90.7		20	Mississippi	84.8
4	Massachusetts	89.1		21	Vermont	84.7
18	Michigan	84.9		22	North Dakota	84.4
18	Minnesota	84.9		23	Pennsylvania	84.3
20	Mississippi	84.8		24	Alabama	84.2
25	Missouri	84.0		25	Missouri	84.0
34	Montana	80.9		26	Nebraska	83.7
26	Nebraska	83.7		27	Tennessee	83.6
47	Nevada	73.5		28	Georgia	82.6
5	New Hampshire	87.5		28	Illinois	82.6
10	New Jersey	86.1		30	South Dakota	82.3
50	New Mexico	64.6		31	Florida	82.2
38	New York	79.9		32	Kentucky	81.6
12	North Carolina	85.8		33	Washington	81.0
22	North Dakota	84.4		34	Montana	80.9
16	Ohio	85.3		35	South Carolina	80.8
41	Oklahoma	77.9		36	Indiana	80.4
40	Oregon	79.3		37	Colorado	80.1
23	Pennsylvania	84.3		38	New York	79.9
2	Rhode Island	90.4		39	Wyoming	79.8
35	South Carolina	80.8		40	Oregon	79.3
30	South Dakota	82.3		41	Oklahoma	77.9
27	Tennessee	83.6		42	West Virginia	77.5
49	Texas	71.2		43	Arkansas	77.0
11	Utah	86.0		44	Hawaii	76.8
21	Vermont	84.7		44	Idaho	76.8
9	Virginia	86.6		46	California	74.9
33	Washington	81.0		47	Nevada	73.5
42	West Virginia	77.5		48	Arizona	73.0
12	Wisconsin	85.8		49	Texas	71.2
39	Wyoming	79.8		50	New Mexico	64.6
					District of Columbia	87.0

Source: U.S. Department of Health and Human Services, National Center for Health Statistics
"Monthly Vital Statistics Report" (Vol. 43, No. 5, Supplement, October 25, 1994)
*Final data by state of residence.

Percent of Black Mothers Beginning Prenatal Care in First Trimester in 1992

National Percent = 63.9% of Black Mothers*

ALPHA ORDER

RANK ORDER

RANK	STATE	PERCENT	RANK	STATE	PERCENT
35	Alabama	63.7	1	Alaska	81.7
1	Alaska	81.7	2	Montana	81.3
20	Arizona	66.6	3	Maine	80.2
43	Arkansas	57.3	4	Vermont	75.0
11	California	72.3	5	Massachusetts	74.4
18	Colorado	67.6	6	Rhode Island	73.8
8	Connecticut	72.8	7	North Dakota	73.0
40	Delaware	61.3	8	Connecticut	72.8
31	Florida	64.4	8	Maryland	72.8
32	Georgia	64.2	8	New Hampshire	72.8
24	Hawaii	65.9	11	California	72.3
15	Idaho	69.6	12	Iowa	72.0
36	Illinois	63.2	13	Kansas	71.3
39	Indiana	61.7	14	Utah	71.1
12	Iowa	72.0	15	Idaho	69.6
13	Kansas	71.3	16	Washington	68.9
25	Kentucky	65.8	17	Virginia	68.1
34	Louisiana	63.9	18	Colorado	67.6
3	Maine	80.2	19	Tennessee	67.2
8	Maryland	72.8	20	Arizona	66.6
5	Massachusetts	74.4	21	Nebraska	66.4
28	Michigan	65.6	21	Ohio	66.4
50	Minnesota	52.4	23	Wyoming	66.2
30	Mississippi	64.6	24	Hawaii	65.9
33	Missouri	64.0	25	Kentucky	65.8
2	Montana	81.3	25	South Dakota	65.8
21	Nebraska	66.4	27	Oregon	65.7
48	Nevada	54.7	28	Michigan	65.6
8	New Hampshire	72.8	29	North Carolina	64.7
38	New Jersey	62.7	30	Mississippi	64.6
49	New Mexico	53.3	31	Florida	64.4
44	New York	56.9	32	Georgia	64.2
29	North Carolina	64.7	33	Missouri	64.0
7	North Dakota	73.0	34	Louisiana	63.9
21	Ohio	66.4	35	Alabama	63.7
42	Oklahoma	58.9	36	Illinois	63.2
27	Oregon	65.7	37	Texas	62.8
47	Pennsylvania	54.8	38	New Jersey	62.7
6	Rhode Island	73.8	39	Indiana	61.7
45	South Carolina	56.1	40	Delaware	61.3
25	South Dakota	65.8	41	Wisconsin	60.2
19	Tennessee	67.2	42	Oklahoma	58.9
37	Texas	62.8	43	Arkansas	57.3
14	Utah	71.1	44	New York	56.9
4	Vermont	75.0	45	South Carolina	56.1
17	Virginia	68.1	46	West Virginia	55.4
16	Washington	68.9	47	Pennsylvania	54.8
46	West Virginia	55.4	48	Nevada	54.7
41	Wisconsin	60.2	49	New Mexico	53.3
23	Wyoming	66.2	50	Minnesota	52.4
				District of Columbia	52.3

Source: U.S. Department of Health and Human Services, National Center for Health Statistics
"Monthly Vital Statistics Report" (Vol. 43, No. 5, Supplement, October 25, 1994)
*Final data by state of residence.

Percent of Mothers Receiving Late or No Prenatal Care in 1992

National Percent = 5.2% of Mothers*

ALPHA ORDER			RANK ORDER		
RANK	**STATE**	**PERCENT**	**RANK**	**STATE**	**PERCENT**
20	Alabama	4.7	1	New Mexico	9.9
41	Alaska	3.0	2	Texas	9.2
3	Arizona	8.1	3	Arizona	8.1
7	Arkansas	6.5	4	Nevada	7.8
12	California	5.3	5	South Carolina	6.9
18	Colorado	4.9	6	New York	6.8
44	Connecticut	2.6	7	Arkansas	6.5
20	Delaware	4.7	8	Oklahoma	6.4
22	Florida	4.6	9	Louisiana	5.8
11	Georgia	5.4	10	Hawaii	5.7
10	Hawaii	5.7	11	Georgia	5.4
13	Idaho	5.2	12	California	5.3
15	Illinois	5.0	13	Idaho	5.2
18	Indiana	4.9	13	Pennsylvania	5.2
46	Iowa	2.4	15	Illinois	5.0
39	Kansas	3.2	15	Mississippi	5.0
25	Kentucky	4.2	15	South Dakota	5.0
9	Louisiana	5.8	18	Colorado	4.9
50	Maine	1.8	18	Indiana	4.9
34	Maryland	3.7	20	Alabama	4.7
47	Massachusetts	2.1	20	Delaware	4.7
34	Michigan	3.7	22	Florida	4.6
38	Minnesota	3.5	22	New Jersey	4.6
15	Mississippi	5.0	24	Wyoming	4.3
25	Missouri	4.2	25	Kentucky	4.2
25	Montana	4.2	25	Missouri	4.2
39	Nebraska	3.2	25	Montana	4.2
4	Nevada	7.8	25	North Carolina	4.2
47	New Hampshire	2.1	25	West Virginia	4.2
22	New Jersey	4.6	30	Oregon	4.0
1	New Mexico	9.9	30	Tennessee	4.0
6	New York	6.8	30	Washington	4.0
25	North Carolina	4.2	33	Ohio	3.9
42	North Dakota	2.8	34	Maryland	3.7
33	Ohio	3.9	34	Michigan	3.7
8	Oklahoma	6.4	34	Virginia	3.7
30	Oregon	4.0	37	Wisconsin	3.6
13	Pennsylvania	5.2	38	Minnesota	3.5
49	Rhode Island	2.0	39	Kansas	3.2
5	South Carolina	6.9	39	Nebraska	3.2
15	South Dakota	5.0	41	Alaska	3.0
30	Tennessee	4.0	42	North Dakota	2.8
2	Texas	9.2	43	Vermont	2.7
45	Utah	2.5	44	Connecticut	2.6
43	Vermont	2.7	45	Utah	2.5
34	Virginia	3.7	46	Iowa	2.4
30	Washington	4.0	47	Massachusetts	2.1
25	West Virginia	4.2	47	New Hampshire	2.1
37	Wisconsin	3.6	49	Rhode Island	2.0
24	Wyoming	4.3	50	Maine	1.8
				District of Columbia	13.9

Source: U.S. Department of Health and Human Services, National Center for Health Statistics
"Monthly Vital Statistics Report" (Vol. 43, No. 5, Supplement, October 25, 1994)
*Final data by state of residence. "Late" means care begun in third trimester.

Percent of White Mothers Receiving Late or No Prenatal Care in 1992

National Percent = 4.2% of White Mothers*

<table>
<tr><td colspan="3">ALPHA ORDER</td><td colspan="3">RANK ORDER</td></tr>
<tr><td>RANK</td><td>STATE</td><td>PERCENT</td><td>RANK</td><td>STATE</td><td>PERCENT</td></tr>
<tr><td>32</td><td>Alabama</td><td>2.6</td><td>1</td><td>Texas</td><td>8.9</td></tr>
<tr><td>41</td><td>Alaska</td><td>2.2</td><td>2</td><td>New Mexico</td><td>8.6</td></tr>
<tr><td>3</td><td>Arizona</td><td>7.5</td><td>3</td><td>Arizona</td><td>7.5</td></tr>
<tr><td>9</td><td>Arkansas</td><td>4.7</td><td>4</td><td>Nevada</td><td>7.0</td></tr>
<tr><td>5</td><td>California</td><td>5.4</td><td>5</td><td>California</td><td>5.4</td></tr>
<tr><td>10</td><td>Colorado</td><td>4.5</td><td>6</td><td>Idaho</td><td>5.1</td></tr>
<tr><td>46</td><td>Connecticut</td><td>1.9</td><td>6</td><td>Oklahoma</td><td>5.1</td></tr>
<tr><td>32</td><td>Delaware</td><td>2.6</td><td>8</td><td>New York</td><td>4.8</td></tr>
<tr><td>20</td><td>Florida</td><td>3.5</td><td>9</td><td>Arkansas</td><td>4.7</td></tr>
<tr><td>20</td><td>Georgia</td><td>3.5</td><td>10</td><td>Colorado</td><td>4.5</td></tr>
<tr><td>16</td><td>Hawaii</td><td>3.7</td><td>11</td><td>Indiana</td><td>4.2</td></tr>
<tr><td>6</td><td>Idaho</td><td>5.1</td><td>12</td><td>South Carolina</td><td>3.9</td></tr>
<tr><td>16</td><td>Illinois</td><td>3.7</td><td>12</td><td>West Virginia</td><td>3.9</td></tr>
<tr><td>11</td><td>Indiana</td><td>4.2</td><td>12</td><td>Wyoming</td><td>3.9</td></tr>
<tr><td>41</td><td>Iowa</td><td>2.2</td><td>15</td><td>Oregon</td><td>3.8</td></tr>
<tr><td>25</td><td>Kansas</td><td>2.8</td><td>16</td><td>Hawaii</td><td>3.7</td></tr>
<tr><td>16</td><td>Kentucky</td><td>3.7</td><td>16</td><td>Illinois</td><td>3.7</td></tr>
<tr><td>29</td><td>Louisiana</td><td>2.7</td><td>16</td><td>Kentucky</td><td>3.7</td></tr>
<tr><td>47</td><td>Maine</td><td>1.8</td><td>16</td><td>Washington</td><td>3.7</td></tr>
<tr><td>47</td><td>Maryland</td><td>1.8</td><td>20</td><td>Florida</td><td>3.5</td></tr>
<tr><td>49</td><td>Massachusetts</td><td>1.7</td><td>20</td><td>Georgia</td><td>3.5</td></tr>
<tr><td>35</td><td>Michigan</td><td>2.5</td><td>22</td><td>Montana</td><td>3.2</td></tr>
<tr><td>37</td><td>Minnesota</td><td>2.4</td><td>23</td><td>Pennsylvania</td><td>3.1</td></tr>
<tr><td>37</td><td>Mississippi</td><td>2.4</td><td>24</td><td>Missouri</td><td>2.9</td></tr>
<tr><td>24</td><td>Missouri</td><td>2.9</td><td>25</td><td>Kansas</td><td>2.8</td></tr>
<tr><td>22</td><td>Montana</td><td>3.2</td><td>25</td><td>Nebraska</td><td>2.8</td></tr>
<tr><td>25</td><td>Nebraska</td><td>2.8</td><td>25</td><td>New Jersey</td><td>2.8</td></tr>
<tr><td>4</td><td>Nevada</td><td>7.0</td><td>25</td><td>South Dakota</td><td>2.8</td></tr>
<tr><td>44</td><td>New Hampshire</td><td>2.0</td><td>29</td><td>Louisiana</td><td>2.7</td></tr>
<tr><td>25</td><td>New Jersey</td><td>2.8</td><td>29</td><td>Ohio</td><td>2.7</td></tr>
<tr><td>2</td><td>New Mexico</td><td>8.6</td><td>29</td><td>Tennessee</td><td>2.7</td></tr>
<tr><td>8</td><td>New York</td><td>4.8</td><td>32</td><td>Alabama</td><td>2.6</td></tr>
<tr><td>37</td><td>North Carolina</td><td>2.4</td><td>32</td><td>Delaware</td><td>2.6</td></tr>
<tr><td>44</td><td>North Dakota</td><td>2.0</td><td>32</td><td>Vermont</td><td>2.6</td></tr>
<tr><td>29</td><td>Ohio</td><td>2.7</td><td>35</td><td>Michigan</td><td>2.5</td></tr>
<tr><td>6</td><td>Oklahoma</td><td>5.1</td><td>35</td><td>Wisconsin</td><td>2.5</td></tr>
<tr><td>15</td><td>Oregon</td><td>3.8</td><td>37</td><td>Minnesota</td><td>2.4</td></tr>
<tr><td>23</td><td>Pennsylvania</td><td>3.1</td><td>37</td><td>Mississippi</td><td>2.4</td></tr>
<tr><td>50</td><td>Rhode Island</td><td>1.5</td><td>37</td><td>North Carolina</td><td>2.4</td></tr>
<tr><td>12</td><td>South Carolina</td><td>3.9</td><td>37</td><td>Virginia</td><td>2.4</td></tr>
<tr><td>25</td><td>South Dakota</td><td>2.8</td><td>41</td><td>Alaska</td><td>2.2</td></tr>
<tr><td>29</td><td>Tennessee</td><td>2.7</td><td>41</td><td>Iowa</td><td>2.2</td></tr>
<tr><td>1</td><td>Texas</td><td>8.9</td><td>43</td><td>Utah</td><td>2.1</td></tr>
<tr><td>43</td><td>Utah</td><td>2.1</td><td>44</td><td>New Hampshire</td><td>2.0</td></tr>
<tr><td>32</td><td>Vermont</td><td>2.6</td><td>44</td><td>North Dakota</td><td>2.0</td></tr>
<tr><td>37</td><td>Virginia</td><td>2.4</td><td>46</td><td>Connecticut</td><td>1.9</td></tr>
<tr><td>16</td><td>Washington</td><td>3.7</td><td>47</td><td>Maine</td><td>1.8</td></tr>
<tr><td>12</td><td>West Virginia</td><td>3.9</td><td>47</td><td>Maryland</td><td>1.8</td></tr>
<tr><td>35</td><td>Wisconsin</td><td>2.5</td><td>49</td><td>Massachusetts</td><td>1.7</td></tr>
<tr><td>12</td><td>Wyoming</td><td>3.9</td><td>50</td><td>Rhode Island</td><td>1.5</td></tr>
<tr><td></td><td></td><td></td><td></td><td>District of Columbia</td><td>3.1</td></tr>
</table>

Source: U.S. Department of Health and Human Services, National Center for Health Statistics
"Monthly Vital Statistics Report" (Vol. 43, No. 5, Supplement, October 25, 1994)
*Final data by state of residence. "Late" means care begun in third trimester.

Percent of Black Mothers Receiving Late or No Prenatal Care in 1992

National Percent = 9.9% of Black Mothers*

ALPHA ORDER				RANK ORDER		
RANK	STATE	PERCENT		RANK	STATE	PERCENT
21	Alabama	8.7		1	Pennsylvania	16.9
NA	Alaska**	NA		2	Minnesota	13.8
16	Arizona	10.1		2	Nevada	13.8
7	Arkansas	12.2		2	New York	13.8
36	California	6.3		5	West Virginia	13.2
20	Colorado	8.8		6	New Mexico	12.7
34	Connecticut	7.0		7	Arkansas	12.2
12	Delaware	11.2		8	Oklahoma	12.1
27	Florida	8.0		8	Texas	12.1
22	Georgia	8.6		10	New Jersey	11.8
40	Hawaii	4.7		10	South Carolina	11.8
NA	Idaho**	NA		12	Delaware	11.2
19	Illinois	9.6		13	Wisconsin	10.7
15	Indiana	10.4		14	Missouri	10.6
37	Iowa	5.6		15	Indiana	10.4
34	Kansas	7.0		16	Arizona	10.1
23	Kentucky	8.4		16	Louisiana	10.1
16	Louisiana	10.1		16	Ohio	10.1
NA	Maine**	NA		19	Illinois	9.6
31	Maryland	7.7		20	Colorado	8.8
39	Massachusetts	5.2		21	Alabama	8.7
23	Michigan	8.4		22	Georgia	8.6
2	Minnesota	13.8		23	Kentucky	8.4
31	Mississippi	7.7		23	Michigan	8.4
14	Missouri	10.6		23	North Carolina	8.4
NA	Montana**	NA		26	Oregon	8.3
28	Nebraska	7.9		27	Florida	8.0
2	Nevada	13.8		28	Nebraska	7.9
NA	New Hampshire**	NA		29	Tennessee	7.8
10	New Jersey	11.8		29	Washington	7.8
6	New Mexico	12.7		31	Maryland	7.7
2	New York	13.8		31	Mississippi	7.7
23	North Carolina	8.4		33	Virginia	7.6
NA	North Dakota**	NA		34	Connecticut	7.0
16	Ohio	10.1		34	Kansas	7.0
8	Oklahoma	12.1		36	California	6.3
26	Oregon	8.3		37	Iowa	5.6
1	Pennsylvania	16.9		38	Rhode Island	5.5
38	Rhode Island	5.5		39	Massachusetts	5.2
10	South Carolina	11.8		40	Hawaii	4.7
NA	South Dakota**	NA		NA	Alaska**	NA
29	Tennessee	7.8		NA	Idaho**	NA
8	Texas	12.1		NA	Maine**	NA
NA	Utah**	NA		NA	Montana**	NA
NA	Vermont**	NA		NA	New Hampshire**	NA
33	Virginia	7.6		NA	North Dakota**	NA
29	Washington	7.8		NA	South Dakota**	NA
5	West Virginia	13.2		NA	Utah**	NA
13	Wisconsin	10.7		NA	Vermont**	NA
NA	Wyoming**	NA		NA	Wyoming**	NA
					District of Columbia	16.0

Source: U.S. Department of Health and Human Services, National Center for Health Statistics
   "Monthly Vital Statistics Report" (Vol. 43, No. 5, Supplement, October 25, 1994)
*Final data by state of residence. "Late" means care begun in third trimester.
**Insufficient data.

Median Weight Gain During Pregnancy in 1992

National Median = 30.5 Pounds

ALPHA ORDER

RANK	STATE	POUNDS
44	Alabama	30.2
2	Alaska	31.0
13	Arizona	30.7
44	Arkansas	30.2
NA	California*	NA
8	Colorado	30.8
13	Connecticut	30.7
47	Delaware	30.1
8	Florida	30.8
40	Georgia	30.3
5	Hawaii	30.9
27	Idaho	30.5
27	Illinois	30.5
8	Indiana	30.8
36	Iowa	30.4
2	Kansas	31.0
40	Kentucky	30.3
49	Louisiana	27.9
21	Maine	30.6
13	Maryland	30.7
36	Massachusetts	30.4
13	Michigan	30.7
21	Minnesota	30.6
48	Mississippi	29.4
5	Missouri	30.9
21	Montana	30.6
27	Nebraska	30.5
8	Nevada	30.8
2	New Hampshire	31.0
40	New Jersey	30.3
13	New Mexico	30.7
21	New York	30.6
27	North Carolina	30.5
13	North Dakota	30.7
5	Ohio	30.9
27	Oklahoma	30.5
13	Oregon	30.7
36	Pennsylvania	30.4
1	Rhode Island	31.7
44	South Carolina	30.2
27	South Dakota	30.5
36	Tennessee	30.4
27	Texas	30.5
21	Utah	30.6
8	Vermont	30.8
27	Virginia	30.5
27	Washington	30.5
40	West Virginia	30.3
13	Wisconsin	30.7
21	Wyoming	30.6

RANK ORDER

RANK	STATE	POUNDS
1	Rhode Island	31.7
2	Alaska	31.0
2	Kansas	31.0
2	New Hampshire	31.0
5	Hawaii	30.9
5	Missouri	30.9
5	Ohio	30.9
8	Colorado	30.8
8	Florida	30.8
8	Indiana	30.8
8	Nevada	30.8
8	Vermont	30.8
13	Arizona	30.7
13	Connecticut	30.7
13	Maryland	30.7
13	Michigan	30.7
13	New Mexico	30.7
13	North Dakota	30.7
13	Oregon	30.7
13	Wisconsin	30.7
21	Maine	30.6
21	Minnesota	30.6
21	Montana	30.6
21	New York	30.6
21	Utah	30.6
21	Wyoming	30.6
27	Idaho	30.5
27	Illinois	30.5
27	Nebraska	30.5
27	North Carolina	30.5
27	Oklahoma	30.5
27	South Dakota	30.5
27	Texas	30.5
27	Virginia	30.5
27	Washington	30.5
36	Iowa	30.4
36	Massachusetts	30.4
36	Pennsylvania	30.4
36	Tennessee	30.4
40	Georgia	30.3
40	Kentucky	30.3
40	New Jersey	30.3
40	West Virginia	30.3
44	Alabama	30.2
44	Arkansas	30.2
44	South Carolina	30.2
47	Delaware	30.1
48	Mississippi	29.4
49	Louisiana	27.9
NA	California*	NA
	District of Columbia	28.3

Source: U.S. Department of Health and Human Services, National Center for Health Statistics
   (unpublished data, table 1-226)
*Not available.

Percent of Births to Women Considered Alcoholic Drinkers During Pregnancy in 1992

National Percent = 2.6% of Live Births*

ALPHA ORDER				RANK ORDER		
RANK	STATE	PERCENT		RANK	STATE	PERCENT
38	Alabama	1.7		1	Massachusetts	11.1
2	Alaska	8.6		2	Alaska	8.6
17	Arizona	2.7		3	Wisconsin	5.3
35	Arkansas	1.8		4	Montana	4.1
NA	California**	NA		5	Wyoming	4.0
20	Colorado	2.5		6	Oregon	3.9
26	Connecticut	2.1		7	Pennsylvania	3.4
29	Delaware	2.0		8	Iowa	3.3
31	Florida	1.9		8	Nevada	3.3
31	Georgia	1.9		8	Washington	3.3
31	Hawaii	1.9		11	New Hampshire	3.1
12	Idaho	2.9		12	Idaho	2.9
42	Illinois	1.5		12	Maryland	2.9
35	Indiana	1.8		14	New Mexico	2.8
8	Iowa	3.3		14	Ohio	2.8
46	Kansas	1.1		14	Rhode Island	2.8
23	Kentucky	2.4		17	Arizona	2.7
46	Louisiana	1.1		17	Nebraska	2.7
35	Maine	1.8		19	Minnesota	2.6
12	Maryland	2.9		20	Colorado	2.5
1	Massachusetts	11.1		20	Michigan	2.5
20	Michigan	2.5		20	North Dakota	2.5
19	Minnesota	2.6		23	Kentucky	2.4
45	Mississippi	1.2		23	Missouri	2.4
23	Missouri	2.4		25	Virginia	2.2
4	Montana	4.1		26	Connecticut	2.1
17	Nebraska	2.7		26	New Jersey	2.1
8	Nevada	3.3		26	Vermont	2.1
11	New Hampshire	3.1		29	Delaware	2.0
26	New Jersey	2.1		29	North Carolina	2.0
14	New Mexico	2.8		31	Florida	1.9
NA	New York**	NA		31	Georgia	1.9
29	North Carolina	2.0		31	Hawaii	1.9
20	North Dakota	2.5		31	Oklahoma	1.9
14	Ohio	2.8		35	Arkansas	1.8
31	Oklahoma	1.9		35	Indiana	1.8
6	Oregon	3.9		35	Maine	1.8
7	Pennsylvania	3.4		38	Alabama	1.7
14	Rhode Island	2.8		38	Tennessee	1.7
42	South Carolina	1.5		40	Texas	1.6
NA	South Dakota**	NA		40	West Virginia	1.6
38	Tennessee	1.7		42	Illinois	1.5
40	Texas	1.6		42	South Carolina	1.5
42	Utah	1.5		42	Utah	1.5
26	Vermont	2.1		45	Mississippi	1.2
25	Virginia	2.2		46	Kansas	1.1
8	Washington	3.3		46	Louisiana	1.1
40	West Virginia	1.6		NA	California**	NA
3	Wisconsin	5.3		NA	New York**	NA
5	Wyoming	4.0		NA	South Dakota**	NA
					District of Columbia	6.2

Source: U.S. Department of Health and Human Services, National Center for Health Statistics
(unpublished data, table 1-215)
*HHS defines "Drinker" as averaging at least one drink or less per week.
**Not available.

54

Percent of Births to Women Who Smoked During Pregnancy in 1992

National Percent = 16.9% of Live Births*

<u>ALPHA ORDER</u>

RANK	STATE	PERCENT
33	Alabama	15.1
5	Alaska	23.3
40	Arizona	12.6
10	Arkansas	21.1
NA	California**	NA
31	Colorado	15.5
39	Connecticut	12.9
27	Delaware	16.4
28	Florida	16.3
38	Georgia	13.4
43	Hawaii	11.4
29	Idaho	15.7
30	Illinois	15.6
14	Indiana	20.5
NA	Iowa**	NA
36	Kansas	13.8
1	Kentucky	27.0
41	Louisiana	12.4
12	Maine	20.7
37	Maryland	13.7
5	Massachusetts	23.3
9	Michigan	21.2
32	Minnesota	15.2
34	Mississippi	14.9
4	Missouri	23.4
18	Montana	20.2
19	Nebraska	19.9
21	Nevada	19.6
21	New Hampshire	19.6
44	New Jersey	10.3
42	New Mexico	11.8
NA	New York**	NA
24	North Carolina	18.6
13	North Dakota	20.6
7	Ohio	23.2
25	Oklahoma	18.2
14	Oregon	20.5
14	Pennsylvania	20.5
17	Rhode Island	20.4
26	South Carolina	17.1
NA	South Dakota**	NA
11	Tennessee	20.8
46	Texas	9.3
45	Utah	10.1
23	Vermont	18.9
34	Virginia	14.9
19	Washington	19.9
1	West Virginia	27.0
8	Wisconsin	21.7
3	Wyoming	23.6

<u>RANK ORDER</u>

RANK	STATE	PERCENT
1	Kentucky	27.0
1	West Virginia	27.0
3	Wyoming	23.6
4	Missouri	23.4
5	Alaska	23.3
5	Massachusetts	23.3
7	Ohio	23.2
8	Wisconsin	21.7
9	Michigan	21.2
10	Arkansas	21.1
11	Tennessee	20.8
12	Maine	20.7
13	North Dakota	20.6
14	Indiana	20.5
14	Oregon	20.5
14	Pennsylvania	20.5
17	Rhode Island	20.4
18	Montana	20.2
19	Nebraska	19.9
19	Washington	19.9
21	Nevada	19.6
21	New Hampshire	19.6
23	Vermont	18.9
24	North Carolina	18.6
25	Oklahoma	18.2
26	South Carolina	17.1
27	Delaware	16.4
28	Florida	16.3
29	Idaho	15.7
30	Illinois	15.6
31	Colorado	15.5
32	Minnesota	15.2
33	Alabama	15.1
34	Mississippi	14.9
34	Virginia	14.9
36	Kansas	13.8
37	Maryland	13.7
38	Georgia	13.4
39	Connecticut	12.9
40	Arizona	12.6
41	Louisiana	12.4
42	New Mexico	11.8
43	Hawaii	11.4
44	New Jersey	10.3
45	Utah	10.1
46	Texas	9.3
NA	California**	NA
NA	Iowa**	NA
NA	New York**	NA
NA	South Dakota**	NA
	District of Columbia	13.0

Source: U.S. Department of Health and Human Services, National Center for Health Statistics
(unpublished data, table 1-211)

*HHS defines "Smoker" as averaging at least one cigarette a day.

**Not available.

Percent of Births Not in a Hospital in 1992

National Percent = 1.06% of Live Births*

<table>
<tr><td colspan="3">ALPHA ORDER</td><td colspan="3">RANK ORDER</td></tr>
<tr><td>RANK</td><td>STATE</td><td>PERCENT</td><td>RANK</td><td>STATE</td><td>PERCENT</td></tr>
<tr><td>46</td><td>Alabama</td><td>0.37</td><td>1</td><td>Alaska</td><td>3.83</td></tr>
<tr><td>1</td><td>Alaska</td><td>3.83</td><td>2</td><td>Idaho</td><td>3.80</td></tr>
<tr><td>14</td><td>Arizona</td><td>1.35</td><td>3</td><td>Nevada</td><td>3.38</td></tr>
<tr><td>27</td><td>Arkansas</td><td>0.77</td><td>4</td><td>Montana</td><td>3.13</td></tr>
<tr><td>16</td><td>California</td><td>1.03</td><td>5</td><td>Utah</td><td>2.71</td></tr>
<tr><td>26</td><td>Colorado</td><td>0.80</td><td>6</td><td>Oregon</td><td>2.40</td></tr>
<tr><td>44</td><td>Connecticut</td><td>0.42</td><td>7</td><td>Vermont</td><td>2.33</td></tr>
<tr><td>9</td><td>Delaware</td><td>1.93</td><td>8</td><td>Texas</td><td>1.97</td></tr>
<tr><td>13</td><td>Florida</td><td>1.56</td><td>9</td><td>Delaware</td><td>1.93</td></tr>
<tr><td>37</td><td>Georgia</td><td>0.58</td><td>10</td><td>Washington</td><td>1.88</td></tr>
<tr><td>19</td><td>Hawaii</td><td>0.98</td><td>11</td><td>Pennsylvania</td><td>1.82</td></tr>
<tr><td>2</td><td>Idaho</td><td>3.80</td><td>12</td><td>New Mexico</td><td>1.62</td></tr>
<tr><td>31</td><td>Illinois</td><td>0.67</td><td>13</td><td>Florida</td><td>1.56</td></tr>
<tr><td>23</td><td>Indiana</td><td>0.85</td><td>14</td><td>Arizona</td><td>1.35</td></tr>
<tr><td>38</td><td>Iowa</td><td>0.56</td><td>15</td><td>New Hampshire</td><td>1.18</td></tr>
<tr><td>33</td><td>Kansas</td><td>0.63</td><td>16</td><td>California</td><td>1.03</td></tr>
<tr><td>40</td><td>Kentucky</td><td>0.48</td><td>16</td><td>Maine</td><td>1.03</td></tr>
<tr><td>41</td><td>Louisiana</td><td>0.45</td><td>18</td><td>Oklahoma</td><td>1.00</td></tr>
<tr><td>16</td><td>Maine</td><td>1.03</td><td>19</td><td>Hawaii</td><td>0.98</td></tr>
<tr><td>20</td><td>Maryland</td><td>0.97</td><td>20</td><td>Maryland</td><td>0.97</td></tr>
<tr><td>41</td><td>Massachusetts</td><td>0.45</td><td>21</td><td>Ohio</td><td>0.92</td></tr>
<tr><td>28</td><td>Michigan</td><td>0.72</td><td>22</td><td>Wisconsin</td><td>0.87</td></tr>
<tr><td>39</td><td>Minnesota</td><td>0.51</td><td>23</td><td>Indiana</td><td>0.85</td></tr>
<tr><td>47</td><td>Mississippi</td><td>0.32</td><td>23</td><td>Missouri</td><td>0.85</td></tr>
<tr><td>23</td><td>Missouri</td><td>0.85</td><td>25</td><td>New York</td><td>0.83</td></tr>
<tr><td>4</td><td>Montana</td><td>3.13</td><td>26</td><td>Colorado</td><td>0.80</td></tr>
<tr><td>48</td><td>Nebraska</td><td>0.31</td><td>27</td><td>Arkansas</td><td>0.77</td></tr>
<tr><td>3</td><td>Nevada</td><td>3.38</td><td>28</td><td>Michigan</td><td>0.72</td></tr>
<tr><td>15</td><td>New Hampshire</td><td>1.18</td><td>29</td><td>North Carolina</td><td>0.71</td></tr>
<tr><td>35</td><td>New Jersey</td><td>0.60</td><td>30</td><td>Tennessee</td><td>0.69</td></tr>
<tr><td>12</td><td>New Mexico</td><td>1.62</td><td>31</td><td>Illinois</td><td>0.67</td></tr>
<tr><td>25</td><td>New York</td><td>0.83</td><td>32</td><td>Virginia</td><td>0.64</td></tr>
<tr><td>29</td><td>North Carolina</td><td>0.71</td><td>33</td><td>Kansas</td><td>0.63</td></tr>
<tr><td>49</td><td>North Dakota</td><td>0.28</td><td>34</td><td>Wyoming</td><td>0.61</td></tr>
<tr><td>21</td><td>Ohio</td><td>0.92</td><td>35</td><td>New Jersey</td><td>0.60</td></tr>
<tr><td>18</td><td>Oklahoma</td><td>1.00</td><td>35</td><td>West Virginia</td><td>0.60</td></tr>
<tr><td>6</td><td>Oregon</td><td>2.40</td><td>37</td><td>Georgia</td><td>0.58</td></tr>
<tr><td>11</td><td>Pennsylvania</td><td>1.82</td><td>38</td><td>Iowa</td><td>0.56</td></tr>
<tr><td>50</td><td>Rhode Island</td><td>0.15</td><td>39</td><td>Minnesota</td><td>0.51</td></tr>
<tr><td>41</td><td>South Carolina</td><td>0.45</td><td>40</td><td>Kentucky</td><td>0.48</td></tr>
<tr><td>45</td><td>South Dakota</td><td>0.40</td><td>41</td><td>Louisiana</td><td>0.45</td></tr>
<tr><td>30</td><td>Tennessee</td><td>0.69</td><td>41</td><td>Massachusetts</td><td>0.45</td></tr>
<tr><td>8</td><td>Texas</td><td>1.97</td><td>41</td><td>South Carolina</td><td>0.45</td></tr>
<tr><td>5</td><td>Utah</td><td>2.71</td><td>44</td><td>Connecticut</td><td>0.42</td></tr>
<tr><td>7</td><td>Vermont</td><td>2.33</td><td>45</td><td>South Dakota</td><td>0.40</td></tr>
<tr><td>32</td><td>Virginia</td><td>0.64</td><td>46</td><td>Alabama</td><td>0.37</td></tr>
<tr><td>10</td><td>Washington</td><td>1.88</td><td>47</td><td>Mississippi</td><td>0.32</td></tr>
<tr><td>35</td><td>West Virginia</td><td>0.60</td><td>48</td><td>Nebraska</td><td>0.31</td></tr>
<tr><td>22</td><td>Wisconsin</td><td>0.87</td><td>49</td><td>North Dakota</td><td>0.28</td></tr>
<tr><td>34</td><td>Wyoming</td><td>0.61</td><td>50</td><td>Rhode Island</td><td>0.15</td></tr>
<tr><td></td><td></td><td></td><td></td><td>District of Columbia</td><td>1.61</td></tr>
</table>

Source: Morgan Quitno Press using data from US Dept of Health & Human Services, National Center for Health Statistics
(unpublished data, table 1-279)
*Includes free-standing birthing centers, clinics, doctor's offices, residences and other.

Percent of Births Attended by Midwives in 1992

National Percent = 4.90% of Live Births*

ALPHA ORDER

ALPHA ORDER

RANK	STATE	PERCENT
24	Alabama	4.24
2	Alaska	13.95
9	Arizona	7.92
43	Arkansas	0.96
13	California	6.91
20	Colorado	5.62
23	Connecticut	4.62
10	Delaware	7.87
5	Florida	11.45
7	Georgia	8.88
36	Hawaii	2.53
31	Idaho	2.89
45	Illinois	0.84
44	Indiana	0.87
47	Iowa	0.61
48	Kansas	0.41
29	Kentucky	3.11
46	Louisiana	0.64
12	Maine	6.94
11	Maryland	7.41
8	Massachusetts	8.85
32	Michigan	2.86
21	Minnesota	5.54
42	Mississippi	1.21
49	Missouri	0.36
14	Montana	6.85
50	Nebraska	0.11
19	Nevada	5.87
6	New Hampshire	10.24
33	New Jersey	2.72
1	New Mexico	15.65
17	New York	6.39
28	North Carolina	3.25
26	North Dakota	3.89
41	Ohio	1.38
37	Oklahoma	2.38
4	Oregon	11.55
25	Pennsylvania	3.98
17	Rhode Island	6.39
16	South Carolina	6.56
35	South Dakota	2.62
30	Tennessee	2.91
27	Texas	3.64
22	Utah	5.28
3	Vermont	11.87
38	Virginia	2.34
15	Washington	6.68
34	West Virginia	2.67
39	Wisconsin	2.11
40	Wyoming	1.43

RANK ORDER

RANK	STATE	PERCENT
1	New Mexico	15.65
2	Alaska	13.95
3	Vermont	11.87
4	Oregon	11.55
5	Florida	11.45
6	New Hampshire	10.24
7	Georgia	8.88
8	Massachusetts	8.85
9	Arizona	7.92
10	Delaware	7.87
11	Maryland	7.41
12	Maine	6.94
13	California	6.91
14	Montana	6.85
15	Washington	6.68
16	South Carolina	6.56
17	New York	6.39
17	Rhode Island	6.39
19	Nevada	5.87
20	Colorado	5.62
21	Minnesota	5.54
22	Utah	5.28
23	Connecticut	4.62
24	Alabama	4.24
25	Pennsylvania	3.98
26	North Dakota	3.89
27	Texas	3.64
28	North Carolina	3.25
29	Kentucky	3.11
30	Tennessee	2.91
31	Idaho	2.89
32	Michigan	2.86
33	New Jersey	2.72
34	West Virginia	2.67
35	South Dakota	2.62
36	Hawaii	2.53
37	Oklahoma	2.38
38	Virginia	2.34
39	Wisconsin	2.11
40	Wyoming	1.43
41	Ohio	1.38
42	Mississippi	1.21
43	Arkansas	0.96
44	Indiana	0.87
45	Illinois	0.84
46	Louisiana	0.64
47	Iowa	0.61
48	Kansas	0.41
49	Missouri	0.36
50	Nebraska	0.11

District of Columbia — 9.22

Source: Morgan Quitno Press using data from US Dept of Health & Human Services, National Center for Health Statistics (unpublished data, table 1-278)

*Includes certified nurse midwives and other midwives.

Reported Legal Abortions in 1990

National Total = 1,429,577 Reported Legal Abortions*

ALPHA ORDER					RANK ORDER			
RANK	STATE	ABORTIONS	% of USA		RANK	STATE	ABORTIONS	% of USA
22	Alabama	15,012	1.05%		1	California	357,579	25.01%
47	Alaska	1,489	0.10%		2	New York	159,098	11.13%
21	Arizona	15,783	1.10%		3	Texas	92,580	6.48%
36	Arkansas	5,953	0.42%		4	Illinois	67,350	4.71%
1	California	357,579	25.01%		5	Florida	66,071	4.62%
27	Colorado	12,679	0.89%		6	Pennsylvania	52,143	3.65%
17	Connecticut	18,776	1.31%		7	New Jersey	41,358	2.89%
37	Delaware	5,557	0.39%		8	Massachusetts	39,739	2.78%
5	Florida	66,071	4.62%		9	Georgia	39,245	2.75%
9	Georgia	39,245	2.75%		10	North Carolina	36,494	2.55%
40	Hawaii	4,748	0.33%		11	Michigan	36,183	2.53%
48	Idaho	1,390	0.10%		12	Virginia	32,992	2.31%
4	Illinois	67,350	4.71%		13	Ohio	32,165	2.25%
23	Indiana	14,351	1.00%		14	Washington	31,443	2.20%
33	Iowa	7,166	0.50%		15	Maryland	22,425	1.57%
31	Kansas	7,516	0.53%		16	Tennessee	21,144	1.48%
28	Kentucky	10,921	0.76%		17	Connecticut	18,776	1.31%
26	Louisiana	13,020	0.91%		18	Minnesota	17,156	1.20%
41	Maine	4,607	0.32%		19	Wisconsin	16,848	1.18%
15	Maryland	22,425	1.57%		20	Missouri	16,366	1.14%
8	Massachusetts	39,739	2.78%		21	Arizona	15,783	1.10%
11	Michigan	36,183	2.53%		22	Alabama	15,012	1.05%
18	Minnesota	17,156	1.20%		23	Indiana	14,351	1.00%
34	Mississippi	6,842	0.48%		24	Oregon	13,658	0.96%
20	Missouri	16,366	1.14%		25	South Carolina	13,285	0.93%
43	Montana	3,365	0.24%		26	Louisiana	13,020	0.91%
35	Nebraska	6,346	0.44%		27	Colorado	12,679	0.89%
32	Nevada	7,226	0.51%		28	Kentucky	10,921	0.76%
42	New Hampshire	4,259	0.30%		29	Oklahoma	10,708	0.75%
7	New Jersey	41,358	2.89%		30	Rhode Island	7,782	0.54%
38	New Mexico	5,288	0.37%		31	Kansas	7,516	0.53%
2	New York	159,098	11.13%		32	Nevada	7,226	0.51%
10	North Carolina	36,494	2.55%		33	Iowa	7,166	0.50%
46	North Dakota	1,723	0.12%		34	Mississippi	6,842	0.48%
13	Ohio	32,165	2.25%		35	Nebraska	6,346	0.44%
29	Oklahoma	10,708	0.75%		36	Arkansas	5,953	0.42%
24	Oregon	13,658	0.96%		37	Delaware	5,557	0.39%
6	Pennsylvania	52,143	3.65%		38	New Mexico	5,288	0.37%
30	Rhode Island	7,782	0.54%		39	Utah	4,786	0.33%
25	South Carolina	13,285	0.93%		40	Hawaii	4,748	0.33%
49	South Dakota	946	0.07%		41	Maine	4,607	0.32%
16	Tennessee	21,144	1.48%		42	New Hampshire	4,259	0.30%
3	Texas	92,580	6.48%		43	Montana	3,365	0.24%
39	Utah	4,786	0.33%		44	Vermont	3,184	0.22%
44	Vermont	3,184	0.22%		45	West Virginia	2,500	0.17%
12	Virginia	32,992	2.31%		46	North Dakota	1,723	0.12%
14	Washington	31,443	2.20%		47	Alaska	1,489	0.10%
45	West Virginia	2,500	0.17%		48	Idaho	1,390	0.10%
19	Wisconsin	16,848	1.18%		49	South Dakota	946	0.07%
50	Wyoming	363	0.03%		50	Wyoming	363	0.03%
						District of Columbia	19,969	1.40%

Source: U.S. Department of Health and Human Services, Centers for Disease Control and Prevention
"Abortion Surveillance-United States, 1990" (Morbidity and Mortality Weekly Report, Vol. 42, No. SS-6, 12/17/93)
*By state of occurrence.

Reported Legal Abortions per 1,000 Live Births in 1990

National Rate = 345 Reported Legal Abortions per 1,000 Live Births*

ALPHA ORDER				RANK ORDER		
RANK	**STATE**	**RATE**		**RANK**	**STATE**	**RATE**
26	Alabama	237		1	California	585
46	Alaska	125		2	New York	545
31	Arizona	229		3	Rhode Island	512
43	Arkansas	163		4	Delaware	500
1	California	585		5	Massachusetts	430
26	Colorado	237		6	Washington	397
8	Connecticut	375		7	Vermont	384
4	Delaware	500		8	Connecticut	375
14	Florida	332		9	Georgia	349
9	Georgia	349		9	North Carolina	349
29	Hawaii	232		11	Illinois	345
49	Idaho	85		12	New Jersey	337
11	Illinois	345		13	Virginia	334
42	Indiana	167		14	Florida	332
40	Iowa	182		15	Nevada	331
37	Kansas	193		16	Oregon	319
35	Kentucky	202		17	Pennsylvania	305
41	Louisiana	181		18	Texas	293
22	Maine	266		19	Montana	290
21	Maryland	279		20	Tennessee	282
5	Massachusetts	430		21	Maryland	279
28	Michigan	236		22	Maine	266
24	Minnesota	252		23	Nebraska	260
44	Mississippi	157		24	Minnesota	252
34	Missouri	207		25	New Hampshire	243
19	Montana	290		26	Alabama	237
23	Nebraska	260		26	Colorado	237
15	Nevada	331		28	Michigan	236
25	New Hampshire	243		29	Hawaii	232
12	New Jersey	337		29	Wisconsin	232
36	New Mexico	194		31	Arizona	229
2	New York	545		32	South Carolina	227
9	North Carolina	349		33	Oklahoma	225
39	North Dakota	186		34	Missouri	207
37	Ohio	193		35	Kentucky	202
33	Oklahoma	225		36	New Mexico	194
16	Oregon	319		37	Kansas	193
17	Pennsylvania	305		37	Ohio	193
3	Rhode Island	512		39	North Dakota	186
32	South Carolina	227		40	Iowa	182
48	South Dakota	86		41	Louisiana	181
20	Tennessee	282		42	Indiana	167
18	Texas	293		43	Arkansas	163
45	Utah	132		44	Mississippi	157
7	Vermont	384		45	Utah	132
13	Virginia	334		46	Alaska	125
6	Washington	397		47	West Virginia	111
47	West Virginia	111		48	South Dakota	86
29	Wisconsin	232		49	Idaho	85
50	Wyoming	52		50	Wyoming	52
				District of Columbia**		NA

Source: U.S. Department of Health and Human Services, Centers for Disease Control and Prevention

   "Abortion Surveillance–United States, 1990" (Morbidity and Mortality Weekly Report, Vol. 42, No. SS-6, 12/17/93)

*By state of occurrence.

**The District of Columbia's ratio was not listed but was noted as being greater than 1,000 abortions per 1,000 live births.

Reported Legal Abortions per 1,000 Women Ages 15 to 44 in 1990

National Rate = 24 Reported Legal Abortions per 1,000 Women Ages 15 to 44*

ALPHA ORDER

RANK	STATE	RATE
26	Alabama	16
43	Alaska	11
18	Arizona	19
43	Arkansas	11
1	California	50
26	Colorado	16
9	Connecticut	24
3	Delaware	34
9	Florida	24
9	Georgia	24
22	Hawaii	18
47	Idaho	6
8	Illinois	25
43	Indiana	11
40	Iowa	12
35	Kansas	14
37	Kentucky	13
37	Louisiana	13
26	Maine	16
18	Maryland	19
5	Massachusetts	27
26	Michigan	16
25	Minnesota	17
43	Mississippi	11
35	Missouri	14
18	Montana	19
22	Nebraska	18
7	Nevada	26
26	New Hampshire	16
12	New Jersey	23
32	New Mexico	15
2	New York	37
12	North Carolina	23
40	North Dakota	12
37	Ohio	13
32	Oklahoma	15
16	Oregon	21
18	Pennsylvania	19
4	Rhode Island	33
26	South Carolina	16
47	South Dakota	6
22	Tennessee	18
12	Texas	23
40	Utah	12
12	Vermont	23
16	Virginia	21
5	Washington	27
47	West Virginia	6
32	Wisconsin	15
50	Wyoming	4

RANK ORDER

RANK	STATE	RATE
1	California	50
2	New York	37
3	Delaware	34
4	Rhode Island	33
5	Massachusetts	27
5	Washington	27
7	Nevada	26
8	Illinois	25
9	Connecticut	24
9	Florida	24
9	Georgia	24
12	New Jersey	23
12	North Carolina	23
12	Texas	23
12	Vermont	23
16	Oregon	21
16	Virginia	21
18	Arizona	19
18	Maryland	19
18	Montana	19
18	Pennsylvania	19
22	Hawaii	18
22	Nebraska	18
22	Tennessee	18
25	Minnesota	17
26	Alabama	16
26	Colorado	16
26	Maine	16
26	Michigan	16
26	New Hampshire	16
26	South Carolina	16
32	New Mexico	15
32	Oklahoma	15
32	Wisconsin	15
35	Kansas	14
35	Missouri	14
37	Kentucky	13
37	Louisiana	13
37	Ohio	13
40	Iowa	12
40	North Dakota	12
40	Utah	12
43	Alaska	11
43	Arkansas	11
43	Indiana	11
43	Mississippi	11
47	Idaho	6
47	South Dakota	6
47	West Virginia	6
50	Wyoming	4

District of Columbia**   NA

Source: U.S. Department of Health and Human Services, Centers for Disease Control and Prevention
"Abortion Surveillance-United States, 1990" (Morbidity and Mortality Weekly Report, Vol. 42, No. SS-6, 12/17/93)
*By state of occurrence.
**The District of Columbia's ratio was not listed but was noted as being greater than 1,000 abortions per 1,000 women ages 15 to 44..

Percent of Reported Legal Abortions Obtained by Out-Of-State Residents in 1990

Reporting States Percent = 8.2% of Reported Legal Abortions*

<table>
<tr><td colspan="3">ALPHA ORDER</td><td colspan="3">RANK ORDER</td></tr>
<tr><td>RANK</td><td>STATE</td><td>PERCENT</td><td>RANK</td><td>STATE</td><td>PERCENT</td></tr>
<tr><td>NA</td><td>Alabama**</td><td>NA</td><td>1</td><td>Kansas</td><td>46.5</td></tr>
<tr><td>NA</td><td>Alaska**</td><td>NA</td><td>2</td><td>North Dakota</td><td>38.2</td></tr>
<tr><td>38</td><td>Arizona</td><td>2.5</td><td>3</td><td>Vermont</td><td>29.8</td></tr>
<tr><td>36</td><td>Arkansas</td><td>3.2</td><td>4</td><td>Kentucky</td><td>29.3</td></tr>
<tr><td>NA</td><td>California**</td><td>NA</td><td>5</td><td>Montana</td><td>23.6</td></tr>
<tr><td>23</td><td>Colorado</td><td>8.2</td><td>6</td><td>Mississippi</td><td>22.7</td></tr>
<tr><td>NA</td><td>Connecticut**</td><td>NA</td><td>7</td><td>Rhode Island</td><td>21.7</td></tr>
<tr><td>NA</td><td>Delaware**</td><td>NA</td><td>8</td><td>Nebraska</td><td>20.2</td></tr>
<tr><td>NA</td><td>Florida**</td><td>NA</td><td>9</td><td>South Dakota</td><td>19.4</td></tr>
<tr><td>21</td><td>Georgia</td><td>8.3</td><td>10</td><td>Tennessee</td><td>17.4</td></tr>
<tr><td>39</td><td>Hawaii</td><td>0.8</td><td>11</td><td>Utah</td><td>15.2</td></tr>
<tr><td>20</td><td>Idaho</td><td>9.0</td><td>12</td><td>Maine</td><td>12.6</td></tr>
<tr><td>NA</td><td>Illinois**</td><td>NA</td><td>13</td><td>Wyoming</td><td>12.4</td></tr>
<tr><td>34</td><td>Indiana</td><td>3.6</td><td>14</td><td>West Virginia</td><td>11.7</td></tr>
<tr><td>NA</td><td>Iowa**</td><td>NA</td><td>15</td><td>Nevada</td><td>11.2</td></tr>
<tr><td>1</td><td>Kansas</td><td>46.5</td><td>16</td><td>Missouri</td><td>10.8</td></tr>
<tr><td>4</td><td>Kentucky</td><td>29.3</td><td>17</td><td>Minnesota</td><td>10.7</td></tr>
<tr><td>NA</td><td>Louisiana**</td><td>NA</td><td>18</td><td>Ohio</td><td>9.7</td></tr>
<tr><td>12</td><td>Maine</td><td>12.6</td><td>19</td><td>Oregon</td><td>9.6</td></tr>
<tr><td>24</td><td>Maryland</td><td>6.8</td><td>20</td><td>Idaho</td><td>9.0</td></tr>
<tr><td>31</td><td>Massachusetts</td><td>3.9</td><td>21</td><td>Georgia</td><td>8.3</td></tr>
<tr><td>30</td><td>Michigan</td><td>4.2</td><td>21</td><td>North Carolina</td><td>8.3</td></tr>
<tr><td>17</td><td>Minnesota</td><td>10.7</td><td>23</td><td>Colorado</td><td>8.2</td></tr>
<tr><td>6</td><td>Mississippi</td><td>22.7</td><td>24</td><td>Maryland</td><td>6.8</td></tr>
<tr><td>16</td><td>Missouri</td><td>10.8</td><td>25</td><td>South Carolina</td><td>6.1</td></tr>
<tr><td>5</td><td>Montana</td><td>23.6</td><td>25</td><td>Wisconsin</td><td>6.1</td></tr>
<tr><td>8</td><td>Nebraska</td><td>20.2</td><td>27</td><td>Virginia</td><td>6.0</td></tr>
<tr><td>15</td><td>Nevada</td><td>11.2</td><td>28</td><td>Pennsylvania</td><td>5.9</td></tr>
<tr><td>NA</td><td>New Hampshire**</td><td>NA</td><td>29</td><td>Washington</td><td>4.9</td></tr>
<tr><td>37</td><td>New Jersey</td><td>3.0</td><td>30</td><td>Michigan</td><td>4.2</td></tr>
<tr><td>31</td><td>New Mexico</td><td>3.9</td><td>31</td><td>Massachusetts</td><td>3.9</td></tr>
<tr><td>35</td><td>New York</td><td>3.4</td><td>31</td><td>New Mexico</td><td>3.9</td></tr>
<tr><td>21</td><td>North Carolina</td><td>8.3</td><td>31</td><td>Texas</td><td>3.9</td></tr>
<tr><td>2</td><td>North Dakota</td><td>38.2</td><td>34</td><td>Indiana</td><td>3.6</td></tr>
<tr><td>18</td><td>Ohio</td><td>9.7</td><td>35</td><td>New York</td><td>3.4</td></tr>
<tr><td>NA</td><td>Oklahoma**</td><td>NA</td><td>36</td><td>Arkansas</td><td>3.2</td></tr>
<tr><td>19</td><td>Oregon</td><td>9.6</td><td>37</td><td>New Jersey</td><td>3.0</td></tr>
<tr><td>28</td><td>Pennsylvania</td><td>5.9</td><td>38</td><td>Arizona</td><td>2.5</td></tr>
<tr><td>7</td><td>Rhode Island</td><td>21.7</td><td>39</td><td>Hawaii</td><td>0.8</td></tr>
<tr><td>25</td><td>South Carolina</td><td>6.1</td><td>NA</td><td>Alabama**</td><td>NA</td></tr>
<tr><td>9</td><td>South Dakota</td><td>19.4</td><td>NA</td><td>Alaska**</td><td>NA</td></tr>
<tr><td>10</td><td>Tennessee</td><td>17.4</td><td>NA</td><td>California**</td><td>NA</td></tr>
<tr><td>31</td><td>Texas</td><td>3.9</td><td>NA</td><td>Connecticut**</td><td>NA</td></tr>
<tr><td>11</td><td>Utah</td><td>15.2</td><td>NA</td><td>Delaware**</td><td>NA</td></tr>
<tr><td>3</td><td>Vermont</td><td>29.8</td><td>NA</td><td>Florida**</td><td>NA</td></tr>
<tr><td>27</td><td>Virginia</td><td>6.0</td><td>NA</td><td>Illinois**</td><td>NA</td></tr>
<tr><td>29</td><td>Washington</td><td>4.9</td><td>NA</td><td>Iowa**</td><td>NA</td></tr>
<tr><td>14</td><td>West Virginia</td><td>11.7</td><td>NA</td><td>Louisiana**</td><td>NA</td></tr>
<tr><td>25</td><td>Wisconsin</td><td>6.1</td><td>NA</td><td>New Hampshire**</td><td>NA</td></tr>
<tr><td>13</td><td>Wyoming</td><td>12.4</td><td>NA</td><td>Oklahoma**</td><td>NA</td></tr>
<tr><td></td><td></td><td></td><td></td><td>District of Columbia</td><td>52.9</td></tr>
</table>

Source: U.S. Department of Health and Human Services, Centers for Disease Control and Prevention
"Abortion Surveillance-United States, 1990" (Morbidity and Mortality Weekly Report, Vol. 42, No. SS-6, 12/17/93)
*By state of occurrence.
**Not reported.

Percent of Legal Abortions Obtained by White Women in 1990

Reporting States Percent = 63.5% of Reported Legal Abortions*

ALPHA ORDER			RANK ORDER		
RANK	STATE	PERCENT	RANK	STATE	PERCENT
NA	Alabama**	NA	1	Vermont	98.3
NA	Alaska**	NA	2	Maine	96.2
14	Arizona	80.8	3	Idaho	96.0
19	Arkansas	70.0	4	North Dakota	91.8
NA	California**	NA	5	Utah	91.6
NA	Colorado**	NA	6	South Dakota	91.4
NA	Connecticut**	NA	7	Nevada	90.0
NA	Delaware**	NA	8	New Mexico	89.4
NA	Florida**	NA	9	Oregon	87.8
28	Georgia	52.4	10	West Virginia	87.2
NA	Hawaii**	NA	11	Minnesota	86.5
3	Idaho	96.0	12	Kansas	82.8
NA	Illinois**	NA	13	Rhode Island	82.6
18	Indiana	73.9	14	Arizona	80.8
NA	Iowa**	NA	15	Kentucky	80.2
12	Kansas	82.8	16	Wisconsin	78.4
15	Kentucky	80.2	17	Texas	76.4
25	Louisiana	55.8	18	Indiana	73.9
2	Maine	96.2	19	Arkansas	70.0
30	Maryland	47.9	20	Tennessee	65.2
NA	Massachusetts**	NA	21	Missouri	63.2
NA	Michigan**	NA	22	Virginia	61.9
11	Minnesota	86.5	23	North Carolina	57.5
29	Mississippi	48.7	24	South Carolina	56.5
21	Missouri	63.2	25	Louisiana	55.8
NA	Montana**	NA	26	New Jersey	55.3
NA	Nebraska**	NA	27	New York	53.9
7	Nevada	90.0	28	Georgia	52.4
NA	New Hampshire**	NA	29	Mississippi	48.7
26	New Jersey	55.3	30	Maryland	47.9
8	New Mexico	89.4	NA	Alabama**	NA
27	New York	53.9	NA	Alaska**	NA
23	North Carolina	57.5	NA	California**	NA
4	North Dakota	91.8	NA	Colorado**	NA
NA	Ohio**	NA	NA	Connecticut**	NA
NA	Oklahoma**	NA	NA	Delaware**	NA
9	Oregon	87.8	NA	Florida**	NA
NA	Pennsylvania**	NA	NA	Hawaii**	NA
13	Rhode Island	82.6	NA	Illinois**	NA
24	South Carolina	56.5	NA	Iowa**	NA
6	South Dakota	91.4	NA	Massachusetts**	NA
20	Tennessee	65.2	NA	Michigan**	NA
17	Texas	76.4	NA	Montana**	NA
5	Utah	91.6	NA	Nebraska**	NA
1	Vermont	98.3	NA	New Hampshire**	NA
22	Virginia	61.9	NA	Ohio**	NA
NA	Washington**	NA	NA	Oklahoma**	NA
10	West Virginia	87.2	NA	Pennsylvania**	NA
16	Wisconsin	78.4	NA	Washington**	NA
NA	Wyoming**	NA	NA	Wyoming**	NA
				District of Columbia	22.8

Source: U.S. Department of Health and Human Services, Centers for Disease Control and Prevention
"Abortion Surveillance–United States, 1990" (Morbidity and Mortality Weekly Report, Vol. 42, No. SS-6, 12/17/93)
*By state of occurrence. Includes those of Hispanic ethnicity. National percent is for reporting states only.
**Not reported.

Percent of Reported Legal Abortions Obtained by Black Women in 1990

Reporting States Percent = 31.2% of Reported Legal Abortions*

ALPHA ORDER

RANK	STATE	PERCENT
NA	Alabama**	NA
NA	Alaska**	NA
22	Arizona	4.9
12	Arkansas	28.0
NA	California**	NA
NA	Colorado**	NA
NA	Connecticut**	NA
NA	Delaware**	NA
NA	Florida**	NA
3	Georgia	43.9
NA	Hawaii**	NA
29	Idaho	0.4
NA	Illinois**	NA
13	Indiana	21.9
NA	Iowa**	NA
17	Kansas	14.2
16	Kentucky	16.7
4	Louisiana	42.5
28	Maine	1.2
2	Maryland	46.6
NA	Massachusetts**	NA
NA	Michigan**	NA
21	Minnesota	6.5
1	Mississippi	50.3
9	Missouri	34.7
NA	Montana**	NA
NA	Nebraska**	NA
20	Nevada	7.4
NA	New Hampshire**	NA
6	New Jersey	40.4
24	New Mexico	2.3
7	New York	39.3
8	North Carolina	36.5
26	North Dakota	1.3
NA	Ohio**	NA
NA	Oklahoma**	NA
23	Oregon	4.2
NA	Pennsylvania**	NA
19	Rhode Island	11.7
5	South Carolina	42.1
26	South Dakota	1.3
11	Tennessee	32.5
14	Texas	19.9
25	Utah	2.1
29	Vermont	0.4
10	Virginia	34.6
NA	Washington**	NA
18	West Virginia	12.0
15	Wisconsin	18.9
NA	Wyoming**	NA

RANK ORDER

RANK	STATE	PERCENT
1	Mississippi	50.3
2	Maryland	46.6
3	Georgia	43.9
4	Louisiana	42.5
5	South Carolina	42.1
6	New Jersey	40.4
7	New York	39.3
8	North Carolina	36.5
9	Missouri	34.7
10	Virginia	34.6
11	Tennessee	32.5
12	Arkansas	28.0
13	Indiana	21.9
14	Texas	19.9
15	Wisconsin	18.9
16	Kentucky	16.7
17	Kansas	14.2
18	West Virginia	12.0
19	Rhode Island	11.7
20	Nevada	7.4
21	Minnesota	6.5
22	Arizona	4.9
23	Oregon	4.2
24	New Mexico	2.3
25	Utah	2.1
26	North Dakota	1.3
26	South Dakota	1.3
28	Maine	1.2
29	Idaho	0.4
29	Vermont	0.4
NA	Alabama**	NA
NA	Alaska**	NA
NA	California**	NA
NA	Colorado**	NA
NA	Connecticut**	NA
NA	Delaware**	NA
NA	Florida**	NA
NA	Hawaii**	NA
NA	Illinois**	NA
NA	Iowa**	NA
NA	Massachusetts**	NA
NA	Michigan**	NA
NA	Montana**	NA
NA	Nebraska**	NA
NA	New Hampshire**	NA
NA	Ohio**	NA
NA	Oklahoma**	NA
NA	Pennsylvania**	NA
NA	Washington**	NA
NA	Wyoming**	NA

District of Columbia	61.3

Source: U.S. Department of Health and Human Services, Centers for Disease Control and Prevention
"Abortion Surveillance-United States, 1990" (Morbidity and Mortality Weekly Report, Vol. 42, No. SS-6, 12/17/93)
*By state of occurrence. National percent is for reporting states only.
**Not reported.

Percent of Reported Legal Abortions Obtained by Married Women in 1990

Reporting States Percent = 21.2% of Reported Legal Abortions*

<table>
<tr><td colspan="3">ALPHA ORDER</td><td colspan="3">RANK ORDER</td></tr>
<tr><td>RANK</td><td>STATE</td><td>PERCENT</td><td>RANK</td><td>STATE</td><td>PERCENT</td></tr>
<tr><td>NA</td><td>Alabama**</td><td>NA</td><td>1</td><td>Utah</td><td>37.8</td></tr>
<tr><td>NA</td><td>Alaska**</td><td>NA</td><td>2</td><td>Nevada</td><td>25.9</td></tr>
<tr><td>NA</td><td>Arizona**</td><td>NA</td><td>3</td><td>Hawaii</td><td>25.2</td></tr>
<tr><td>19</td><td>Arkansas</td><td>20.6</td><td>4</td><td>Wyoming</td><td>25.1</td></tr>
<tr><td>NA</td><td>California**</td><td>NA</td><td>5</td><td>Oregon</td><td>24.4</td></tr>
<tr><td>24</td><td>Colorado</td><td>19.7</td><td>6</td><td>Texas</td><td>24.1</td></tr>
<tr><td>NA</td><td>Connecticut**</td><td>NA</td><td>7</td><td>Idaho</td><td>23.7</td></tr>
<tr><td>NA</td><td>Delaware**</td><td>NA</td><td>8</td><td>North Carolina</td><td>23.4</td></tr>
<tr><td>NA</td><td>Florida**</td><td>NA</td><td>9</td><td>Rhode Island</td><td>23.1</td></tr>
<tr><td>20</td><td>Georgia</td><td>20.5</td><td>10</td><td>New York</td><td>22.0</td></tr>
<tr><td>3</td><td>Hawaii</td><td>25.2</td><td>11</td><td>Vermont</td><td>21.9</td></tr>
<tr><td>7</td><td>Idaho</td><td>23.7</td><td>12</td><td>Missouri</td><td>21.6</td></tr>
<tr><td>NA</td><td>Illinois**</td><td>NA</td><td>13</td><td>Massachusetts</td><td>21.4</td></tr>
<tr><td>26</td><td>Indiana</td><td>19.5</td><td>14</td><td>Maryland</td><td>21.2</td></tr>
<tr><td>NA</td><td>Iowa**</td><td>NA</td><td>14</td><td>South Carolina</td><td>21.2</td></tr>
<tr><td>28</td><td>Kansas</td><td>19.1</td><td>14</td><td>West Virginia</td><td>21.2</td></tr>
<tr><td>32</td><td>Kentucky</td><td>17.8</td><td>17</td><td>New Jersey</td><td>21.0</td></tr>
<tr><td>NA</td><td>Louisiana**</td><td>NA</td><td>18</td><td>Tennessee</td><td>20.8</td></tr>
<tr><td>21</td><td>Maine</td><td>20.4</td><td>19</td><td>Arkansas</td><td>20.6</td></tr>
<tr><td>14</td><td>Maryland</td><td>21.2</td><td>20</td><td>Georgia</td><td>20.5</td></tr>
<tr><td>13</td><td>Massachusetts</td><td>21.4</td><td>21</td><td>Maine</td><td>20.4</td></tr>
<tr><td>32</td><td>Michigan</td><td>17.8</td><td>22</td><td>South Dakota</td><td>20.1</td></tr>
<tr><td>29</td><td>Minnesota</td><td>18.8</td><td>23</td><td>New Mexico</td><td>20.0</td></tr>
<tr><td>27</td><td>Mississippi</td><td>19.3</td><td>24</td><td>Colorado</td><td>19.7</td></tr>
<tr><td>12</td><td>Missouri</td><td>21.6</td><td>24</td><td>North Dakota</td><td>19.7</td></tr>
<tr><td>29</td><td>Montana</td><td>18.8</td><td>26</td><td>Indiana</td><td>19.5</td></tr>
<tr><td>NA</td><td>Nebraska**</td><td>NA</td><td>27</td><td>Mississippi</td><td>19.3</td></tr>
<tr><td>2</td><td>Nevada</td><td>25.9</td><td>28</td><td>Kansas</td><td>19.1</td></tr>
<tr><td>NA</td><td>New Hampshire**</td><td>NA</td><td>29</td><td>Minnesota</td><td>18.8</td></tr>
<tr><td>17</td><td>New Jersey</td><td>21.0</td><td>29</td><td>Montana</td><td>18.8</td></tr>
<tr><td>23</td><td>New Mexico</td><td>20.0</td><td>31</td><td>Virginia</td><td>18.5</td></tr>
<tr><td>10</td><td>New York</td><td>22.0</td><td>32</td><td>Kentucky</td><td>17.8</td></tr>
<tr><td>8</td><td>North Carolina</td><td>23.4</td><td>32</td><td>Michigan</td><td>17.8</td></tr>
<tr><td>24</td><td>North Dakota</td><td>19.7</td><td>34</td><td>Ohio</td><td>17.1</td></tr>
<tr><td>34</td><td>Ohio</td><td>17.1</td><td>35</td><td>Wisconsin</td><td>15.0</td></tr>
<tr><td>NA</td><td>Oklahoma**</td><td>NA</td><td>NA</td><td>Alabama**</td><td>NA</td></tr>
<tr><td>5</td><td>Oregon</td><td>24.4</td><td>NA</td><td>Alaska**</td><td>NA</td></tr>
<tr><td>NA</td><td>Pennsylvania**</td><td>NA</td><td>NA</td><td>Arizona**</td><td>NA</td></tr>
<tr><td>9</td><td>Rhode Island</td><td>23.1</td><td>NA</td><td>California**</td><td>NA</td></tr>
<tr><td>14</td><td>South Carolina</td><td>21.2</td><td>NA</td><td>Connecticut**</td><td>NA</td></tr>
<tr><td>22</td><td>South Dakota</td><td>20.1</td><td>NA</td><td>Delaware**</td><td>NA</td></tr>
<tr><td>18</td><td>Tennessee</td><td>20.8</td><td>NA</td><td>Florida**</td><td>NA</td></tr>
<tr><td>6</td><td>Texas</td><td>24.1</td><td>NA</td><td>Illinois**</td><td>NA</td></tr>
<tr><td>1</td><td>Utah</td><td>37.8</td><td>NA</td><td>Iowa**</td><td>NA</td></tr>
<tr><td>11</td><td>Vermont</td><td>21.9</td><td>NA</td><td>Louisiana**</td><td>NA</td></tr>
<tr><td>31</td><td>Virginia</td><td>18.5</td><td>NA</td><td>Nebraska**</td><td>NA</td></tr>
<tr><td>NA</td><td>Washington**</td><td>NA</td><td>NA</td><td>New Hampshire**</td><td>NA</td></tr>
<tr><td>14</td><td>West Virginia</td><td>21.2</td><td>NA</td><td>Oklahoma**</td><td>NA</td></tr>
<tr><td>35</td><td>Wisconsin</td><td>15.0</td><td>NA</td><td>Pennsylvania**</td><td>NA</td></tr>
<tr><td>4</td><td>Wyoming</td><td>25.1</td><td>NA</td><td>Washington**</td><td>NA</td></tr>
<tr><td></td><td></td><td></td><td></td><td>District of Columbia**</td><td>NA</td></tr>
</table>

Source: U.S. Department of Health and Human Services, Centers for Disease Control and Prevention
 "Abortion Surveillance-United States, 1990" (Morbidity and Mortality Weekly Report, Vol. 42, No. SS-6, 12/17/93)
*By state of occurrence. National percent is for reporting states only.
**Not reported.

Percent of Reported Legal Abortions Obtained by Unmarried Women in 1990

Reporting States Percent = 76.2% of Reported Legal Abortions*

ALPHA ORDER			RANK ORDER		
RANK	STATE	PERCENT	RANK	STATE	PERCENT
NA	Alabama**	NA	1	Wisconsin	84.5
NA	Alaska**	NA	2	Michigan	81.3
NA	Arizona**	NA	3	Kansas	80.9
19	Arkansas	76.3	4	Kentucky	80.3
NA	California**	NA	5	Mississippi	80.2
11	Colorado	78.6	5	North Dakota	80.2
NA	Connecticut**	NA	7	South Dakota	79.9
NA	Delaware**	NA	8	New Jersey	78.7
NA	Florida**	NA	8	New Mexico	78.7
11	Georgia	78.6	8	West Virginia	78.7
29	Hawaii	73.7	11	Colorado	78.6
20	Idaho	76.0	11	Georgia	78.6
NA	Illinois**	NA	11	Tennessee	78.6
16	Indiana	78.2	14	South Carolina	78.5
NA	Iowa**	NA	15	Virginia	78.4
3	Kansas	80.9	16	Indiana	78.2
4	Kentucky	80.3	17	Minnesota	77.1
NA	Louisiana**	NA	18	Missouri	77.0
24	Maine	74.9	19	Arkansas	76.3
27	Maryland	74.5	20	Idaho	76.0
34	Massachusetts	67.9	20	Rhode Island	76.0
2	Michigan	81.3	22	New York	75.4
17	Minnesota	77.1	23	Texas	75.0
5	Mississippi	80.2	24	Maine	74.9
18	Missouri	77.0	24	Wyoming	74.9
31	Montana	73.6	26	Ohio	74.8
NA	Nebraska**	NA	27	Maryland	74.5
32	Nevada	72.7	28	Oregon	74.2
NA	New Hampshire**	NA	29	Hawaii	73.7
8	New Jersey	78.7	29	North Carolina	73.7
8	New Mexico	78.7	31	Montana	73.6
22	New York	75.4	32	Nevada	72.7
29	North Carolina	73.7	33	Vermont	70.7
5	North Dakota	80.2	34	Massachusetts	67.9
26	Ohio	74.8	35	Utah	62.2
NA	Oklahoma**	NA	NA	Alabama**	NA
28	Oregon	74.2	NA	Alaska**	NA
NA	Pennsylvania**	NA	NA	Arizona**	NA
20	Rhode Island	76.0	NA	California**	NA
14	South Carolina	78.5	NA	Connecticut**	NA
7	South Dakota	79.9	NA	Delaware**	NA
11	Tennessee	78.6	NA	Florida**	NA
23	Texas	75.0	NA	Illinois**	NA
35	Utah	62.2	NA	Iowa**	NA
33	Vermont	70.7	NA	Louisiana**	NA
15	Virginia	78.4	NA	Nebraska**	NA
NA	Washington**	NA	NA	New Hampshire**	NA
8	West Virginia	78.7	NA	Oklahoma**	NA
1	Wisconsin	84.5	NA	Pennsylvania**	NA
24	Wyoming	74.9	NA	Washington**	NA
				District of Columbia**	NA

Source: U.S. Department of Health and Human Services, Centers for Disease Control and Prevention
   "Abortion Surveillance–United States, 1990" (Morbidity and Mortality Weekly Report, Vol. 42, No. SS-6, 12/17/93)
By state of occurrence. National percent is for reporting states only.
**Not reported.*

Reported Legal Abortions Obtained by Teenagers in 1990

Reporting States Total = 185,867 Legal Abortions Obtained by Teenagers*

ALPHA ORDER				RANK ORDER			
RANK	STATE	ABORTIONS	% of USA	RANK	STATE	ABORTIONS	% of USA
NA	Alabama**	NA	NA	1	New York	30,831	16.59%
NA	Alaska**	NA	NA	2	Texas	18,015	9.69%
20	Arizona	3,231	1.74%	3	Pennsylvania	12,536	6.74%
26	Arkansas	1,653	0.89%	4	North Carolina	9,725	5.23%
NA	California**	NA	NA	5	Michigan	9,296	5.00%
22	Colorado	3,075	1.65%	6	Georgia	8,998	4.84%
NA	Connecticut**	NA	NA	7	New Jersey	8,948	4.81%
NA	Delaware**	NA	NA	8	Massachusetts	7,617	4.10%
NA	Florida**	NA	NA	9	Virginia	7,430	4.00%
6	Georgia	8,998	4.84%	10	Washington	6,849	3.68%
32	Hawaii	979	0.53%	11	Ohio	6,148	3.31%
37	Idaho	334	0.18%	12	Tennessee	5,499	2.96%
NA	Illinois**	NA	NA	13	Maryland	5,022	2.70%
17	Indiana	3,413	1.84%	14	Minnesota	3,830	2.06%
NA	Iowa**	NA	NA	15	Missouri	3,680	1.98%
23	Kansas	2,164	1.16%	16	Kentucky	3,415	1.84%
16	Kentucky	3,415	1.84%	17	Indiana	3,413	1.84%
21	Louisiana	3,084	1.66%	18	South Carolina	3,342	1.80%
31	Maine	1,114	0.60%	19	Oregon	3,267	1.76%
13	Maryland	5,022	2.70%	20	Arizona	3,231	1.74%
8	Massachusetts	7,617	4.10%	21	Louisiana	3,084	1.66%
5	Michigan	9,296	5.00%	22	Colorado	3,075	1.65%
14	Minnesota	3,830	2.06%	23	Kansas	2,164	1.16%
24	Mississippi	1,966	1.06%	24	Mississippi	1,966	1.06%
15	Missouri	3,680	1.98%	25	Nebraska	1,813	0.98%
33	Montana	935	0.50%	26	Arkansas	1,653	0.89%
25	Nebraska	1,813	0.98%	27	Rhode Island	1,610	0.87%
29	Nevada	1,264	0.68%	28	New Mexico	1,289	0.69%
NA	New Hampshire**	NA	NA	29	Nevada	1,264	0.68%
7	New Jersey	8,948	4.81%	30	Utah	1,142	0.61%
28	New Mexico	1,289	0.69%	31	Maine	1,114	0.60%
1	New York	30,831	16.59%	32	Hawaii	979	0.53%
4	North Carolina	9,725	5.23%	33	Montana	935	0.50%
36	North Dakota	475	0.26%	34	Vermont	799	0.43%
11	Ohio	6,148	3.31%	35	West Virginia	717	0.39%
NA	Oklahoma**	NA	NA	36	North Dakota	475	0.26%
19	Oregon	3,267	1.76%	37	Idaho	334	0.18%
3	Pennsylvania	12,536	6.74%	38	South Dakota	260	0.14%
27	Rhode Island	1,610	0.87%	39	Wyoming	102	0.05%
18	South Carolina	3,342	1.80%	NA	Alabama**	NA	NA
38	South Dakota	260	0.14%	NA	Alaska**	NA	NA
12	Tennessee	5,499	2.96%	NA	California**	NA	NA
2	Texas	18,015	9.69%	NA	Connecticut**	NA	NA
30	Utah	1,142	0.61%	NA	Delaware**	NA	NA
34	Vermont	799	0.43%	NA	Florida**	NA	NA
9	Virginia	7,430	4.00%	NA	Illinois**	NA	NA
10	Washington	6,849	3.68%	NA	Iowa**	NA	NA
35	West Virginia	717	0.39%	NA	New Hampshire**	NA	NA
NA	Wisconsin**	NA	NA	NA	Oklahoma**	NA	NA
39	Wyoming	102	0.05%	NA	Wisconsin**	NA	NA
					District of Columbia**	NA	NA

Source: U.S. Department of Health and Human Services, Centers for Disease Control and Prevention
"Abortion Surveillance–United States, 1990" (Morbidity and Mortality Weekly Report, Vol. 42, No. SS-6, 12/17/93)
*By state of occurrence. National total is for reporting states only.
**Not reported.

Percent of Reported Legal Abortions Obtained by Teenagers in 1990

Reporting States Percent = 22.16% of Legal Abortions Obtained by Teenagers*

ALPHA ORDER

RANK ORDER

RANK	STATE	PERCENT
NA	Alabama**	NA
NA	Alaska**	NA
34	Arizona	20.47
8	Arkansas	27.77
NA	California**	NA
17	Colorado	24.25
NA	Connecticut**	NA
NA	Delaware**	NA
NA	Florida**	NA
25	Georgia	22.93
33	Hawaii	20.62
20	Idaho	24.03
NA	Illinois**	NA
23	Indiana	23.78
NA	Iowa**	NA
2	Kansas	28.79
1	Kentucky	31.27
24	Louisiana	23.69
18	Maine	24.18
28	Maryland	22.39
37	Massachusetts	19.17
13	Michigan	25.69
29	Minnesota	22.32
3	Mississippi	28.73
27	Missouri	22.49
7	Montana	27.79
5	Nebraska	28.57
39	Nevada	17.49
NA	New Hampshire**	NA
31	New Jersey	21.64
16	New Mexico	24.38
36	New York	19.38
11	North Carolina	26.65
9	North Dakota	27.57
38	Ohio	19.11
NA	Oklahoma**	NA
21	Oregon	23.92
19	Pennsylvania	24.04
32	Rhode Island	20.69
14	South Carolina	25.16
10	South Dakota	27.48
12	Tennessee	26.01
35	Texas	19.46
22	Utah	23.86
15	Vermont	25.09
26	Virginia	22.52
30	Washington	21.78
4	West Virginia	28.68
NA	Wisconsin**	NA
6	Wyoming	28.10

RANK	STATE	PERCENT
1	Kentucky	31.27
2	Kansas	28.79
3	Mississippi	28.73
4	West Virginia	28.68
5	Nebraska	28.57
6	Wyoming	28.10
7	Montana	27.79
8	Arkansas	27.77
9	North Dakota	27.57
10	South Dakota	27.48
11	North Carolina	26.65
12	Tennessee	26.01
13	Michigan	25.69
14	South Carolina	25.16
15	Vermont	25.09
16	New Mexico	24.38
17	Colorado	24.25
18	Maine	24.18
19	Pennsylvania	24.04
20	Idaho	24.03
21	Oregon	23.92
22	Utah	23.86
23	Indiana	23.78
24	Louisiana	23.69
25	Georgia	22.93
26	Virginia	22.52
27	Missouri	22.49
28	Maryland	22.39
29	Minnesota	22.32
30	Washington	21.78
31	New Jersey	21.64
32	Rhode Island	20.69
33	Hawaii	20.62
34	Arizona	20.47
35	Texas	19.46
36	New York	19.38
37	Massachusetts	19.17
38	Ohio	19.11
39	Nevada	17.49
NA	Alabama**	NA
NA	Alaska**	NA
NA	California**	NA
NA	Connecticut**	NA
NA	Delaware**	NA
NA	Florida**	NA
NA	Illinois**	NA
NA	Iowa**	NA
NA	New Hampshire**	NA
NA	Oklahoma**	NA
NA	Wisconsin**	NA
	District of Columbia**	NA

Source: Morgan Quitno Press using data from US Dept of Health & Human Serv's, Centers for Disease Control-Prevention "Abortion Surveillance-United States, 1990" (Morbidity and Mortality Weekly Report, Vol. 42, No. SS-6, 12/17/93)
*By state of occurrence. National percent is for reporting states only.
**Not reported.

Reported Legal Abortions Obtained by Teenagers 17 Years and Younger in 1990

Reporting States Total = 72,731 Reported Legal Abortions*

ALPHA ORDER					RANK ORDER			
RANK	STATE	ABORTIONS	% of USA		RANK	STATE	ABORTIONS	% of USA
NA	Alabama**	NA	NA		1	New York	12,410	17.06%
NA	Alaska**	NA	NA		2	Texas	6,532	8.98%
20	Arizona	1,158	1.59%		3	Pennsylvania	4,974	6.84%
26	Arkansas	560	0.77%		4	North Carolina	4,058	5.58%
NA	California**	NA	NA		5	Georgia	3,836	5.27%
17	Colorado	1,344	1.85%		6	Michigan	3,820	5.25%
NA	Connecticut**	NA	NA		7	New Jersey	3,534	4.86%
NA	Delaware**	NA	NA		8	Virginia	2,908	4.00%
NA	Florida**	NA	NA		9	Washington	2,764	3.80%
5	Georgia	3,836	5.27%		10	Massachusetts	2,468	3.39%
31	Hawaii	466	0.64%		11	Tennessee	2,295	3.16%
36	Idaho	135	0.19%		12	Maryland	2,076	2.85%
NA	Illinois**	NA	NA		13	Ohio	2,069	2.84%
21	Indiana	1,125	1.55%		14	Kentucky	1,559	2.14%
NA	Iowa**	NA	NA		15	Minnesota	1,389	1.91%
23	Kansas	992	1.36%		16	Oregon	1,360	1.87%
14	Kentucky	1,559	2.14%		17	Colorado	1,344	1.85%
22	Louisiana	1,045	1.44%		18	South Carolina	1,303	1.79%
30	Maine	467	0.64%		19	Missouri	1,265	1.74%
12	Maryland	2,076	2.85%		20	Arizona	1,158	1.59%
10	Massachusetts	2,468	3.39%		21	Indiana	1,125	1.55%
6	Michigan	3,820	5.25%		22	Louisiana	1,045	1.44%
15	Minnesota	1,389	1.91%		23	Kansas	992	1.36%
24	Mississippi	921	1.27%		24	Mississippi	921	1.27%
19	Missouri	1,265	1.74%		25	Nebraska	708	0.97%
33	Montana	392	0.54%		26	Arkansas	560	0.77%
25	Nebraska	708	0.97%		27	New Mexico	550	0.76%
28	Nevada	500	0.69%		28	Nevada	500	0.69%
NA	New Hampshire**	NA	NA		29	Rhode Island	481	0.66%
7	New Jersey	3,534	4.86%		30	Maine	467	0.64%
27	New Mexico	550	0.76%		31	Hawaii	466	0.64%
1	New York	12,410	17.06%		32	Utah	409	0.56%
4	North Carolina	4,058	5.58%		33	Montana	392	0.54%
37	North Dakota	122	0.17%		34	Vermont	314	0.43%
13	Ohio	2,069	2.84%		35	West Virginia	269	0.37%
NA	Oklahoma**	NA	NA		36	Idaho	135	0.19%
16	Oregon	1,360	1.87%		37	North Dakota	122	0.17%
3	Pennsylvania	4,974	6.84%		38	South Dakota	119	0.16%
29	Rhode Island	481	0.66%		39	Wyoming	34	0.05%
18	South Carolina	1,303	1.79%		NA	Alabama**	NA	NA
38	South Dakota	119	0.16%		NA	Alaska**	NA	NA
11	Tennessee	2,295	3.16%		NA	California**	NA	NA
2	Texas	6,532	8.98%		NA	Connecticut**	NA	NA
32	Utah	409	0.56%		NA	Delaware**	NA	NA
34	Vermont	314	0.43%		NA	Florida**	NA	NA
8	Virginia	2,908	4.00%		NA	Illinois**	NA	NA
9	Washington	2,764	3.80%		NA	Iowa**	NA	NA
35	West Virginia	269	0.37%		NA	New Hampshire**	NA	NA
NA	Wisconsin**	NA	NA		NA	Oklahoma**	NA	NA
39	Wyoming	34	0.05%		NA	Wisconsin**	NA	NA
						District of Columbia**	NA	NA

Source: Morgan Quitno Press using data from US Dept of Health & Human Serv's, Centers for Disease Control-Prevention "Abortion Surveillance-United States, 1990" (Morbidity and Mortality Weekly Report, Vol. 42, No. SS-6, 12/17/93)

*By state of occurrence. National total is for reporting states only.

**Not reported.

Percent of Reported Legal Abortions Obtained
By Teenagers 17 Years and Younger in 1990
Reporting States Percent = 8.67% of Reported Legal Abortions*

ALPHA ORDER

RANK	STATE	PERCENT
NA	Alabama**	NA
NA	Alaska**	NA
33	Arizona	7.34
21	Arkansas	9.41
NA	California**	NA
10	Colorado	10.60
NA	Connecticut**	NA
NA	Delaware**	NA
NA	Florida**	NA
18	Georgia	9.77
16	Hawaii	9.81
19	Idaho	9.71
NA	Illinois**	NA
30	Indiana	7.84
NA	Iowa**	NA
3	Kansas	13.20
1	Kentucky	14.28
29	Louisiana	8.03
13	Maine	10.14
23	Maryland	9.26
38	Massachusetts	6.21
11	Michigan	10.56
28	Minnesota	8.10
2	Mississippi	13.46
32	Missouri	7.73
5	Montana	11.65
6	Nebraska	11.16
36	Nevada	6.92
NA	New Hampshire**	NA
27	New Jersey	8.54
12	New Mexico	10.40
31	New York	7.80
7	North Carolina	11.12
34	North Dakota	7.08
37	Ohio	6.43
NA	Oklahoma**	NA
14	Oregon	9.96
20	Pennsylvania	9.54
39	Rhode Island	6.18
16	South Carolina	9.81
4	South Dakota	12.58
8	Tennessee	10.85
35	Texas	7.06
26	Utah	8.55
15	Vermont	9.86
24	Virginia	8.81
25	Washington	8.79
9	West Virginia	10.76
NA	Wisconsin**	NA
22	Wyoming	9.37

RANK ORDER

RANK	STATE	PERCENT
1	Kentucky	14.28
2	Mississippi	13.46
3	Kansas	13.20
4	South Dakota	12.58
5	Montana	11.65
6	Nebraska	11.16
7	North Carolina	11.12
8	Tennessee	10.85
9	West Virginia	10.76
10	Colorado	10.60
11	Michigan	10.56
12	New Mexico	10.40
13	Maine	10.14
14	Oregon	9.96
15	Vermont	9.86
16	Hawaii	9.81
16	South Carolina	9.81
18	Georgia	9.77
19	Idaho	9.71
20	Pennsylvania	9.54
21	Arkansas	9.41
22	Wyoming	9.37
23	Maryland	9.26
24	Virginia	8.81
25	Washington	8.79
26	Utah	8.55
27	New Jersey	8.54
28	Minnesota	8.10
29	Louisiana	8.03
30	Indiana	7.84
31	New York	7.80
32	Missouri	7.73
33	Arizona	7.34
34	North Dakota	7.08
35	Texas	7.06
36	Nevada	6.92
37	Ohio	6.43
38	Massachusetts	6.21
39	Rhode Island	6.18
NA	Alabama**	NA
NA	Alaska**	NA
NA	California**	NA
NA	Connecticut**	NA
NA	Delaware**	NA
NA	Florida**	NA
NA	Illinois**	NA
NA	Iowa**	NA
NA	New Hampshire**	NA
NA	Oklahoma**	NA
NA	Wisconsin**	NA
	District of Columbia**	NA

Source: Morgan Quitno Press using data from US Dept of Health & Human Serv's, Centers for Disease Control-Prevention "Abortion Surveillance-United States, 1990" (Morbidity and Mortality Weekly Report, Vol. 42, No. SS-6, 12/17/93)
*By state of occurrence. National percent is for reporting states only.
**Not reported.

Percent of Teenage Abortions Obtained by Teenagers 17 Years and Younger in 1990

Reporting States Percent = 39.13% of Teenage Abortions*

ALPHA ORDER

RANK	STATE	PERCENT
NA	Alabama**	NA
NA	Alaska**	NA
29	Arizona	35.84
32	Arkansas	33.88
NA	California**	NA
6	Colorado	43.71
NA	Connecticut**	NA
NA	Delaware**	NA
NA	Florida**	NA
8	Georgia	42.63
1	Hawaii	47.60
16	Idaho	40.42
NA	Illinois**	NA
36	Indiana	32.96
NA	Iowa**	NA
3	Kansas	45.84
5	Kentucky	45.65
32	Louisiana	33.88
10	Maine	41.92
14	Maryland	41.34
37	Massachusetts	32.40
15	Michigan	41.09
27	Minnesota	36.27
2	Mississippi	46.85
31	Missouri	34.38
9	Montana	41.93
24	Nebraska	39.05
20	Nevada	39.56
NA	New Hampshire**	NA
21	New Jersey	39.49
7	New Mexico	42.67
18	New York	40.25
11	North Carolina	41.73
39	North Dakota	25.68
34	Ohio	33.65
NA	Oklahoma**	NA
13	Oregon	41.63
19	Pennsylvania	39.68
38	Rhode Island	29.88
25	South Carolina	38.99
4	South Dakota	45.77
11	Tennessee	41.73
28	Texas	36.26
30	Utah	35.81
22	Vermont	39.30
23	Virginia	39.14
17	Washington	40.36
26	West Virginia	37.52
NA	Wisconsin**	NA
35	Wyoming	33.33

RANK ORDER

RANK	STATE	PERCENT
1	Hawaii	47.60
2	Mississippi	46.85
3	Kansas	45.84
4	South Dakota	45.77
5	Kentucky	45.65
6	Colorado	43.71
7	New Mexico	42.67
8	Georgia	42.63
9	Montana	41.93
10	Maine	41.92
11	North Carolina	41.73
11	Tennessee	41.73
13	Oregon	41.63
14	Maryland	41.34
15	Michigan	41.09
16	Idaho	40.42
17	Washington	40.36
18	New York	40.25
19	Pennsylvania	39.68
20	Nevada	39.56
21	New Jersey	39.49
22	Vermont	39.30
23	Virginia	39.14
24	Nebraska	39.05
25	South Carolina	38.99
26	West Virginia	37.52
27	Minnesota	36.27
28	Texas	36.26
29	Arizona	35.84
30	Utah	35.81
31	Missouri	34.38
32	Arkansas	33.88
32	Louisiana	33.88
34	Ohio	33.65
35	Wyoming	33.33
36	Indiana	32.96
37	Massachusetts	32.40
38	Rhode Island	29.88
39	North Dakota	25.68
NA	Alabama**	NA
NA	Alaska**	NA
NA	California**	NA
NA	Connecticut**	NA
NA	Delaware**	NA
NA	Florida**	NA
NA	Illinois**	NA
NA	Iowa**	NA
NA	New Hampshire**	NA
NA	Oklahoma**	NA
NA	Wisconsin**	NA
	District of Columbia**	NA

Source: Morgan Quitno Press using data from US Dept of Health & Human Serv's, Centers for Disease Control-Prevention "Abortion Surveillance-United States, 1990" (Morbidity and Mortality Weekly Report, Vol. 42, No. SS-6, 12/17/93)
*By state of occurrence. National percent is for reporting states only.
**Not reported.

Reported Legal Abortions Performed at 12 Weeks or Less of Gestation in 1990

Reporting States Total = 682,489 Abortions*

<table>
<tr><td colspan="4">ALPHA ORDER</td><td colspan="4">RANK ORDER</td></tr>
<tr><td>RANK</td><td>STATE</td><td>ABORTIONS</td><td>% of USA</td><td>RANK</td><td>STATE</td><td>ABORTIONS</td><td>% of USA</td></tr>
<tr><td>NA</td><td>Alabama**</td><td>NA</td><td>NA</td><td>1</td><td>New York</td><td>135,708</td><td>19.88%</td></tr>
<tr><td>NA</td><td>Alaska**</td><td>NA</td><td>NA</td><td>2</td><td>Texas</td><td>80,791</td><td>11.84%</td></tr>
<tr><td>NA</td><td>Arizona**</td><td>NA</td><td>NA</td><td>3</td><td>Pennsylvania</td><td>46,605</td><td>6.83%</td></tr>
<tr><td>25</td><td>Arkansas</td><td>5,354</td><td>0.78%</td><td>4</td><td>New Jersey</td><td>33,193</td><td>4.86%</td></tr>
<tr><td>NA</td><td>California**</td><td>NA</td><td>NA</td><td>5</td><td>Michigan</td><td>32,116</td><td>4.71%</td></tr>
<tr><td>19</td><td>Colorado</td><td>11,135</td><td>1.63%</td><td>6</td><td>Georgia</td><td>31,693</td><td>4.64%</td></tr>
<tr><td>NA</td><td>Connecticut**</td><td>NA</td><td>NA</td><td>7</td><td>Virginia</td><td>31,650</td><td>4.64%</td></tr>
<tr><td>NA</td><td>Delaware**</td><td>NA</td><td>NA</td><td>8</td><td>North Carolina</td><td>31,562</td><td>4.62%</td></tr>
<tr><td>NA</td><td>Florida**</td><td>NA</td><td>NA</td><td>9</td><td>Washington</td><td>28,698</td><td>4.20%</td></tr>
<tr><td>6</td><td>Georgia</td><td>31,693</td><td>4.64%</td><td>10</td><td>Maryland</td><td>20,388</td><td>2.99%</td></tr>
<tr><td>29</td><td>Hawaii</td><td>3,824</td><td>0.56%</td><td>11</td><td>Tennessee</td><td>19,472</td><td>2.85%</td></tr>
<tr><td>34</td><td>Idaho</td><td>1,365</td><td>0.20%</td><td>12</td><td>Minnesota</td><td>15,024</td><td>2.20%</td></tr>
<tr><td>NA</td><td>Illinois**</td><td>NA</td><td>NA</td><td>13</td><td>Wisconsin</td><td>14,723</td><td>2.16%</td></tr>
<tr><td>15</td><td>Indiana</td><td>13,863</td><td>2.03%</td><td>14</td><td>Missouri</td><td>14,546</td><td>2.13%</td></tr>
<tr><td>NA</td><td>Iowa**</td><td>NA</td><td>NA</td><td>15</td><td>Indiana</td><td>13,863</td><td>2.03%</td></tr>
<tr><td>24</td><td>Kansas</td><td>5,779</td><td>0.85%</td><td>16</td><td>South Carolina</td><td>12,791</td><td>1.87%</td></tr>
<tr><td>20</td><td>Kentucky</td><td>8,548</td><td>1.25%</td><td>17</td><td>Oregon</td><td>11,936</td><td>1.75%</td></tr>
<tr><td>18</td><td>Louisiana</td><td>11,209</td><td>1.64%</td><td>18</td><td>Louisiana</td><td>11,209</td><td>1.64%</td></tr>
<tr><td>27</td><td>Maine</td><td>4,217</td><td>0.62%</td><td>19</td><td>Colorado</td><td>11,135</td><td>1.63%</td></tr>
<tr><td>10</td><td>Maryland</td><td>20,388</td><td>2.99%</td><td>20</td><td>Kentucky</td><td>8,548</td><td>1.25%</td></tr>
<tr><td>NA</td><td>Massachusetts**</td><td>NA</td><td>NA</td><td>21</td><td>Rhode Island</td><td>7,123</td><td>1.04%</td></tr>
<tr><td>5</td><td>Michigan</td><td>32,116</td><td>4.71%</td><td>22</td><td>Nevada</td><td>6,578</td><td>0.96%</td></tr>
<tr><td>12</td><td>Minnesota</td><td>15,024</td><td>2.20%</td><td>23</td><td>Mississippi</td><td>6,123</td><td>0.90%</td></tr>
<tr><td>23</td><td>Mississippi</td><td>6,123</td><td>0.90%</td><td>24</td><td>Kansas</td><td>5,779</td><td>0.85%</td></tr>
<tr><td>14</td><td>Missouri</td><td>14,546</td><td>2.13%</td><td>25</td><td>Arkansas</td><td>5,354</td><td>0.78%</td></tr>
<tr><td>31</td><td>Montana</td><td>3,014</td><td>0.44%</td><td>26</td><td>Utah</td><td>4,310</td><td>0.63%</td></tr>
<tr><td>NA</td><td>Nebraska**</td><td>NA</td><td>NA</td><td>27</td><td>Maine</td><td>4,217</td><td>0.62%</td></tr>
<tr><td>22</td><td>Nevada</td><td>6,578</td><td>0.96%</td><td>28</td><td>New Mexico</td><td>4,079</td><td>0.60%</td></tr>
<tr><td>NA</td><td>New Hampshire**</td><td>NA</td><td>NA</td><td>29</td><td>Hawaii</td><td>3,824</td><td>0.56%</td></tr>
<tr><td>4</td><td>New Jersey</td><td>33,193</td><td>4.86%</td><td>30</td><td>Vermont</td><td>3,034</td><td>0.44%</td></tr>
<tr><td>28</td><td>New Mexico</td><td>4,079</td><td>0.60%</td><td>31</td><td>Montana</td><td>3,014</td><td>0.44%</td></tr>
<tr><td>1</td><td>New York</td><td>135,708</td><td>19.88%</td><td>32</td><td>West Virginia</td><td>2,252</td><td>0.33%</td></tr>
<tr><td>8</td><td>North Carolina</td><td>31,562</td><td>4.62%</td><td>33</td><td>North Dakota</td><td>1,550</td><td>0.23%</td></tr>
<tr><td>33</td><td>North Dakota</td><td>1,550</td><td>0.23%</td><td>34</td><td>Idaho</td><td>1,365</td><td>0.20%</td></tr>
<tr><td>NA</td><td>Ohio**</td><td>NA</td><td>NA</td><td>35</td><td>South Dakota</td><td>942</td><td>0.14%</td></tr>
<tr><td>NA</td><td>Oklahoma**</td><td>NA</td><td>NA</td><td>36</td><td>Wyoming</td><td>362</td><td>0.05%</td></tr>
<tr><td>17</td><td>Oregon</td><td>11,936</td><td>1.75%</td><td>NA</td><td>Alabama**</td><td>NA</td><td>NA</td></tr>
<tr><td>3</td><td>Pennsylvania</td><td>46,605</td><td>6.83%</td><td>NA</td><td>Alaska**</td><td>NA</td><td>NA</td></tr>
<tr><td>21</td><td>Rhode Island</td><td>7,123</td><td>1.04%</td><td>NA</td><td>Arizona**</td><td>NA</td><td>NA</td></tr>
<tr><td>16</td><td>South Carolina</td><td>12,791</td><td>1.87%</td><td>NA</td><td>California**</td><td>NA</td><td>NA</td></tr>
<tr><td>35</td><td>South Dakota</td><td>942</td><td>0.14%</td><td>NA</td><td>Connecticut**</td><td>NA</td><td>NA</td></tr>
<tr><td>11</td><td>Tennessee</td><td>19,472</td><td>2.85%</td><td>NA</td><td>Delaware**</td><td>NA</td><td>NA</td></tr>
<tr><td>2</td><td>Texas</td><td>80,791</td><td>11.84%</td><td>NA</td><td>Florida**</td><td>NA</td><td>NA</td></tr>
<tr><td>26</td><td>Utah</td><td>4,310</td><td>0.63%</td><td>NA</td><td>Illinois**</td><td>NA</td><td>NA</td></tr>
<tr><td>30</td><td>Vermont</td><td>3,034</td><td>0.44%</td><td>NA</td><td>Iowa**</td><td>NA</td><td>NA</td></tr>
<tr><td>7</td><td>Virginia</td><td>31,650</td><td>4.64%</td><td>NA</td><td>Massachusetts**</td><td>NA</td><td>NA</td></tr>
<tr><td>9</td><td>Washington</td><td>28,698</td><td>4.20%</td><td>NA</td><td>Nebraska**</td><td>NA</td><td>NA</td></tr>
<tr><td>32</td><td>West Virginia</td><td>2,252</td><td>0.33%</td><td>NA</td><td>New Hampshire**</td><td>NA</td><td>NA</td></tr>
<tr><td>13</td><td>Wisconsin</td><td>14,723</td><td>2.16%</td><td>NA</td><td>Ohio**</td><td>NA</td><td>NA</td></tr>
<tr><td>36</td><td>Wyoming</td><td>362</td><td>0.05%</td><td>NA</td><td>Oklahoma**</td><td>NA</td><td>NA</td></tr>
<tr><td colspan="4"></td><td colspan="2">District of Columbia</td><td>16,932</td><td>2.48%</td></tr>
</table>

Source: Morgan Quitno Press using data from US Dept of Health & Human Serv's, Centers for Disease Control-Prevention "Abortion Surveillance-United States, 1990" (Morbidity and Mortality Weekly Report, Vol. 42, No. SS-6, 12/17/93)
*By state of occurrence. National total is for reporting states only.
**Not reported.

Percent of Reported Legal Abortions Performed at 12 Weeks or Less of Gestation: 1990

Reporting States Percent = 87.36% of Reported Legal Abortions*

ALPHA ORDER			RANK ORDER		
RANK	STATE	PERCENT	RANK	STATE	PERCENT
NA	Alabama**	NA	1	Wyoming	99.72
NA	Alaska**	NA	2	South Dakota	99.58
NA	Arizona**	NA	3	Idaho	98.20
17	Arkansas	89.94	4	Indiana	96.60
NA	California**	NA	5	South Carolina	96.28
23	Colorado	87.82	6	Virginia	95.93
NA	Connecticut**	NA	7	Vermont	95.29
NA	Delaware**	NA	8	Tennessee	92.09
NA	Florida**	NA	9	Maine	91.53
31	Georgia	80.76	9	Rhode Island	91.53
32	Hawaii	80.54	11	Washington	91.27
3	Idaho	98.20	12	Nevada	91.03
NA	Illinois**	NA	13	Maryland	90.92
4	Indiana	96.60	14	West Virginia	90.08
NA	Iowa**	NA	15	Utah	90.05
36	Kansas	76.89	16	North Dakota	89.96
34	Kentucky	78.27	17	Arkansas	89.94
29	Louisiana	86.09	18	Montana	89.57
9	Maine	91.53	19	Mississippi	89.49
13	Maryland	90.92	20	Pennsylvania	89.38
NA	Massachusetts**	NA	21	Missouri	88.88
22	Michigan	88.76	22	Michigan	88.76
24	Minnesota	87.57	23	Colorado	87.82
19	Mississippi	89.49	24	Minnesota	87.57
21	Missouri	88.88	25	Oregon	87.39
18	Montana	89.57	25	Wisconsin	87.39
NA	Nebraska**	NA	27	Texas	87.27
12	Nevada	91.03	28	North Carolina	86.49
NA	New Hampshire**	NA	29	Louisiana	86.09
33	New Jersey	80.26	30	New York	85.30
35	New Mexico	77.14	31	Georgia	80.76
30	New York	85.30	32	Hawaii	80.54
28	North Carolina	86.49	33	New Jersey	80.26
16	North Dakota	89.96	34	Kentucky	78.27
NA	Ohio**	NA	35	New Mexico	77.14
NA	Oklahoma**	NA	36	Kansas	76.89
25	Oregon	87.39	NA	Alabama**	NA
20	Pennsylvania	89.38	NA	Alaska**	NA
9	Rhode Island	91.53	NA	Arizona**	NA
5	South Carolina	96.28	NA	California**	NA
2	South Dakota	99.58	NA	Connecticut**	NA
8	Tennessee	92.09	NA	Delaware**	NA
27	Texas	87.27	NA	Florida**	NA
15	Utah	90.05	NA	Illinois**	NA
7	Vermont	95.29	NA	Iowa**	NA
6	Virginia	95.93	NA	Massachusetts**	NA
11	Washington	91.27	NA	Nebraska**	NA
14	West Virginia	90.08	NA	New Hampshire**	NA
25	Wisconsin	87.39	NA	Ohio**	NA
1	Wyoming	99.72	NA	Oklahoma**	NA

District of Columbia   84.79

Source: Morgan Quitno Press using data from US Dept of Health & Human Serv's, Centers for Disease Control-Prevention "Abortion Surveillance-United States, 1990" (Morbidity and Mortality Weekly Report, Vol. 42, No. SS-6, 12/17/93)
*By state of occurrence. National percent is for reporting states only.
**Not reported.

Reported Legal Abortions Performed At or After 21 Weeks of Gestation in 1990

Reporting States Total = 7,604 Reported Legal Abortions*

ALPHA ORDER				RANK ORDER			
RANK	STATE	ABORTIONS	% of USA	RANK	STATE	ABORTIONS	% of USA
NA	Alabama**	NA	NA	1	New York	2,081	27.37%
NA	Alaska**	NA	NA	2	Texas	1,294	17.02%
NA	Arizona**	NA	NA	3	New Jersey	758	9.97%
21	Arkansas	19	0.25%	4	Georgia	746	9.81%
NA	California**	NA	NA	5	Pennsylvania	420	5.52%
13	Colorado	126	1.66%	6	Kentucky	379	4.98%
NA	Connecticut**	NA	NA	7	Washington	284	3.73%
NA	Delaware**	NA	NA	8	Kansas	272	3.58%
NA	Florida**	NA	NA	9	Oregon	221	2.91%
4	Georgia	746	9.81%	10	Wisconsin	185	2.43%
17	Hawaii	54	0.71%	11	Louisiana	141	1.85%
29	Idaho	1	0.01%	12	Virginia	128	1.68%
NA	Illinois**	NA	NA	13	Colorado	126	1.66%
32	Indiana	0	0.00%	14	Michigan	92	1.21%
NA	Iowa**	NA	NA	15	Minnesota	85	1.12%
8	Kansas	272	3.58%	16	North Carolina	73	0.96%
6	Kentucky	379	4.98%	17	Hawaii	54	0.71%
11	Louisiana	141	1.85%	18	Missouri	47	0.62%
32	Maine	0	0.00%	19	South Carolina	32	0.42%
21	Maryland	19	0.25%	20	New Mexico	31	0.41%
NA	Massachusetts**	NA	NA	21	Arkansas	19	0.25%
14	Michigan	92	1.21%	21	Maryland	19	0.25%
15	Minnesota	85	1.12%	23	Tennessee	18	0.24%
25	Mississippi	10	0.13%	24	Rhode Island	11	0.14%
18	Missouri	47	0.62%	25	Mississippi	10	0.13%
32	Montana	0	0.00%	26	West Virginia	9	0.12%
NA	Nebraska**	NA	NA	27	Vermont	6	0.08%
29	Nevada	1	0.01%	28	Utah	4	0.05%
NA	New Hampshire**	NA	NA	29	Idaho	1	0.01%
3	New Jersey	758	9.97%	29	Nevada	1	0.01%
20	New Mexico	31	0.41%	29	Wyoming	1	0.01%
1	New York	2,081	27.37%	32	Indiana	0	0.00%
16	North Carolina	73	0.96%	32	Maine	0	0.00%
32	North Dakota	0	0.00%	32	Montana	0	0.00%
NA	Ohio**	NA	NA	32	North Dakota	0	0.00%
NA	Oklahoma**	NA	NA	32	South Dakota	0	0.00%
9	Oregon	221	2.91%	NA	Alabama**	NA	NA
5	Pennsylvania	420	5.52%	NA	Alaska**	NA	NA
24	Rhode Island	11	0.14%	NA	Arizona**	NA	NA
19	South Carolina	32	0.42%	NA	California**	NA	NA
32	South Dakota	0	0.00%	NA	Connecticut**	NA	NA
23	Tennessee	18	0.24%	NA	Delaware**	NA	NA
2	Texas	1,294	17.02%	NA	Florida**	NA	NA
28	Utah	4	0.05%	NA	Illinois**	NA	NA
27	Vermont	6	0.08%	NA	Iowa**	NA	NA
12	Virginia	128	1.68%	NA	Massachusetts**	NA	NA
7	Washington	284	3.73%	NA	Nebraska**	NA	NA
26	West Virginia	9	0.12%	NA	New Hampshire**	NA	NA
10	Wisconsin	185	2.43%	NA	Ohio**	NA	NA
29	Wyoming	1	0.01%	NA	Oklahoma**	NA	NA
					District of Columbia	56	0.74%

Source: U.S. Department of Health and Human Services, Centers for Disease Control and Prevention
   "Abortion Surveillance-United States, 1990" (Morbidity and Mortality Weekly Report, Vol. 42, No. SS-6, 12/17/93)
*By state of occurrence. National total is for reporting states only.
**Not reported.

Percent of Reported Legal Abortions Performed At or After 21 Weeks of Gestation: 1990

Reporting States Percent = 0.97% of Reported Legal Abortions*

ALPHA ORDER

RANK	STATE	PERCENT
NA	Alabama**	NA
NA	Alaska**	NA
NA	Arizona**	NA
18	Arkansas	0.32
NA	California**	NA
11	Colorado	0.99
NA	Connecticut**	NA
NA	Delaware**	NA
NA	Florida**	NA
3	Georgia	1.90
8	Hawaii	1.14
30	Idaho	0.07
NA	Illinois**	NA
32	Indiana	0.00
NA	Iowa**	NA
1	Kansas	3.62
2	Kentucky	3.47
10	Louisiana	1.08
32	Maine	0.00
28	Maryland	0.08
NA	Massachusetts**	NA
21	Michigan	0.25
15	Minnesota	0.50
25	Mississippi	0.15
19	Missouri	0.29
32	Montana	0.00
NA	Nebraska**	NA
31	Nevada	0.01
NA	New Hampshire**	NA
4	New Jersey	1.83
14	New Mexico	0.59
7	New York	1.31
23	North Carolina	0.20
32	North Dakota	0.00
NA	Ohio**	NA
NA	Oklahoma**	NA
5	Oregon	1.62
13	Pennsylvania	0.81
26	Rhode Island	0.14
22	South Carolina	0.24
32	South Dakota	0.00
27	Tennessee	0.09
6	Texas	1.40
28	Utah	0.08
24	Vermont	0.19
16	Virginia	0.39
12	Washington	0.90
17	West Virginia	0.36
9	Wisconsin	1.10
20	Wyoming	0.28

RANK ORDER

RANK	STATE	PERCENT
1	Kansas	3.62
2	Kentucky	3.47
3	Georgia	1.90
4	New Jersey	1.83
5	Oregon	1.62
6	Texas	1.40
7	New York	1.31
8	Hawaii	1.14
9	Wisconsin	1.10
10	Louisiana	1.08
11	Colorado	0.99
12	Washington	0.90
13	Pennsylvania	0.81
14	New Mexico	0.59
15	Minnesota	0.50
16	Virginia	0.39
17	West Virginia	0.36
18	Arkansas	0.32
19	Missouri	0.29
20	Wyoming	0.28
21	Michigan	0.25
22	South Carolina	0.24
23	North Carolina	0.20
24	Vermont	0.19
25	Mississippi	0.15
26	Rhode Island	0.14
27	Tennessee	0.09
28	Maryland	0.08
28	Utah	0.08
30	Idaho	0.07
31	Nevada	0.01
32	Indiana	0.00
32	Maine	0.00
32	Montana	0.00
32	North Dakota	0.00
32	South Dakota	0.00
NA	Alabama**	NA
NA	Alaska**	NA
NA	Arizona**	NA
NA	California**	NA
NA	Connecticut**	NA
NA	Delaware**	NA
NA	Florida**	NA
NA	Illinois**	NA
NA	Iowa**	NA
NA	Massachusetts**	NA
NA	Nebraska**	NA
NA	New Hampshire**	NA
NA	Ohio**	NA
NA	Oklahoma**	NA

District of Columbia   0.28

Source: Morgan Quitno Press using data from US Dept of Health & Human Serv's, Centers for Disease Control-Prevention "Abortion Surveillance-United States, 1990" (Morbidity and Mortality Weekly Report, Vol. 42, No. SS-6, 12/17/93)
*By state of occurrence. National percent is for reporting states only.
**Not reported.

II. DEATHS

II. DEATHS (Continued)

Deaths in 1993

National Total = 2,268,000 Deaths*

ALPHA ORDER

RANK	STATE	DEATHS	% of USA
20	Alabama	41,540	1.83%
50	Alaska	2,247	0.10%
25	Arizona	32,090	1.41%
31	Arkansas	26,371	1.16%
1	California	217,559	9.59%
32	Colorado	23,722	1.05%
27	Connecticut	29,057	1.28%
46	Delaware	6,116	0.27%
3	Florida	146,309	6.45%
13	Georgia	55,851	2.46%
44	Hawaii	7,280	0.32%
42	Idaho	8,345	0.37%
6	Illinois	107,563	4.74%
14	Indiana	52,210	2.30%
28	Iowa	27,862	1.23%
33	Kansas	23,337	1.03%
22	Kentucky	36,921	1.63%
21	Louisiana	40,117	1.77%
37	Maine	11,479	0.51%
18	Maryland	43,087	1.90%
11	Massachusetts	56,460	2.49%
8	Michigan	82,651	3.64%
23	Minnesota	36,236	1.60%
30	Mississippi	26,575	1.17%
12	Missouri	56,305	2.48%
43	Montana	7,502	0.33%
35	Nebraska	15,401	0.68%
38	Nevada	10,886	0.48%
41	New Hampshire	8,919	0.39%
9	New Jersey	72,776	3.21%
36	New Mexico	11,861	0.52%
2	New York	170,203	7.50%
10	North Carolina	62,580	2.76%
47	North Dakota	5,925	0.26%
7	Ohio	100,678	4.44%
24	Oklahoma	32,574	1.44%
29	Oregon	27,275	1.20%
5	Pennsylvania	126,977	5.60%
40	Rhode Island	9,709	0.43%
26	South Carolina	31,404	1.38%
45	South Dakota	6,863	0.30%
16	Tennessee	49,628	2.19%
4	Texas	135,603	5.98%
39	Utah	10,193	0.45%
48	Vermont	4,868	0.21%
15	Virginia	51,773	2.28%
19	Washington	41,986	1.85%
34	West Virginia	19,929	0.88%
17	Wisconsin	44,033	1.94%
49	Wyoming	3,544	0.16%

RANK ORDER

RANK	STATE	DEATHS	% of USA
1	California	217,559	9.59%
2	New York	170,203	7.50%
3	Florida	146,309	6.45%
4	Texas	135,603	5.98%
5	Pennsylvania	126,977	5.60%
6	Illinois	107,563	4.74%
7	Ohio	100,678	4.44%
8	Michigan	82,651	3.64%
9	New Jersey	72,776	3.21%
10	North Carolina	62,580	2.76%
11	Massachusetts	56,460	2.49%
12	Missouri	56,305	2.48%
13	Georgia	55,851	2.46%
14	Indiana	52,210	2.30%
15	Virginia	51,773	2.28%
16	Tennessee	49,628	2.19%
17	Wisconsin	44,033	1.94%
18	Maryland	43,087	1.90%
19	Washington	41,986	1.85%
20	Alabama	41,540	1.83%
21	Louisiana	40,117	1.77%
22	Kentucky	36,921	1.63%
23	Minnesota	36,236	1.60%
24	Oklahoma	32,574	1.44%
25	Arizona	32,090	1.41%
26	South Carolina	31,404	1.38%
27	Connecticut	29,057	1.28%
28	Iowa	27,862	1.23%
29	Oregon	27,275	1.20%
30	Mississippi	26,575	1.17%
31	Arkansas	26,371	1.16%
32	Colorado	23,722	1.05%
33	Kansas	23,337	1.03%
34	West Virginia	19,929	0.88%
35	Nebraska	15,401	0.68%
36	New Mexico	11,861	0.52%
37	Maine	11,479	0.51%
38	Nevada	10,886	0.48%
39	Utah	10,193	0.45%
40	Rhode Island	9,709	0.43%
41	New Hampshire	8,919	0.39%
42	Idaho	8,345	0.37%
43	Montana	7,502	0.33%
44	Hawaii	7,280	0.32%
45	South Dakota	6,863	0.30%
46	Delaware	6,116	0.27%
47	North Dakota	5,925	0.26%
48	Vermont	4,868	0.21%
49	Wyoming	3,544	0.16%
50	Alaska	2,247	0.10%
	District of Columbia	6,713	0.30%

Source: U.S. Department of Health and Human Services, National Center for Health Statistics
"Monthly Vital Statistics Report" (Vol. 42, No. 13, October 11, 1994)
*Provisional data. By state of residence.

Death Rate in 1993

National Rate = 8.8 Deaths per 1,000 Population*

ALPHA ORDER

RANK ORDER

RANK	STATE	RATE		RANK	STATE	RATE
8	Alabama	9.9		1	West Virginia	11.0
50	Alaska	3.8		2	Arkansas	10.9
35	Arizona	8.2		3	Missouri	10.8
2	Arkansas	10.9		4	Florida	10.7
46	California	7.0		5	Pennsylvania	10.5
47	Colorado	6.7		6	Mississippi	10.1
27	Connecticut	8.9		6	Oklahoma	10.1
29	Delaware	8.7		8	Alabama	9.9
4	Florida	10.7		8	Iowa	9.9
36	Georgia	8.1		10	Kentucky	9.7
48	Hawaii	6.2		10	Rhode Island	9.7
42	Idaho	7.6		10	Tennessee	9.7
20	Illinois	9.2		13	Nebraska	9.6
23	Indiana	9.1		13	South Dakota	9.6
8	Iowa	9.9		15	Massachusetts	9.4
20	Kansas	9.2		15	New York	9.4
10	Kentucky	9.7		17	Louisiana	9.3
17	Louisiana	9.3		17	Maine	9.3
17	Maine	9.3		17	North Dakota	9.3
29	Maryland	8.7		20	Illinois	9.2
15	Massachusetts	9.4		20	Kansas	9.2
29	Michigan	8.7		20	New Jersey	9.2
37	Minnesota	8.0		23	Indiana	9.1
6	Mississippi	10.1		23	Ohio	9.1
3	Missouri	10.8		25	North Carolina	9.0
27	Montana	8.9		25	Oregon	9.0
13	Nebraska	9.6		27	Connecticut	8.9
41	Nevada	7.8		27	Montana	8.9
40	New Hampshire	7.9		29	Delaware	8.7
20	New Jersey	9.2		29	Maryland	8.7
45	New Mexico	7.3		29	Michigan	8.7
15	New York	9.4		29	Wisconsin	8.7
25	North Carolina	9.0		33	South Carolina	8.6
17	North Dakota	9.3		34	Vermont	8.5
23	Ohio	9.1		35	Arizona	8.2
6	Oklahoma	10.1		36	Georgia	8.1
25	Oregon	9.0		37	Minnesota	8.0
5	Pennsylvania	10.5		37	Virginia	8.0
10	Rhode Island	9.7		37	Washington	8.0
33	South Carolina	8.6		40	New Hampshire	7.9
13	South Dakota	9.6		41	Nevada	7.8
10	Tennessee	9.7		42	Idaho	7.6
43	Texas	7.5		43	Texas	7.5
49	Utah	5.5		43	Wyoming	7.5
34	Vermont	8.5		45	New Mexico	7.3
37	Virginia	8.0		46	California	7.0
37	Washington	8.0		47	Colorado	6.7
1	West Virginia	11.0		48	Hawaii	6.2
29	Wisconsin	8.7		49	Utah	5.5
43	Wyoming	7.5		50	Alaska	3.8
					District of Columbia	11.6

Source: U.S. Department of Health and Human Services, National Center for Health Statistics
"Monthly Vital Statistics Report" (Vol. 42, No. 13, October 11, 1994)
*Provisional data. By state of residence.

Births to Deaths Ratio in 1993

National Ratio = 1.78 Births for Every Death in 1993*

ALPHA ORDER			RANK ORDER		
RANK	STATE	RATIO	RANK	STATE	RATIO
36	Alabama	1.52	1	Alaska	4.70
1	Alaska	4.70	2	Utah	3.58
8	Arizona	2.21	3	California	2.71
48	Arkansas	1.30	4	Hawaii	2.69
3	California	2.71	5	Texas	2.44
7	Colorado	2.31	6	New Mexico	2.33
29	Connecticut	1.58	7	Colorado	2.31
19	Delaware	1.73	8	Arizona	2.21
46	Florida	1.32	9	Idaho	2.06
10	Georgia	2.01	10	Georgia	2.01
4	Hawaii	2.69	11	Nevada	1.94
9	Idaho	2.06	12	Wyoming	1.88
14	Illinois	1.78	13	Virginia	1.84
26	Indiana	1.62	14	Illinois	1.78
45	Iowa	1.33	15	Minnesota	1.76
25	Kansas	1.63	16	Maryland	1.75
43	Kentucky	1.42	17	Louisiana	1.74
17	Louisiana	1.74	17	Michigan	1.74
47	Maine	1.31	19	Delaware	1.73
16	Maryland	1.75	20	South Carolina	1.72
34	Massachusetts	1.53	21	Washington	1.70
17	Michigan	1.74	22	New Jersey	1.69
15	Minnesota	1.76	23	New Hampshire	1.68
28	Mississippi	1.59	24	New York	1.64
44	Missouri	1.38	25	Kansas	1.63
34	Montana	1.53	26	Indiana	1.62
38	Nebraska	1.48	27	North Carolina	1.61
11	Nevada	1.94	28	Mississippi	1.59
23	New Hampshire	1.68	29	Connecticut	1.58
22	New Jersey	1.69	29	South Dakota	1.58
6	New Mexico	2.33	31	Wisconsin	1.57
24	New York	1.64	32	Ohio	1.56
27	North Carolina	1.61	33	Oregon	1.55
38	North Dakota	1.48	34	Massachusetts	1.53
32	Ohio	1.56	34	Montana	1.53
42	Oklahoma	1.43	36	Alabama	1.52
33	Oregon	1.55	37	Vermont	1.50
49	Pennsylvania	1.25	38	Nebraska	1.48
41	Rhode Island	1.47	38	North Dakota	1.48
20	South Carolina	1.72	38	Tennessee	1.48
29	South Dakota	1.58	41	Rhode Island	1.47
38	Tennessee	1.48	42	Oklahoma	1.43
5	Texas	2.44	43	Kentucky	1.42
2	Utah	3.58	44	Missouri	1.38
37	Vermont	1.50	45	Iowa	1.33
13	Virginia	1.84	46	Florida	1.32
21	Washington	1.70	47	Maine	1.31
50	West Virginia	1.11	48	Arkansas	1.30
31	Wisconsin	1.57	49	Pennsylvania	1.25
12	Wyoming	1.88	50	West Virginia	1.11
				District of Columbia	1.46

Source: Morgan Quitno Press using data from US Dept of Health & Human Services, National Center for Health Statistics "Monthly Vital Statistics Report" (Vol. 42, No. 13, October 11, 1994)
*Provisional data. By state of residence.

77

Deaths in 1990

National Total = 2,148,463 Deaths*

ALPHA ORDER					RANK ORDER			
RANK	STATE	DEATHS	% of USA		RANK	STATE	DEATHS	% of USA
18	Alabama	39,381	1.83%		1	California	214,369	9.98%
50	Alaska	2,188	0.10%		2	New York	168,936	7.86%
26	Arizona	28,789	1.34%		3	Florida	134,385	6.25%
31	Arkansas	24,652	1.15%		4	Texas	125,479	5.84%
1	California	214,369	9.98%		5	Pennsylvania	121,951	5.68%
33	Colorado	21,583	1.00%		6	Illinois	103,006	4.79%
27	Connecticut	27,607	1.28%		7	Ohio	98,822	4.60%
46	Delaware	5,764	0.27%		8	Michigan	78,744	3.67%
3	Florida	134,385	6.25%		9	New Jersey	70,383	3.28%
12	Georgia	51,810	2.41%		10	North Carolina	57,315	2.67%
44	Hawaii	6,782	0.32%		11	Massachusetts	53,179	2.48%
42	Idaho	7,452	0.35%		12	Georgia	51,810	2.41%
6	Illinois	103,006	4.79%		13	Missouri	50,377	2.34%
14	Indiana	49,569	2.31%		14	Indiana	49,569	2.31%
28	Iowa	26,884	1.25%		15	Virginia	48,013	2.23%
32	Kansas	22,279	1.04%		16	Tennessee	46,315	2.16%
22	Kentucky	35,078	1.63%		17	Wisconsin	42,733	1.99%
20	Louisiana	37,571	1.75%		18	Alabama	39,381	1.83%
36	Maine	11,106	0.52%		19	Maryland	38,413	1.79%
19	Maryland	38,413	1.79%		20	Louisiana	37,571	1.75%
11	Massachusetts	53,179	2.48%		21	Washington	37,087	1.73%
8	Michigan	78,744	3.67%		22	Kentucky	35,078	1.63%
23	Minnesota	34,776	1.62%		23	Minnesota	34,776	1.62%
30	Mississippi	25,127	1.17%		24	Oklahoma	30,378	1.41%
13	Missouri	50,377	2.34%		25	South Carolina	29,715	1.38%
43	Montana	6,861	0.32%		26	Arizona	28,789	1.34%
35	Nebraska	14,769	0.69%		27	Connecticut	27,607	1.28%
39	Nevada	9,318	0.43%		28	Iowa	26,884	1.25%
41	New Hampshire	8,488	0.40%		29	Oregon	25,136	1.17%
9	New Jersey	70,383	3.28%		30	Mississippi	25,127	1.17%
37	New Mexico	10,625	0.49%		31	Arkansas	24,652	1.15%
2	New York	168,936	7.86%		32	Kansas	22,279	1.04%
10	North Carolina	57,315	2.67%		33	Colorado	21,583	1.00%
47	North Dakota	5,678	0.26%		34	West Virginia	19,385	0.90%
7	Ohio	98,822	4.60%		35	Nebraska	14,769	0.69%
24	Oklahoma	30,378	1.41%		36	Maine	11,106	0.52%
29	Oregon	25,136	1.17%		37	New Mexico	10,625	0.49%
5	Pennsylvania	121,951	5.68%		38	Rhode Island	9,576	0.45%
38	Rhode Island	9,576	0.45%		39	Nevada	9,318	0.43%
25	South Carolina	29,715	1.38%		40	Utah	9,192	0.43%
45	South Dakota	6,326	0.29%		41	New Hampshire	8,488	0.40%
16	Tennessee	46,315	2.16%		42	Idaho	7,452	0.35%
4	Texas	125,479	5.84%		43	Montana	6,861	0.32%
40	Utah	9,192	0.43%		44	Hawaii	6,782	0.32%
48	Vermont	4,595	0.21%		45	South Dakota	6,326	0.29%
15	Virginia	48,013	2.23%		46	Delaware	5,764	0.27%
21	Washington	37,087	1.73%		47	North Dakota	5,678	0.26%
34	West Virginia	19,385	0.90%		48	Vermont	4,595	0.21%
17	Wisconsin	42,733	1.99%		49	Wyoming	3,203	0.15%
49	Wyoming	3,203	0.15%		50	Alaska	2,188	0.10%
					District of Columbia		7,313	0.34%

Source: U.S. Department of Health and Human Services, National Center for Health Statistics
"Monthly Vital Statistics Report" (Vol. 41, No. 7(S), January 7, 1993)
*Final data by state of residence.

Death Rate in 1990

National Rate = 8.63 Deaths per 1,000 Population*

ALPHA ORDER				RANK ORDER		
RANK	STATE	RATE		RANK	STATE	RATE
7	Alabama	9.74		1	West Virginia	10.80
50	Alaska	3.98		2	Arkansas	10.48
37	Arizona	7.84		3	Florida	10.38
2	Arkansas	10.48		4	Pennsylvania	10.26
44	California	7.19		5	Missouri	9.84
47	Colorado	6.55		6	Mississippi	9.76
32	Connecticut	8.40		7	Alabama	9.74
27	Delaware	8.64		8	Iowa	9.68
3	Florida	10.38		9	Oklahoma	9.66
35	Georgia	7.99		10	Rhode Island	9.54
48	Hawaii	6.11		11	Kentucky	9.51
42	Idaho	7.40		12	Tennessee	9.49
19	Illinois	9.00		13	New York	9.38
21	Indiana	8.94		14	Nebraska	9.36
8	Iowa	9.68		15	Ohio	9.11
20	Kansas	8.99		16	New Jersey	9.10
11	Kentucky	9.51		17	South Dakota	9.09
22	Louisiana	8.90		18	Maine	9.05
18	Maine	9.05		19	Illinois	9.00
34	Maryland	8.03		20	Kansas	8.99
24	Massachusetts	8.84		21	Indiana	8.94
31	Michigan	8.47		22	Louisiana	8.90
36	Minnesota	7.95		22	North Dakota	8.90
6	Mississippi	9.76		24	Massachusetts	8.84
5	Missouri	9.84		24	Oregon	8.84
29	Montana	8.59		26	Wisconsin	8.74
14	Nebraska	9.36		27	Delaware	8.64
38	Nevada	7.75		27	North Carolina	8.64
40	New Hampshire	7.65		29	Montana	8.59
16	New Jersey	9.10		30	South Carolina	8.52
46	New Mexico	7.01		31	Michigan	8.47
13	New York	9.38		32	Connecticut	8.40
27	North Carolina	8.64		33	Vermont	8.17
22	North Dakota	8.90		34	Maryland	8.03
15	Ohio	9.11		35	Georgia	7.99
9	Oklahoma	9.66		36	Minnesota	7.95
24	Oregon	8.84		37	Arizona	7.84
4	Pennsylvania	10.26		38	Nevada	7.75
10	Rhode Island	9.54		38	Virginia	7.75
30	South Carolina	8.52		40	New Hampshire	7.65
17	South Dakota	9.09		41	Washington	7.62
12	Tennessee	9.49		42	Idaho	7.40
43	Texas	7.38		43	Texas	7.38
49	Utah	5.33		44	California	7.19
33	Vermont	8.17		45	Wyoming	7.06
38	Virginia	7.75		46	New Mexico	7.01
41	Washington	7.62		47	Colorado	6.55
1	West Virginia	10.80		48	Hawaii	6.11
26	Wisconsin	8.74		49	Utah	5.33
45	Wyoming	7.06		50	Alaska	3.98
					District of Columbia	12.00

Source: U.S. Department of Health and Human Services, National Center for Health Statistics
"Monthly Vital Statistics Report" (Vol. 41, No. 7(S), January 7, 1993)
*Final data by state of residence.

Deaths in 1980

National Total = 1,989,841 Deaths*

ALPHA ORDER				RANK ORDER			
RANK	STATE	DEATHS	% of USA	RANK	STATE	DEATHS	% of USA
19	Alabama	35,542	1.79%	1	California	186,624	9.38%
50	Alaska	1,714	0.09%	2	New York	172,853	8.69%
32	Arizona	21,367	1.07%	3	Pennsylvania	123,594	6.21%
29	Arkansas	22,744	1.14%	4	Texas	108,180	5.44%
1	California	186,624	9.38%	5	Florida	104,670	5.26%
34	Colorado	18,956	0.95%	6	Illinois	102,935	5.17%
25	Connecticut	27,275	1.37%	7	Ohio	98,421	4.95%
46	Delaware	5,044	0.25%	8	Michigan	75,187	3.78%
5	Florida	104,670	5.26%	9	New Jersey	68,943	3.46%
14	Georgia	44,262	2.22%	10	Massachusetts	55,070	2.77%
47	Hawaii	4,981	0.25%	11	Missouri	49,660	2.50%
41	Idaho	6,763	0.34%	12	North Carolina	48,440	2.43%
6	Illinois	102,935	5.17%	13	Indiana	47,345	2.38%
13	Indiana	47,345	2.38%	14	Georgia	44,262	2.22%
26	Iowa	27,120	1.36%	15	Virginia	42,506	2.14%
30	Kansas	22,034	1.11%	16	Wisconsin	40,838	2.05%
21	Kentucky	33,796	1.70%	17	Tennessee	40,774	2.05%
18	Louisiana	35,651	1.79%	18	Louisiana	35,651	1.79%
36	Maine	10,800	0.54%	19	Alabama	35,542	1.79%
20	Maryland	34,016	1.71%	20	Maryland	34,016	1.71%
10	Massachusetts	55,070	2.77%	21	Kentucky	33,796	1.70%
8	Michigan	75,187	3.78%	22	Minnesota	33,366	1.68%
22	Minnesota	33,366	1.68%	23	Washington	32,007	1.61%
28	Mississippi	23,656	1.19%	24	Oklahoma	28,234	1.42%
11	Missouri	49,660	2.50%	25	Connecticut	27,275	1.37%
42	Montana	6,666	0.34%	26	Iowa	27,120	1.36%
35	Nebraska	14,474	0.73%	27	South Carolina	25,154	1.26%
44	Nevada	5,896	0.30%	28	Mississippi	23,656	1.19%
40	New Hampshire	7,647	0.38%	29	Arkansas	22,744	1.14%
9	New Jersey	68,943	3.46%	30	Kansas	22,034	1.11%
38	New Mexico	9,093	0.46%	31	Oregon	21,798	1.10%
2	New York	172,853	8.69%	32	Arizona	21,367	1.07%
12	North Carolina	48,440	2.43%	33	West Virginia	19,237	0.97%
45	North Dakota	5,596	0.28%	34	Colorado	18,956	0.95%
7	Ohio	98,421	4.95%	35	Nebraska	14,474	0.73%
24	Oklahoma	28,234	1.42%	36	Maine	10,800	0.54%
31	Oregon	21,798	1.10%	37	Rhode Island	9,325	0.47%
3	Pennsylvania	123,594	6.21%	38	New Mexico	9,093	0.46%
37	Rhode Island	9,325	0.47%	39	Utah	8,120	0.41%
27	South Carolina	25,154	1.26%	40	New Hampshire	7,647	0.38%
43	South Dakota	6,556	0.33%	41	Idaho	6,763	0.34%
17	Tennessee	40,774	2.05%	42	Montana	6,666	0.34%
4	Texas	108,180	5.44%	43	South Dakota	6,556	0.33%
39	Utah	8,120	0.41%	44	Nevada	5,896	0.30%
48	Vermont	4,582	0.23%	45	North Dakota	5,596	0.28%
15	Virginia	42,506	2.14%	46	Delaware	5,044	0.25%
23	Washington	32,007	1.61%	47	Hawaii	4,981	0.25%
33	West Virginia	19,237	0.97%	48	Vermont	4,582	0.23%
16	Wisconsin	40,838	2.05%	49	Wyoming	3,221	0.16%
49	Wyoming	3,221	0.16%	50	Alaska	1,714	0.09%
					District of Columbia	7,108	0.36%

Source: U.S. Department of Health and Human Services, National Center for Health Statistics
"Vital Statistics of the United States 1980" and "Monthly Vital Statistics Report"
*Final data by state of residence.

Death Rate in 1980

National Rate = 8.77 Deaths per 1,000 Population*

ALPHA ORDER			RANK ORDER		
RANK	STATE	RATE	RANK	STATE	RATE
18	Alabama	9.12	1	Florida	10.72
50	Alaska	4.25	2	Pennsylvania	10.41
40	Arizona	7.84	3	Missouri	10.08
4	Arkansas	9.94	4	Arkansas	9.94
39	California	7.86	5	West Virginia	9.87
47	Colorado	6.54	6	New York	9.84
23	Connecticut	8.77	6	Rhode Island	9.84
27	Delaware	8.47	8	Maine	9.60
1	Florida	10.72	9	Massachusetts	9.59
35	Georgia	8.09	10	South Dakota	9.47
49	Hawaii	5.15	11	Mississippi	9.37
44	Idaho	7.15	12	New Jersey	9.36
20	Illinois	8.99	13	Oklahoma	9.32
25	Indiana	8.62	14	Iowa	9.30
14	Iowa	9.30	14	Kansas	9.30
14	Kansas	9.30	16	Kentucky	9.22
16	Kentucky	9.22	17	Nebraska	9.20
28	Louisiana	8.46	18	Alabama	9.12
8	Maine	9.60	19	Ohio	9.11
36	Maryland	8.06	20	Illinois	8.99
9	Massachusetts	9.59	21	Vermont	8.95
34	Michigan	8.11	22	Tennessee	8.87
33	Minnesota	8.17	23	Connecticut	8.77
11	Mississippi	9.37	24	Wisconsin	8.67
3	Missouri	10.08	25	Indiana	8.62
28	Montana	8.46	26	North Dakota	8.56
17	Nebraska	9.20	27	Delaware	8.47
43	Nevada	7.35	28	Louisiana	8.46
30	New Hampshire	8.30	28	Montana	8.46
12	New Jersey	9.36	30	New Hampshire	8.30
45	New Mexico	6.96	31	Oregon	8.27
6	New York	9.84	32	North Carolina	8.23
32	North Carolina	8.23	33	Minnesota	8.17
26	North Dakota	8.56	34	Michigan	8.11
19	Ohio	9.11	35	Georgia	8.09
13	Oklahoma	9.32	36	Maryland	8.06
31	Oregon	8.27	37	South Carolina	8.05
2	Pennsylvania	10.41	38	Virginia	7.94
6	Rhode Island	9.84	39	California	7.86
37	South Carolina	8.05	40	Arizona	7.84
10	South Dakota	9.47	41	Washington	7.73
22	Tennessee	8.87	42	Texas	7.58
42	Texas	7.58	43	Nevada	7.35
48	Utah	5.54	44	Idaho	7.15
21	Vermont	8.95	45	New Mexico	6.96
38	Virginia	7.94	46	Wyoming	6.84
41	Washington	7.73	47	Colorado	6.54
5	West Virginia	9.87	48	Utah	5.54
24	Wisconsin	8.67	49	Hawaii	5.15
46	Wyoming	6.84	50	Alaska	4.25
				District of Columbia	11.09

Source: U.S. Department of Health and Human Services, National Center for Health Statistics
"Vital Statistics of the United States 1980" and "Monthly Vital Statistics Report"
Final data by state of residence.

Infant Deaths in 1994

National Total = 32,000 Infant Deaths*

ALPHA ORDER

RANK	STATE	DEATHS	% of USA
17	Alabama	633	1.98%
NA	Alaska**	NA	NA
19	Arizona	539	1.68%
29	Arkansas	312	0.98%
1	California	3,874	12.11%
28	Colorado	374	1.17%
NA	Connecticut**	NA	NA
45	Delaware	80	0.25%
5	Florida	1,565	4.89%
9	Georgia	1,151	3.60%
38	Hawaii	127	0.40%
39	Idaho	126	0.39%
4	Illinois	1,838	5.74%
12	Indiana	755	2.36%
33	Iowa	233	0.73%
30	Kansas	307	0.96%
25	Kentucky	429	1.34%
14	Louisiana	660	2.06%
44	Maine	86	0.27%
15	Maryland	656	2.05%
27	Massachusetts	422	1.32%
8	Michigan	1,205	3.77%
22	Minnesota	466	1.46%
26	Mississippi	423	1.32%
18	Missouri	624	1.95%
41	Montana	97	0.30%
35	Nebraska	186	0.58%
37	Nevada	128	0.40%
42	New Hampshire	94	0.29%
11	New Jersey	972	3.04%
32	New Mexico	270	0.84%
3	New York	2,375	7.42%
10	North Carolina	1,008	3.15%
46	North Dakota	62	0.19%
6	Ohio	1,466	4.58%
24	Oklahoma	441	1.38%
31	Oregon	286	0.89%
7	Pennsylvania	1,260	3.94%
43	Rhode Island	93	0.29%
21	South Carolina	489	1.53%
40	South Dakota	122	0.38%
16	Tennessee	637	1.99%
2	Texas	2,440	7.63%
34	Utah	204	0.64%
48	Vermont	32	0.10%
13	Virginia	727	2.27%
23	Washington	455	1.42%
36	West Virginia	153	0.48%
20	Wisconsin	523	1.63%
47	Wyoming	39	0.12%

RANK ORDER

RANK	STATE	DEATHS	% of USA
1	California	3,874	12.11%
2	Texas	2,440	7.63%
3	New York	2,375	7.42%
4	Illinois	1,838	5.74%
5	Florida	1,565	4.89%
6	Ohio	1,466	4.58%
7	Pennsylvania	1,260	3.94%
8	Michigan	1,205	3.77%
9	Georgia	1,151	3.60%
10	North Carolina	1,008	3.15%
11	New Jersey	972	3.04%
12	Indiana	755	2.36%
13	Virginia	727	2.27%
14	Louisiana	660	2.06%
15	Maryland	656	2.05%
16	Tennessee	637	1.99%
17	Alabama	633	1.98%
18	Missouri	624	1.95%
19	Arizona	539	1.68%
20	Wisconsin	523	1.63%
21	South Carolina	489	1.53%
22	Minnesota	466	1.46%
23	Washington	455	1.42%
24	Oklahoma	441	1.38%
25	Kentucky	429	1.34%
26	Mississippi	423	1.32%
27	Massachusetts	422	1.32%
28	Colorado	374	1.17%
29	Arkansas	312	0.98%
30	Kansas	307	0.96%
31	Oregon	286	0.89%
32	New Mexico	270	0.84%
33	Iowa	233	0.73%
34	Utah	204	0.64%
35	Nebraska	186	0.58%
36	West Virginia	153	0.48%
37	Nevada	128	0.40%
38	Hawaii	127	0.40%
39	Idaho	126	0.39%
40	South Dakota	122	0.38%
41	Montana	97	0.30%
42	New Hampshire	94	0.29%
43	Rhode Island	93	0.29%
44	Maine	86	0.27%
45	Delaware	80	0.25%
46	North Dakota	62	0.19%
47	Wyoming	39	0.12%
48	Vermont	32	0.10%
NA	Alaska**	NA	NA
NA	Connecticut**	NA	NA
	District of Columbia	157	0.49%

Source: U.S. Department of Health and Human Services, National Center for Health Statistics
"Monthly Vital Statistics Report" (Vol. 43, No. 7, December 19, 1994)
For 12 months ending July 1994. Provisional data. Deaths under 1 year old by state of residence. Total includes states not shown separately.
***Not available.*

Infant Mortality Rate in 1994

National Rate = 8.0 Infant Deaths per 1,000 Live Births*

ALPHA ORDER

RANK	STATE	RATE
2	Alabama	10.4
NA	Alaska**	NA
26	Arizona	7.8
13	Arkansas	9.1
38	California	6.6
34	Colorado	6.9
NA	Connecticut**	NA
28	Delaware	7.7
23	Florida	8.1
2	Georgia	10.4
39	Hawaii	6.5
31	Idaho	7.3
6	Illinois	9.7
12	Indiana	9.2
40	Iowa	6.4
20	Kansas	8.2
19	Kentucky	8.3
6	Louisiana	9.7
44	Maine	5.8
14	Maryland	9.0
47	Massachusetts	5.0
15	Michigan	8.7
31	Minnesota	7.3
4	Mississippi	10.1
24	Missouri	8.0
15	Montana	8.7
20	Nebraska	8.2
42	Nevada	5.9
41	New Hampshire	6.2
20	New Jersey	8.2
8	New Mexico	9.6
17	New York	8.5
5	North Carolina	10.0
33	North Dakota	7.1
10	Ohio	9.3
9	Oklahoma	9.4
37	Oregon	6.7
24	Pennsylvania	8.0
34	Rhode Island	6.9
10	South Carolina	9.3
1	South Dakota	11.4
17	Tennessee	8.5
29	Texas	7.5
46	Utah	5.4
48	Vermont	4.6
26	Virginia	7.8
44	Washington	5.8
34	West Virginia	6.9
29	Wisconsin	7.5
42	Wyoming	5.9

RANK ORDER

RANK	STATE	RATE
1	South Dakota	11.4
2	Alabama	10.4
2	Georgia	10.4
4	Mississippi	10.1
5	North Carolina	10.0
6	Illinois	9.7
6	Louisiana	9.7
8	New Mexico	9.6
9	Oklahoma	9.4
10	Ohio	9.3
10	South Carolina	9.3
12	Indiana	9.2
13	Arkansas	9.1
14	Maryland	9.0
15	Michigan	8.7
15	Montana	8.7
17	New York	8.5
17	Tennessee	8.5
19	Kentucky	8.3
20	Kansas	8.2
20	Nebraska	8.2
20	New Jersey	8.2
23	Florida	8.1
24	Missouri	8.0
24	Pennsylvania	8.0
26	Arizona	7.8
26	Virginia	7.8
28	Delaware	7.7
29	Texas	7.5
29	Wisconsin	7.5
31	Idaho	7.3
31	Minnesota	7.3
33	North Dakota	7.1
34	Colorado	6.9
34	Rhode Island	6.9
34	West Virginia	6.9
37	Oregon	6.7
38	California	6.6
39	Hawaii	6.5
40	Iowa	6.4
41	New Hampshire	6.2
42	Nevada	5.9
42	Wyoming	5.9
44	Maine	5.8
44	Washington	5.8
46	Utah	5.4
47	Massachusetts	5.0
48	Vermont	4.6
NA	Alaska**	NA
NA	Connecticut**	NA

| | District of Columbia | 16.8 |

Source: U.S. Department of Health and Human Services, National Center for Health Statistics
   "Monthly Vital Statistics Report" (Vol. 43, No. 7, December 19, 1994)
For 12 months ending July 1994. Provisional data. Deaths under 1 year old by state of residence. Total includes states not shown separately.
**Not available.*

Infant Deaths in 1993

National Total = 33,300 Infant Deaths*

ALPHA ORDER

RANK ORDER

RANK	STATE	DEATHS	% of USA		RANK	STATE	DEATHS	% of USA
18	Alabama	629	1.89%		1	California	3,925	11.79%
46	Alaska	79	0.24%		2	Texas	2,510	7.54%
22	Arizona	497	1.49%		3	New York	2,312	6.94%
30	Arkansas	324	0.97%		4	Illinois	1,975	5.93%
1	California	3,925	11.79%		5	Florida	1,674	5.03%
28	Colorado	413	1.24%		6	Ohio	1,386	4.16%
29	Connecticut	327	0.98%		7	Pennsylvania	1,381	4.15%
45	Delaware	88	0.26%		8	Michigan	1,338	4.02%
5	Florida	1,674	5.03%		9	Georgia	1,140	3.42%
9	Georgia	1,140	3.42%		10	North Carolina	1,032	3.10%
39	Hawaii	132	0.40%		11	New Jersey	980	2.94%
40	Idaho	128	0.38%		12	Virginia	812	2.44%
4	Illinois	1,975	5.93%		13	Indiana	790	2.37%
13	Indiana	790	2.37%		14	Tennessee	726	2.18%
33	Iowa	257	0.77%		15	Maryland	709	2.13%
31	Kansas	312	0.94%		16	Louisiana	686	2.06%
26	Kentucky	462	1.39%		17	Missouri	656	1.97%
16	Louisiana	686	2.06%		18	Alabama	629	1.89%
43	Maine	99	0.30%		19	Wisconsin	557	1.67%
15	Maryland	709	2.13%		20	South Carolina	510	1.53%
24	Massachusetts	484	1.45%		21	Mississippi	501	1.50%
8	Michigan	1,338	4.02%		22	Arizona	497	1.49%
25	Minnesota	464	1.39%		23	Washington	494	1.48%
21	Mississippi	501	1.50%		24	Massachusetts	484	1.45%
17	Missouri	656	1.97%		25	Minnesota	464	1.39%
44	Montana	91	0.27%		26	Kentucky	462	1.39%
37	Nebraska	202	0.61%		27	Oklahoma	430	1.29%
38	Nevada	140	0.42%		28	Colorado	413	1.24%
47	New Hampshire	72	0.22%		29	Connecticut	327	0.98%
11	New Jersey	980	2.94%		30	Arkansas	324	0.97%
34	New Mexico	256	0.77%		31	Kansas	312	0.94%
3	New York	2,312	6.94%		32	Oregon	282	0.85%
10	North Carolina	1,032	3.10%		33	Iowa	257	0.77%
48	North Dakota	62	0.19%		34	New Mexico	256	0.77%
6	Ohio	1,386	4.16%		35	Utah	217	0.65%
27	Oklahoma	430	1.29%		36	West Virginia	204	0.61%
32	Oregon	282	0.85%		37	Nebraska	202	0.61%
7	Pennsylvania	1,381	4.15%		38	Nevada	140	0.42%
41	Rhode Island	121	0.36%		39	Hawaii	132	0.40%
20	South Carolina	510	1.53%		40	Idaho	128	0.38%
42	South Dakota	114	0.34%		41	Rhode Island	121	0.36%
14	Tennessee	726	2.18%		42	South Dakota	114	0.34%
2	Texas	2,510	7.54%		43	Maine	99	0.30%
35	Utah	217	0.65%		44	Montana	91	0.27%
50	Vermont	36	0.11%		45	Delaware	88	0.26%
12	Virginia	812	2.44%		46	Alaska	79	0.24%
23	Washington	494	1.48%		47	New Hampshire	72	0.22%
36	West Virginia	204	0.61%		48	North Dakota	62	0.19%
19	Wisconsin	557	1.67%		49	Wyoming	54	0.16%
49	Wyoming	54	0.16%		50	Vermont	36	0.11%
						District of Columbia	181	0.54%

Source: U.S. Department of Health and Human Services, National Center for Health Statistics
   "Monthly Vital Statistics Report" (Vol. 42, No. 13, October 11, 1994)
*Provisional data. Deaths under 1 year old by state of residence.

Infant Mortality Rate in 1993

National Rate = 8.3 Infant Deaths per 1,000 Live Births*

ALPHA ORDER			RANK ORDER		
RANK	STATE	RATE	RANK	STATE	RATE
6	Alabama	9.9	1	Mississippi	11.9
33	Alaska	7.5	2	South Dakota	10.5
39	Arizona	7.0	3	Illinois	10.3
9	Arkansas	9.5	3	North Carolina	10.3
42	California	6.7	5	Georgia	10.1
33	Colorado	7.5	6	Alabama	9.9
37	Connecticut	7.1	6	Tennessee	9.9
25	Delaware	8.3	8	Louisiana	9.8
20	Florida	8.7	9	Arkansas	9.5
5	Georgia	10.1	10	Maryland	9.4
42	Hawaii	6.7	10	South Carolina	9.4
33	Idaho	7.5	12	Indiana	9.3
3	Illinois	10.3	12	Michigan	9.3
12	Indiana	9.3	12	New Mexico	9.3
40	Iowa	6.9	12	West Virginia	9.3
27	Kansas	8.2	16	Oklahoma	9.2
17	Kentucky	8.8	17	Kentucky	8.8
8	Louisiana	9.8	17	Nebraska	8.8
45	Maine	6.6	17	Ohio	8.8
10	Maryland	9.4	20	Florida	8.7
48	Massachusetts	5.6	20	Pennsylvania	8.7
12	Michigan	9.3	22	Missouri	8.5
36	Minnesota	7.3	22	Rhode Island	8.5
1	Mississippi	11.9	22	Virginia	8.5
22	Missouri	8.5	25	Delaware	8.3
31	Montana	7.9	25	New York	8.3
17	Nebraska	8.8	27	Kansas	8.2
45	Nevada	6.6	28	Wyoming	8.1
50	New Hampshire	4.8	29	New Jersey	8.0
29	New Jersey	8.0	29	Wisconsin	8.0
12	New Mexico	9.3	31	Montana	7.9
25	New York	8.3	32	Texas	7.6
3	North Carolina	10.3	33	Alaska	7.5
37	North Dakota	7.1	33	Colorado	7.5
17	Ohio	8.8	33	Idaho	7.5
16	Oklahoma	9.2	36	Minnesota	7.3
42	Oregon	6.7	37	Connecticut	7.1
20	Pennsylvania	8.7	37	North Dakota	7.1
22	Rhode Island	8.5	39	Arizona	7.0
10	South Carolina	9.4	40	Iowa	6.9
2	South Dakota	10.5	40	Washington	6.9
6	Tennessee	9.9	42	California	6.7
32	Texas	7.6	42	Hawaii	6.7
47	Utah	6.0	42	Oregon	6.7
49	Vermont	4.9	45	Maine	6.6
22	Virginia	8.5	45	Nevada	6.6
40	Washington	6.9	47	Utah	6.0
12	West Virginia	9.3	48	Massachusetts	5.6
29	Wisconsin	8.0	49	Vermont	4.9
28	Wyoming	8.1	50	New Hampshire	4.8
				District of Columbia	18.5

Source: U.S. Department of Health and Human Services, National Center for Health Statistics
   "Monthly Vital Statistics Report" (Vol. 42, No. 13, October 11, 1994)
*Provisional data. Deaths under 1 year old by state of residence.

Infant Deaths in 1990

National Total = 38,351 Infant Deaths*

ALPHA ORDER

RANK ORDER

RANK	STATE	DEATHS	% of USA		RANK	STATE	DEATHS	% of USA
18	Alabama	688	1.79%		1	California	4,844	12.63%
41	Alaska	125	0.33%		2	New York	2,851	7.43%
22	Arizona	610	1.59%		3	Texas	2,552	6.65%
31	Arkansas	336	0.88%		4	Illinois	2,104	5.49%
1	California	4,844	12.63%		5	Florida	1,918	5.00%
26	Colorado	472	1.23%		6	Pennsylvania	1,643	4.28%
29	Connecticut	398	1.04%		7	Michigan	1,641	4.28%
44	Delaware	112	0.29%		8	Ohio	1,640	4.28%
5	Florida	1,918	5.00%		9	Georgia	1,392	3.63%
9	Georgia	1,392	3.63%		10	North Carolina	1,109	2.89%
40	Hawaii	138	0.36%		11	New Jersey	1,102	2.87%
39	Idaho	143	0.37%		12	Virginia	1,013	2.64%
4	Illinois	2,104	5.49%		13	Indiana	831	2.17%
13	Indiana	831	2.17%		14	Louisiana	799	2.08%
33	Iowa	319	0.83%		15	Tennessee	771	2.01%
32	Kansas	329	0.86%		16	Maryland	766	2.00%
27	Kentucky	461	1.20%		17	Missouri	748	1.95%
14	Louisiana	799	2.08%		18	Alabama	688	1.79%
46	Maine	108	0.28%		19	South Carolina	683	1.78%
16	Maryland	766	2.00%		20	Massachusetts	650	1.69%
20	Massachusetts	650	1.69%		21	Washington	621	1.62%
7	Michigan	1,641	4.28%		22	Arizona	610	1.59%
25	Minnesota	496	1.29%		23	Wisconsin	598	1.56%
24	Mississippi	529	1.38%		24	Mississippi	529	1.38%
17	Missouri	748	1.95%		25	Minnesota	496	1.29%
47	Montana	105	0.27%		26	Colorado	472	1.23%
37	Nebraska	202	0.53%		27	Kentucky	461	1.20%
38	Nevada	181	0.47%		28	Oklahoma	438	1.14%
41	New Hampshire	125	0.33%		29	Connecticut	398	1.04%
11	New Jersey	1,102	2.87%		30	Oregon	354	0.92%
35	New Mexico	246	0.64%		31	Arkansas	336	0.88%
2	New York	2,851	7.43%		32	Kansas	329	0.86%
10	North Carolina	1,109	2.89%		33	Iowa	319	0.83%
48	North Dakota	74	0.19%		34	Utah	271	0.71%
8	Ohio	1,640	4.28%		35	New Mexico	246	0.64%
28	Oklahoma	438	1.14%		36	West Virginia	223	0.58%
30	Oregon	354	0.92%		37	Nebraska	202	0.53%
6	Pennsylvania	1,643	4.28%		38	Nevada	181	0.47%
43	Rhode Island	123	0.32%		39	Idaho	143	0.37%
19	South Carolina	683	1.78%		40	Hawaii	138	0.36%
45	South Dakota	111	0.29%		41	Alaska	125	0.33%
15	Tennessee	771	2.01%		41	New Hampshire	125	0.33%
3	Texas	2,552	6.65%		43	Rhode Island	123	0.32%
34	Utah	271	0.71%		44	Delaware	112	0.29%
50	Vermont	53	0.14%		45	South Dakota	111	0.29%
12	Virginia	1,013	2.64%		46	Maine	108	0.28%
21	Washington	621	1.62%		47	Montana	105	0.27%
36	West Virginia	223	0.58%		48	North Dakota	74	0.19%
23	Wisconsin	598	1.56%		49	Wyoming	60	0.16%
49	Wyoming	60	0.16%		50	Vermont	53	0.14%
					District of Columbia	245	0.64%

Source: U.S. Department of Health and Human Services, National Center for Health Statistics
"Monthly Vital Statistics Report" (Vol. 41, No. 7(S), January 7, 1993)
*Final data by state of residence. Infant deaths are those under 1 year old.

Infant Mortality Rate in 1990

National Rate = 9.22 Infant Deaths per 1,000 Live Births*

ALPHA ORDER

RANK	STATE	RATE
5	Alabama	10.84
9	Alaska	10.50
27	Arizona	8.84
22	Arkansas	9.22
42	California	7.91
28	Colorado	8.82
41	Connecticut	7.94
13	Delaware	10.08
17	Florida	9.62
1	Georgia	12.36
48	Hawaii	6.74
29	Idaho	8.70
6	Illinois	10.75
16	Indiana	9.64
37	Iowa	8.09
32	Kansas	8.43
31	Kentucky	8.48
4	Louisiana	11.07
50	Maine	6.22
19	Maryland	9.55
47	Massachusetts	7.02
7	Michigan	10.68
45	Minnesota	7.29
2	Mississippi	12.14
21	Missouri	9.44
24	Montana	9.04
34	Nebraska	8.29
33	Nevada	8.38
46	New Hampshire	7.11
25	New Jersey	9.01
26	New Mexico	8.98
18	New York	9.58
8	North Carolina	10.61
40	North Dakota	8.00
15	Ohio	9.83
23	Oklahoma	9.19
35	Oregon	8.25
19	Pennsylvania	9.55
37	Rhode Island	8.09
3	South Carolina	11.65
12	South Dakota	10.09
10	Tennessee	10.29
39	Texas	8.07
44	Utah	7.47
49	Vermont	6.41
11	Virginia	10.20
43	Washington	7.84
14	West Virginia	9.87
36	Wisconsin	8.20
30	Wyoming	8.59

RANK ORDER

RANK	STATE	RATE
1	Georgia	12.36
2	Mississippi	12.14
3	South Carolina	11.65
4	Louisiana	11.07
5	Alabama	10.84
6	Illinois	10.75
7	Michigan	10.68
8	North Carolina	10.61
9	Alaska	10.50
10	Tennessee	10.29
11	Virginia	10.20
12	South Dakota	10.09
13	Delaware	10.08
14	West Virginia	9.87
15	Ohio	9.83
16	Indiana	9.64
17	Florida	9.62
18	New York	9.58
19	Maryland	9.55
19	Pennsylvania	9.55
21	Missouri	9.44
22	Arkansas	9.22
23	Oklahoma	9.19
24	Montana	9.04
25	New Jersey	9.01
26	New Mexico	8.98
27	Arizona	8.84
28	Colorado	8.82
29	Idaho	8.70
30	Wyoming	8.59
31	Kentucky	8.48
32	Kansas	8.43
33	Nevada	8.38
34	Nebraska	8.29
35	Oregon	8.25
36	Wisconsin	8.20
37	Iowa	8.09
37	Rhode Island	8.09
39	Texas	8.07
40	North Dakota	8.00
41	Connecticut	7.94
42	California	7.91
43	Washington	7.84
44	Utah	7.47
45	Minnesota	7.29
46	New Hampshire	7.11
47	Massachusetts	7.02
48	Hawaii	6.74
49	Vermont	6.41
50	Maine	6.22
	District of Columbia	20.68

Source: U.S. Department of Health and Human Services, National Center for Health Statistics
"Monthly Vital Statistics Report" (Vol. 41, No. 7(S), January 7, 1993)
*Final data by state of residence. Infant deaths are those under 1 year old.

Infant Deaths in 1980

National Total = 45,526 Infant Deaths*

ALPHA ORDER					RANK ORDER			
RANK	STATE		DEATHS	% of USA	RANK	STATE	DEATHS	% of USA
16	Alabama		962	2.11%	1	California	4,454	9.78%
48	Alaska		117	0.26%	2	Texas	3,326	7.31%
27	Arizona		620	1.36%	3	New York	2,994	6.58%
31	Arkansas		472	1.04%	4	Illinois	2,812	6.18%
1	California		4,454	9.78%	5	Ohio	2,160	4.74%
30	Colorado		501	1.10%	6	Pennsylvania	2,101	4.61%
33	Connecticut		433	0.95%	7	Florida	1,921	4.22%
47	Delaware		131	0.29%	8	Michigan	1,862	4.09%
7	Florida		1,921	4.22%	9	Georgia	1,337	2.94%
9	Georgia		1,337	2.94%	10	North Carolina	1,224	2.69%
39	Hawaii		187	0.41%	11	New Jersey	1,215	2.67%
38	Idaho		216	0.47%	12	Louisiana	1,178	2.59%
4	Illinois		2,812	6.18%	13	Virginia	1,067	2.34%
14	Indiana		1,050	2.31%	14	Indiana	1,050	2.31%
28	Iowa		565	1.24%	15	Missouri	980	2.15%
34	Kansas		424	0.93%	16	Alabama	962	2.11%
23	Kentucky		766	1.68%	17	Tennessee	935	2.05%
12	Louisiana		1,178	2.59%	18	Maryland	842	1.85%
41	Maine		152	0.33%	19	Mississippi	814	1.79%
18	Maryland		842	1.85%	20	South Carolina	812	1.78%
24	Massachusetts		763	1.68%	21	Washington	798	1.75%
8	Michigan		1,862	4.09%	22	Wisconsin	770	1.69%
25	Minnesota		678	1.49%	23	Kentucky	766	1.68%
19	Mississippi		814	1.79%	24	Massachusetts	763	1.68%
15	Missouri		980	2.15%	25	Minnesota	678	1.49%
40	Montana		176	0.39%	26	Oklahoma	663	1.46%
36	Nebraska		314	0.69%	27	Arizona	620	1.36%
44	Nevada		143	0.31%	28	Iowa	565	1.24%
45	New Hampshire		136	0.30%	29	Oregon	525	1.15%
11	New Jersey		1,215	2.67%	30	Colorado	501	1.10%
37	New Mexico		301	0.66%	31	Arkansas	472	1.04%
3	New York		2,994	6.58%	32	Utah	436	0.96%
10	North Carolina		1,224	2.69%	33	Connecticut	433	0.95%
42	North Dakota		145	0.32%	34	Kansas	424	0.93%
5	Ohio		2,160	4.74%	35	West Virginia	348	0.76%
26	Oklahoma		663	1.46%	36	Nebraska	314	0.69%
29	Oregon		525	1.15%	37	New Mexico	301	0.66%
6	Pennsylvania		2,101	4.61%	38	Idaho	216	0.47%
46	Rhode Island		134	0.29%	39	Hawaii	187	0.41%
20	South Carolina		812	1.78%	40	Montana	176	0.39%
42	South Dakota		145	0.32%	41	Maine	152	0.33%
17	Tennessee		935	2.05%	42	North Dakota	145	0.32%
2	Texas		3,326	7.31%	42	South Dakota	145	0.32%
32	Utah		436	0.96%	44	Nevada	143	0.31%
50	Vermont		84	0.18%	45	New Hampshire	136	0.30%
13	Virginia		1,067	2.34%	46	Rhode Island	134	0.29%
21	Washington		798	1.75%	47	Delaware	131	0.29%
35	West Virginia		348	0.76%	48	Alaska	117	0.26%
22	Wisconsin		770	1.69%	49	Wyoming	103	0.23%
49	Wyoming		103	0.23%	50	Vermont	84	0.18%
						District of Columbia	234	0.51%

Source: U.S. Department of Health and Human Services, National Center for Health Statistics
"Monthly Vital Statistics Report"
*Final data by state of residence. Deaths under 1 year old, exclusive of fetal deaths.

Infant Mortality Rate in 1980

National Rate = 12.60 Infant Deaths per 1,000 Live Births*

ALPHA ORDER

RANK ORDER

RANK	STATE	RATE		RANK	STATE	RATE
3	Alabama	15.15		1	Mississippi	17.01
24	Alaska	12.28		2	South Carolina	15.62
22	Arizona	12.39		3	Alabama	15.15
18	Arkansas	12.66		4	Illinois	14.80
35	California	11.05		5	Florida	14.58
46	Colorado	10.07		6	North Carolina	14.49
34	Connecticut	11.17		7	Georgia	14.48
10	Delaware	13.92		8	Louisiana	14.34
5	Florida	14.58		9	Maryland	14.05
7	Georgia	14.48		10	Delaware	13.92
44	Hawaii	10.30		11	Virginia	13.60
39	Idaho	10.71		12	Tennessee	13.51
4	Illinois	14.80		13	Pennsylvania	13.23
28	Indiana	11.87		14	Kentucky	12.86
29	Iowa	11.82		15	Michigan	12.80
43	Kansas	10.41		16	Ohio	12.77
14	Kentucky	12.86		17	Oklahoma	12.72
8	Louisiana	14.34		18	Arkansas	12.66
50	Maine	9.23		19	New Jersey	12.54
9	Maryland	14.05		20	New York	12.53
41	Massachusetts	10.51		21	Missouri	12.42
15	Michigan	12.80		22	Arizona	12.39
47	Minnesota	10.00		22	Montana	12.39
1	Mississippi	17.01		24	Alaska	12.28
21	Missouri	12.42		25	Oregon	12.17
22	Montana	12.39		26	Texas	12.16
33	Nebraska	11.48		27	North Dakota	12.10
38	Nevada	10.74		28	Indiana	11.87
48	New Hampshire	9.89		29	Iowa	11.82
19	New Jersey	12.54		30	West Virginia	11.81
32	New Mexico	11.53		31	Washington	11.76
20	New York	12.53		32	New Mexico	11.53
6	North Carolina	14.49		33	Nebraska	11.48
27	North Dakota	12.10		34	Connecticut	11.17
16	Ohio	12.77		35	California	11.05
17	Oklahoma	12.72		36	Rhode Island	10.99
25	Oregon	12.17		37	South Dakota	10.92
13	Pennsylvania	13.23		38	Nevada	10.74
36	Rhode Island	10.99		39	Idaho	10.71
2	South Carolina	15.62		40	Vermont	10.65
37	South Dakota	10.92		41	Massachusetts	10.51
12	Tennessee	13.51		42	Utah	10.43
26	Texas	12.16		43	Kansas	10.41
42	Utah	10.43		44	Hawaii	10.30
40	Vermont	10.65		45	Wisconsin	10.29
11	Virginia	13.60		46	Colorado	10.07
31	Washington	11.76		47	Minnesota	10.00
30	West Virginia	11.81		48	New Hampshire	9.89
45	Wisconsin	10.29		49	Wyoming	9.75
49	Wyoming	9.75		50	Maine	9.23
					District of Columbia	25.00

Source: U.S. Department of Health and Human Services, National Center for Health Statistics
"Monthly Vital Statistics Report"

*Final data by state of residence. Deaths under 1 year old, exclusive of fetal deaths.

Percent Change in Infant Mortality Rate: 1980 to 1990

National Percent Change = 26.83% Decrease in Infant Mortality Rate*

<table>
<tr><td colspan="3">ALPHA ORDER</td><td colspan="3">RANK ORDER</td></tr>
<tr><th>RANK</th><th>STATE</th><th>RATE</th><th>RANK</th><th>STATE</th><th>RATE</th></tr>
<tr><td>35</td><td>Alabama</td><td>(28.45)</td><td>1</td><td>South Dakota</td><td>(7.60)</td></tr>
<tr><td>4</td><td>Alaska</td><td>(14.50)</td><td>2</td><td>Wyoming</td><td>(11.90)</td></tr>
<tr><td>37</td><td>Arizona</td><td>(28.65)</td><td>3</td><td>Colorado</td><td>(12.41)</td></tr>
<tr><td>25</td><td>Arkansas</td><td>(27.17)</td><td>4</td><td>Alaska</td><td>(14.50)</td></tr>
<tr><td>34</td><td>California</td><td>(28.42)</td><td>5</td><td>Georgia</td><td>(14.64)</td></tr>
<tr><td>3</td><td>Colorado</td><td>(12.41)</td><td>6</td><td>West Virginia</td><td>(16.43)</td></tr>
<tr><td>38</td><td>Connecticut</td><td>(28.92)</td><td>7</td><td>Michigan</td><td>(16.56)</td></tr>
<tr><td>27</td><td>Delaware</td><td>(27.59)</td><td>8</td><td>Idaho</td><td>(18.77)</td></tr>
<tr><td>47</td><td>Florida</td><td>(34.02)</td><td>9</td><td>Indiana</td><td>(18.79)</td></tr>
<tr><td>5</td><td>Georgia</td><td>(14.64)</td><td>10</td><td>Kansas</td><td>(19.02)</td></tr>
<tr><td>49</td><td>Hawaii</td><td>(34.56)</td><td>11</td><td>Wisconsin</td><td>(20.31)</td></tr>
<tr><td>8</td><td>Idaho</td><td>(18.77)</td><td>12</td><td>Nevada</td><td>(21.97)</td></tr>
<tr><td>26</td><td>Illinois</td><td>(27.36)</td><td>13</td><td>New Mexico</td><td>(22.12)</td></tr>
<tr><td>9</td><td>Indiana</td><td>(18.79)</td><td>14</td><td>Louisiana</td><td>(22.80)</td></tr>
<tr><td>39</td><td>Iowa</td><td>(31.56)</td><td>15</td><td>Ohio</td><td>(23.02)</td></tr>
<tr><td>10</td><td>Kansas</td><td>(19.02)</td><td>16</td><td>New York</td><td>(23.54)</td></tr>
<tr><td>48</td><td>Kentucky</td><td>(34.06)</td><td>17</td><td>Tennessee</td><td>(23.83)</td></tr>
<tr><td>14</td><td>Louisiana</td><td>(22.80)</td><td>18</td><td>Missouri</td><td>(23.99)</td></tr>
<tr><td>42</td><td>Maine</td><td>(32.61)</td><td>19</td><td>Virginia</td><td>(25.00)</td></tr>
<tr><td>40</td><td>Maryland</td><td>(32.03)</td><td>20</td><td>South Carolina</td><td>(25.42)</td></tr>
<tr><td>43</td><td>Massachusetts</td><td>(33.21)</td><td>21</td><td>Rhode Island</td><td>(26.39)</td></tr>
<tr><td>7</td><td>Michigan</td><td>(16.56)</td><td>22</td><td>North Carolina</td><td>(26.78)</td></tr>
<tr><td>24</td><td>Minnesota</td><td>(27.10)</td><td>23</td><td>Montana</td><td>(27.04)</td></tr>
<tr><td>36</td><td>Mississippi</td><td>(28.63)</td><td>24</td><td>Minnesota</td><td>(27.10)</td></tr>
<tr><td>18</td><td>Missouri</td><td>(23.99)</td><td>25</td><td>Arkansas</td><td>(27.17)</td></tr>
<tr><td>23</td><td>Montana</td><td>(27.04)</td><td>26</td><td>Illinois</td><td>(27.36)</td></tr>
<tr><td>29</td><td>Nebraska</td><td>(27.79)</td><td>27</td><td>Delaware</td><td>(27.59)</td></tr>
<tr><td>12</td><td>Nevada</td><td>(21.97)</td><td>28</td><td>Oklahoma</td><td>(27.75)</td></tr>
<tr><td>31</td><td>New Hampshire</td><td>(28.11)</td><td>29</td><td>Nebraska</td><td>(27.79)</td></tr>
<tr><td>32</td><td>New Jersey</td><td>(28.15)</td><td>30</td><td>Pennsylvania</td><td>(27.82)</td></tr>
<tr><td>13</td><td>New Mexico</td><td>(22.12)</td><td>31</td><td>New Hampshire</td><td>(28.11)</td></tr>
<tr><td>16</td><td>New York</td><td>(23.54)</td><td>32</td><td>New Jersey</td><td>(28.15)</td></tr>
<tr><td>22</td><td>North Carolina</td><td>(26.78)</td><td>33</td><td>Utah</td><td>(28.38)</td></tr>
<tr><td>46</td><td>North Dakota</td><td>(33.88)</td><td>34</td><td>California</td><td>(28.42)</td></tr>
<tr><td>15</td><td>Ohio</td><td>(23.02)</td><td>35</td><td>Alabama</td><td>(28.45)</td></tr>
<tr><td>28</td><td>Oklahoma</td><td>(27.75)</td><td>36</td><td>Mississippi</td><td>(28.63)</td></tr>
<tr><td>41</td><td>Oregon</td><td>(32.21)</td><td>37</td><td>Arizona</td><td>(28.65)</td></tr>
<tr><td>30</td><td>Pennsylvania</td><td>(27.82)</td><td>38</td><td>Connecticut</td><td>(28.92)</td></tr>
<tr><td>21</td><td>Rhode Island</td><td>(26.39)</td><td>39</td><td>Iowa</td><td>(31.56)</td></tr>
<tr><td>20</td><td>South Carolina</td><td>(25.42)</td><td>40</td><td>Maryland</td><td>(32.03)</td></tr>
<tr><td>1</td><td>South Dakota</td><td>(7.60)</td><td>41</td><td>Oregon</td><td>(32.21)</td></tr>
<tr><td>17</td><td>Tennessee</td><td>(23.83)</td><td>42</td><td>Maine</td><td>(32.61)</td></tr>
<tr><td>45</td><td>Texas</td><td>(33.63)</td><td>43</td><td>Massachusetts</td><td>(33.21)</td></tr>
<tr><td>33</td><td>Utah</td><td>(28.38)</td><td>44</td><td>Washington</td><td>(33.33)</td></tr>
<tr><td>50</td><td>Vermont</td><td>(39.81)</td><td>45</td><td>Texas</td><td>(33.63)</td></tr>
<tr><td>19</td><td>Virginia</td><td>(25.00)</td><td>46</td><td>North Dakota</td><td>(33.88)</td></tr>
<tr><td>44</td><td>Washington</td><td>(33.33)</td><td>47</td><td>Florida</td><td>(34.02)</td></tr>
<tr><td>6</td><td>West Virginia</td><td>(16.43)</td><td>48</td><td>Kentucky</td><td>(34.06)</td></tr>
<tr><td>11</td><td>Wisconsin</td><td>(20.31)</td><td>49</td><td>Hawaii</td><td>(34.56)</td></tr>
<tr><td>2</td><td>Wyoming</td><td>(11.90)</td><td>50</td><td>Vermont</td><td>(39.81)</td></tr>
<tr><td></td><td></td><td></td><td></td><td>District of Columbia</td><td>(17.28)</td></tr>
</table>

Source: Morgan Quitno Press using data from US Dept of Health & Human Services, National Center for Health Statistics
"Monthly Vital Statistics Report" (Vol. 41, No. 7(S), January 7, 1993)
"Vital Statistics of the United States, 1980" (Vol. I–Natality, issued 1984) and unpublished data
*Final data by state of residence. Infant deaths are those occurring under 1 year, exclusive of fetal deaths.

White Infant Deaths in 1992

National Total = 22,164 White Infant Deaths*

ALPHA ORDER

RANK	STATE	DEATHS	% of USA
24	Alabama	306	1.38%
45	Alaska	58	0.26%
14	Arizona	465	2.10%
32	Arkansas	227	1.02%
1	California	3,119	14.07%
22	Colorado	356	1.61%
30	Connecticut	251	1.13%
49	Delaware	46	0.21%
6	Florida	999	4.51%
12	Georgia	491	2.22%
50	Hawaii	18	0.08%
37	Idaho	148	0.67%
5	Illinois	1,052	4.75%
9	Indiana	594	2.68%
26	Iowa	280	1.26%
29	Kansas	252	1.14%
20	Kentucky	381	1.72%
27	Louisiana	275	1.24%
42	Maine	87	0.39%
23	Maryland	332	1.50%
16	Massachusetts	435	1.96%
8	Michigan	783	3.53%
21	Minnesota	369	1.66%
35	Mississippi	173	0.78%
17	Missouri	429	1.94%
44	Montana	67	0.30%
38	Nebraska	143	0.65%
39	Nevada	111	0.50%
40	New Hampshire	91	0.41%
10	New Jersey	535	2.41%
36	New Mexico	157	0.71%
3	New York	1,510	6.81%
11	North Carolina	514	2.32%
45	North Dakota	58	0.26%
4	Ohio	1,056	4.76%
25	Oklahoma	293	1.32%
28	Oregon	266	1.20%
7	Pennsylvania	943	4.25%
41	Rhode Island	88	0.40%
31	South Carolina	241	1.09%
43	South Dakota	70	0.32%
19	Tennessee	386	1.74%
2	Texas	1,850	8.35%
33	Utah	213	0.96%
48	Vermont	56	0.25%
13	Virginia	485	2.19%
15	Washington	448	2.02%
34	West Virginia	190	0.86%
18	Wisconsin	389	1.76%
47	Wyoming	57	0.26%

RANK ORDER

RANK	STATE	DEATHS	% of USA
1	California	3,119	14.07%
2	Texas	1,850	8.35%
3	New York	1,510	6.81%
4	Ohio	1,056	4.76%
5	Illinois	1,052	4.75%
6	Florida	999	4.51%
7	Pennsylvania	943	4.25%
8	Michigan	783	3.53%
9	Indiana	594	2.68%
10	New Jersey	535	2.41%
11	North Carolina	514	2.32%
12	Georgia	491	2.22%
13	Virginia	485	2.19%
14	Arizona	465	2.10%
15	Washington	448	2.02%
16	Massachusetts	435	1.96%
17	Missouri	429	1.94%
18	Wisconsin	389	1.76%
19	Tennessee	386	1.74%
20	Kentucky	381	1.72%
21	Minnesota	369	1.66%
22	Colorado	356	1.61%
23	Maryland	332	1.50%
24	Alabama	306	1.38%
25	Oklahoma	293	1.32%
26	Iowa	280	1.26%
27	Louisiana	275	1.24%
28	Oregon	266	1.20%
29	Kansas	252	1.14%
30	Connecticut	251	1.13%
31	South Carolina	241	1.09%
32	Arkansas	227	1.02%
33	Utah	213	0.96%
34	West Virginia	190	0.86%
35	Mississippi	173	0.78%
36	New Mexico	157	0.71%
37	Idaho	148	0.67%
38	Nebraska	143	0.65%
39	Nevada	111	0.50%
40	New Hampshire	91	0.41%
41	Rhode Island	88	0.40%
42	Maine	87	0.39%
43	South Dakota	70	0.32%
44	Montana	67	0.30%
45	Alaska	58	0.26%
45	North Dakota	58	0.26%
47	Wyoming	57	0.26%
48	Vermont	56	0.25%
49	Delaware	46	0.21%
50	Hawaii	18	0.08%
	District of Columbia	21	0.09%

Source: U.S. Department of Health and Human Services, National Center for Health Statistics
  "Monthly Vital Statistics Report" (Vol. 43, No. 6(S), December 8, 1994)
*Final data. Deaths of infants under 1 year old, exclusive of fetal deaths. Based on race of the mother.

White Infant Mortality Rate in 1992

National Rate = 6.9 White Infant Deaths per 1,000 White Live Births*

ALPHA ORDER			RANK ORDER		
RANK	STATE	RATE	RANK	STATE	RATE
13	Alabama	7.6	1	Wyoming	9.0
17	Alaska	7.3	2	West Virginia	8.9
10	Arizona	7.8	3	Idaho	8.8
4	Arkansas	8.6	4	Arkansas	8.6
40	California	6.3	5	Indiana	8.0
20	Colorado	7.2	5	Mississippi	8.0
41	Connecticut	6.2	7	Kentucky	7.9
46	Delaware	5.8	7	Ohio	7.9
24	Florida	7.0	7	Oklahoma	7.9
21	Georgia	7.1	10	Arizona	7.8
50	Hawaii**	3.1	11	Iowa	7.7
3	Idaho	8.8	11	South Dakota	7.7
15	Illinois	7.4	13	Alabama	7.6
5	Indiana	8.0	14	Kansas	7.5
11	Iowa	7.7	15	Illinois	7.4
14	Kansas	7.5	15	North Dakota	7.4
7	Kentucky	7.9	17	Alaska	7.3
27	Louisiana	6.9	17	North Carolina	7.3
49	Maine	5.5	17	Vermont	7.3
35	Maryland	6.7	20	Colorado	7.2
46	Massachusetts	5.8	21	Georgia	7.1
24	Michigan	7.0	21	New York	7.1
41	Minnesota	6.2	21	South Carolina	7.1
5	Mississippi	8.0	24	Florida	7.0
27	Missouri	6.9	24	Michigan	7.0
35	Montana	6.7	24	Tennessee	7.0
35	Nebraska	6.7	27	Louisiana	6.9
44	Nevada	5.9	27	Missouri	6.9
46	New Hampshire	5.8	27	Pennsylvania	6.9
44	New Jersey	5.9	27	Rhode Island	6.9
32	New Mexico	6.8	27	Virginia	6.9
21	New York	7.1	32	New Mexico	6.8
17	North Carolina	7.3	32	Oregon	6.8
15	North Dakota	7.4	32	Texas	6.8
7	Ohio	7.9	35	Maryland	6.7
7	Oklahoma	7.9	35	Montana	6.7
32	Oregon	6.8	35	Nebraska	6.7
27	Pennsylvania	6.9	38	Washington	6.4
27	Rhode Island	6.9	38	Wisconsin	6.4
21	South Carolina	7.1	40	California	6.3
11	South Dakota	7.7	41	Connecticut	6.2
24	Tennessee	7.0	41	Minnesota	6.2
32	Texas	6.8	43	Utah	6.0
43	Utah	6.0	44	Nevada	5.9
17	Vermont	7.3	44	New Jersey	5.9
27	Virginia	6.9	46	Delaware	5.8
38	Washington	6.4	46	Massachusetts	5.8
2	West Virginia	8.9	46	New Hampshire	5.8
38	Wisconsin	6.4	49	Maine	5.5
1	Wyoming	9.0	50	Hawaii**	3.1

District of Columbia	13.1

Source: U.S. Department of Health and Human Services, National Center for Health Statistics
"Monthly Vital Statistics Report" (Vol. 43, No. 6(S), December 8, 1994)
*Final data. Deaths of infants under 1 year old, exclusive of fetal deaths. Based on race of the mother.
**Calculated by Morgan Quitno Press. Based on fewer than 20 white infant deaths.

Black Infant Deaths in 1992

National Total = 11,348 Black Infant Deaths*

ALPHA ORDER

RANK ORDER

RANK	STATE	DEATHS	% of USA	RANK	STATE	DEATHS	% of USA
15	Alabama	349	3.08%	1	New York	961	8.47%
40	Alaska	7	0.06%	2	Illinois	849	7.48%
32	Arizona	41	0.36%	3	California	782	6.89%
21	Arkansas	132	1.16%	4	Florida	681	6.00%
3	California	782	6.89%	5	Michigan	657	5.79%
31	Colorado	44	0.39%	6	Georgia	644	5.68%
23	Connecticut	106	0.93%	7	Texas	612	5.39%
30	Delaware	46	0.41%	8	Pennsylvania	519	4.57%
4	Florida	681	6.00%	9	North Carolina	499	4.40%
6	Georgia	644	5.68%	10	Ohio	467	4.12%
41	Hawaii	6	0.05%	11	New Jersey	438	3.86%
42	Idaho	3	0.03%	12	Virginia	422	3.72%
2	Illinois	849	7.48%	13	Maryland	419	3.69%
20	Indiana	191	1.68%	14	Louisiana	389	3.43%
35	Iowa	23	0.20%	15	Alabama	349	3.08%
26	Kansas	72	0.63%	16	South Carolina	345	3.04%
27	Kentucky	66	0.58%	17	Mississippi	330	2.91%
14	Louisiana	389	3.43%	18	Tennessee	305	2.69%
46	Maine	1	0.01%	19	Missouri	212	1.87%
13	Maryland	419	3.69%	20	Indiana	191	1.68%
22	Massachusetts	116	1.02%	21	Arkansas	132	1.16%
5	Michigan	657	5.79%	22	Massachusetts	116	1.02%
28	Minnesota	51	0.45%	23	Connecticut	106	0.93%
17	Mississippi	330	2.91%	24	Wisconsin	99	0.87%
19	Missouri	212	1.87%	25	Oklahoma	87	0.77%
44	Montana	2	0.02%	26	Kansas	72	0.63%
34	Nebraska	26	0.23%	27	Kentucky	66	0.58%
33	Nevada	36	0.32%	28	Minnesota	51	0.45%
42	New Hampshire	3	0.03%	29	Washington	50	0.44%
11	New Jersey	438	3.86%	30	Delaware	46	0.41%
37	New Mexico	15	0.13%	31	Colorado	44	0.39%
1	New York	961	8.47%	32	Arizona	41	0.36%
9	North Carolina	499	4.40%	33	Nevada	36	0.32%
47	North Dakota	0	0.00%	34	Nebraska	26	0.23%
10	Ohio	467	4.12%	35	Iowa	23	0.20%
25	Oklahoma	87	0.77%	36	Oregon	22	0.19%
36	Oregon	22	0.19%	37	New Mexico	15	0.13%
8	Pennsylvania	519	4.57%	37	Rhode Island	15	0.13%
37	Rhode Island	15	0.13%	39	West Virginia	12	0.11%
16	South Carolina	345	3.04%	40	Alaska	7	0.06%
47	South Dakota	0	0.00%	41	Hawaii	6	0.05%
18	Tennessee	305	2.69%	42	Idaho	3	0.03%
7	Texas	612	5.39%	42	New Hampshire	3	0.03%
44	Utah	2	0.02%	44	Montana	2	0.02%
47	Vermont	0	0.00%	44	Utah	2	0.02%
12	Virginia	422	3.72%	46	Maine	1	0.01%
29	Washington	50	0.44%	47	North Dakota	0	0.00%
39	West Virginia	12	0.11%	47	South Dakota	0	0.00%
24	Wisconsin	99	0.87%	47	Vermont	0	0.00%
47	Wyoming	0	0.00%	47	Wyoming	0	0.00%
					District of Columbia	194	1.71%

Source: U.S. Department of Health and Human Services, National Center for Health Statistics
"Monthly Vital Statistics Report" (Vol. 43, No. 6(S), December 8, 1994)
*Final data. Deaths of infants under 1 year old, exclusive of fetal deaths. Based on race of the mother.

Black Infant Mortality Rate in 1992

National Rate = 16.8 Black Infant Deaths per 1,000 Black Live Births*

ALPHA ORDER

RANK	STATE	RATE
26	Alabama	16.2
41	Alaska**	12.9
22	Arizona	16.7
26	Arkansas	16.2
20	California	16.8
36	Colorado	14.6
19	Connecticut	17.2
14	Delaware	18.0
34	Florida	15.1
30	Georgia	15.9
45	Hawaii**	8.8
1	Idaho**	51.7
10	Illinois	19.8
9	Indiana	20.3
12	Iowa	19.4
7	Kansas	21.7
42	Kentucky	12.7
40	Louisiana	13.0
44	Maine**	12.2
24	Maryland	16.5
39	Massachusetts	13.4
6	Michigan	22.1
17	Minnesota	17.5
28	Mississippi	16.1
30	Missouri	15.9
2	Montana**	40.8
10	Nebraska	19.8
23	Nevada	16.6
4	New Hampshire**	27.5
13	New Jersey	18.7
3	New Mexico**	29.2
33	New York	15.8
24	North Carolina	16.5
47	North Dakota**	0.0
14	Ohio	18.0
20	Oklahoma	16.8
5	Oregon	23.0
8	Pennsylvania	20.4
43	Rhode Island**	12.6
29	South Carolina	16.0
47	South Dakota**	0.0
18	Tennessee	17.4
37	Texas	14.2
46	Utah**	8.2
47	Vermont**	0.0
16	Virginia	17.7
30	Washington	15.9
35	West Virginia**	14.7
38	Wisconsin	13.5
47	Wyoming**	0.0

RANK ORDER

RANK	STATE	RATE
1	Idaho**	51.7
2	Montana**	40.8
3	New Mexico**	29.2
4	New Hampshire**	27.5
5	Oregon	23.0
6	Michigan	22.1
7	Kansas	21.7
8	Pennsylvania	20.4
9	Indiana	20.3
10	Illinois	19.8
10	Nebraska	19.8
12	Iowa	19.4
13	New Jersey	18.7
14	Delaware	18.0
14	Ohio	18.0
16	Virginia	17.7
17	Minnesota	17.5
18	Tennessee	17.4
19	Connecticut	17.2
20	California	16.8
20	Oklahoma	16.8
22	Arizona	16.7
23	Nevada	16.6
24	Maryland	16.5
24	North Carolina	16.5
26	Alabama	16.2
26	Arkansas	16.2
28	Mississippi	16.1
29	South Carolina	16.0
30	Georgia	15.9
30	Missouri	15.9
30	Washington	15.9
33	New York	15.8
34	Florida	15.1
35	West Virginia**	14.7
36	Colorado	14.6
37	Texas	14.2
38	Wisconsin	13.5
39	Massachusetts	13.4
40	Louisiana	13.0
41	Alaska**	12.9
42	Kentucky	12.7
43	Rhode Island**	12.6
44	Maine**	12.2
45	Hawaii**	8.8
46	Utah**	8.2
47	North Dakota**	0.0
47	South Dakota**	0.0
47	Vermont**	0.0
47	Wyoming**	0.0
	District of Columbia	22.0

Source: U.S. Department of Health and Human Services, National Center for Health Statistics
  "Monthly Vital Statistics Report" (Vol. 43, No. 6(S), December 8, 1994)
*Final data. Deaths of infants under 1 year old, exclusive of fetal deaths. Based on race of the mother.
**Calculated by Morgan Quitno Press. Based on fewer than 20 black infant deaths.*

White Infant Mortality Rate in 1980

National Rate = 10.86 White Infant Deaths per 1,000 Live Births*

ALPHA ORDER			RANK ORDER		
RANK	**STATE**	**RATE**	**RANK**	**STATE**	**RATE**
8	Alabama	11.62	1	North Carolina	12.01
49	Alaska	8.89	2	Oregon	11.97
12	Arizona	11.54	3	Kentucky	11.96
35	Arkansas	10.27	4	Tennessee	11.84
34	California	10.35	5	Virginia	11.75
43	Colorado	9.62	6	Pennsylvania	11.74
37	Connecticut	10.06	7	Florida	11.73
41	Delaware	9.75	8	Alabama	11.62
7	Florida	11.73	8	North Dakota	11.62
26	Georgia	10.69	10	Oklahoma	11.60
50	Hawaii	8.50	11	Illinois	11.56
28	Idaho	10.63	12	Arizona	11.54
11	Illinois	11.56	13	Montana	11.51
31	Indiana	10.46	14	Maryland	11.41
15	Iowa	11.40	15	Iowa	11.40
45	Kansas	9.38	16	West Virginia	11.39
3	Kentucky	11.96	17	Washington	11.26
31	Louisiana	10.46	18	New Mexico	11.17
46	Maine	9.36	19	Ohio	11.08
14	Maryland	11.41	19	Texas	11.08
38	Massachusetts	10.02	21	Mississippi	11.05
30	Michigan	10.51	22	Missouri	10.96
44	Minnesota	9.53	23	Rhode Island	10.81
21	Mississippi	11.05	24	South Carolina	10.79
22	Missouri	10.96	25	Vermont	10.71
13	Montana	11.51	26	Georgia	10.69
28	Nebraska	10.63	27	New York	10.67
40	Nevada	9.78	28	Idaho	10.63
39	New Hampshire	9.86	28	Nebraska	10.63
36	New Jersey	10.22	30	Michigan	10.51
18	New Mexico	11.17	31	Indiana	10.46
27	New York	10.67	31	Louisiana	10.46
1	North Carolina	12.01	33	Utah	10.39
8	North Dakota	11.62	34	California	10.35
19	Ohio	11.08	35	Arkansas	10.27
10	Oklahoma	11.60	36	New Jersey	10.22
2	Oregon	11.97	37	Connecticut	10.06
6	Pennsylvania	11.74	38	Massachusetts	10.02
23	Rhode Island	10.81	39	New Hampshire	9.86
24	South Carolina	10.79	40	Nevada	9.78
48	South Dakota	8.91	41	Delaware	9.75
4	Tennessee	11.84	42	Wisconsin	9.67
19	Texas	11.08	43	Colorado	9.62
33	Utah	10.39	44	Minnesota	9.53
25	Vermont	10.71	45	Kansas	9.38
5	Virginia	11.75	46	Maine	9.36
17	Washington	11.26	47	Wyoming	9.23
16	West Virginia	11.39	48	South Dakota	8.91
42	Wisconsin	9.67	49	Alaska	8.89
47	Wyoming	9.23	50	Hawaii	8.50
				District of Columbia	16.90

Source: U.S. Department of Health and Human Services, National Center for Health Statistics,
"Vital Statistics of the United States, 1980" (Vol. I–Natality, issued 1984) and unpublished data
*Deaths of infants under 1 year old, exclusive of fetal deaths. Final data by state of residence.

Black Infant Mortality Rate in 1980

National Rate = 22.19 Black Infant Deaths per 1,000 Live Births*

ALPHA ORDER			RANK ORDER		
RANK	STATE	RATE	RANK	STATE	RATE
27	Alabama	21.65	1	Utah**	40.54
12	Alaska**	24.79	2	North Dakota**	38.96
19	Arizona	23.19	3	Wyoming**	38.46
39	Arkansas	20.07	4	New Hampshire**	37.04
35	California	20.34	5	Iowa	32.06
25	Colorado	22.50	6	Delaware	28.37
34	Connecticut	20.42	7	Nebraska	28.16
6	Delaware	28.37	8	New Mexico**	27.57
18	Florida	23.30	9	Illinois	27.08
30	Georgia	21.16	10	Minnesota	26.29
45	Hawaii**	17.16	11	Michigan	24.86
46	Idaho**	0.00	12	Alaska**	24.79
9	Illinois	27.08	13	Pennsylvania	24.46
14	Indiana	24.37	14	Indiana	24.37
5	Iowa	32.06	15	Ohio	24.13
24	Kansas	22.70	16	Mississippi	23.78
22	Kentucky	22.81	17	West Virginia	23.68
32	Louisiana	20.74	18	Florida	23.30
46	Maine**	0.00	19	Arizona	23.19
31	Maryland	21.01	20	South Carolina	22.98
44	Massachusetts	18.78	21	Oklahoma	22.92
11	Michigan	24.86	22	Kentucky	22.81
10	Minnesota	26.29	23	New Jersey	22.78
16	Mississippi	23.78	24	Kansas	22.70
28	Missouri	21.41	25	Colorado	22.50
46	Montana**	0.00	26	Nevada	22.24
7	Nebraska	28.16	27	Alabama	21.65
26	Nevada	22.24	28	Missouri	21.41
4	New Hampshire**	37.04	29	Washington	21.27
23	New Jersey	22.78	30	Georgia	21.16
8	New Mexico**	27.57	31	Maryland	21.01
33	New York	20.66	32	Louisiana	20.74
36	North Carolina	20.28	33	New York	20.66
2	North Dakota**	38.96	34	Connecticut	20.42
15	Ohio	24.13	35	California	20.34
21	Oklahoma	22.92	36	North Carolina	20.28
38	Oregon**	20.23	37	Virginia	20.26
13	Pennsylvania	24.46	38	Oregon**	20.23
43	Rhode Island**	19.06	39	Arkansas	20.07
20	South Carolina	22.98	40	Wisconsin	19.47
46	South Dakota**	0.00	41	Tennessee	19.41
41	Tennessee	19.41	42	Texas	19.40
42	Texas	19.40	43	Rhode Island**	19.06
1	Utah**	40.54	44	Massachusetts	18.78
46	Vermont**	0.00	45	Hawaii**	17.16
37	Virginia	20.26	46	Idaho**	0.00
29	Washington	21.27	46	Maine**	0.00
17	West Virginia	23.68	46	Montana**	0.00
40	Wisconsin	19.47	46	South Dakota**	0.00
3	Wyoming**	38.46	46	Vermont**	0.00
				District of Columbia	26.91

Source: U.S. Department of Health and Human Services, National Center for Health Statistics
"Vital Statistics of the United States, 1980" (Vol. I-Natality, issued 1984) and unpublished data
Deaths of infants under 1 year old, exclusive of fetal deaths. Final data by state of residence.
**Based on fewer than 20 black infant deaths.*

Neonatal Deaths in 1992

National Total = 21,849 Neonatal Deaths*

ALPHA ORDER

RANK	STATE	DEATHS	% of USA
15	Alabama	432	1.98%
46	Alaska	47	0.22%
21	Arizona	331	1.51%
30	Arkansas	207	0.95%
1	California	2,564	11.74%
29	Colorado	230	1.05%
26	Connecticut	260	1.19%
42	Delaware	63	0.29%
5	Florida	1,125	5.15%
9	Georgia	745	3.41%
40	Hawaii	77	0.35%
37	Idaho	91	0.42%
4	Illinois	1,242	5.68%
14	Indiana	502	2.30%
32	Iowa	181	0.83%
31	Kansas	200	0.92%
27	Kentucky	246	1.13%
18	Louisiana	402	1.84%
43	Maine	57	0.26%
13	Maryland	521	2.38%
17	Massachusetts	416	1.90%
7	Michigan	961	4.40%
24	Minnesota	293	1.34%
22	Mississippi	320	1.46%
19	Missouri	398	1.82%
48	Montana	34	0.16%
37	Nebraska	91	0.42%
41	Nevada	65	0.30%
45	New Hampshire	54	0.25%
11	New Jersey	679	3.11%
36	New Mexico	109	0.50%
2	New York	1,691	7.74%
10	North Carolina	712	3.26%
47	North Dakota	44	0.20%
8	Ohio	956	4.38%
28	Oklahoma	242	1.11%
33	Oregon	159	0.73%
6	Pennsylvania	984	4.50%
39	Rhode Island	78	0.36%
20	South Carolina	386	1.77%
44	South Dakota	56	0.26%
16	Tennessee	420	1.92%
3	Texas	1,512	6.92%
34	Utah	132	0.60%
49	Vermont	31	0.14%
12	Virginia	615	2.81%
25	Washington	292	1.34%
35	West Virginia	124	0.57%
23	Wisconsin	304	1.39%
50	Wyoming	27	0.12%

RANK ORDER

RANK	STATE	DEATHS	% of USA
1	California	2,564	11.74%
2	New York	1,691	7.74%
3	Texas	1,512	6.92%
4	Illinois	1,242	5.68%
5	Florida	1,125	5.15%
6	Pennsylvania	984	4.50%
7	Michigan	961	4.40%
8	Ohio	956	4.38%
9	Georgia	745	3.41%
10	North Carolina	712	3.26%
11	New Jersey	679	3.11%
12	Virginia	615	2.81%
13	Maryland	521	2.38%
14	Indiana	502	2.30%
15	Alabama	432	1.98%
16	Tennessee	420	1.92%
17	Massachusetts	416	1.90%
18	Louisiana	402	1.84%
19	Missouri	398	1.82%
20	South Carolina	386	1.77%
21	Arizona	331	1.51%
22	Mississippi	320	1.46%
23	Wisconsin	304	1.39%
24	Minnesota	293	1.34%
25	Washington	292	1.34%
26	Connecticut	260	1.19%
27	Kentucky	246	1.13%
28	Oklahoma	242	1.11%
29	Colorado	230	1.05%
30	Arkansas	207	0.95%
31	Kansas	200	0.92%
32	Iowa	181	0.83%
33	Oregon	159	0.73%
34	Utah	132	0.60%
35	West Virginia	124	0.57%
36	New Mexico	109	0.50%
37	Idaho	91	0.42%
37	Nebraska	91	0.42%
39	Rhode Island	78	0.36%
40	Hawaii	77	0.35%
41	Nevada	65	0.30%
42	Delaware	63	0.29%
43	Maine	57	0.26%
44	South Dakota	56	0.26%
45	New Hampshire	54	0.25%
46	Alaska	47	0.22%
47	North Dakota	44	0.20%
48	Montana	34	0.16%
49	Vermont	31	0.14%
50	Wyoming	27	0.12%
	District of Columbia	141	0.65%

Source: U.S. Department of Health and Human Services, National Center for Health Statistics
"Monthly Vital Statistics Report" (Vol. 43, No. 6(S), December 8, 1994)
*Final data. Deaths of infants under 28 days, exclusive of fetal deaths.

Neonatal Death Rate in 1992

National Rate = 5.4 Neonatal Deaths per 1,000 Live Births*

ALPHA ORDER			RANK ORDER		
RANK	STATE	RATE	RANK	STATE	RATE
2	Alabama	6.9	1	Mississippi	7.5
38	Alaska	4.0	2	Alabama	6.9
29	Arizona	4.8	2	South Carolina	6.9
12	Arkansas	5.9	4	North Carolina	6.8
35	California	4.3	5	Georgia	6.7
37	Colorado	4.2	5	Maryland	6.7
21	Connecticut	5.5	5	Michigan	6.7
12	Delaware	5.9	8	Illinois	6.5
12	Florida	5.9	9	Virginia	6.3
5	Georgia	6.7	10	Indiana	6.0
41	Hawaii	3.9	10	Pennsylvania	6.0
24	Idaho	5.2	12	Arkansas	5.9
8	Illinois	6.5	12	Delaware	5.9
10	Indiana	6.0	12	Florida	5.9
31	Iowa	4.7	12	New York	5.9
23	Kansas	5.3	12	Ohio	5.9
33	Kentucky	4.6	17	Louisiana	5.7
17	Louisiana	5.7	17	New Jersey	5.7
46	Maine	3.5	17	Tennessee	5.7
5	Maryland	6.7	20	West Virginia	5.6
29	Massachusetts	4.8	21	Connecticut	5.5
5	Michigan	6.7	22	Rhode Island	5.4
34	Minnesota	4.5	23	Kansas	5.3
1	Mississippi	7.5	24	Idaho	5.2
24	Missouri	5.2	24	Missouri	5.2
49	Montana	3.0	26	Oklahoma	5.1
41	Nebraska	3.9	26	South Dakota	5.1
50	Nevada	2.9	28	North Dakota	5.0
48	New Hampshire	3.4	29	Arizona	4.8
17	New Jersey	5.7	29	Massachusetts	4.8
41	New Mexico	3.9	31	Iowa	4.7
12	New York	5.9	31	Texas	4.7
4	North Carolina	6.8	33	Kentucky	4.6
28	North Dakota	5.0	34	Minnesota	4.5
12	Ohio	5.9	35	California	4.3
26	Oklahoma	5.1	35	Wisconsin	4.3
44	Oregon	3.8	37	Colorado	4.2
10	Pennsylvania	6.0	38	Alaska	4.0
22	Rhode Island	5.4	38	Vermont	4.0
2	South Carolina	6.9	38	Wyoming	4.0
26	South Dakota	5.1	41	Hawaii	3.9
17	Tennessee	5.7	41	Nebraska	3.9
31	Texas	4.7	41	New Mexico	3.9
46	Utah	3.5	44	Oregon	3.8
38	Vermont	4.0	45	Washington	3.7
9	Virginia	6.3	46	Maine	3.5
45	Washington	3.7	46	Utah	3.5
20	West Virginia	5.6	48	New Hampshire	3.4
35	Wisconsin	4.3	49	Montana	3.0
38	Wyoming	4.0	50	Nevada	2.9
				District of Columbia	12.9

Source: U.S. Department of Health and Human Services, National Center for Health Statistics
    "Monthly Vital Statistics Report" (Vol. 43, No. 6(S), December 8, 1994)
*Final data. Deaths of infants under 28 days, exclusive of fetal deaths.

White Neonatal Deaths in 1992

National Total = 13,915 White Neonatal Deaths*

<u>ALPHA ORDER</u>

RANK	STATE	DEATHS	% of USA
23	Alabama	203	1.46%
48	Alaska	26	0.19%
15	Arizona	270	1.94%
32	Arkansas	130	0.93%
1	California	1,898	13.64%
24	Colorado	197	1.42%
25	Connecticut	179	1.29%
45	Delaware	35	0.25%
5	Florida	675	4.85%
14	Georgia	297	2.13%
50	Hawaii	10	0.07%
36	Idaho	90	0.65%
4	Illinois	703	5.05%
10	Indiana	369	2.65%
27	Iowa	166	1.19%
30	Kansas	153	1.10%
22	Kentucky	206	1.48%
27	Louisiana	166	1.19%
40	Maine	55	0.40%
20	Maryland	232	1.67%
12	Massachusetts	322	2.31%
8	Michigan	497	3.57%
19	Minnesota	236	1.70%
35	Mississippi	98	0.70%
16	Missouri	258	1.85%
47	Montana	29	0.21%
38	Nebraska	79	0.57%
41	Nevada	53	0.38%
42	New Hampshire	52	0.37%
9	New Jersey	382	2.75%
37	New Mexico	87	0.63%
3	New York	1,044	7.50%
11	North Carolina	350	2.52%
44	North Dakota	40	0.29%
6	Ohio	665	4.78%
26	Oklahoma	169	1.21%
31	Oregon	142	1.02%
7	Pennsylvania	638	4.58%
39	Rhode Island	61	0.44%
29	South Carolina	160	1.15%
43	South Dakota	44	0.32%
21	Tennessee	212	1.52%
2	Texas	1,132	8.14%
33	Utah	129	0.93%
46	Vermont	31	0.22%
13	Virginia	307	2.21%
17	Washington	243	1.75%
34	West Virginia	118	0.85%
18	Wisconsin	237	1.70%
49	Wyoming	24	0.17%

<u>RANK ORDER</u>

RANK	STATE	DEATHS	% of USA
1	California	1,898	13.64%
2	Texas	1,132	8.14%
3	New York	1,044	7.50%
4	Illinois	703	5.05%
5	Florida	675	4.85%
6	Ohio	665	4.78%
7	Pennsylvania	638	4.58%
8	Michigan	497	3.57%
9	New Jersey	382	2.75%
10	Indiana	369	2.65%
11	North Carolina	350	2.52%
12	Massachusetts	322	2.31%
13	Virginia	307	2.21%
14	Georgia	297	2.13%
15	Arizona	270	1.94%
16	Missouri	258	1.85%
17	Washington	243	1.75%
18	Wisconsin	237	1.70%
19	Minnesota	236	1.70%
20	Maryland	232	1.67%
21	Tennessee	212	1.52%
22	Kentucky	206	1.48%
23	Alabama	203	1.46%
24	Colorado	197	1.42%
25	Connecticut	179	1.29%
26	Oklahoma	169	1.21%
27	Iowa	166	1.19%
27	Louisiana	166	1.19%
29	South Carolina	160	1.15%
30	Kansas	153	1.10%
31	Oregon	142	1.02%
32	Arkansas	130	0.93%
33	Utah	129	0.93%
34	West Virginia	118	0.85%
35	Mississippi	98	0.70%
36	Idaho	90	0.65%
37	New Mexico	87	0.63%
38	Nebraska	79	0.57%
39	Rhode Island	61	0.44%
40	Maine	55	0.40%
41	Nevada	53	0.38%
42	New Hampshire	52	0.37%
43	South Dakota	44	0.32%
44	North Dakota	40	0.29%
45	Delaware	35	0.25%
46	Vermont	31	0.22%
47	Montana	29	0.21%
48	Alaska	26	0.19%
49	Wyoming	24	0.17%
50	Hawaii	10	0.07%
	District of Columbia	16	0.11%

*Source: U.S. Department of Health and Human Services, National Center for Health Statistics
"Monthly Vital Statistics Report" (Vol. 43, No. 6(S), December 8, 1994)*
*Final data. Deaths of infants under 28 days, exclusive of fetal deaths. Based on race of the mother.

White Neonatal Death Rate in 1992

National Rate = 4.3 White Neonatal Deaths per 1,000 Live White Births*

ALPHA ORDER			RANK ORDER		
RANK	STATE	RATE	RANK	STATE	RATE
3	Alabama	5.1	1	West Virginia	5.6
46	Alaska	3.3	2	Idaho	5.3
17	Arizona	4.5	3	Alabama	5.1
6	Arkansas	4.9	3	North Dakota	5.1
36	California	3.9	5	Indiana	5.0
34	Colorado	4.0	6	Arkansas	4.9
22	Connecticut	4.4	6	Illinois	4.9
22	Delaware	4.4	6	New York	4.9
13	Florida	4.7	6	North Carolina	4.9
26	Georgia	4.3	6	Ohio	4.9
50	Hawaii**	1.7	11	Rhode Island	4.8
2	Idaho	5.3	11	South Dakota	4.8
6	Illinois	4.9	13	Florida	4.7
5	Indiana	5.0	13	Maryland	4.7
17	Iowa	4.5	13	Pennsylvania	4.7
17	Kansas	4.5	13	South Carolina	4.7
26	Kentucky	4.3	17	Arizona	4.5
29	Louisiana	4.2	17	Iowa	4.5
44	Maine	3.5	17	Kansas	4.5
13	Maryland	4.7	17	Mississippi	4.5
26	Massachusetts	4.3	17	Oklahoma	4.5
22	Michigan	4.4	22	Connecticut	4.4
34	Minnesota	4.0	22	Delaware	4.4
17	Mississippi	4.5	22	Michigan	4.4
29	Missouri	4.2	22	Virginia	4.4
48	Montana	2.9	26	Georgia	4.3
41	Nebraska	3.7	26	Kentucky	4.3
49	Nevada	2.8	26	Massachusetts	4.3
46	New Hampshire	3.3	29	Louisiana	4.2
29	New Jersey	4.2	29	Missouri	4.2
38	New Mexico	3.8	29	New Jersey	4.2
6	New York	4.9	29	Texas	4.2
6	North Carolina	4.9	33	Vermont	4.1
3	North Dakota	5.1	34	Colorado	4.0
6	Ohio	4.9	34	Minnesota	4.0
17	Oklahoma	4.5	36	California	3.9
43	Oregon	3.6	36	Wisconsin	3.9
13	Pennsylvania	4.7	38	New Mexico	3.8
11	Rhode Island	4.8	38	Tennessee	3.8
13	South Carolina	4.7	38	Wyoming	3.8
11	South Dakota	4.8	41	Nebraska	3.7
38	Tennessee	3.8	41	Utah	3.7
29	Texas	4.2	43	Oregon	3.6
41	Utah	3.7	44	Maine	3.5
33	Vermont	4.1	44	Washington	3.5
22	Virginia	4.4	46	Alaska	3.3
44	Washington	3.5	46	New Hampshire	3.3
1	West Virginia	5.6	48	Montana	2.9
36	Wisconsin	3.9	49	Nevada	2.8
38	Wyoming	3.8	50	Hawaii**	1.7
				District of Columbia**	10.0

Source: U.S. Department of Health and Human Services, National Center for Health Statistics
   "Monthly Vital Statistics Report" (Vol. 43, No. 6(S), December 8, 1994)
*Final data. Deaths of infants under 28 days, exclusive of fetal deaths. Based on race of the mother.
**Calculated by Morgan Quitno Press. Based on fewer than 20 white neonatal deaths.

Black Neonatal Deaths in 1992

National Total = 7,296 Black Neonatal Deaths*

ALPHA ORDER					RANK ORDER			
RANK	STATE	DEATHS	% of USA		RANK	STATE	DEATHS	% of USA
15	Alabama	229	3.14%		1	New York	605	8.29%
41	Alaska	3	0.04%		2	Illinois	519	7.11%
32	Arizona	21	0.29%		3	California	495	6.78%
23	Arkansas	76	1.04%		4	Michigan	451	6.18%
3	California	495	6.78%		5	Florida	440	6.03%
31	Colorado	24	0.33%		5	Georgia	440	6.03%
22	Connecticut	78	1.07%		7	Texas	366	5.02%
30	Delaware	28	0.38%		8	North Carolina	341	4.67%
5	Florida	440	6.03%		9	Pennsylvania	338	4.63%
5	Georgia	440	6.03%		10	Virginia	299	4.10%
40	Hawaii	4	0.05%		11	Ohio	286	3.92%
43	Idaho	1	0.01%		12	Maryland	282	3.87%
2	Illinois	519	7.11%		13	New Jersey	280	3.84%
20	Indiana	128	1.75%		14	Louisiana	234	3.21%
34	Iowa	12	0.16%		15	Alabama	229	3.14%
26	Kansas	43	0.59%		16	South Carolina	226	3.10%
27	Kentucky	40	0.55%		17	Mississippi	220	3.02%
14	Louisiana	234	3.21%		18	Tennessee	204	2.80%
45	Maine	0	0.00%		19	Missouri	137	1.88%
12	Maryland	282	3.87%		20	Indiana	128	1.75%
21	Massachusetts	82	1.12%		21	Massachusetts	82	1.12%
4	Michigan	451	6.18%		22	Connecticut	78	1.07%
28	Minnesota	37	0.51%		23	Arkansas	76	1.04%
17	Mississippi	220	3.02%		24	Wisconsin	54	0.74%
19	Missouri	137	1.88%		25	Oklahoma	52	0.71%
45	Montana	0	0.00%		26	Kansas	43	0.59%
34	Nebraska	12	0.16%		27	Kentucky	40	0.55%
36	Nevada	11	0.15%		28	Minnesota	37	0.51%
42	New Hampshire	2	0.03%		29	Washington	36	0.49%
13	New Jersey	280	3.84%		30	Delaware	28	0.38%
38	New Mexico	5	0.07%		31	Colorado	24	0.33%
1	New York	605	8.29%		32	Arizona	21	0.29%
8	North Carolina	341	4.67%		33	Rhode Island	14	0.19%
45	North Dakota	0	0.00%		34	Iowa	12	0.16%
11	Ohio	286	3.92%		34	Nebraska	12	0.16%
25	Oklahoma	52	0.71%		36	Nevada	11	0.15%
37	Oregon	10	0.14%		37	Oregon	10	0.14%
9	Pennsylvania	338	4.63%		38	New Mexico	5	0.07%
33	Rhode Island	14	0.19%		38	West Virginia	5	0.07%
16	South Carolina	226	3.10%		40	Hawaii	4	0.05%
45	South Dakota	0	0.00%		41	Alaska	3	0.04%
18	Tennessee	204	2.80%		42	New Hampshire	2	0.03%
7	Texas	366	5.02%		43	Idaho	1	0.01%
43	Utah	1	0.01%		43	Utah	1	0.01%
45	Vermont	0	0.00%		45	Maine	0	0.00%
10	Virginia	299	4.10%		45	Montana	0	0.00%
29	Washington	36	0.49%		45	North Dakota	0	0.00%
38	West Virginia	5	0.07%		45	South Dakota	0	0.00%
24	Wisconsin	54	0.74%		45	Vermont	0	0.00%
45	Wyoming	0	0.00%		45	Wyoming	0	0.00%
						District of Columbia	125	1.71%

Source: U.S. Department of Health and Human Services, National Center for Health Statistics
"Monthly Vital Statistics Report" (Vol. 43, No. 6(S), December 8, 1994)
*Final data. Deaths of infants under 28 days, exclusive of fetal deaths. Based on race of the mother.

Black Neonatal Death Rate in 1992

National Rate = 10.8 Black Neonatal Deaths per 1,000 Live Black Births*

ALPHA ORDER

RANK	STATE	RATE
21	Alabama	10.6
42	Alaska**	5.5
34	Arizona	8.6
32	Arkansas	9.3
21	California	10.6
36	Colorado	8.0
7	Connecticut	12.7
17	Delaware	11.0
29	Florida	9.8
19	Georgia	10.9
41	Hawaii**	5.8
2	Idaho**	17.2
10	Illinois	12.1
4	Indiana	13.6
26	Iowa**	10.1
6	Kansas	13.0
38	Kentucky	7.7
37	Louisiana	7.8
45	Maine**	0.0
16	Maryland	11.1
31	Massachusetts	9.5
3	Michigan	15.2
7	Minnesota	12.7
20	Mississippi	10.7
25	Missouri	10.3
45	Montana**	0.0
33	Nebraska**	9.1
43	Nevada**	5.1
1	New Hampshire**	18.3
11	New Jersey	12.0
30	New Mexico**	9.7
28	New York	9.9
15	North Carolina	11.2
45	North Dakota**	0.0
17	Ohio	11.0
26	Oklahoma	10.1
23	Oregon**	10.5
5	Pennsylvania	13.3
12	Rhode Island**	11.8
23	South Carolina	10.5
45	South Dakota**	0.0
13	Tennessee	11.7
35	Texas	8.5
44	Utah**	4.1
45	Vermont**	0.0
9	Virginia	12.5
14	Washington	11.4
40	West Virginia**	6.1
39	Wisconsin	7.4
45	Wyoming**	0.0

RANK ORDER

RANK	STATE	RATE
1	New Hampshire**	18.3
2	Idaho**	17.2
3	Michigan	15.2
4	Indiana	13.6
5	Pennsylvania	13.3
6	Kansas	13.0
7	Connecticut	12.7
7	Minnesota	12.7
9	Virginia	12.5
10	Illinois	12.1
11	New Jersey	12.0
12	Rhode Island**	11.8
13	Tennessee	11.7
14	Washington	11.4
15	North Carolina	11.2
16	Maryland	11.1
17	Delaware	11.0
17	Ohio	11.0
19	Georgia	10.9
20	Mississippi	10.7
21	Alabama	10.6
21	California	10.6
23	Oregon**	10.5
23	South Carolina	10.5
25	Missouri	10.3
26	Iowa**	10.1
26	Oklahoma	10.1
28	New York	9.9
29	Florida	9.8
30	New Mexico**	9.7
31	Massachusetts	9.5
32	Arkansas	9.3
33	Nebraska**	9.1
34	Arizona	8.6
35	Texas	8.5
36	Colorado	8.0
37	Louisiana	7.8
38	Kentucky	7.7
39	Wisconsin	7.4
40	West Virginia**	6.1
41	Hawaii**	5.8
42	Alaska**	5.5
43	Nevada**	5.1
44	Utah**	4.1
45	Maine**	0.0
45	Montana**	0.0
45	North Dakota**	0.0
45	South Dakota**	0.0
45	Vermont**	0.0
45	Wyoming**	0.0

District of Columbia	14.2

Source: U.S. Department of Health and Human Services, National Center for Health Statistics
"Monthly Vital Statistics Report" (Vol. 43, No. 6(S), December 8, 1994)
*Final data. Deaths of infants under 28 days, exclusive of fetal deaths. Based on race of the mother.
**Calculated by Morgan Quitno Press. Based on fewer than 20 black neonatal deaths.

Deaths by AIDS Through 1993

National Total = 197,727 Deaths*

RANK	STATE	DEATHS	% of USA
24	Alabama	1,268	0.64%
46	Alaska	82	0.04%
20	Arizona	1,731	0.88%
34	Arkansas	590	0.30%
2	California	38,447	19.44%
19	Colorado	2,089	1.06%
18	Connecticut	2,250	1.14%
37	Delaware	440	0.22%
3	Florida	18,929	9.57%
8	Georgia	5,318	2.69%
31	Hawaii	752	0.38%
44	Idaho	118	0.06%
6	Illinois	6,591	3.33%
23	Indiana	1,376	0.70%
39	Iowa	305	0.15%
33	Kansas	652	0.33%
32	Kentucky	735	0.37%
12	Louisiana	2,954	1.49%
42	Maine	206	0.10%
9	Maryland	4,259	2.15%
10	Massachusetts	4,089	2.07%
14	Michigan	2,684	1.36%
26	Minnesota	1,030	0.52%
30	Mississippi	838	0.42%
17	Missouri	2,325	1.18%
46	Montana	82	0.04%
40	Nebraska	250	0.13%
28	Nevada	910	0.46%
43	New Hampshire	194	0.10%
5	New Jersey	11,823	5.98%
38	New Mexico	426	0.22%
1	New York	43,253	21.88%
16	North Carolina	2,336	1.18%
50	North Dakota	23	0.01%
11	Ohio	3,040	1.54%
27	Oklahoma	961	0.49%
25	Oregon	1,235	0.62%
7	Pennsylvania	5,540	2.80%
35	Rhode Island	480	0.24%
21	South Carolina	1,507	0.76%
49	South Dakota	32	0.02%
22	Tennessee	1,438	0.73%
4	Texas	13,819	6.99%
36	Utah	448	0.23%
45	Vermont	93	0.05%
13	Virginia	2,810	1.42%
15	Washington	2,672	1.35%
41	West Virginia	233	0.12%
29	Wisconsin	868	0.44%
48	Wyoming	47	0.02%

RANK	STATE	DEATHS	% of USA
1	New York	43,253	21.88%
2	California	38,447	19.44%
3	Florida	18,929	9.57%
4	Texas	13,819	6.99%
5	New Jersey	11,823	5.98%
6	Illinois	6,591	3.33%
7	Pennsylvania	5,540	2.80%
8	Georgia	5,318	2.69%
9	Maryland	4,259	2.15%
10	Massachusetts	4,089	2.07%
11	Ohio	3,040	1.54%
12	Louisiana	2,954	1.49%
13	Virginia	2,810	1.42%
14	Michigan	2,684	1.36%
15	Washington	2,672	1.35%
16	North Carolina	2,336	1.18%
17	Missouri	2,325	1.18%
18	Connecticut	2,250	1.14%
19	Colorado	2,089	1.06%
20	Arizona	1,731	0.88%
21	South Carolina	1,507	0.76%
22	Tennessee	1,438	0.73%
23	Indiana	1,376	0.70%
24	Alabama	1,268	0.64%
25	Oregon	1,235	0.62%
26	Minnesota	1,030	0.52%
27	Oklahoma	961	0.49%
28	Nevada	910	0.46%
29	Wisconsin	868	0.44%
30	Mississippi	838	0.42%
31	Hawaii	752	0.38%
32	Kentucky	735	0.37%
33	Kansas	652	0.33%
34	Arkansas	590	0.30%
35	Rhode Island	480	0.24%
36	Utah	448	0.23%
37	Delaware	440	0.22%
38	New Mexico	426	0.22%
39	Iowa	305	0.15%
40	Nebraska	250	0.13%
41	West Virginia	233	0.12%
42	Maine	206	0.10%
43	New Hampshire	194	0.10%
44	Idaho	118	0.06%
45	Vermont	93	0.05%
46	Alaska	82	0.04%
46	Montana	82	0.04%
48	Wyoming	47	0.02%
49	South Dakota	32	0.02%
50	North Dakota	23	0.01%
	District of Columbia	3,149	1.59%

Source: U.S. Department of Health and Human Services, Public Health Service
"Health, United States 1993" (DHHS Pub. No.: ((PHS) 94-1232, May 1994)
*Cumulative deaths through September 30, 1993. However, due to reporting delays, these totals should increase. AIDS is Acquired Immunodeficiency Syndrome.

Deaths by AIDS in 1993

National Preliminary Total = 16,885 Deaths*

ALPHA ORDER					RANK ORDER			
RANK	**STATE**		**DEATHS**	**% of USA**	**RANK**	**STATE**	**DEATHS**	**% of USA**
22	Alabama		168	0.99%	1	California	3,514	20.81%
43	Alaska		16	0.09%	2	Florida	2,138	12.66%
29	Arizona		103	0.61%	3	New York	1,952	11.56%
31	Arkansas		88	0.52%	4	Texas	1,012	5.99%
1	California		3,514	20.81%	5	Illinois	820	4.86%
16	Colorado		257	1.52%	6	New Jersey	701	4.15%
23	Connecticut		165	0.98%	7	Pennsylvania	455	2.69%
34	Delaware		83	0.49%	8	Maryland	429	2.54%
2	Florida		2,138	12.66%	9	Georgia	382	2.26%
9	Georgia		382	2.26%	10	Michigan	372	2.20%
32	Hawaii		86	0.51%	11	Ohio	371	2.20%
41	Idaho		24	0.14%	12	Washington	353	2.09%
5	Illinois		820	4.86%	13	Louisiana	315	1.87%
20	Indiana		176	1.04%	14	Missouri	274	1.62%
39	Iowa		30	0.18%	15	North Carolina	268	1.59%
35	Kansas		75	0.44%	16	Colorado	257	1.52%
33	Kentucky		85	0.50%	17	Massachusetts	236	1.40%
13	Louisiana		315	1.87%	18	Tennessee	227	1.34%
47	Maine		8	0.05%	19	Virginia	220	1.30%
8	Maryland		429	2.54%	20	Indiana	176	1.04%
17	Massachusetts		236	1.40%	20	Wisconsin	176	1.04%
10	Michigan		372	2.20%	22	Alabama	168	0.99%
27	Minnesota		125	0.74%	23	Connecticut	165	0.98%
30	Mississippi		92	0.54%	24	Nevada	142	0.84%
14	Missouri		274	1.62%	25	Oregon	137	0.81%
45	Montana		13	0.08%	26	South Carolina	128	0.76%
40	Nebraska		28	0.17%	27	Minnesota	125	0.74%
24	Nevada		142	0.84%	28	Oklahoma	107	0.63%
45	New Hampshire		13	0.08%	29	Arizona	103	0.61%
6	New Jersey		701	4.15%	30	Mississippi	92	0.54%
37	New Mexico		56	0.33%	31	Arkansas	88	0.52%
3	New York		1,952	11.56%	32	Hawaii	86	0.51%
15	North Carolina		268	1.59%	33	Kentucky	85	0.50%
50	North Dakota		0	0.00%	34	Delaware	83	0.49%
11	Ohio		371	2.20%	35	Kansas	75	0.44%
28	Oklahoma		107	0.63%	36	Utah	60	0.36%
25	Oregon		137	0.81%	37	New Mexico	56	0.33%
7	Pennsylvania		455	2.69%	38	Rhode Island	41	0.24%
38	Rhode Island		41	0.24%	39	Iowa	30	0.18%
26	South Carolina		128	0.76%	40	Nebraska	28	0.17%
48	South Dakota		4	0.02%	41	Idaho	24	0.14%
18	Tennessee		227	1.34%	42	West Virginia	23	0.14%
4	Texas		1,012	5.99%	43	Alaska	16	0.09%
36	Utah		60	0.36%	44	Vermont	14	0.08%
44	Vermont		14	0.08%	45	Montana	13	0.08%
19	Virginia		220	1.30%	45	New Hampshire	13	0.08%
12	Washington		353	2.09%	47	Maine	8	0.05%
42	West Virginia		23	0.14%	48	South Dakota	4	0.02%
20	Wisconsin		176	1.04%	48	Wyoming	4	0.02%
48	Wyoming		4	0.02%	50	North Dakota	0	0.00%
						District of Columbia	319	1.89%

*Source: U.S. Department of Health and Human Services, Public Health Service
"Health, United States 1993" (DHHS Pub. No.: ((PHS) 94-1232, May 1994)*
Deaths for January through September 1993. However, due to reporting delays, these totals should increase. AIDS is Acquired Immunodeficiency Syndrome.

Deaths by AIDS in 1992

National Total = 33,566 Deaths*

ALPHA ORDER

RANK	STATE	DEATHS	% of USA
25	Alabama	224	0.67%
45	Alaska	20	0.06%
21	Arizona	340	1.01%
35	Arkansas	90	0.27%
2	California	6,029	17.96%
20	Colorado	373	1.11%
18	Connecticut	403	1.20%
37	Delaware	65	0.19%
3	Florida	3,111	9.27%
6	Georgia	1,162	3.46%
33	Hawaii	111	0.33%
43	Idaho	32	0.10%
7	Illinois	1,113	3.32%
23	Indiana	264	0.79%
39	Iowa	58	0.17%
32	Kansas	128	0.38%
31	Kentucky	130	0.39%
15	Louisiana	574	1.71%
41	Maine	49	0.15%
9	Maryland	762	2.27%
10	Massachusetts	702	2.09%
14	Michigan	580	1.73%
28	Minnesota	170	0.51%
29	Mississippi	157	0.47%
17	Missouri	415	1.24%
46	Montana	18	0.05%
40	Nebraska	55	0.16%
30	Nevada	134	0.40%
43	New Hampshire	32	0.10%
5	New Jersey	1,926	5.74%
34	New Mexico	102	0.30%
1	New York	6,495	19.35%
11	North Carolina	686	2.04%
49	North Dakota	7	0.02%
12	Ohio	615	1.83%
26	Oklahoma	193	0.57%
24	Oregon	227	0.68%
8	Pennsylvania	994	2.96%
36	Rhode Island	81	0.24%
19	South Carolina	390	1.16%
49	South Dakota	7	0.02%
22	Tennessee	279	0.83%
4	Texas	2,398	7.14%
38	Utah	59	0.18%
46	Vermont	18	0.05%
13	Virginia	586	1.75%
16	Washington	447	1.33%
42	West Virginia	38	0.11%
27	Wisconsin	192	0.57%
48	Wyoming	13	0.04%

RANK ORDER

RANK	STATE	DEATHS	% of USA
1	New York	6,495	19.35%
2	California	6,029	17.96%
3	Florida	3,111	9.27%
4	Texas	2,398	7.14%
5	New Jersey	1,926	5.74%
6	Georgia	1,162	3.46%
7	Illinois	1,113	3.32%
8	Pennsylvania	994	2.96%
9	Maryland	762	2.27%
10	Massachusetts	702	2.09%
11	North Carolina	686	2.04%
12	Ohio	615	1.83%
13	Virginia	586	1.75%
14	Michigan	580	1.73%
15	Louisiana	574	1.71%
16	Washington	447	1.33%
17	Missouri	415	1.24%
18	Connecticut	403	1.20%
19	South Carolina	390	1.16%
20	Colorado	373	1.11%
21	Arizona	340	1.01%
22	Tennessee	279	0.83%
23	Indiana	264	0.79%
24	Oregon	227	0.68%
25	Alabama	224	0.67%
26	Oklahoma	193	0.57%
27	Wisconsin	192	0.57%
28	Minnesota	170	0.51%
29	Mississippi	157	0.47%
30	Nevada	134	0.40%
31	Kentucky	130	0.39%
32	Kansas	128	0.38%
33	Hawaii	111	0.33%
34	New Mexico	102	0.30%
35	Arkansas	90	0.27%
36	Rhode Island	81	0.24%
37	Delaware	65	0.19%
38	Utah	59	0.18%
39	Iowa	58	0.17%
40	Nebraska	55	0.16%
41	Maine	49	0.15%
42	West Virginia	38	0.11%
43	Idaho	32	0.10%
43	New Hampshire	32	0.10%
45	Alaska	20	0.06%
46	Montana	18	0.05%
46	Vermont	18	0.05%
48	Wyoming	13	0.04%
49	North Dakota	7	0.02%
49	South Dakota	7	0.02%
	District of Columbia	512	1.53%

Source: U.S. Department of Health and Human Services, National Center for Health Statistics
"Monthly Vital Statistics Report" (Vol. 43, No. 6(S), December 8, 1994)
Updated numbers. AIDS is Acquired Immunodeficiency Syndrome.

Death Rate by AIDS in 1992

National Rate = 13.2 Deaths by AIDS per 100,000 Population*

ALPHA ORDER

RANK	STATE	RATE
31	Alabama	5.4
39	Alaska	3.4
19	Arizona	8.9
35	Arkansas	3.8
4	California	19.5
11	Colorado	10.8
9	Connecticut	12.3
17	Delaware	9.4
3	Florida	23.1
5	Georgia	17.2
15	Hawaii	9.6
43	Idaho	3.0
15	Illinois	9.6
33	Indiana	4.7
47	Iowa	2.1
32	Kansas	5.1
38	Kentucky	3.5
8	Louisiana	13.4
34	Maine	4.0
6	Maryland	15.5
10	Massachusetts	11.7
26	Michigan	6.1
35	Minnesota	3.8
27	Mississippi	6.0
23	Missouri	8.0
46	Montana**	2.2
39	Nebraska	3.4
13	Nevada	10.0
44	New Hampshire	2.9
2	New Jersey	24.6
25	New Mexico	6.4
1	New York	35.9
13	North Carolina	10.0
49	North Dakota**	1.1
29	Ohio	5.6
27	Oklahoma	6.0
24	Oregon	7.6
21	Pennsylvania	8.3
22	Rhode Island	8.1
11	South Carolina	10.8
50	South Dakota**	1.0
29	Tennessee	5.6
7	Texas	13.6
41	Utah	3.3
42	Vermont**	3.2
18	Virginia	9.2
20	Washington	8.7
47	West Virginia	2.1
35	Wisconsin	3.8
45	Wyoming**	2.8

RANK ORDER

RANK	STATE	RATE
1	New York	35.9
2	New Jersey	24.6
3	Florida	23.1
4	California	19.5
5	Georgia	17.2
6	Maryland	15.5
7	Texas	13.6
8	Louisiana	13.4
9	Connecticut	12.3
10	Massachusetts	11.7
11	Colorado	10.8
11	South Carolina	10.8
13	Nevada	10.0
13	North Carolina	10.0
15	Hawaii	9.6
15	Illinois	9.6
17	Delaware	9.4
18	Virginia	9.2
19	Arizona	8.9
20	Washington	8.7
21	Pennsylvania	8.3
22	Rhode Island	8.1
23	Missouri	8.0
24	Oregon	7.6
25	New Mexico	6.4
26	Michigan	6.1
27	Mississippi	6.0
27	Oklahoma	6.0
29	Ohio	5.6
29	Tennessee	5.6
31	Alabama	5.4
32	Kansas	5.1
33	Indiana	4.7
34	Maine	4.0
35	Arkansas	3.8
35	Minnesota	3.8
35	Wisconsin	3.8
38	Kentucky	3.5
39	Alaska	3.4
39	Nebraska	3.4
41	Utah	3.3
42	Vermont**	3.2
43	Idaho	3.0
44	New Hampshire	2.9
45	Wyoming**	2.8
46	Montana**	2.2
47	Iowa	2.1
47	West Virginia	2.1
49	North Dakota**	1.1
50	South Dakota**	1.0

	District of Columbia	87.5

Source: U.S. Department of Health and Human Services, National Center for Health Statistics
"Monthly Vital Statistics Report" (Vol. 43, No. 6(S), December 8, 1994)
Updated numbers. AIDS is Acquired Immunodeficiency Syndrome.
**Rates for North Dakota, South Dakota, Montana, Vermont and Wyoming were calculated by the editors.*

Estimated Deaths by Cancer in 1995

National Estimated Total = 547,000 Deaths

ALPHA ORDER

RANK	STATE	DEATHS	% of USA
22	Alabama	9,100	1.66%
50	Alaska	500	0.09%
24	Arizona	8,300	1.52%
30	Arkansas	6,100	1.12%
1	California	51,200	9.36%
32	Colorado	6,000	1.10%
26	Connecticut	7,000	1.28%
45	Delaware	1,700	0.31%
2	Florida	39,100	7.15%
15	Georgia	12,200	2.23%
43	Hawaii	1,800	0.33%
42	Idaho	1,900	0.35%
6	Illinois	25,900	4.73%
14	Indiana	12,500	2.29%
29	Iowa	6,500	1.19%
33	Kansas	5,600	1.02%
20	Kentucky	9,300	1.70%
21	Louisiana	9,200	1.68%
36	Maine	3,200	0.59%
18	Maryland	10,500	1.92%
11	Massachusetts	13,800	2.52%
8	Michigan	20,200	3.69%
23	Minnesota	8,800	1.61%
30	Mississippi	6,100	1.12%
13	Missouri	12,600	2.30%
43	Montana	1,800	0.33%
35	Nebraska	3,400	0.62%
37	Nevada	2,900	0.53%
39	New Hampshire	2,400	0.44%
9	New Jersey	18,700	3.42%
38	New Mexico	2,600	0.48%
3	New York	38,500	7.04%
10	North Carolina	15,300	2.80%
46	North Dakota	1,500	0.27%
7	Ohio	25,000	4.57%
27	Oklahoma	6,900	1.26%
27	Oregon	6,900	1.26%
5	Pennsylvania	31,200	5.70%
39	Rhode Island	2,400	0.44%
25	South Carolina	7,800	1.43%
46	South Dakota	1,500	0.27%
16	Tennessee	11,400	2.08%
4	Texas	33,100	6.05%
41	Utah	2,200	0.40%
48	Vermont	1,100	0.20%
12	Virginia	12,800	2.34%
19	Washington	10,300	1.88%
34	West Virginia	4,700	0.86%
17	Wisconsin	11,100	2.03%
49	Wyoming	800	0.15%

RANK ORDER

RANK	STATE	DEATHS	% of USA
1	California	51,200	9.36%
2	Florida	39,100	7.15%
3	New York	38,500	7.04%
4	Texas	33,100	6.05%
5	Pennsylvania	31,200	5.70%
6	Illinois	25,900	4.73%
7	Ohio	25,000	4.57%
8	Michigan	20,200	3.69%
9	New Jersey	18,700	3.42%
10	North Carolina	15,300	2.80%
11	Massachusetts	13,800	2.52%
12	Virginia	12,800	2.34%
13	Missouri	12,600	2.30%
14	Indiana	12,500	2.29%
15	Georgia	12,200	2.23%
16	Tennessee	11,400	2.08%
17	Wisconsin	11,100	2.03%
18	Maryland	10,500	1.92%
19	Washington	10,300	1.88%
20	Kentucky	9,300	1.70%
21	Louisiana	9,200	1.68%
22	Alabama	9,100	1.66%
23	Minnesota	8,800	1.61%
24	Arizona	8,300	1.52%
25	South Carolina	7,800	1.43%
26	Connecticut	7,000	1.28%
27	Oklahoma	6,900	1.26%
27	Oregon	6,900	1.26%
29	Iowa	6,500	1.19%
30	Arkansas	6,100	1.12%
30	Mississippi	6,100	1.12%
32	Colorado	6,000	1.10%
33	Kansas	5,600	1.02%
34	West Virginia	4,700	0.86%
35	Nebraska	3,400	0.62%
36	Maine	3,200	0.59%
37	Nevada	2,900	0.53%
38	New Mexico	2,600	0.48%
39	New Hampshire	2,400	0.44%
39	Rhode Island	2,400	0.44%
41	Utah	2,200	0.40%
42	Idaho	1,900	0.35%
43	Hawaii	1,800	0.33%
43	Montana	1,800	0.33%
45	Delaware	1,700	0.31%
46	North Dakota	1,500	0.27%
46	South Dakota	1,500	0.27%
48	Vermont	1,100	0.20%
49	Wyoming	800	0.15%
50	Alaska	500	0.09%
	District of Columbia	1,600	0.29%

Source: American Cancer Society
"Cancer Facts & Figures-1995" (Copyright 1995, Reprinted with permission from the American Cancer Society)

Estimated Death Rate by Cancer in 1995

National Rate = 210.1 Deaths by Cancer per 100,000 Population*

ALPHA ORDER				RANK ORDER		
RANK	**STATE**	**RATE**		**RANK**	**STATE**	**RATE**
23	Alabama	215.7		1	Florida	280.2
50	Alaska	82.5		2	Pennsylvania	258.9
35	Arizona	203.7		3	Maine	258.1
5	Arkansas	248.7		4	West Virginia	258.0
46	California	162.9		5	Arkansas	248.7
45	Colorado	164.1		6	Kentucky	243.0
24	Connecticut	213.7		7	Delaware	240.8
7	Delaware	240.8		8	Rhode Island	240.7
1	Florida	280.2		9	Missouri	238.7
42	Georgia	172.9		10	New Jersey	236.6
48	Hawaii	152.7		11	North Dakota	235.1
44	Idaho	167.7		12	Iowa	229.8
17	Illinois	220.4		13	Mississippi	228.6
21	Indiana	217.3		14	Massachusetts	228.4
12	Iowa	229.8		15	Ohio	225.2
19	Kansas	219.3		16	Oregon	223.6
6	Kentucky	243.0		17	Illinois	220.4
25	Louisiana	213.2		18	Tennessee	220.3
3	Maine	258.1		19	Kansas	219.3
32	Maryland	209.7		20	Wisconsin	218.4
14	Massachusetts	228.4		21	Indiana	217.3
27	Michigan	212.7		22	North Carolina	216.4
39	Minnesota	192.7		23	Alabama	215.7
13	Mississippi	228.6		24	Connecticut	213.7
9	Missouri	238.7		25	Louisiana	213.2
31	Montana	210.3		26	South Carolina	212.9
33	Nebraska	209.5		27	Michigan	212.7
36	Nevada	199.0		28	New York	211.9
30	New Hampshire	211.1		29	Oklahoma	211.8
10	New Jersey	236.6		30	New Hampshire	211.1
47	New Mexico	157.2		31	Montana	210.3
28	New York	211.9		32	Maryland	209.7
22	North Carolina	216.4		33	Nebraska	209.5
11	North Dakota	235.1		34	South Dakota	208.0
15	Ohio	225.2		35	Arizona	203.7
29	Oklahoma	211.8		36	Nevada	199.0
16	Oregon	223.6		37	Virginia	195.4
2	Pennsylvania	258.9		38	Washington	192.8
8	Rhode Island	240.7		39	Minnesota	192.7
26	South Carolina	212.9		40	Vermont	189.7
34	South Dakota	208.0		41	Texas	180.1
18	Tennessee	220.3		42	Georgia	172.9
41	Texas	180.1		43	Wyoming	168.1
49	Utah	115.3		44	Idaho	167.7
40	Vermont	189.7		45	Colorado	164.1
37	Virginia	195.4		46	California	162.9
38	Washington	192.8		47	New Mexico	157.2
4	West Virginia	258.0		48	Hawaii	152.7
20	Wisconsin	218.4		49	Utah	115.3
43	Wyoming	168.1		50	Alaska	82.5
					District of Columbia	280.7

Source: Morgan Quitno Press using data from American Cancer Society
    "Cancer Facts & Figures-1995" (Copyright 1995, Reprinted with permission from the American Cancer Society)
*Rates calculated using 1994 Census resident population estimates.

Estimated Deaths by Bladder Cancer in 1995

National Estimated Total = 11,200 Deaths

RANK	STATE	DEATHS	% of USA
27	Alabama	140	1.25%
49	Alaska	10	0.09%
21	Arizona	180	1.61%
28	Arkansas	120	1.07%
1	California	1,100	9.82%
25	Colorado	150	1.34%
22	Connecticut	170	1.52%
36	Delaware	60	0.54%
2	Florida	900	8.04%
18	Georgia	190	1.70%
47	Hawaii	20	0.18%
44	Idaho	30	0.27%
8	Illinois	460	4.11%
13	Indiana	270	2.41%
23	Iowa	160	1.43%
33	Kansas	70	0.63%
25	Kentucky	150	1.34%
32	Louisiana	110	0.98%
33	Maine	70	0.63%
17	Maryland	210	1.88%
10	Massachusetts	380	3.39%
8	Michigan	460	4.11%
23	Minnesota	160	1.43%
36	Mississippi	60	0.54%
14	Missouri	230	2.05%
41	Montana	40	0.36%
40	Nebraska	50	0.45%
47	Nevada	20	0.18%
33	New Hampshire	70	0.63%
7	New Jersey	490	4.38%
41	New Mexico	40	0.36%
3	New York	850	7.59%
11	North Carolina	300	2.68%
44	North Dakota	30	0.27%
6	Ohio	520	4.64%
28	Oklahoma	120	1.07%
28	Oregon	120	1.07%
4	Pennsylvania	680	6.07%
36	Rhode Island	60	0.54%
18	South Carolina	190	1.70%
36	South Dakota	60	0.54%
18	Tennessee	190	1.70%
5	Texas	560	5.00%
41	Utah	40	0.36%
44	Vermont	30	0.27%
15	Virginia	220	1.96%
15	Washington	220	1.96%
28	West Virginia	120	1.07%
12	Wisconsin	280	2.50%
49	Wyoming	10	0.09%

RANK	STATE	DEATHS	% of USA
1	California	1,100	9.82%
2	Florida	900	8.04%
3	New York	850	7.59%
4	Pennsylvania	680	6.07%
5	Texas	560	5.00%
6	Ohio	520	4.64%
7	New Jersey	490	4.38%
8	Illinois	460	4.11%
8	Michigan	460	4.11%
10	Massachusetts	380	3.39%
11	North Carolina	300	2.68%
12	Wisconsin	280	2.50%
13	Indiana	270	2.41%
14	Missouri	230	2.05%
15	Virginia	220	1.96%
15	Washington	220	1.96%
17	Maryland	210	1.88%
18	Georgia	190	1.70%
18	South Carolina	190	1.70%
18	Tennessee	190	1.70%
21	Arizona	180	1.61%
22	Connecticut	170	1.52%
23	Iowa	160	1.43%
23	Minnesota	160	1.43%
25	Colorado	150	1.34%
25	Kentucky	150	1.34%
27	Alabama	140	1.25%
28	Arkansas	120	1.07%
28	Oklahoma	120	1.07%
28	Oregon	120	1.07%
28	West Virginia	120	1.07%
32	Louisiana	110	0.98%
33	Kansas	70	0.63%
33	Maine	70	0.63%
33	New Hampshire	70	0.63%
36	Delaware	60	0.54%
36	Mississippi	60	0.54%
36	Rhode Island	60	0.54%
36	South Dakota	60	0.54%
40	Nebraska	50	0.45%
41	Montana	40	0.36%
41	New Mexico	40	0.36%
41	Utah	40	0.36%
44	Idaho	30	0.27%
44	North Dakota	30	0.27%
44	Vermont	30	0.27%
47	Hawaii	20	0.18%
47	Nevada	20	0.18%
49	Alaska	10	0.09%
49	Wyoming	10	0.09%
	District of Columbia	30	0.27%

Source: American Cancer Society
"Cancer Facts & Figures–1995" (Copyright 1995, Reprinted with permission from the American Cancer Society)

Estimated Death Rate by Bladder Cancer in 1995

National Estimated Rate = 4.3 Deaths by Bladder Cancer per 100,000 Population*

ALPHA ORDER			RANK ORDER		
RANK	**STATE**	**RATE**	**RANK**	**STATE**	**RATE**
37	Alabama	3.3	1	Delaware	8.5
48	Alaska	1.7	2	South Dakota	8.3
23	Arizona	4.4	3	West Virginia	6.6
16	Arkansas	4.9	4	Florida	6.5
34	California	3.5	5	Massachusetts	6.3
27	Colorado	4.1	6	New Hampshire	6.2
13	Connecticut	5.2	6	New Jersey	6.2
1	Delaware	8.5	8	Rhode Island	6.0
4	Florida	6.5	9	Iowa	5.7
40	Georgia	2.7	10	Maine	5.6
48	Hawaii	1.7	10	Pennsylvania	5.6
42	Idaho	2.6	12	Wisconsin	5.5
29	Illinois	3.9	13	Connecticut	5.2
18	Indiana	4.7	13	South Carolina	5.2
9	Iowa	5.7	13	Vermont	5.2
40	Kansas	2.7	16	Arkansas	4.9
29	Kentucky	3.9	17	Michigan	4.8
43	Louisiana	2.5	18	Indiana	4.7
10	Maine	5.6	18	Montana	4.7
25	Maryland	4.2	18	New York	4.7
5	Massachusetts	6.3	18	North Dakota	4.7
17	Michigan	4.8	18	Ohio	4.7
34	Minnesota	3.5	23	Arizona	4.4
45	Mississippi	2.2	23	Missouri	4.4
23	Missouri	4.4	25	Maryland	4.2
18	Montana	4.7	25	North Carolina	4.2
38	Nebraska	3.1	27	Colorado	4.1
50	Nevada	1.4	27	Washington	4.1
6	New Hampshire	6.2	29	Illinois	3.9
6	New Jersey	6.2	29	Kentucky	3.9
44	New Mexico	2.4	29	Oregon	3.9
18	New York	4.7	32	Oklahoma	3.7
25	North Carolina	4.2	32	Tennessee	3.7
18	North Dakota	4.7	34	California	3.5
18	Ohio	4.7	34	Minnesota	3.5
32	Oklahoma	3.7	36	Virginia	3.4
29	Oregon	3.9	37	Alabama	3.3
10	Pennsylvania	5.6	38	Nebraska	3.1
8	Rhode Island	6.0	39	Texas	3.0
13	South Carolina	5.2	40	Georgia	2.7
2	South Dakota	8.3	40	Kansas	2.7
32	Tennessee	3.7	42	Idaho	2.6
39	Texas	3.0	43	Louisiana	2.5
46	Utah	2.1	44	New Mexico	2.4
13	Vermont	5.2	45	Mississippi	2.2
36	Virginia	3.4	46	Utah	2.1
27	Washington	4.1	46	Wyoming	2.1
3	West Virginia	6.6	48	Alaska	1.7
12	Wisconsin	5.5	48	Hawaii	1.7
46	Wyoming	2.1	50	Nevada	1.4
				District of Columbia	5.3

Source: Morgan Quitno Press using data from American Cancer Society
"Cancer Facts & Figures–1995" (Copyright 1995, Reprinted with permission from the American Cancer Society)
Rates calculated using 1994 Census resident population estimates.

Estimated Deaths by Female Breast Cancer in 1995

National Estimated Total = 46,000 Deaths*

ALPHA ORDER

RANK	STATE	DEATHS	% of USA
22	Alabama	710	1.54%
50	Alaska	40	0.09%
24	Arizona	630	1.37%
30	Arkansas	480	1.04%
1	California	4,400	9.57%
28	Colorado	560	1.22%
27	Connecticut	580	1.26%
43	Delaware	150	0.33%
3	Florida	2,900	6.30%
15	Georgia	970	2.11%
47	Hawaii	110	0.24%
41	Idaho	190	0.41%
6	Illinois	2,400	5.22%
13	Indiana	1,000	2.17%
26	Iowa	590	1.28%
30	Kansas	480	1.04%
25	Kentucky	610	1.33%
20	Louisiana	810	1.76%
36	Maine	250	0.54%
18	Maryland	870	1.89%
10	Massachusetts	1,200	2.61%
9	Michigan	1,600	3.48%
21	Minnesota	780	1.70%
33	Mississippi	470	1.02%
13	Missouri	1,000	2.17%
44	Montana	130	0.28%
35	Nebraska	320	0.70%
41	Nevada	190	0.41%
38	New Hampshire	230	0.50%
8	New Jersey	1,800	3.91%
40	New Mexico	210	0.46%
2	New York	3,700	8.04%
10	North Carolina	1,200	2.61%
44	North Dakota	130	0.28%
7	Ohio	2,100	4.57%
29	Oklahoma	500	1.09%
30	Oregon	480	1.04%
4	Pennsylvania	2,800	6.09%
37	Rhode Island	240	0.52%
23	South Carolina	690	1.50%
46	South Dakota	120	0.26%
17	Tennessee	880	1.91%
5	Texas	2,600	5.65%
39	Utah	220	0.48%
47	Vermont	110	0.24%
10	Virginia	1,200	2.61%
19	Washington	850	1.85%
34	West Virginia	330	0.72%
16	Wisconsin	950	2.07%
49	Wyoming	80	0.17%

RANK ORDER

RANK	STATE	DEATHS	% of USA
1	California	4,400	9.57%
2	New York	3,700	8.04%
3	Florida	2,900	6.30%
4	Pennsylvania	2,800	6.09%
5	Texas	2,600	5.65%
6	Illinois	2,400	5.22%
7	Ohio	2,100	4.57%
8	New Jersey	1,800	3.91%
9	Michigan	1,600	3.48%
10	Massachusetts	1,200	2.61%
10	North Carolina	1,200	2.61%
10	Virginia	1,200	2.61%
13	Indiana	1,000	2.17%
13	Missouri	1,000	2.17%
15	Georgia	970	2.11%
16	Wisconsin	950	2.07%
17	Tennessee	880	1.91%
18	Maryland	870	1.89%
19	Washington	850	1.85%
20	Louisiana	810	1.76%
21	Minnesota	780	1.70%
22	Alabama	710	1.54%
23	South Carolina	690	1.50%
24	Arizona	630	1.37%
25	Kentucky	610	1.33%
26	Iowa	590	1.28%
27	Connecticut	580	1.26%
28	Colorado	560	1.22%
29	Oklahoma	500	1.09%
30	Arkansas	480	1.04%
30	Kansas	480	1.04%
30	Oregon	480	1.04%
33	Mississippi	470	1.02%
34	West Virginia	330	0.72%
35	Nebraska	320	0.70%
36	Maine	250	0.54%
37	Rhode Island	240	0.52%
38	New Hampshire	230	0.50%
39	Utah	220	0.48%
40	New Mexico	210	0.46%
41	Idaho	190	0.41%
41	Nevada	190	0.41%
43	Delaware	150	0.33%
44	Montana	130	0.28%
44	North Dakota	130	0.28%
46	South Dakota	120	0.26%
47	Hawaii	110	0.24%
47	Vermont	110	0.24%
49	Wyoming	80	0.17%
50	Alaska	40	0.09%
	District of Columbia	160	0.35%

Source: American Cancer Society
"Cancer Facts & Figures–1995" (Copyright 1995, Reprinted with permission from the American Cancer Society)

Estimated Death Rate by Female Breast Cancer in 1995

National Estimated Rate = 34.5 Deaths per 100,000 Female Population*

ALPHA ORDER

RANK	STATE	RATE
35	Alabama	32.3
50	Alaska	14.0
39	Arizona	30.6
14	Arkansas	37.8
43	California	28.0
40	Colorado	30.4
24	Connecticut	34.4
4	Delaware	41.3
7	Florida	40.3
45	Georgia	26.8
49	Hawaii	18.9
30	Idaho	33.4
8	Illinois	39.8
25	Indiana	33.8
5	Iowa	40.6
16	Kansas	37.0
37	Kentucky	30.9
21	Louisiana	36.2
10	Maine	39.3
25	Maryland	33.8
13	Massachusetts	38.3
32	Michigan	32.8
29	Minnesota	33.6
25	Mississippi	33.8
18	Missouri	36.6
41	Montana	30.2
12	Nebraska	38.5
46	Nevada	26.6
9	New Hampshire	39.7
3	New Jersey	44.1
47	New Mexico	25.0
11	New York	39.2
31	North Carolina	33.0
5	North Dakota	40.6
18	Ohio	36.6
42	Oklahoma	30.0
38	Oregon	30.7
2	Pennsylvania	44.7
1	Rhode Island	46.3
20	South Carolina	36.4
32	South Dakota	32.8
32	Tennessee	32.8
44	Texas	27.9
48	Utah	22.9
15	Vermont	37.3
22	Virginia	35.9
36	Washington	31.6
23	West Virginia	34.9
17	Wisconsin	36.7
25	Wyoming	33.8

RANK ORDER

RANK	STATE	RATE
1	Rhode Island	46.3
2	Pennsylvania	44.7
3	New Jersey	44.1
4	Delaware	41.3
5	Iowa	40.6
5	North Dakota	40.6
7	Florida	40.3
8	Illinois	39.8
9	New Hampshire	39.7
10	Maine	39.3
11	New York	39.2
12	Nebraska	38.5
13	Massachusetts	38.3
14	Arkansas	37.8
15	Vermont	37.3
16	Kansas	37.0
17	Wisconsin	36.7
18	Missouri	36.6
18	Ohio	36.6
20	South Carolina	36.4
21	Louisiana	36.2
22	Virginia	35.9
23	West Virginia	34.9
24	Connecticut	34.4
25	Indiana	33.8
25	Maryland	33.8
25	Mississippi	33.8
25	Wyoming	33.8
29	Minnesota	33.6
30	Idaho	33.4
31	North Carolina	33.0
32	Michigan	32.8
32	South Dakota	32.8
32	Tennessee	32.8
35	Alabama	32.3
36	Washington	31.6
37	Kentucky	30.9
38	Oregon	30.7
39	Arizona	30.6
40	Colorado	30.4
41	Montana	30.2
42	Oklahoma	30.0
43	California	28.0
44	Texas	27.9
45	Georgia	26.8
46	Nevada	26.6
47	New Mexico	25.0
48	Utah	22.9
49	Hawaii	18.9
50	Alaska	14.0
	District of Columbia	52.6

Source: Morgan Quitno Press using data from American Cancer Society
"Cancer Facts & Figures-1995" (Copyright 1995, Reprinted with permission from the American Cancer Society)
Rates calculated using 1994 Census resident female population estimates.

Estimated Deaths by Colon and Rectum Cancer in 1995

National Estimated Total = 55,300 Deaths

ALPHA ORDER

RANK	STATE	DEATHS	% of USA
23	Alabama	800	1.45%
50	Alaska	50	0.09%
27	Arizona	710	1.28%
29	Arkansas	630	1.14%
1	California	4,900	8.86%
29	Colorado	630	1.14%
26	Connecticut	760	1.37%
42	Delaware	190	0.34%
3	Florida	3,600	6.51%
18	Georgia	980	1.77%
42	Hawaii	190	0.34%
42	Idaho	190	0.34%
6	Illinois	2,800	5.06%
13	Indiana	1,200	2.17%
24	Iowa	780	1.41%
32	Kansas	610	1.10%
19	Kentucky	950	1.72%
22	Louisiana	860	1.56%
36	Maine	300	0.54%
16	Maryland	1,100	1.99%
10	Massachusetts	1,700	3.07%
8	Michigan	2,300	4.16%
19	Minnesota	950	1.72%
31	Mississippi	620	1.12%
12	Missouri	1,300	2.35%
45	Montana	180	0.33%
35	Nebraska	350	0.63%
39	Nevada	210	0.38%
40	New Hampshire	200	0.36%
9	New Jersey	2,000	3.62%
40	New Mexico	200	0.36%
2	New York	4,200	7.59%
11	North Carolina	1,500	2.71%
45	North Dakota	180	0.33%
7	Ohio	2,600	4.70%
28	Oklahoma	660	1.19%
33	Oregon	590	1.07%
4	Pennsylvania	3,300	5.97%
37	Rhode Island	290	0.52%
25	South Carolina	770	1.39%
47	South Dakota	150	0.27%
13	Tennessee	1,200	2.17%
4	Texas	3,300	5.97%
38	Utah	230	0.42%
48	Vermont	120	0.22%
13	Virginia	1,200	2.17%
21	Washington	870	1.57%
34	West Virginia	520	0.94%
16	Wisconsin	1,100	1.99%
49	Wyoming	80	0.14%

RANK ORDER

RANK	STATE	DEATHS	% of USA
1	California	4,900	8.86%
2	New York	4,200	7.59%
3	Florida	3,600	6.51%
4	Pennsylvania	3,300	5.97%
4	Texas	3,300	5.97%
6	Illinois	2,800	5.06%
7	Ohio	2,600	4.70%
8	Michigan	2,300	4.16%
9	New Jersey	2,000	3.62%
10	Massachusetts	1,700	3.07%
11	North Carolina	1,500	2.71%
12	Missouri	1,300	2.35%
13	Indiana	1,200	2.17%
13	Tennessee	1,200	2.17%
13	Virginia	1,200	2.17%
16	Maryland	1,100	1.99%
16	Wisconsin	1,100	1.99%
18	Georgia	980	1.77%
19	Kentucky	950	1.72%
19	Minnesota	950	1.72%
21	Washington	870	1.57%
22	Louisiana	860	1.56%
23	Alabama	800	1.45%
24	Iowa	780	1.41%
25	South Carolina	770	1.39%
26	Connecticut	760	1.37%
27	Arizona	710	1.28%
28	Oklahoma	660	1.19%
29	Arkansas	630	1.14%
29	Colorado	630	1.14%
31	Mississippi	620	1.12%
32	Kansas	610	1.10%
33	Oregon	590	1.07%
34	West Virginia	520	0.94%
35	Nebraska	350	0.63%
36	Maine	300	0.54%
37	Rhode Island	290	0.52%
38	Utah	230	0.42%
39	Nevada	210	0.38%
40	New Hampshire	200	0.36%
40	New Mexico	200	0.36%
42	Delaware	190	0.34%
42	Hawaii	190	0.34%
42	Idaho	190	0.34%
45	Montana	180	0.33%
45	North Dakota	180	0.33%
47	South Dakota	150	0.27%
48	Vermont	120	0.22%
49	Wyoming	80	0.14%
50	Alaska	50	0.09%
	District of Columbia	200	0.36%

Source: American Cancer Society
"Cancer Facts & Figures-1995" (Copyright 1995, Reprinted with permission from the American Cancer Society)

Estimated Death Rate by Colon and Rectum Cancer in 1995

National Estimated Rate = 21.2 Deaths per 100,000 Population*

<table>
<tr><td colspan="3"><u>ALPHA ORDER</u></td><td colspan="3"><u>RANK ORDER</u></td></tr>
<tr><td>RANK</td><td>STATE</td><td>RATE</td><td>RANK</td><td>STATE</td><td>RATE</td></tr>
<tr><td>35</td><td>Alabama</td><td>19.0</td><td>1</td><td>Rhode Island</td><td>29.1</td></tr>
<tr><td>50</td><td>Alaska</td><td>8.3</td><td>2</td><td>West Virginia</td><td>28.5</td></tr>
<tr><td>39</td><td>Arizona</td><td>17.4</td><td>3</td><td>North Dakota</td><td>28.2</td></tr>
<tr><td>9</td><td>Arkansas</td><td>25.7</td><td>4</td><td>Massachusetts</td><td>28.1</td></tr>
<tr><td>45</td><td>California</td><td>15.6</td><td>5</td><td>Iowa</td><td>27.6</td></tr>
<tr><td>40</td><td>Colorado</td><td>17.2</td><td>6</td><td>Pennsylvania</td><td>27.4</td></tr>
<tr><td>18</td><td>Connecticut</td><td>23.2</td><td>7</td><td>Delaware</td><td>26.9</td></tr>
<tr><td>7</td><td>Delaware</td><td>26.9</td><td>8</td><td>Florida</td><td>25.8</td></tr>
<tr><td>8</td><td>Florida</td><td>25.8</td><td>9</td><td>Arkansas</td><td>25.7</td></tr>
<tr><td>47</td><td>Georgia</td><td>13.9</td><td>10</td><td>New Jersey</td><td>25.3</td></tr>
<tr><td>44</td><td>Hawaii</td><td>16.1</td><td>11</td><td>Kentucky</td><td>24.8</td></tr>
<tr><td>41</td><td>Idaho</td><td>16.8</td><td>12</td><td>Missouri</td><td>24.6</td></tr>
<tr><td>16</td><td>Illinois</td><td>23.8</td><td>13</td><td>Maine</td><td>24.2</td></tr>
<tr><td>28</td><td>Indiana</td><td>20.9</td><td>13</td><td>Michigan</td><td>24.2</td></tr>
<tr><td>5</td><td>Iowa</td><td>27.6</td><td>15</td><td>Kansas</td><td>23.9</td></tr>
<tr><td>15</td><td>Kansas</td><td>23.9</td><td>16</td><td>Illinois</td><td>23.8</td></tr>
<tr><td>11</td><td>Kentucky</td><td>24.8</td><td>17</td><td>Ohio</td><td>23.4</td></tr>
<tr><td>33</td><td>Louisiana</td><td>19.9</td><td>18</td><td>Connecticut</td><td>23.2</td></tr>
<tr><td>13</td><td>Maine</td><td>24.2</td><td>18</td><td>Mississippi</td><td>23.2</td></tr>
<tr><td>22</td><td>Maryland</td><td>22.0</td><td>18</td><td>Tennessee</td><td>23.2</td></tr>
<tr><td>4</td><td>Massachusetts</td><td>28.1</td><td>21</td><td>New York</td><td>23.1</td></tr>
<tr><td>13</td><td>Michigan</td><td>24.2</td><td>22</td><td>Maryland</td><td>22.0</td></tr>
<tr><td>29</td><td>Minnesota</td><td>20.8</td><td>23</td><td>Nebraska</td><td>21.6</td></tr>
<tr><td>18</td><td>Mississippi</td><td>23.2</td><td>23</td><td>Wisconsin</td><td>21.6</td></tr>
<tr><td>12</td><td>Missouri</td><td>24.6</td><td>25</td><td>North Carolina</td><td>21.2</td></tr>
<tr><td>26</td><td>Montana</td><td>21.0</td><td>26</td><td>Montana</td><td>21.0</td></tr>
<tr><td>23</td><td>Nebraska</td><td>21.6</td><td>26</td><td>South Carolina</td><td>21.0</td></tr>
<tr><td>46</td><td>Nevada</td><td>14.4</td><td>28</td><td>Indiana</td><td>20.9</td></tr>
<tr><td>38</td><td>New Hampshire</td><td>17.6</td><td>29</td><td>Minnesota</td><td>20.8</td></tr>
<tr><td>10</td><td>New Jersey</td><td>25.3</td><td>29</td><td>South Dakota</td><td>20.8</td></tr>
<tr><td>48</td><td>New Mexico</td><td>12.1</td><td>31</td><td>Vermont</td><td>20.7</td></tr>
<tr><td>21</td><td>New York</td><td>23.1</td><td>32</td><td>Oklahoma</td><td>20.3</td></tr>
<tr><td>25</td><td>North Carolina</td><td>21.2</td><td>33</td><td>Louisiana</td><td>19.9</td></tr>
<tr><td>3</td><td>North Dakota</td><td>28.2</td><td>34</td><td>Oregon</td><td>19.1</td></tr>
<tr><td>17</td><td>Ohio</td><td>23.4</td><td>35</td><td>Alabama</td><td>19.0</td></tr>
<tr><td>32</td><td>Oklahoma</td><td>20.3</td><td>36</td><td>Virginia</td><td>18.3</td></tr>
<tr><td>34</td><td>Oregon</td><td>19.1</td><td>37</td><td>Texas</td><td>18.0</td></tr>
<tr><td>6</td><td>Pennsylvania</td><td>27.4</td><td>38</td><td>New Hampshire</td><td>17.6</td></tr>
<tr><td>1</td><td>Rhode Island</td><td>29.1</td><td>39</td><td>Arizona</td><td>17.4</td></tr>
<tr><td>26</td><td>South Carolina</td><td>21.0</td><td>40</td><td>Colorado</td><td>17.2</td></tr>
<tr><td>29</td><td>South Dakota</td><td>20.8</td><td>41</td><td>Idaho</td><td>16.8</td></tr>
<tr><td>18</td><td>Tennessee</td><td>23.2</td><td>41</td><td>Wyoming</td><td>16.8</td></tr>
<tr><td>37</td><td>Texas</td><td>18.0</td><td>43</td><td>Washington</td><td>16.3</td></tr>
<tr><td>48</td><td>Utah</td><td>12.1</td><td>44</td><td>Hawaii</td><td>16.1</td></tr>
<tr><td>31</td><td>Vermont</td><td>20.7</td><td>45</td><td>California</td><td>15.6</td></tr>
<tr><td>36</td><td>Virginia</td><td>18.3</td><td>46</td><td>Nevada</td><td>14.4</td></tr>
<tr><td>43</td><td>Washington</td><td>16.3</td><td>47</td><td>Georgia</td><td>13.9</td></tr>
<tr><td>2</td><td>West Virginia</td><td>28.5</td><td>48</td><td>New Mexico</td><td>12.1</td></tr>
<tr><td>23</td><td>Wisconsin</td><td>21.6</td><td>48</td><td>Utah</td><td>12.1</td></tr>
<tr><td>41</td><td>Wyoming</td><td>16.8</td><td>50</td><td>Alaska</td><td>8.3</td></tr>
<tr><td></td><td></td><td></td><td></td><td>District of Columbia</td><td>35.1</td></tr>
</table>

Source: Morgan Quitno Press using data from American Cancer Society
   "Cancer Facts & Figures–1995" (Copyright 1995, Reprinted with permission from the American Cancer Society)
Rates calculated using 1994 Census resident population estimates.

Estimated Deaths by Leukemia in 1995

National Estimated Total = 20,400 Deaths

<u>ALPHA ORDER</u>

RANK	STATE	DEATHS	% of USA
20	Alabama	360	1.76%
50	Alaska	10	0.05%
20	Arizona	360	1.76%
28	Arkansas	250	1.23%
1	California	2,000	9.80%
29	Colorado	230	1.13%
27	Connecticut	260	1.27%
45	Delaware	50	0.25%
2	Florida	1,400	6.86%
12	Georgia	490	2.40%
45	Hawaii	50	0.25%
40	Idaho	80	0.39%
5	Illinois	1,100	5.39%
14	Indiana	450	2.21%
26	Iowa	270	1.32%
29	Kansas	230	1.13%
22	Kentucky	350	1.72%
22	Louisiana	350	1.72%
37	Maine	100	0.49%
24	Maryland	340	1.67%
15	Massachusetts	430	2.11%
8	Michigan	820	4.02%
15	Minnesota	430	2.11%
32	Mississippi	210	1.03%
11	Missouri	500	2.45%
42	Montana	70	0.34%
35	Nebraska	120	0.59%
38	Nevada	90	0.44%
42	New Hampshire	70	0.34%
9	New Jersey	600	2.94%
35	New Mexico	120	0.59%
3	New York	1,300	6.37%
10	North Carolina	550	2.70%
45	North Dakota	50	0.25%
7	Ohio	970	4.75%
29	Oklahoma	230	1.13%
25	Oregon	280	1.37%
5	Pennsylvania	1,100	5.39%
38	Rhode Island	90	0.44%
32	South Carolina	210	1.03%
44	South Dakota	60	0.29%
18	Tennessee	410	2.01%
3	Texas	1,300	6.37%
40	Utah	80	0.39%
48	Vermont	40	0.20%
13	Virginia	470	2.30%
18	Washington	410	2.01%
34	West Virginia	150	0.74%
15	Wisconsin	430	2.11%
49	Wyoming	30	0.15%

<u>RANK ORDER</u>

RANK	STATE	DEATHS	% of USA
1	California	2,000	9.80%
2	Florida	1,400	6.86%
3	New York	1,300	6.37%
3	Texas	1,300	6.37%
5	Illinois	1,100	5.39%
5	Pennsylvania	1,100	5.39%
7	Ohio	970	4.75%
8	Michigan	820	4.02%
9	New Jersey	600	2.94%
10	North Carolina	550	2.70%
11	Missouri	500	2.45%
12	Georgia	490	2.40%
13	Virginia	470	2.30%
14	Indiana	450	2.21%
15	Massachusetts	430	2.11%
15	Minnesota	430	2.11%
15	Wisconsin	430	2.11%
18	Tennessee	410	2.01%
18	Washington	410	2.01%
20	Alabama	360	1.76%
20	Arizona	360	1.76%
22	Kentucky	350	1.72%
22	Louisiana	350	1.72%
24	Maryland	340	1.67%
25	Oregon	280	1.37%
26	Iowa	270	1.32%
27	Connecticut	260	1.27%
28	Arkansas	250	1.23%
29	Colorado	230	1.13%
29	Kansas	230	1.13%
29	Oklahoma	230	1.13%
32	Mississippi	210	1.03%
32	South Carolina	210	1.03%
34	West Virginia	150	0.74%
35	Nebraska	120	0.59%
35	New Mexico	120	0.59%
37	Maine	100	0.49%
38	Nevada	90	0.44%
38	Rhode Island	90	0.44%
40	Idaho	80	0.39%
40	Utah	80	0.39%
42	Montana	70	0.34%
42	New Hampshire	70	0.34%
44	South Dakota	60	0.29%
45	Delaware	50	0.25%
45	Hawaii	50	0.25%
45	North Dakota	50	0.25%
48	Vermont	40	0.20%
49	Wyoming	30	0.15%
50	Alaska	10	0.05%
	District of Columbia	50	0.25%

Source: American Cancer Society
"Cancer Facts & Figures-1995" (Copyright 1995, Reprinted with permission from the American Cancer Society)

Estimated Death Rate by Leukemia in 1995

National Estimated Rate = 7.8 Deaths by Leukemia per 100,000 Population*

ALPHA ORDER			RANK ORDER		
RANK	STATE	RATE	RANK	STATE	RATE
15	Alabama	8.5	1	Arkansas	10.2
50	Alaska	1.7	2	Florida	10.0
12	Arizona	8.8	3	Iowa	9.5
1	Arkansas	10.2	3	Missouri	9.5
42	California	6.4	5	Illinois	9.4
43	Colorado	6.3	5	Minnesota	9.4
22	Connecticut	7.9	7	Kentucky	9.1
34	Delaware	7.1	7	Oregon	9.1
2	Florida	10.0	7	Pennsylvania	9.1
39	Georgia	6.9	10	Kansas	9.0
48	Hawaii	4.2	10	Rhode Island	9.0
34	Idaho	7.1	12	Arizona	8.8
5	Illinois	9.4	13	Ohio	8.7
25	Indiana	7.8	14	Michigan	8.6
3	Iowa	9.5	15	Alabama	8.5
10	Kansas	9.0	15	Wisconsin	8.5
7	Kentucky	9.1	17	South Dakota	8.3
20	Louisiana	8.1	18	Montana	8.2
20	Maine	8.1	18	West Virginia	8.2
41	Maryland	6.8	20	Louisiana	8.1
34	Massachusetts	7.1	20	Maine	8.1
14	Michigan	8.6	22	Connecticut	7.9
5	Minnesota	9.4	22	Mississippi	7.9
22	Mississippi	7.9	22	Tennessee	7.9
3	Missouri	9.5	25	Indiana	7.8
18	Montana	8.2	25	North Carolina	7.8
30	Nebraska	7.4	25	North Dakota	7.8
45	Nevada	6.2	28	Washington	7.7
45	New Hampshire	6.2	29	New Jersey	7.6
29	New Jersey	7.6	30	Nebraska	7.4
31	New Mexico	7.3	31	New Mexico	7.3
32	New York	7.2	32	New York	7.2
25	North Carolina	7.8	32	Virginia	7.2
25	North Dakota	7.8	34	Delaware	7.1
13	Ohio	8.7	34	Idaho	7.1
34	Oklahoma	7.1	34	Massachusetts	7.1
7	Oregon	9.1	34	Oklahoma	7.1
7	Pennsylvania	9.1	34	Texas	7.1
10	Rhode Island	9.0	39	Georgia	6.9
47	South Carolina	5.7	39	Vermont	6.9
17	South Dakota	8.3	41	Maryland	6.8
22	Tennessee	7.9	42	California	6.4
34	Texas	7.1	43	Colorado	6.3
48	Utah	4.2	43	Wyoming	6.3
39	Vermont	6.9	45	Nevada	6.2
32	Virginia	7.2	45	New Hampshire	6.2
28	Washington	7.7	47	South Carolina	5.7
18	West Virginia	8.2	48	Hawaii	4.2
15	Wisconsin	8.5	48	Utah	4.2
43	Wyoming	6.3	50	Alaska	1.7
				District of Columbia	8.8

Source: Morgan Quitno Press using data from American Cancer Society
"Cancer Facts & Figures-1995" (Copyright 1995, Reprinted with permission from the American Cancer Society)
Rates calculated using 1994 Census resident population estimates.

Estimated Deaths by Lung Cancer in 1995

National Estimated Total = 157,400 Deaths

ALPHA ORDER

RANK ORDER

RANK	STATE	DEATHS	% of USA
21	Alabama	2,800	1.78%
50	Alaska	170	0.11%
23	Arizona	2,400	1.52%
26	Arkansas	2,100	1.33%
1	California	14,000	8.89%
34	Colorado	1,400	0.89%
29	Connecticut	2,000	1.27%
41	Delaware	540	0.34%
2	Florida	12,200	7.75%
13	Georgia	3,800	2.41%
43	Hawaii	510	0.32%
44	Idaho	440	0.28%
7	Illinois	6,900	4.38%
11	Indiana	4,000	2.54%
30	Iowa	1,800	1.14%
32	Kansas	1,600	1.02%
17	Kentucky	3,300	2.10%
20	Louisiana	2,900	1.84%
35	Maine	1,000	0.64%
18	Maryland	3,100	1.97%
15	Massachusetts	3,600	2.29%
8	Michigan	5,500	3.49%
26	Minnesota	2,100	1.33%
31	Mississippi	1,700	1.08%
11	Missouri	4,000	2.54%
42	Montana	520	0.33%
37	Nebraska	880	0.56%
35	Nevada	1,000	0.64%
39	New Hampshire	650	0.41%
9	New Jersey	4,800	3.05%
38	New Mexico	670	0.43%
3	New York	10,500	6.67%
10	North Carolina	4,600	2.92%
47	North Dakota	340	0.22%
6	Ohio	7,400	4.70%
25	Oklahoma	2,200	1.40%
26	Oregon	2,100	1.33%
5	Pennsylvania	8,500	5.40%
39	Rhode Island	650	0.41%
23	South Carolina	2,400	1.52%
46	South Dakota	350	0.22%
14	Tennessee	3,700	2.35%
4	Texas	10,200	6.48%
45	Utah	410	0.26%
48	Vermont	310	0.20%
15	Virginia	3,600	2.29%
19	Washington	3,000	1.91%
32	West Virginia	1,600	1.02%
22	Wisconsin	2,600	1.65%
49	Wyoming	200	0.13%

RANK	STATE	DEATHS	% of USA
1	California	14,000	8.89%
2	Florida	12,200	7.75%
3	New York	10,500	6.67%
4	Texas	10,200	6.48%
5	Pennsylvania	8,500	5.40%
6	Ohio	7,400	4.70%
7	Illinois	6,900	4.38%
8	Michigan	5,500	3.49%
9	New Jersey	4,800	3.05%
10	North Carolina	4,600	2.92%
11	Indiana	4,000	2.54%
11	Missouri	4,000	2.54%
13	Georgia	3,800	2.41%
14	Tennessee	3,700	2.35%
15	Massachusetts	3,600	2.29%
15	Virginia	3,600	2.29%
17	Kentucky	3,300	2.10%
18	Maryland	3,100	1.97%
19	Washington	3,000	1.91%
20	Louisiana	2,900	1.84%
21	Alabama	2,800	1.78%
22	Wisconsin	2,600	1.65%
23	Arizona	2,400	1.52%
23	South Carolina	2,400	1.52%
25	Oklahoma	2,200	1.40%
26	Arkansas	2,100	1.33%
26	Minnesota	2,100	1.33%
26	Oregon	2,100	1.33%
29	Connecticut	2,000	1.27%
30	Iowa	1,800	1.14%
31	Mississippi	1,700	1.08%
32	Kansas	1,600	1.02%
32	West Virginia	1,600	1.02%
34	Colorado	1,400	0.89%
35	Maine	1,000	0.64%
35	Nevada	1,000	0.64%
37	Nebraska	880	0.56%
38	New Mexico	670	0.43%
39	New Hampshire	650	0.41%
39	Rhode Island	650	0.41%
41	Delaware	540	0.34%
42	Montana	520	0.33%
43	Hawaii	510	0.32%
44	Idaho	440	0.28%
45	Utah	410	0.26%
46	South Dakota	350	0.22%
47	North Dakota	340	0.22%
48	Vermont	310	0.20%
49	Wyoming	200	0.13%
50	Alaska	170	0.11%
	District of Columbia	360	0.23%

Source: American Cancer Society
"Cancer Facts & Figures–1995" (Copyright 1995, Reprinted with permission from the American Cancer Society)

Estimated Death Rate by Lung Cancer in 1995

National Estimated Rate = 60.5 Deaths by Lung Cancer per 100,000 Population*

ALPHA ORDER			RANK ORDER		
RANK	STATE		RANK	STATE	RATE
16	Alabama	66.4	1	West Virginia	87.8
49	Alaska	28.1	2	Florida	87.4
28	Arizona	58.9	3	Kentucky	86.2
4	Arkansas	85.6	4	Arkansas	85.6
43	California	44.5	5	Maine	80.6
48	Colorado	38.3	6	Delaware	76.5
24	Connecticut	61.1	7	Missouri	75.8
6	Delaware	76.5	8	Tennessee	71.5
2	Florida	87.4	9	Pennsylvania	70.5
37	Georgia	53.9	10	Indiana	69.5
44	Hawaii	43.3	11	Nevada	68.6
47	Idaho	38.8	12	Oregon	68.0
29	Illinois	58.7	13	Oklahoma	67.5
10	Indiana	69.5	14	Louisiana	67.2
21	Iowa	63.6	15	Ohio	66.7
22	Kansas	62.6	16	Alabama	66.4
3	Kentucky	86.2	17	South Carolina	65.5
14	Louisiana	67.2	18	Rhode Island	65.2
5	Maine	80.6	19	North Carolina	65.1
23	Maryland	61.9	20	Mississippi	63.7
27	Massachusetts	59.6	21	Iowa	63.6
30	Michigan	57.9	22	Kansas	62.6
42	Minnesota	46.0	23	Maryland	61.9
20	Mississippi	63.7	24	Connecticut	61.1
7	Missouri	75.8	25	Montana	60.7
25	Montana	60.7	25	New Jersey	60.7
36	Nebraska	54.2	27	Massachusetts	59.6
11	Nevada	68.6	28	Arizona	58.9
32	New Hampshire	57.2	29	Illinois	58.7
25	New Jersey	60.7	30	Michigan	57.9
46	New Mexico	40.5	31	New York	57.8
31	New York	57.8	32	New Hampshire	57.2
19	North Carolina	65.1	33	Washington	56.1
39	North Dakota	53.3	34	Texas	55.5
15	Ohio	66.7	35	Virginia	54.9
13	Oklahoma	67.5	36	Nebraska	54.2
12	Oregon	68.0	37	Georgia	53.9
9	Pennsylvania	70.5	38	Vermont	53.4
18	Rhode Island	65.2	39	North Dakota	53.3
17	South Carolina	65.5	40	Wisconsin	51.2
41	South Dakota	48.5	41	South Dakota	48.5
8	Tennessee	71.5	42	Minnesota	46.0
34	Texas	55.5	43	California	44.5
50	Utah	21.5	44	Hawaii	43.3
38	Vermont	53.4	45	Wyoming	42.0
35	Virginia	54.9	46	New Mexico	40.5
33	Washington	56.1	47	Idaho	38.8
1	West Virginia	87.8	48	Colorado	38.3
40	Wisconsin	51.2	49	Alaska	28.1
45	Wyoming	42.0	50	Utah	21.5
				District of Columbia	63.2

Source: Morgan Quitno Press using data from American Cancer Society
    "Cancer Facts & Figures–1995" (Copyright 1995, Reprinted with permission from the American Cancer Society)
*Rates calculated using 1994 Census resident population estimates.

Estimated Deaths by Oral Cancer in 1995

National Estimated Total = 8,370 Deaths

ALPHA ORDER					RANK ORDER			
RANK	STATE		DEATHS	% of USA	RANK	STATE	DEATHS	% of USA
26	Alabama		110	1.31%	1	California	830	9.92%
46	Alaska		10	0.12%	2	Florida	680	8.12%
29	Arizona		100	1.19%	3	Texas	630	7.53%
31	Arkansas		80	0.96%	4	New York	580	6.93%
1	California		830	9.92%	5	Illinois	450	5.38%
26	Colorado		110	1.31%	6	Pennsylvania	380	4.54%
22	Connecticut		130	1.55%	7	Ohio	320	3.82%
38	Delaware		50	0.60%	8	New Jersey	290	3.46%
2	Florida		680	8.12%	9	Michigan	270	3.23%
12	Georgia		200	2.39%	9	North Carolina	270	3.23%
40	Hawaii		30	0.36%	11	Massachusetts	250	2.99%
40	Idaho		30	0.36%	12	Georgia	200	2.39%
5	Illinois		450	5.38%	13	Virginia	180	2.15%
15	Indiana		160	1.91%	14	Wisconsin	170	2.03%
33	Iowa		70	0.84%	15	Indiana	160	1.91%
30	Kansas		90	1.08%	15	Louisiana	160	1.91%
22	Kentucky		130	1.55%	15	Washington	160	1.91%
15	Louisiana		160	1.91%	18	Maryland	150	1.79%
35	Maine		60	0.72%	19	Missouri	140	1.67%
18	Maryland		150	1.79%	19	South Carolina	140	1.67%
11	Massachusetts		250	2.99%	19	Tennessee	140	1.67%
9	Michigan		270	3.23%	22	Connecticut	130	1.55%
24	Minnesota		120	1.43%	22	Kentucky	130	1.55%
24	Mississippi		120	1.43%	24	Minnesota	120	1.43%
19	Missouri		140	1.67%	24	Mississippi	120	1.43%
46	Montana		10	0.12%	26	Alabama	110	1.31%
35	Nebraska		60	0.72%	26	Colorado	110	1.31%
40	Nevada		30	0.36%	26	Oregon	110	1.31%
39	New Hampshire		40	0.48%	29	Arizona	100	1.19%
8	New Jersey		290	3.46%	30	Kansas	90	1.08%
35	New Mexico		60	0.72%	31	Arkansas	80	0.96%
4	New York		580	6.93%	31	West Virginia	80	0.96%
9	North Carolina		270	3.23%	33	Iowa	70	0.84%
44	North Dakota		20	0.24%	33	Oklahoma	70	0.84%
7	Ohio		320	3.82%	35	Maine	60	0.72%
33	Oklahoma		70	0.84%	35	Nebraska	60	0.72%
26	Oregon		110	1.31%	35	New Mexico	60	0.72%
6	Pennsylvania		380	4.54%	38	Delaware	50	0.60%
40	Rhode Island		30	0.36%	39	New Hampshire	40	0.48%
19	South Carolina		140	1.67%	40	Hawaii	30	0.36%
46	South Dakota		10	0.12%	40	Idaho	30	0.36%
19	Tennessee		140	1.67%	40	Nevada	30	0.36%
3	Texas		630	7.53%	40	Rhode Island	30	0.36%
44	Utah		20	0.24%	44	North Dakota	20	0.24%
46	Vermont		10	0.12%	44	Utah	20	0.24%
13	Virginia		180	2.15%	46	Alaska	10	0.12%
15	Washington		160	1.91%	46	Montana	10	0.12%
31	West Virginia		80	0.96%	46	South Dakota	10	0.12%
14	Wisconsin		170	2.03%	46	Vermont	10	0.12%
46	Wyoming		10	0.12%	46	Wyoming	10	0.12%
					District of Columbia		20	0.24%

Source: American Cancer Society
"Cancer Facts & Figures-1995" (Copyright 1995, Reprinted with permission from the American Cancer Society)

119

Estimated Death Rate by Oral Cancer in 1995

National Estimated Rate = 3.2 Deaths by Oral Cancer per 100,000 Population*

ALPHA ORDER			RANK ORDER		
RANK	STATE	RATE	RANK	STATE	RATE
36	Alabama	2.6	1	Delaware	7.1
46	Alaska	1.7	2	Florida	4.9
40	Arizona	2.5	3	Maine	4.8
20	Arkansas	3.3	4	Mississippi	4.5
36	California	2.6	5	West Virginia	4.4
25	Colorado	3.0	6	Massachusetts	4.1
7	Connecticut	4.0	7	Connecticut	4.0
1	Delaware	7.1	8	Illinois	3.8
2	Florida	4.9	8	North Carolina	3.8
30	Georgia	2.8	8	South Carolina	3.8
40	Hawaii	2.5	11	Louisiana	3.7
36	Idaho	2.6	11	Nebraska	3.7
8	Illinois	3.8	11	New Jersey	3.7
30	Indiana	2.8	14	New Mexico	3.6
40	Iowa	2.5	14	Oregon	3.6
16	Kansas	3.5	16	Kansas	3.5
18	Kentucky	3.4	16	New Hampshire	3.5
11	Louisiana	3.7	18	Kentucky	3.4
3	Maine	4.8	18	Texas	3.4
25	Maryland	3.0	20	Arkansas	3.3
6	Massachusetts	4.1	20	Wisconsin	3.3
30	Michigan	2.8	22	New York	3.2
36	Minnesota	2.6	22	Pennsylvania	3.2
4	Mississippi	4.5	24	North Dakota	3.1
33	Missouri	2.7	25	Colorado	3.0
49	Montana	1.2	25	Maryland	3.0
11	Nebraska	3.7	25	Rhode Island	3.0
43	Nevada	2.1	25	Washington	3.0
16	New Hampshire	3.5	29	Ohio	2.9
11	New Jersey	3.7	30	Georgia	2.8
14	New Mexico	3.6	30	Indiana	2.8
22	New York	3.2	30	Michigan	2.8
8	North Carolina	3.8	33	Missouri	2.7
24	North Dakota	3.1	33	Tennessee	2.7
29	Ohio	2.9	33	Virginia	2.7
43	Oklahoma	2.1	36	Alabama	2.6
14	Oregon	3.6	36	California	2.6
22	Pennsylvania	3.2	36	Idaho	2.6
25	Rhode Island	3.0	36	Minnesota	2.6
8	South Carolina	3.8	40	Arizona	2.5
48	South Dakota	1.4	40	Hawaii	2.5
33	Tennessee	2.7	40	Iowa	2.5
18	Texas	3.4	43	Nevada	2.1
50	Utah	1.0	43	Oklahoma	2.1
46	Vermont	1.7	43	Wyoming	2.1
33	Virginia	2.7	46	Alaska	1.7
25	Washington	3.0	46	Vermont	1.7
5	West Virginia	4.4	48	South Dakota	1.4
20	Wisconsin	3.3	49	Montana	1.2
43	Wyoming	2.1	50	Utah	1.0
				District of Columbia	3.5

Source: Morgan Quitno Press using data from American Cancer Society
"Cancer Facts & Figures-1995" (Copyright 1995, Reprinted with permission from the American Cancer Society)
*Rates calculated using 1994 Census resident population estimates.

Estimated Deaths by Prostate Cancer in 1995

National Estimated Total = 40,400 Deaths

ALPHA ORDER					RANK ORDER			
RANK	STATE		DEATHS	% of USA	RANK	STATE	DEATHS	% of USA
24	Alabama		590	1.46%	1	California	3,700	9.16%
50	Alaska		30	0.07%	2	Florida	3,100	7.67%
22	Arizona		680	1.68%	3	New York	2,600	6.44%
27	Arkansas		530	1.31%	4	Pennsylvania	2,400	5.94%
1	California		3,700	9.16%	5	Texas	2,200	5.45%
27	Colorado		530	1.31%	6	Illinois	1,900	4.70%
29	Connecticut		520	1.29%	7	Ohio	1,800	4.46%
47	Delaware		90	0.22%	8	Michigan	1,500	3.71%
2	Florida		3,100	7.67%	9	New Jersey	1,300	3.22%
14	Georgia		920	2.28%	9	North Carolina	1,300	3.22%
43	Hawaii		140	0.35%	11	Massachusetts	970	2.40%
41	Idaho		170	0.42%	12	Virginia	950	2.35%
6	Illinois		1,900	4.70%	13	Wisconsin	930	2.30%
17	Indiana		790	1.96%	14	Georgia	920	2.28%
29	Iowa		520	1.29%	15	Maryland	830	2.05%
33	Kansas		410	1.01%	16	Missouri	800	1.98%
25	Kentucky		570	1.41%	17	Indiana	790	1.96%
21	Louisiana		710	1.76%	17	Washington	790	1.96%
37	Maine		220	0.54%	19	Tennessee	780	1.93%
15	Maryland		830	2.05%	20	Minnesota	770	1.91%
11	Massachusetts		970	2.40%	21	Louisiana	710	1.76%
8	Michigan		1,500	3.71%	22	Arizona	680	1.68%
20	Minnesota		770	1.91%	23	South Carolina	640	1.58%
32	Mississippi		490	1.21%	24	Alabama	590	1.46%
16	Missouri		800	1.98%	25	Kentucky	570	1.41%
44	Montana		130	0.32%	26	Oregon	540	1.34%
35	Nebraska		260	0.64%	27	Arkansas	530	1.31%
38	Nevada		200	0.50%	27	Colorado	530	1.31%
39	New Hampshire		190	0.47%	29	Connecticut	520	1.29%
9	New Jersey		1,300	3.22%	29	Iowa	520	1.29%
40	New Mexico		180	0.45%	29	Oklahoma	520	1.29%
3	New York		2,600	6.44%	32	Mississippi	490	1.21%
9	North Carolina		1,300	3.22%	33	Kansas	410	1.01%
41	North Dakota		170	0.42%	34	West Virginia	280	0.69%
7	Ohio		1,800	4.46%	35	Nebraska	260	0.64%
29	Oklahoma		520	1.29%	36	Utah	240	0.59%
26	Oregon		540	1.34%	37	Maine	220	0.54%
4	Pennsylvania		2,400	5.94%	38	Nevada	200	0.50%
44	Rhode Island		130	0.32%	39	New Hampshire	190	0.47%
23	South Carolina		640	1.58%	40	New Mexico	180	0.45%
44	South Dakota		130	0.32%	41	Idaho	170	0.42%
19	Tennessee		780	1.93%	41	North Dakota	170	0.42%
5	Texas		2,200	5.45%	43	Hawaii	140	0.35%
36	Utah		240	0.59%	44	Montana	130	0.32%
48	Vermont		80	0.20%	44	Rhode Island	130	0.32%
12	Virginia		950	2.35%	44	South Dakota	130	0.32%
17	Washington		790	1.96%	47	Delaware	90	0.22%
34	West Virginia		280	0.69%	48	Vermont	80	0.20%
13	Wisconsin		930	2.30%	49	Wyoming	60	0.15%
49	Wyoming		60	0.15%	50	Alaska	30	0.07%
						District of Columbia	120	0.30%

Source: American Cancer Society
"Cancer Facts & Figures-1995" (Copyright 1995, Reprinted with permission from the American Cancer Society)

Estimated Death Rate by Prostate Cancer in 1995

National Estimated Rate = 31.8 Deaths per 100,000 Male Population*

ALPHA ORDER				RANK ORDER		
RANK	STATE	RATE		RANK	STATE	RATE
37	Alabama	29.2		1	North Dakota	53.5
50	Alaska	9.4		2	Florida	45.9
18	Arizona	33.8		3	Arkansas	44.8
3	Arkansas	44.8		4	Pennsylvania	41.5
47	California	23.5		5	Mississippi	38.3
36	Colorado	29.3		6	North Carolina	37.9
22	Connecticut	32.8		7	Iowa	37.8
43	Delaware	26.2		8	Wisconsin	37.3
2	Florida	45.9		9	South Dakota	36.6
42	Georgia	26.8		10	Maine	36.4
47	Hawaii	23.5		11	South Carolina	36.2
32	Idaho	30.1		12	Oregon	35.5
21	Illinois	33.2		13	Minnesota	34.3
38	Indiana	28.3		14	Louisiana	34.2
7	Iowa	37.8		15	Maryland	34.1
24	Kansas	32.7		15	New Hampshire	34.1
30	Kentucky	30.7		17	New Jersey	34.0
14	Louisiana	34.2		18	Arizona	33.8
10	Maine	36.4		19	Ohio	33.6
15	Maryland	34.1		20	Massachusetts	33.4
20	Massachusetts	33.4		21	Illinois	33.2
26	Michigan	32.5		22	Connecticut	32.8
13	Minnesota	34.3		22	Nebraska	32.8
5	Mississippi	38.3		24	Kansas	32.7
28	Missouri	31.4		24	Oklahoma	32.7
31	Montana	30.6		26	Michigan	32.5
22	Nebraska	32.8		27	West Virginia	31.9
41	Nevada	27.0		28	Missouri	31.4
15	New Hampshire	34.1		29	Tennessee	31.3
17	New Jersey	34.0		30	Kentucky	30.7
49	New Mexico	22.1		31	Montana	30.6
33	New York	29.8		32	Idaho	30.1
6	North Carolina	37.9		33	New York	29.8
1	North Dakota	53.5		33	Washington	29.8
19	Ohio	33.6		35	Virginia	29.6
24	Oklahoma	32.7		36	Colorado	29.3
12	Oregon	35.5		37	Alabama	29.2
4	Pennsylvania	41.5		38	Indiana	28.3
40	Rhode Island	27.1		39	Vermont	28.1
11	South Carolina	36.2		40	Rhode Island	27.1
9	South Dakota	36.6		41	Nevada	27.0
29	Tennessee	31.3		42	Georgia	26.8
46	Texas	24.3		43	Delaware	26.2
44	Utah	25.3		44	Utah	25.3
39	Vermont	28.1		45	Wyoming	25.1
35	Virginia	29.6		46	Texas	24.3
33	Washington	29.8		47	California	23.5
27	West Virginia	31.9		47	Hawaii	23.5
8	Wisconsin	37.3		49	New Mexico	22.1
45	Wyoming	25.1		50	Alaska	9.4
					District of Columbia	45.1

Source: Morgan Quitno Press using data from American Cancer Society
"Cancer Facts & Figures-1995" (Copyright 1995, Reprinted with permission from the American Cancer Society)
*Rates calculated using 1994 Census resident male population estimates.

Estimated Deaths by Skin Melanoma in 1995

National Estimated Total = 7,200 Deaths

ALPHA ORDER

RANK	STATE	DEATHS	% of USA
18	Alabama	140	1.94%
48	Alaska	10	0.14%
18	Arizona	140	1.94%
33	Arkansas	70	0.97%
1	California	950	13.19%
26	Colorado	100	1.39%
29	Connecticut	90	1.25%
41	Delaware	30	0.42%
2	Florida	490	6.81%
15	Georgia	150	2.08%
48	Hawaii	10	0.14%
43	Idaho	20	0.28%
6	Illinois	300	4.17%
20	Indiana	130	1.81%
26	Iowa	100	1.39%
22	Kansas	110	1.53%
20	Kentucky	130	1.81%
29	Louisiana	90	1.25%
38	Maine	40	0.56%
22	Maryland	110	1.53%
11	Massachusetts	180	2.50%
9	Michigan	210	2.92%
22	Minnesota	110	1.53%
33	Mississippi	70	0.97%
11	Missouri	180	2.50%
43	Montana	20	0.28%
41	Nebraska	30	0.42%
35	Nevada	50	0.69%
38	New Hampshire	40	0.56%
9	New Jersey	210	2.92%
35	New Mexico	50	0.69%
3	New York	450	6.25%
8	North Carolina	220	3.06%
43	North Dakota	20	0.28%
7	Ohio	240	3.33%
26	Oklahoma	100	1.39%
22	Oregon	110	1.53%
5	Pennsylvania	340	4.72%
38	Rhode Island	40	0.56%
29	South Carolina	90	1.25%
43	South Dakota	20	0.28%
11	Tennessee	180	2.50%
4	Texas	390	5.42%
32	Utah	80	1.11%
43	Vermont	20	0.28%
14	Virginia	170	2.36%
15	Washington	150	2.08%
35	West Virginia	50	0.69%
15	Wisconsin	150	2.08%
48	Wyoming	10	0.14%

RANK ORDER

RANK	STATE	DEATHS	% of USA
1	California	950	13.19%
2	Florida	490	6.81%
3	New York	450	6.25%
4	Texas	390	5.42%
5	Pennsylvania	340	4.72%
6	Illinois	300	4.17%
7	Ohio	240	3.33%
8	North Carolina	220	3.06%
9	Michigan	210	2.92%
9	New Jersey	210	2.92%
11	Massachusetts	180	2.50%
11	Missouri	180	2.50%
11	Tennessee	180	2.50%
14	Virginia	170	2.36%
15	Georgia	150	2.08%
15	Washington	150	2.08%
15	Wisconsin	150	2.08%
18	Alabama	140	1.94%
18	Arizona	140	1.94%
20	Indiana	130	1.81%
20	Kentucky	130	1.81%
22	Kansas	110	1.53%
22	Maryland	110	1.53%
22	Minnesota	110	1.53%
22	Oregon	110	1.53%
26	Colorado	100	1.39%
26	Iowa	100	1.39%
26	Oklahoma	100	1.39%
29	Connecticut	90	1.25%
29	Louisiana	90	1.25%
29	South Carolina	90	1.25%
32	Utah	80	1.11%
33	Arkansas	70	0.97%
33	Mississippi	70	0.97%
35	Nevada	50	0.69%
35	New Mexico	50	0.69%
35	West Virginia	50	0.69%
38	Maine	40	0.56%
38	New Hampshire	40	0.56%
38	Rhode Island	40	0.56%
41	Delaware	30	0.42%
41	Nebraska	30	0.42%
43	Idaho	20	0.28%
43	Montana	20	0.28%
43	North Dakota	20	0.28%
43	South Dakota	20	0.28%
43	Vermont	20	0.28%
48	Alaska	10	0.14%
48	Hawaii	10	0.14%
48	Wyoming	10	0.14%
	District of Columbia	10	0.14%

Source: American Cancer Society
"Cancer Facts & Figures–1995" (Copyright 1995, Reprinted with permission from the American Cancer Society)

Estimated Death Rate by Skin Melanoma in 1995

National Estimated Rate = 2.8 Deaths by Skin Melanoma per 100,000 Population*

ALPHA ORDER

RANK	STATE	RATE
15	Alabama	3.3
49	Alaska	1.7
10	Arizona	3.4
24	Arkansas	2.9
20	California	3.0
28	Colorado	2.7
28	Connecticut	2.7
2	Delaware	4.2
6	Florida	3.5
43	Georgia	2.1
50	Hawaii	0.8
47	Idaho	1.8
32	Illinois	2.6
38	Indiana	2.3
6	Iowa	3.5
1	Kansas	4.3
10	Kentucky	3.4
43	Louisiana	2.1
16	Maine	3.2
40	Maryland	2.2
20	Massachusetts	3.0
40	Michigan	2.2
37	Minnesota	2.4
32	Mississippi	2.6
10	Missouri	3.4
38	Montana	2.3
47	Nebraska	1.8
10	Nevada	3.4
6	New Hampshire	3.5
28	New Jersey	2.7
20	New Mexico	3.0
35	New York	2.5
17	North Carolina	3.1
17	North Dakota	3.1
40	Ohio	2.2
17	Oklahoma	3.1
5	Oregon	3.6
25	Pennsylvania	2.8
4	Rhode Island	4.0
35	South Carolina	2.5
25	South Dakota	2.8
6	Tennessee	3.5
43	Texas	2.1
2	Utah	4.2
10	Vermont	3.4
32	Virginia	2.6
25	Washington	2.8
28	West Virginia	2.7
20	Wisconsin	3.0
43	Wyoming	2.1

RANK ORDER

RANK	STATE	RATE
1	Kansas	4.3
2	Delaware	4.2
2	Utah	4.2
4	Rhode Island	4.0
5	Oregon	3.6
6	Florida	3.5
6	Iowa	3.5
6	New Hampshire	3.5
6	Tennessee	3.5
10	Arizona	3.4
10	Kentucky	3.4
10	Missouri	3.4
10	Nevada	3.4
10	Vermont	3.4
15	Alabama	3.3
16	Maine	3.2
17	North Carolina	3.1
17	North Dakota	3.1
17	Oklahoma	3.1
20	California	3.0
20	Massachusetts	3.0
20	New Mexico	3.0
20	Wisconsin	3.0
24	Arkansas	2.9
25	Pennsylvania	2.8
25	South Dakota	2.8
25	Washington	2.8
28	Colorado	2.7
28	Connecticut	2.7
28	New Jersey	2.7
28	West Virginia	2.7
32	Illinois	2.6
32	Mississippi	2.6
32	Virginia	2.6
35	New York	2.5
35	South Carolina	2.5
37	Minnesota	2.4
38	Indiana	2.3
38	Montana	2.3
40	Maryland	2.2
40	Michigan	2.2
40	Ohio	2.2
43	Georgia	2.1
43	Louisiana	2.1
43	Texas	2.1
43	Wyoming	2.1
47	Idaho	1.8
47	Nebraska	1.8
49	Alaska	1.7
50	Hawaii	0.8
	District of Columbia	1.8

Source: Morgan Quitno Press using data from American Cancer Society
    "Cancer Facts & Figures–1995" (Copyright 1995, Reprinted with permission from the American Cancer Society)
Rates calculated using 1994 Census resident population estimates.

Estimated Deaths by Cancer of the Uterus in 1995

National Estimated Total = 10,700 Deaths

ALPHA ORDER

RANK ORDER

RANK	STATE	DEATHS	% of USA
21	Alabama	160	1.50%
48	Alaska	10	0.09%
30	Arizona	110	1.03%
25	Arkansas	130	1.21%
1	California	1,000	9.35%
25	Colorado	130	1.21%
25	Connecticut	130	1.21%
41	Delaware	30	0.28%
3	Florida	750	7.01%
16	Georgia	200	1.87%
41	Hawaii	30	0.28%
45	Idaho	20	0.19%
6	Illinois	550	5.14%
15	Indiana	210	1.96%
28	Iowa	120	1.12%
30	Kansas	110	1.03%
18	Kentucky	190	1.78%
28	Louisiana	120	1.12%
41	Maine	30	0.28%
14	Maryland	220	2.06%
16	Massachusetts	200	1.87%
8	Michigan	430	4.02%
23	Minnesota	150	1.40%
32	Mississippi	90	0.84%
11	Missouri	280	2.62%
45	Montana	20	0.19%
36	Nebraska	60	0.56%
38	Nevada	40	0.37%
37	New Hampshire	50	0.47%
9	New Jersey	340	3.18%
35	New Mexico	70	0.65%
2	New York	880	8.22%
10	North Carolina	300	2.80%
38	North Dakota	40	0.37%
6	Ohio	550	5.14%
24	Oklahoma	140	1.31%
32	Oregon	90	0.84%
4	Pennsylvania	720	6.73%
41	Rhode Island	30	0.28%
21	South Carolina	160	1.50%
45	South Dakota	20	0.19%
19	Tennessee	180	1.68%
4	Texas	720	6.73%
38	Utah	40	0.37%
48	Vermont	10	0.09%
13	Virginia	250	2.34%
20	Washington	170	1.59%
32	West Virginia	90	0.84%
11	Wisconsin	280	2.62%
48	Wyoming	10	0.09%

RANK	STATE	DEATHS	% of USA
1	California	1,000	9.35%
2	New York	880	8.22%
3	Florida	750	7.01%
4	Pennsylvania	720	6.73%
4	Texas	720	6.73%
6	Illinois	550	5.14%
6	Ohio	550	5.14%
8	Michigan	430	4.02%
9	New Jersey	340	3.18%
10	North Carolina	300	2.80%
11	Missouri	280	2.62%
11	Wisconsin	280	2.62%
13	Virginia	250	2.34%
14	Maryland	220	2.06%
15	Indiana	210	1.96%
16	Georgia	200	1.87%
16	Massachusetts	200	1.87%
18	Kentucky	190	1.78%
19	Tennessee	180	1.68%
20	Washington	170	1.59%
21	Alabama	160	1.50%
21	South Carolina	160	1.50%
23	Minnesota	150	1.40%
24	Oklahoma	140	1.31%
25	Arkansas	130	1.21%
25	Colorado	130	1.21%
25	Connecticut	130	1.21%
28	Iowa	120	1.12%
28	Louisiana	120	1.12%
30	Arizona	110	1.03%
30	Kansas	110	1.03%
32	Mississippi	90	0.84%
32	Oregon	90	0.84%
32	West Virginia	90	0.84%
35	New Mexico	70	0.65%
36	Nebraska	60	0.56%
37	New Hampshire	50	0.47%
38	Nevada	40	0.37%
38	North Dakota	40	0.37%
38	Utah	40	0.37%
41	Delaware	30	0.28%
41	Hawaii	30	0.28%
41	Maine	30	0.28%
41	Rhode Island	30	0.28%
45	Idaho	20	0.19%
45	Montana	20	0.19%
45	South Dakota	20	0.19%
48	Alaska	10	0.09%
48	Vermont	10	0.09%
48	Wyoming	10	0.09%
	District of Columbia	40	0.37%

Source: American Cancer Society

"Cancer Facts & Figures–1995" (Copyright 1995, Reprinted with permission from the American Cancer Society)

Estimated Death Rate by Cancer of the Uterus in 1995

National Estimated Rate = 8.0 Deaths per 100,000 Female Population*

ALPHA ORDER			RANK ORDER		
RANK	**STATE**	**RATE**	**RANK**	**STATE**	**RATE**
26	Alabama	7.3	1	North Dakota	12.5
48	Alaska	3.5	2	Pennsylvania	11.5
42	Arizona	5.3	3	Wisconsin	10.8
6	Arkansas	10.2	4	Florida	10.4
33	California	6.4	5	Missouri	10.3
29	Colorado	7.0	6	Arkansas	10.2
23	Connecticut	7.7	7	Kentucky	9.6
18	Delaware	8.3	7	Ohio	9.6
4	Florida	10.4	9	West Virginia	9.5
39	Georgia	5.5	10	New York	9.3
43	Hawaii	5.2	11	Illinois	9.1
48	Idaho	3.5	12	Michigan	8.8
11	Illinois	9.1	13	New Hampshire	8.6
28	Indiana	7.1	14	Kansas	8.5
18	Iowa	8.3	14	Maryland	8.5
14	Kansas	8.5	16	Oklahoma	8.4
7	Kentucky	9.6	16	South Carolina	8.4
41	Louisiana	5.4	18	Delaware	8.3
44	Maine	4.7	18	Iowa	8.3
14	Maryland	8.5	18	New Jersey	8.3
33	Massachusetts	6.4	18	New Mexico	8.3
12	Michigan	8.8	22	North Carolina	8.2
31	Minnesota	6.5	23	Connecticut	7.7
31	Mississippi	6.5	23	Texas	7.7
5	Missouri	10.3	25	Virginia	7.5
45	Montana	4.6	26	Alabama	7.3
27	Nebraska	7.2	27	Nebraska	7.2
38	Nevada	5.6	28	Indiana	7.1
13	New Hampshire	8.6	29	Colorado	7.0
18	New Jersey	8.3	30	Tennessee	6.7
18	New Mexico	8.3	31	Minnesota	6.5
10	New York	9.3	31	Mississippi	6.5
22	North Carolina	8.2	33	California	6.4
1	North Dakota	12.5	33	Massachusetts	6.4
7	Ohio	9.6	35	Washington	6.3
16	Oklahoma	8.4	36	Oregon	5.8
36	Oregon	5.8	36	Rhode Island	5.8
2	Pennsylvania	11.5	38	Nevada	5.6
36	Rhode Island	5.8	39	Georgia	5.5
16	South Carolina	8.4	39	South Dakota	5.5
39	South Dakota	5.5	41	Louisiana	5.4
30	Tennessee	6.7	42	Arizona	5.3
23	Texas	7.7	43	Hawaii	5.2
46	Utah	4.2	44	Maine	4.7
50	Vermont	3.4	45	Montana	4.6
25	Virginia	7.5	46	Utah	4.2
35	Washington	6.3	46	Wyoming	4.2
9	West Virginia	9.5	48	Alaska	3.5
3	Wisconsin	10.8	48	Idaho	3.5
46	Wyoming	4.2	50	Vermont	3.4
				District of Columbia	13.2

Source: Morgan Quitno Press using data from American Cancer Society
"Cancer Facts & Figures-1995" (Copyright 1995, Reprinted with permission from the American Cancer Society)
*Rates calculated using 1994 Census resident female population estimates.

Deaths by Atherosclerosis in 1992

National Total = 16,831 Deaths*

<u>ALPHA ORDER</u>

RANK	STATE	DEATHS	% of USA
27	Alabama	244	1.45%
50	Alaska	9	0.05%
26	Arizona	259	1.54%
34	Arkansas	166	0.99%
1	California	2,029	12.06%
15	Colorado	387	2.30%
30	Connecticut	189	1.12%
48	Delaware	26	0.15%
3	Florida	949	5.64%
11	Georgia	416	2.47%
47	Hawaii	29	0.17%
45	Idaho	54	0.32%
8	Illinois	620	3.68%
9	Indiana	489	2.91%
16	Iowa	364	2.16%
23	Kansas	304	1.81%
28	Kentucky	209	1.24%
25	Louisiana	280	1.66%
37	Maine	102	0.61%
32	Maryland	174	1.03%
19	Massachusetts	343	2.04%
5	Michigan	780	4.63%
18	Minnesota	348	2.07%
36	Mississippi	119	0.71%
12	Missouri	399	2.37%
40	Montana	73	0.43%
29	Nebraska	202	1.20%
39	Nevada	76	0.45%
38	New Hampshire	93	0.55%
10	New Jersey	454	2.70%
33	New Mexico	167	0.99%
4	New York	811	4.82%
14	North Carolina	389	2.31%
42	North Dakota	69	0.41%
6	Ohio	773	4.59%
20	Oklahoma	332	1.97%
24	Oregon	301	1.79%
7	Pennsylvania	752	4.47%
43	Rhode Island	68	0.40%
35	South Carolina	137	0.81%
44	South Dakota	59	0.35%
16	Tennessee	364	2.16%
2	Texas	1,041	6.19%
41	Utah	71	0.42%
46	Vermont	30	0.18%
21	Virginia	328	1.95%
13	Washington	392	2.33%
31	West Virginia	180	1.07%
22	Wisconsin	312	1.85%
49	Wyoming	18	0.11%

<u>RANK ORDER</u>

RANK	STATE	DEATHS	% of USA
1	California	2,029	12.06%
2	Texas	1,041	6.19%
3	Florida	949	5.64%
4	New York	811	4.82%
5	Michigan	780	4.63%
6	Ohio	773	4.59%
7	Pennsylvania	752	4.47%
8	Illinois	620	3.68%
9	Indiana	489	2.91%
10	New Jersey	454	2.70%
11	Georgia	416	2.47%
12	Missouri	399	2.37%
13	Washington	392	2.33%
14	North Carolina	389	2.31%
15	Colorado	387	2.30%
16	Iowa	364	2.16%
16	Tennessee	364	2.16%
18	Minnesota	348	2.07%
19	Massachusetts	343	2.04%
20	Oklahoma	332	1.97%
21	Virginia	328	1.95%
22	Wisconsin	312	1.85%
23	Kansas	304	1.81%
24	Oregon	301	1.79%
25	Louisiana	280	1.66%
26	Arizona	259	1.54%
27	Alabama	244	1.45%
28	Kentucky	209	1.24%
29	Nebraska	202	1.20%
30	Connecticut	189	1.12%
31	West Virginia	180	1.07%
32	Maryland	174	1.03%
33	New Mexico	167	0.99%
34	Arkansas	166	0.99%
35	South Carolina	137	0.81%
36	Mississippi	119	0.71%
37	Maine	102	0.61%
38	New Hampshire	93	0.55%
39	Nevada	76	0.45%
40	Montana	73	0.43%
41	Utah	71	0.42%
42	North Dakota	69	0.41%
43	Rhode Island	68	0.40%
44	South Dakota	59	0.35%
45	Idaho	54	0.32%
46	Vermont	30	0.18%
47	Hawaii	29	0.17%
48	Delaware	26	0.15%
49	Wyoming	18	0.11%
50	Alaska	9	0.05%
	District of Columbia	51	0.30%

Source: U.S. Department of Health and Human Services, National Center for Health Statistics
unpublished data

*By state of residence. Atherosclerosis is a form of hardening of the arteries.

Death Rate by Atherosclerosis in 1992

National Rate = 6.6 Deaths per 100,000 Population*

ALPHA ORDER				RANK ORDER		
RANK	STATE	RATE		RANK	STATE	RATE
30	Alabama	5.9		1	Iowa	13.0
50	Alaska	1.5		2	Nebraska	12.6
23	Arizona	6.8		3	Kansas	12.1
22	Arkansas	6.9		4	Colorado	11.2
25	California	6.6		5	North Dakota	10.9
4	Colorado	11.2		6	New Mexico	10.6
32	Connecticut	5.8		7	Oklahoma	10.4
46	Delaware	3.8		8	Oregon	10.1
20	Florida	7.0		9	West Virginia	9.9
29	Georgia	6.1		10	Montana	8.9
49	Hawaii	2.5		11	Indiana	8.6
40	Idaho	5.1		12	Michigan	8.3
38	Illinois	5.3		12	New Hampshire	8.3
11	Indiana	8.6		12	South Dakota	8.3
1	Iowa	13.0		15	Maine	8.2
3	Kansas	12.1		16	Minnesota	7.8
37	Kentucky	5.6		17	Missouri	7.7
26	Louisiana	6.5		18	Washington	7.6
15	Maine	8.2		19	Tennessee	7.2
48	Maryland	3.5		20	Florida	7.0
34	Massachusetts	5.7		20	Ohio	7.0
12	Michigan	8.3		22	Arkansas	6.9
16	Minnesota	7.8		23	Arizona	6.8
42	Mississippi	4.5		23	Rhode Island	6.8
17	Missouri	7.7		25	California	6.6
10	Montana	8.9		26	Louisiana	6.5
2	Nebraska	12.6		27	Pennsylvania	6.3
34	Nevada	5.7		28	Wisconsin	6.2
12	New Hampshire	8.3		29	Georgia	6.1
32	New Jersey	5.8		30	Alabama	5.9
6	New Mexico	10.6		30	Texas	5.9
42	New York	4.5		32	Connecticut	5.8
34	North Carolina	5.7		32	New Jersey	5.8
5	North Dakota	10.9		34	Massachusetts	5.7
20	Ohio	7.0		34	Nevada	5.7
7	Oklahoma	10.4		34	North Carolina	5.7
8	Oregon	10.1		37	Kentucky	5.6
27	Pennsylvania	6.3		38	Illinois	5.3
23	Rhode Island	6.8		39	Vermont	5.2
46	South Carolina	3.8		40	Idaho	5.1
12	South Dakota	8.3		40	Virginia	5.1
19	Tennessee	7.2		42	Mississippi	4.5
30	Texas	5.9		42	New York	4.5
44	Utah	3.9		44	Utah	3.9
39	Vermont	5.2		44	Wyoming	3.9
40	Virginia	5.1		46	Delaware	3.8
18	Washington	7.6		46	South Carolina	3.8
9	West Virginia	9.9		48	Maryland	3.5
28	Wisconsin	6.2		49	Hawaii	2.5
44	Wyoming	3.9		50	Alaska	1.5
					District of Columbia	8.7

*Source: U.S. Department of Health and Human Services, National Center for Health Statistics
        unpublished data*

*By state of residence. Atherosclerosis is a form of hardening of the arteries.

Deaths by Cerebrovascular Diseases in 1992

National Total = 143,769 Deaths*

ALPHA ORDER					RANK ORDER			
RANK	STATE	DEATHS	% of USA		RANK	STATE	DEATHS	% of USA
20	Alabama	2,756	1.92%		1	California	15,167	10.55%
50	Alaska	108	0.08%		2	Florida	8,744	6.08%
29	Arizona	1,824	1.27%		3	Texas	8,699	6.05%
28	Arkansas	2,023	1.41%		4	New York	8,323	5.79%
1	California	15,167	10.55%		5	Pennsylvania	7,691	5.35%
33	Colorado	1,430	0.99%		6	Illinois	6,779	4.72%
30	Connecticut	1,753	1.22%		7	Ohio	6,109	4.25%
47	Delaware	324	0.23%		8	Michigan	5,105	3.55%
2	Florida	8,744	6.08%		9	North Carolina	4,576	3.18%
12	Georgia	3,684	2.56%		10	New Jersey	3,878	2.70%
41	Hawaii	557	0.39%		11	Tennessee	3,699	2.57%
38	Idaho	630	0.44%		12	Georgia	3,684	2.56%
6	Illinois	6,779	4.72%		13	Indiana	3,570	2.48%
13	Indiana	3,570	2.48%		14	Missouri	3,451	2.40%
27	Iowa	2,033	1.41%		15	Virginia	3,390	2.36%
32	Kansas	1,626	1.13%		16	Massachusetts	3,332	2.32%
23	Kentucky	2,312	1.61%		17	Wisconsin	3,319	2.31%
22	Louisiana	2,418	1.68%		18	Washington	2,918	2.03%
36	Maine	746	0.52%		19	Minnesota	2,821	1.96%
25	Maryland	2,106	1.46%		20	Alabama	2,756	1.92%
16	Massachusetts	3,332	2.32%		21	South Carolina	2,494	1.73%
8	Michigan	5,105	3.55%		22	Louisiana	2,418	1.68%
19	Minnesota	2,821	1.96%		23	Kentucky	2,312	1.61%
31	Mississippi	1,728	1.20%		24	Oklahoma	2,153	1.50%
14	Missouri	3,451	2.40%		25	Maryland	2,106	1.46%
44	Montana	497	0.35%		26	Oregon	2,102	1.46%
35	Nebraska	1,029	0.72%		27	Iowa	2,033	1.41%
43	Nevada	499	0.35%		28	Arkansas	2,023	1.41%
41	New Hampshire	557	0.39%		29	Arizona	1,824	1.27%
10	New Jersey	3,878	2.70%		30	Connecticut	1,753	1.22%
39	New Mexico	602	0.42%		31	Mississippi	1,728	1.20%
4	New York	8,323	5.79%		32	Kansas	1,626	1.13%
9	North Carolina	4,576	3.18%		33	Colorado	1,430	0.99%
45	North Dakota	481	0.33%		34	West Virginia	1,091	0.76%
7	Ohio	6,109	4.25%		35	Nebraska	1,029	0.72%
24	Oklahoma	2,153	1.50%		36	Maine	746	0.52%
26	Oregon	2,102	1.46%		37	Utah	701	0.49%
5	Pennsylvania	7,691	5.35%		38	Idaho	630	0.44%
40	Rhode Island	586	0.41%		39	New Mexico	602	0.42%
21	South Carolina	2,494	1.73%		40	Rhode Island	586	0.41%
45	South Dakota	481	0.33%		41	Hawaii	557	0.39%
11	Tennessee	3,699	2.57%		41	New Hampshire	557	0.39%
3	Texas	8,699	6.05%		43	Nevada	499	0.35%
37	Utah	701	0.49%		44	Montana	497	0.35%
48	Vermont	288	0.20%		45	North Dakota	481	0.33%
15	Virginia	3,390	2.36%		45	South Dakota	481	0.33%
18	Washington	2,918	2.03%		47	Delaware	324	0.23%
34	West Virginia	1,091	0.76%		48	Vermont	288	0.20%
17	Wisconsin	3,319	2.31%		49	Wyoming	243	0.17%
49	Wyoming	243	0.17%		50	Alaska	108	0.08%
						District of Columbia	336	0.23%

Source: U.S. Department of Health and Human Services, National Center for Health Statistics
"Monthly Vital Statistics Report" (Vol. 43, No. 6(S), March 22, 1995)
*Final data by state of residence. Cerebrovascular diseases include stroke and other disorders of the blood vessels of the brain.

Death Rate by Cerebrovascular Diseases in 1992

National Rate = 56.4 Deaths per 100,000 Population*

ALPHA ORDER			RANK ORDER		
RANK	STATE	RATE	RANK	STATE	RATE
10	Alabama	66.6	1	Arkansas	84.5
50	Alaska	18.4	2	North Dakota	75.9
42	Arizona	47.6	3	Tennessee	73.6
1	Arkansas	84.5	4	Iowa	72.5
40	California	49.1	5	Oregon	70.7
46	Colorado	41.3	6	South Carolina	69.2
33	Connecticut	53.5	7	South Dakota	67.9
43	Delaware	46.9	8	Oklahoma	67.2
14	Florida	64.9	9	North Carolina	66.9
31	Georgia	54.4	10	Alabama	66.6
41	Hawaii	48.2	11	Missouri	66.5
24	Idaho	59.1	11	Wisconsin	66.5
26	Illinois	58.4	13	Mississippi	66.1
18	Indiana	63.1	14	Florida	64.9
4	Iowa	72.5	15	Kansas	64.6
15	Kansas	64.6	16	Nebraska	64.3
20	Kentucky	61.6	17	Pennsylvania	64.1
28	Louisiana	56.5	18	Indiana	63.1
22	Maine	60.3	18	Minnesota	63.1
45	Maryland	42.8	20	Kentucky	61.6
29	Massachusetts	55.6	21	Montana	60.4
32	Michigan	54.1	22	Maine	60.3
18	Minnesota	63.1	22	West Virginia	60.3
13	Mississippi	66.1	24	Idaho	59.1
11	Missouri	66.5	25	Rhode Island	58.5
21	Montana	60.4	26	Illinois	58.4
16	Nebraska	64.3	27	Washington	56.7
49	Nevada	37.3	28	Louisiana	56.5
37	New Hampshire	50.0	29	Massachusetts	55.6
38	New Jersey	49.6	30	Ohio	55.4
48	New Mexico	38.1	31	Georgia	54.4
44	New York	46.0	32	Michigan	54.1
9	North Carolina	66.9	33	Connecticut	53.5
2	North Dakota	75.9	34	Virginia	53.0
30	Ohio	55.4	35	Wyoming	52.3
8	Oklahoma	67.2	36	Vermont	50.4
5	Oregon	70.7	37	New Hampshire	50.0
17	Pennsylvania	64.1	38	New Jersey	49.6
25	Rhode Island	58.5	39	Texas	49.2
6	South Carolina	69.2	40	California	49.1
7	South Dakota	67.9	41	Hawaii	48.2
3	Tennessee	73.6	42	Arizona	47.6
39	Texas	49.2	43	Delaware	46.9
47	Utah	38.7	44	New York	46.0
36	Vermont	50.4	45	Maryland	42.8
34	Virginia	53.0	46	Colorado	41.3
27	Washington	56.7	47	Utah	38.7
22	West Virginia	60.3	48	New Mexico	38.1
11	Wisconsin	66.5	49	Nevada	37.3
35	Wyoming	52.3	50	Alaska	18.4
				District of Columbia	57.4

Source: U.S. Department of Health and Human Services, National Center for Health Statistics
"Monthly Vital Statistics Report" (Vol. 43, No. 6(S), March 22, 1995)
*Final data by state of residence. Cerebrovascular diseases include stroke and other disorders of the blood vessels of the brain.

Deaths by Chronic Liver Disease and Cirrhosis in 1992

National Total = 25,263 Deaths*

<table>
<tr><td colspan="4">ALPHA ORDER</td><td colspan="4">RANK ORDER</td></tr>
<tr><td>RANK</td><td>STATE</td><td>DEATHS</td><td>% of USA</td><td>RANK</td><td>STATE</td><td>DEATHS</td><td>% of USA</td></tr>
<tr><td>20</td><td>Alabama</td><td>380</td><td>1.50%</td><td>1</td><td>California</td><td>3,753</td><td>14.86%</td></tr>
<tr><td>49</td><td>Alaska</td><td>50</td><td>0.20%</td><td>2</td><td>New York</td><td>1,995</td><td>7.90%</td></tr>
<tr><td>15</td><td>Arizona</td><td>456</td><td>1.81%</td><td>3</td><td>Texas</td><td>1,783</td><td>7.06%</td></tr>
<tr><td>34</td><td>Arkansas</td><td>172</td><td>0.68%</td><td>4</td><td>Florida</td><td>1,752</td><td>6.94%</td></tr>
<tr><td>1</td><td>California</td><td>3,753</td><td>14.86%</td><td>5</td><td>Illinois</td><td>1,245</td><td>4.93%</td></tr>
<tr><td>25</td><td>Colorado</td><td>309</td><td>1.22%</td><td>6</td><td>Pennsylvania</td><td>1,208</td><td>4.78%</td></tr>
<tr><td>28</td><td>Connecticut</td><td>277</td><td>1.10%</td><td>7</td><td>Michigan</td><td>950</td><td>3.76%</td></tr>
<tr><td>45</td><td>Delaware</td><td>70</td><td>0.28%</td><td>8</td><td>Ohio</td><td>890</td><td>3.52%</td></tr>
<tr><td>4</td><td>Florida</td><td>1,752</td><td>6.94%</td><td>9</td><td>New Jersey</td><td>854</td><td>3.38%</td></tr>
<tr><td>12</td><td>Georgia</td><td>569</td><td>2.25%</td><td>10</td><td>North Carolina</td><td>730</td><td>2.89%</td></tr>
<tr><td>43</td><td>Hawaii</td><td>73</td><td>0.29%</td><td>11</td><td>Massachusetts</td><td>679</td><td>2.69%</td></tr>
<tr><td>46</td><td>Idaho</td><td>62</td><td>0.25%</td><td>12</td><td>Georgia</td><td>569</td><td>2.25%</td></tr>
<tr><td>5</td><td>Illinois</td><td>1,245</td><td>4.93%</td><td>13</td><td>Virginia</td><td>479</td><td>1.90%</td></tr>
<tr><td>16</td><td>Indiana</td><td>454</td><td>1.80%</td><td>14</td><td>Tennessee</td><td>476</td><td>1.88%</td></tr>
<tr><td>35</td><td>Iowa</td><td>171</td><td>0.68%</td><td>15</td><td>Arizona</td><td>456</td><td>1.81%</td></tr>
<tr><td>36</td><td>Kansas</td><td>156</td><td>0.62%</td><td>16</td><td>Indiana</td><td>454</td><td>1.80%</td></tr>
<tr><td>26</td><td>Kentucky</td><td>301</td><td>1.19%</td><td>16</td><td>Washington</td><td>454</td><td>1.80%</td></tr>
<tr><td>23</td><td>Louisiana</td><td>347</td><td>1.37%</td><td>18</td><td>Maryland</td><td>405</td><td>1.60%</td></tr>
<tr><td>37</td><td>Maine</td><td>129</td><td>0.51%</td><td>19</td><td>Missouri</td><td>386</td><td>1.53%</td></tr>
<tr><td>18</td><td>Maryland</td><td>405</td><td>1.60%</td><td>20</td><td>Alabama</td><td>380</td><td>1.50%</td></tr>
<tr><td>11</td><td>Massachusetts</td><td>679</td><td>2.69%</td><td>21</td><td>Wisconsin</td><td>366</td><td>1.45%</td></tr>
<tr><td>7</td><td>Michigan</td><td>950</td><td>3.76%</td><td>22</td><td>South Carolina</td><td>356</td><td>1.41%</td></tr>
<tr><td>24</td><td>Minnesota</td><td>310</td><td>1.23%</td><td>23</td><td>Louisiana</td><td>347</td><td>1.37%</td></tr>
<tr><td>31</td><td>Mississippi</td><td>226</td><td>0.89%</td><td>24</td><td>Minnesota</td><td>310</td><td>1.23%</td></tr>
<tr><td>19</td><td>Missouri</td><td>386</td><td>1.53%</td><td>25</td><td>Colorado</td><td>309</td><td>1.22%</td></tr>
<tr><td>43</td><td>Montana</td><td>73</td><td>0.29%</td><td>26</td><td>Kentucky</td><td>301</td><td>1.19%</td></tr>
<tr><td>39</td><td>Nebraska</td><td>99</td><td>0.39%</td><td>27</td><td>Oklahoma</td><td>283</td><td>1.12%</td></tr>
<tr><td>33</td><td>Nevada</td><td>177</td><td>0.70%</td><td>28</td><td>Connecticut</td><td>277</td><td>1.10%</td></tr>
<tr><td>41</td><td>New Hampshire</td><td>94</td><td>0.37%</td><td>29</td><td>Oregon</td><td>268</td><td>1.06%</td></tr>
<tr><td>9</td><td>New Jersey</td><td>854</td><td>3.38%</td><td>30</td><td>New Mexico</td><td>228</td><td>0.90%</td></tr>
<tr><td>30</td><td>New Mexico</td><td>228</td><td>0.90%</td><td>31</td><td>Mississippi</td><td>226</td><td>0.89%</td></tr>
<tr><td>2</td><td>New York</td><td>1,995</td><td>7.90%</td><td>32</td><td>West Virginia</td><td>187</td><td>0.74%</td></tr>
<tr><td>10</td><td>North Carolina</td><td>730</td><td>2.89%</td><td>33</td><td>Nevada</td><td>177</td><td>0.70%</td></tr>
<tr><td>47</td><td>North Dakota</td><td>53</td><td>0.21%</td><td>34</td><td>Arkansas</td><td>172</td><td>0.68%</td></tr>
<tr><td>8</td><td>Ohio</td><td>890</td><td>3.52%</td><td>35</td><td>Iowa</td><td>171</td><td>0.68%</td></tr>
<tr><td>27</td><td>Oklahoma</td><td>283</td><td>1.12%</td><td>36</td><td>Kansas</td><td>156</td><td>0.62%</td></tr>
<tr><td>29</td><td>Oregon</td><td>268</td><td>1.06%</td><td>37</td><td>Maine</td><td>129</td><td>0.51%</td></tr>
<tr><td>6</td><td>Pennsylvania</td><td>1,208</td><td>4.78%</td><td>38</td><td>Rhode Island</td><td>109</td><td>0.43%</td></tr>
<tr><td>38</td><td>Rhode Island</td><td>109</td><td>0.43%</td><td>39</td><td>Nebraska</td><td>99</td><td>0.39%</td></tr>
<tr><td>22</td><td>South Carolina</td><td>356</td><td>1.41%</td><td>39</td><td>Utah</td><td>99</td><td>0.39%</td></tr>
<tr><td>42</td><td>South Dakota</td><td>74</td><td>0.29%</td><td>41</td><td>New Hampshire</td><td>94</td><td>0.37%</td></tr>
<tr><td>14</td><td>Tennessee</td><td>476</td><td>1.88%</td><td>42</td><td>South Dakota</td><td>74</td><td>0.29%</td></tr>
<tr><td>3</td><td>Texas</td><td>1,783</td><td>7.06%</td><td>43</td><td>Hawaii</td><td>73</td><td>0.29%</td></tr>
<tr><td>39</td><td>Utah</td><td>99</td><td>0.39%</td><td>43</td><td>Montana</td><td>73</td><td>0.29%</td></tr>
<tr><td>47</td><td>Vermont</td><td>53</td><td>0.21%</td><td>45</td><td>Delaware</td><td>70</td><td>0.28%</td></tr>
<tr><td>13</td><td>Virginia</td><td>479</td><td>1.90%</td><td>46</td><td>Idaho</td><td>62</td><td>0.25%</td></tr>
<tr><td>16</td><td>Washington</td><td>454</td><td>1.80%</td><td>47</td><td>North Dakota</td><td>53</td><td>0.21%</td></tr>
<tr><td>32</td><td>West Virginia</td><td>187</td><td>0.74%</td><td>47</td><td>Vermont</td><td>53</td><td>0.21%</td></tr>
<tr><td>21</td><td>Wisconsin</td><td>366</td><td>1.45%</td><td>49</td><td>Alaska</td><td>50</td><td>0.20%</td></tr>
<tr><td>50</td><td>Wyoming</td><td>41</td><td>0.16%</td><td>50</td><td>Wyoming</td><td>41</td><td>0.16%</td></tr>
<tr><td></td><td></td><td></td><td></td><td></td><td>District of Columbia</td><td>152</td><td>0.60%</td></tr>
</table>

Source: U.S. Department of Health and Human Services, National Center for Health Statistics
  unpublished data
*By state of residence.

Death Rate by Chronic Liver Disease and Cirrhosis in 1992

National Rate = 9.9 Deaths per 100,000 Population*

ALPHA ORDER			RANK ORDER		
RANK	STATE	RATE	RANK	STATE	RATE
22	Alabama	9.2	1	New Mexico	14.4
30	Alaska	8.5	2	Nevada	13.2
5	Arizona	11.9	3	Florida	13.0
43	Arkansas	7.2	4	California	12.1
4	California	12.1	5	Arizona	11.9
24	Colorado	8.9	6	Massachusetts	11.3
31	Connecticut	8.4	7	New York	11.0
15	Delaware	10.1	8	New Jersey	10.9
3	Florida	13.0	8	Rhode Island	10.9
31	Georgia	8.4	10	Illinois	10.7
45	Hawaii	6.3	10	North Carolina	10.7
49	Idaho	5.8	12	Maine	10.4
10	Illinois	10.7	12	South Dakota	10.4
38	Indiana	8.0	14	West Virginia	10.3
48	Iowa	6.1	15	Delaware	10.1
46	Kansas	6.2	15	Michigan	10.1
38	Kentucky	8.0	15	Pennsylvania	10.1
36	Louisiana	8.1	15	Texas	10.1
12	Maine	10.4	19	South Carolina	9.9
35	Maryland	8.2	20	Tennessee	9.5
6	Massachusetts	11.3	21	Vermont	9.3
15	Michigan	10.1	22	Alabama	9.2
44	Minnesota	6.9	23	Oregon	9.0
29	Mississippi	8.6	24	Colorado	8.9
41	Missouri	7.4	24	Montana	8.9
24	Montana	8.9	26	Oklahoma	8.8
46	Nebraska	6.2	26	Washington	8.8
2	Nevada	13.2	26	Wyoming	8.8
31	New Hampshire	8.4	29	Mississippi	8.6
8	New Jersey	10.9	30	Alaska	8.5
1	New Mexico	14.4	31	Connecticut	8.4
7	New York	11.0	31	Georgia	8.4
10	North Carolina	10.7	31	New Hampshire	8.4
31	North Dakota	8.4	31	North Dakota	8.4
36	Ohio	8.1	35	Maryland	8.2
26	Oklahoma	8.8	36	Louisiana	8.1
23	Oregon	9.0	36	Ohio	8.1
15	Pennsylvania	10.1	38	Indiana	8.0
8	Rhode Island	10.9	38	Kentucky	8.0
19	South Carolina	9.9	40	Virginia	7.5
12	South Dakota	10.4	41	Missouri	7.4
20	Tennessee	9.5	42	Wisconsin	7.3
15	Texas	10.1	43	Arkansas	7.2
50	Utah	5.5	44	Minnesota	6.9
21	Vermont	9.3	45	Hawaii	6.3
40	Virginia	7.5	46	Kansas	6.2
26	Washington	8.8	46	Nebraska	6.2
14	West Virginia	10.3	48	Iowa	6.1
42	Wisconsin	7.3	49	Idaho	5.8
26	Wyoming	8.8	50	Utah	5.5
				District of Columbia	25.9

Source: U.S. Department of Health and Human Services, National Center for Health Statistics
    unpublished data
*By state of residence.

Deaths by Chronic Obstructive Pulmonary Diseases in 1992

National Total = 91,938 Deaths*

RANK	STATE	DEATHS	% of USA
22	Alabama	1,456	1.58%
50	Alaska	89	0.10%
19	Arizona	1,696	1.84%
33	Arkansas	940	1.02%
1	California	10,081	10.96%
24	Colorado	1,414	1.54%
30	Connecticut	1,160	1.26%
45	Delaware	248	0.27%
2	Florida	6,546	7.12%
14	Georgia	2,112	2.30%
49	Hawaii	189	0.21%
40	Idaho	429	0.47%
7	Illinois	3,866	4.21%
11	Indiana	2,269	2.47%
29	Iowa	1,172	1.27%
32	Kansas	950	1.03%
18	Kentucky	1,697	1.85%
26	Louisiana	1,268	1.38%
37	Maine	628	0.68%
23	Maryland	1,448	1.57%
13	Massachusetts	2,151	2.34%
8	Michigan	3,085	3.36%
21	Minnesota	1,498	1.63%
34	Mississippi	879	0.96%
12	Missouri	2,220	2.41%
39	Montana	456	0.50%
35	Nebraska	667	0.73%
36	Nevada	636	0.69%
42	New Hampshire	407	0.44%
9	New Jersey	2,421	2.63%
38	New Mexico	535	0.58%
3	New York	5,843	6.36%
10	North Carolina	2,402	2.61%
47	North Dakota	234	0.25%
6	Ohio	4,373	4.76%
25	Oklahoma	1,377	1.50%
28	Oregon	1,255	1.37%
5	Pennsylvania	4,777	5.20%
43	Rhode Island	377	0.41%
27	South Carolina	1,259	1.37%
44	South Dakota	301	0.33%
17	Tennessee	1,922	2.09%
4	Texas	5,383	5.86%
41	Utah	420	0.46%
46	Vermont	242	0.26%
16	Virginia	2,057	2.24%
15	Washington	2,088	2.27%
31	West Virginia	982	1.07%
20	Wisconsin	1,638	1.78%
48	Wyoming	230	0.25%

RANK	STATE	DEATHS	% of USA
1	California	10,081	10.96%
2	Florida	6,546	7.12%
3	New York	5,843	6.36%
4	Texas	5,383	5.86%
5	Pennsylvania	4,777	5.20%
6	Ohio	4,373	4.76%
7	Illinois	3,866	4.21%
8	Michigan	3,085	3.36%
9	New Jersey	2,421	2.63%
10	North Carolina	2,402	2.61%
11	Indiana	2,269	2.47%
12	Missouri	2,220	2.41%
13	Massachusetts	2,151	2.34%
14	Georgia	2,112	2.30%
15	Washington	2,088	2.27%
16	Virginia	2,057	2.24%
17	Tennessee	1,922	2.09%
18	Kentucky	1,697	1.85%
19	Arizona	1,696	1.84%
20	Wisconsin	1,638	1.78%
21	Minnesota	1,498	1.63%
22	Alabama	1,456	1.58%
23	Maryland	1,448	1.57%
24	Colorado	1,414	1.54%
25	Oklahoma	1,377	1.50%
26	Louisiana	1,268	1.38%
27	South Carolina	1,259	1.37%
28	Oregon	1,255	1.37%
29	Iowa	1,172	1.27%
30	Connecticut	1,160	1.26%
31	West Virginia	982	1.07%
32	Kansas	950	1.03%
33	Arkansas	940	1.02%
34	Mississippi	879	0.96%
35	Nebraska	667	0.73%
36	Nevada	636	0.69%
37	Maine	628	0.68%
38	New Mexico	535	0.58%
39	Montana	456	0.50%
40	Idaho	429	0.47%
41	Utah	420	0.46%
42	New Hampshire	407	0.44%
43	Rhode Island	377	0.41%
44	South Dakota	301	0.33%
45	Delaware	248	0.27%
46	Vermont	242	0.26%
47	North Dakota	234	0.25%
48	Wyoming	230	0.25%
49	Hawaii	189	0.21%
50	Alaska	89	0.10%
	District of Columbia	165	0.18%

Source: U.S. Department of Health and Human Services, National Center for Health Statistics
"Monthly Vital Statistics Report" (Vol. 43, No. 6(S), March 22, 1995)
*Final data by state of residence. Includes allied conditions.

Death Rate by Chronic Obstructive Pulmonary Diseases in 1992

National Rate = 36.0 Deaths per 100,000 Population*

ALPHA ORDER

RANK	STATE	RATE
31	Alabama	35.2
50	Alaska	15.1
8	Arizona	44.3
22	Arkansas	39.3
40	California	32.6
16	Colorado	40.8
30	Connecticut	35.4
28	Delaware	35.9
5	Florida	48.6
43	Georgia	31.2
49	Hawaii	16.4
18	Idaho	40.2
37	Illinois	33.3
19	Indiana	40.1
14	Iowa	41.8
24	Kansas	37.8
7	Kentucky	45.2
46	Louisiana	29.6
3	Maine	50.8
47	Maryland	29.4
28	Massachusetts	35.9
39	Michigan	32.7
36	Minnesota	33.5
35	Mississippi	33.6
10	Missouri	42.8
1	Montana	55.5
15	Nebraska	41.7
6	Nevada	47.6
27	New Hampshire	36.5
44	New Jersey	31.0
34	New Mexico	33.8
41	New York	32.3
32	North Carolina	35.1
26	North Dakota	36.9
21	Ohio	39.7
9	Oklahoma	43.0
13	Oregon	42.2
20	Pennsylvania	39.8
25	Rhode Island	37.6
33	South Carolina	34.9
11	South Dakota	42.5
23	Tennessee	38.2
45	Texas	30.4
48	Utah	23.2
12	Vermont	42.4
42	Virginia	32.2
17	Washington	40.6
2	West Virginia	54.3
38	Wisconsin	32.8
4	Wyoming	49.5

RANK ORDER

RANK	STATE	RATE
1	Montana	55.5
2	West Virginia	54.3
3	Maine	50.8
4	Wyoming	49.5
5	Florida	48.6
6	Nevada	47.6
7	Kentucky	45.2
8	Arizona	44.3
9	Oklahoma	43.0
10	Missouri	42.8
11	South Dakota	42.5
12	Vermont	42.4
13	Oregon	42.2
14	Iowa	41.8
15	Nebraska	41.7
16	Colorado	40.8
17	Washington	40.6
18	Idaho	40.2
19	Indiana	40.1
20	Pennsylvania	39.8
21	Ohio	39.7
22	Arkansas	39.3
23	Tennessee	38.2
24	Kansas	37.8
25	Rhode Island	37.6
26	North Dakota	36.9
27	New Hampshire	36.5
28	Delaware	35.9
28	Massachusetts	35.9
30	Connecticut	35.4
31	Alabama	35.2
32	North Carolina	35.1
33	South Carolina	34.9
34	New Mexico	33.8
35	Mississippi	33.6
36	Minnesota	33.5
37	Illinois	33.3
38	Wisconsin	32.8
39	Michigan	32.7
40	California	32.6
41	New York	32.3
42	Virginia	32.2
43	Georgia	31.2
44	New Jersey	31.0
45	Texas	30.4
46	Louisiana	29.6
47	Maryland	29.4
48	Utah	23.2
49	Hawaii	16.4
50	Alaska	15.1
	District of Columbia	28.2

Source: U.S. Department of Health and Human Services, National Center for Health Statistics
"Monthly Vital Statistics Report" (Vol. 43, No. 6(S), March 22, 1995)
Final data by state of residence. Includes allied conditions.

Deaths by Diabetes Mellitus in 1992

National Total = 50,067 Deaths*

ALPHA ORDER					RANK ORDER			

RANK	STATE	DEATHS	% of USA		RANK	STATE	DEATHS	% of USA
20	Alabama	852	1.70%		1	Texas	3,771	7.53%
50	Alaska	47	0.09%		2	California	3,574	7.14%
25	Arizona	659	1.32%		3	Pennsylvania	3,145	6.28%
31	Arkansas	514	1.03%		4	Florida	3,078	6.15%
2	California	3,574	7.14%		5	New York	2,967	5.93%
34	Colorado	437	0.87%		6	Ohio	2,900	5.79%
29	Connecticut	538	1.07%		7	Illinois	2,392	4.78%
41	Delaware	207	0.41%		8	Michigan	2,125	4.24%
4	Florida	3,078	6.15%		9	New Jersey	2,103	4.20%
18	Georgia	984	1.97%		10	North Carolina	1,426	2.85%
44	Hawaii	171	0.34%		11	Indiana	1,255	2.51%
42	Idaho	190	0.38%		12	Massachusetts	1,195	2.39%
7	Illinois	2,392	4.78%		13	Louisiana	1,193	2.38%
11	Indiana	1,255	2.51%		14	Maryland	1,106	2.21%
32	Iowa	506	1.01%		15	Missouri	1,081	2.16%
30	Kansas	515	1.03%		16	Wisconsin	1,042	2.08%
21	Kentucky	817	1.63%		17	Tennessee	1,002	2.00%
13	Louisiana	1,193	2.38%		18	Georgia	984	1.97%
37	Maine	320	0.64%		19	Virginia	963	1.92%
14	Maryland	1,106	2.21%		20	Alabama	852	1.70%
12	Massachusetts	1,195	2.39%		21	Kentucky	817	1.63%
8	Michigan	2,125	4.24%		22	Washington	811	1.62%
24	Minnesota	776	1.55%		23	South Carolina	781	1.56%
33	Mississippi	475	0.95%		24	Minnesota	776	1.55%
15	Missouri	1,081	2.16%		25	Arizona	659	1.32%
46	Montana	160	0.32%		26	Oklahoma	574	1.15%
38	Nebraska	266	0.53%		27	Oregon	561	1.12%
43	Nevada	173	0.35%		28	West Virginia	545	1.09%
39	New Hampshire	240	0.48%		29	Connecticut	538	1.07%
9	New Jersey	2,103	4.20%		30	Kansas	515	1.03%
35	New Mexico	370	0.74%		31	Arkansas	514	1.03%
5	New York	2,967	5.93%		32	Iowa	506	1.01%
10	North Carolina	1,426	2.85%		33	Mississippi	475	0.95%
47	North Dakota	143	0.29%		34	Colorado	437	0.87%
6	Ohio	2,900	5.79%		35	New Mexico	370	0.74%
26	Oklahoma	574	1.15%		36	Utah	359	0.72%
27	Oregon	561	1.12%		37	Maine	320	0.64%
3	Pennsylvania	3,145	6.28%		38	Nebraska	266	0.53%
40	Rhode Island	228	0.46%		39	New Hampshire	240	0.48%
23	South Carolina	781	1.56%		40	Rhode Island	228	0.46%
45	South Dakota	164	0.33%		41	Delaware	207	0.41%
17	Tennessee	1,002	2.00%		42	Idaho	190	0.38%
1	Texas	3,771	7.53%		43	Nevada	173	0.35%
36	Utah	359	0.72%		44	Hawaii	171	0.34%
48	Vermont	125	0.25%		45	South Dakota	164	0.33%
19	Virginia	963	1.92%		46	Montana	160	0.32%
22	Washington	811	1.62%		47	North Dakota	143	0.29%
28	West Virginia	545	1.09%		48	Vermont	125	0.25%
16	Wisconsin	1,042	2.08%		49	Wyoming	68	0.14%
49	Wyoming	68	0.14%		50	Alaska	47	0.09%
						District of Columbia	173	0.35%

Source: U.S. Department of Health and Human Services, National Center for Health Statistics
"Monthly Vital Statistics Report" (Vol. 43, No. 6(S), March 22, 1995)
*Final data by state of residence.

Death Rate by Diabetes Mellitus in 1992

National Rate = 19.6 Deaths per 100,000 Population*

ALPHA ORDER			RANK ORDER		
RANK	STATE	RATE	RANK	STATE	RATE
25	Alabama	20.6	1	West Virginia	30.1
50	Alaska	8.0	2	Delaware	30.0
38	Arizona	17.2	3	Louisiana	27.9
19	Arkansas	21.5	4	New Jersey	26.9
49	California	11.6	5	Ohio	26.3
48	Colorado	12.6	6	Pennsylvania	26.2
40	Connecticut	16.4	7	Maine	25.9
2	Delaware	30.0	8	New Mexico	23.4
10	Florida	22.8	9	South Dakota	23.2
46	Georgia	14.5	10	Florida	22.8
44	Hawaii	14.8	10	Rhode Island	22.8
36	Idaho	17.8	12	North Dakota	22.6
25	Illinois	20.6	13	Maryland	22.5
15	Indiana	22.2	13	Michigan	22.5
34	Iowa	18.1	15	Indiana	22.2
27	Kansas	20.5	16	Vermont	21.9
17	Kentucky	21.8	17	Kentucky	21.8
3	Louisiana	27.9	18	South Carolina	21.7
7	Maine	25.9	19	Arkansas	21.5
13	Maryland	22.5	19	New Hampshire	21.5
28	Massachusetts	19.9	21	Texas	21.3
13	Michigan	22.5	22	North Carolina	20.9
37	Minnesota	17.4	22	Wisconsin	20.9
33	Mississippi	18.2	24	Missouri	20.8
24	Missouri	20.8	25	Alabama	20.6
31	Montana	19.5	25	Illinois	20.6
39	Nebraska	16.6	27	Kansas	20.5
47	Nevada	12.9	28	Massachusetts	19.9
19	New Hampshire	21.5	28	Tennessee	19.9
4	New Jersey	26.9	30	Utah	19.8
8	New Mexico	23.4	31	Montana	19.5
40	New York	16.4	32	Oregon	18.9
22	North Carolina	20.9	33	Mississippi	18.2
12	North Dakota	22.6	34	Iowa	18.1
5	Ohio	26.3	35	Oklahoma	17.9
35	Oklahoma	17.9	36	Idaho	17.8
32	Oregon	18.9	37	Minnesota	17.4
6	Pennsylvania	26.2	38	Arizona	17.2
10	Rhode Island	22.8	39	Nebraska	16.6
18	South Carolina	21.7	40	Connecticut	16.4
9	South Dakota	23.2	40	New York	16.4
28	Tennessee	19.9	42	Washington	15.8
21	Texas	21.3	43	Virginia	15.1
30	Utah	19.8	44	Hawaii	14.8
16	Vermont	21.9	45	Wyoming	14.6
43	Virginia	15.1	46	Georgia	14.5
42	Washington	15.8	47	Nevada	12.9
1	West Virginia	30.1	48	Colorado	12.6
22	Wisconsin	20.9	49	California	11.6
45	Wyoming	14.6	50	Alaska	8.0
				District of Columbia	29.6

Source: U.S. Department of Health and Human Services, National Center for Health Statistics
"Monthly Vital Statistics Report" (Vol. 43, No. 6(S), March 22, 1995)
*Final data by state of residence.

Deaths by Diseases of the Heart in 1992

National Total = 717,706 Deaths*

ALPHA ORDER					RANK ORDER			
RANK	**STATE**		**DEATHS**	**% of USA**	**RANK**	**STATE**	**DEATHS**	**% of USA**
18	Alabama		12,896	1.80%	1	California	67,105	9.35%
50	Alaska		518	0.07%	2	New York	64,110	8.93%
27	Arizona		9,315	1.30%	3	Florida	47,325	6.59%
30	Arkansas		8,237	1.15%	4	Pennsylvania	43,205	6.02%
1	California		67,105	9.35%	5	Texas	40,495	5.64%
34	Colorado		6,169	0.86%	6	Illinois	34,463	4.80%
25	Connecticut		9,659	1.35%	7	Ohio	34,023	4.74%
47	Delaware		1,844	0.26%	8	Michigan	26,895	3.75%
3	Florida		47,325	6.59%	9	New Jersey	23,809	3.32%
14	Georgia		16,483	2.30%	10	North Carolina	18,990	2.65%
44	Hawaii		2,136	0.30%	11	Missouri	17,747	2.47%
42	Idaho		2,325	0.32%	12	Massachusetts	17,068	2.38%
6	Illinois		34,463	4.80%	13	Indiana	16,706	2.33%
13	Indiana		16,706	2.33%	14	Georgia	16,483	2.30%
28	Iowa		9,179	1.28%	15	Virginia	15,500	2.16%
31	Kansas		7,423	1.03%	16	Tennessee	15,015	2.09%
21	Kentucky		11,778	1.64%	17	Wisconsin	14,052	1.96%
19	Louisiana		12,155	1.69%	18	Alabama	12,896	1.80%
36	Maine		3,462	0.48%	19	Louisiana	12,155	1.69%
20	Maryland		11,878	1.65%	20	Maryland	11,878	1.65%
12	Massachusetts		17,068	2.38%	21	Kentucky	11,778	1.64%
8	Michigan		26,895	3.75%	22	Washington	11,183	1.56%
24	Minnesota		10,250	1.43%	23	Oklahoma	10,869	1.51%
29	Mississippi		9,130	1.27%	24	Minnesota	10,250	1.43%
11	Missouri		17,747	2.47%	25	Connecticut	9,659	1.35%
45	Montana		1,907	0.27%	26	South Carolina	9,654	1.35%
35	Nebraska		5,276	0.74%	27	Arizona	9,315	1.30%
38	Nevada		3,102	0.43%	28	Iowa	9,179	1.28%
41	New Hampshire		2,684	0.37%	29	Mississippi	9,130	1.27%
9	New Jersey		23,809	3.32%	30	Arkansas	8,237	1.15%
39	New Mexico		2,966	0.41%	31	Kansas	7,423	1.03%
2	New York		64,110	8.93%	32	Oregon	7,288	1.02%
10	North Carolina		18,990	2.65%	33	West Virginia	6,927	0.97%
46	North Dakota		1,902	0.27%	34	Colorado	6,169	0.86%
7	Ohio		34,023	4.74%	35	Nebraska	5,276	0.74%
23	Oklahoma		10,869	1.51%	36	Maine	3,462	0.48%
32	Oregon		7,288	1.02%	37	Rhode Island	3,234	0.45%
4	Pennsylvania		43,205	6.02%	38	Nevada	3,102	0.43%
37	Rhode Island		3,234	0.45%	39	New Mexico	2,966	0.41%
26	South Carolina		9,654	1.35%	40	Utah	2,750	0.38%
43	South Dakota		2,294	0.32%	41	New Hampshire	2,684	0.37%
16	Tennessee		15,015	2.09%	42	Idaho	2,325	0.32%
5	Texas		40,495	5.64%	43	South Dakota	2,294	0.32%
40	Utah		2,750	0.38%	44	Hawaii	2,136	0.30%
48	Vermont		1,585	0.22%	45	Montana	1,907	0.27%
15	Virginia		15,500	2.16%	46	North Dakota	1,902	0.27%
22	Washington		11,183	1.56%	47	Delaware	1,844	0.26%
33	West Virginia		6,927	0.97%	48	Vermont	1,585	0.22%
17	Wisconsin		14,052	1.96%	49	Wyoming	902	0.13%
49	Wyoming		902	0.13%	50	Alaska	518	0.07%
						District of Columbia	1,838	0.26%

Source: U.S. Department of Health and Human Services, National Center for Health Statistics
"Monthly Vital Statistics Report" (Vol. 43, No. 6(S), March 22, 1995)
*Final data by state of residence.

Death Rate by Diseases of the Heart in 1992

National Rate = 281.4 Deaths per 100,000 Population*

ALPHA ORDER			RANK ORDER		
RANK	STATE	RATE	RANK	STATE	RATE
14	Alabama	311.7	1	West Virginia	382.9
50	Alaska	88.1	2	Pennsylvania	360.2
34	Arizona	243.1	3	New York	354.0
6	Arkansas	344.0	4	Florida	351.0
44	California	217.2	5	Mississippi	349.1
48	Colorado	178.1	6	Arkansas	344.0
22	Connecticut	294.6	7	Missouri	341.9
31	Delaware	266.9	8	Oklahoma	339.1
4	Florida	351.0	9	Nebraska	329.6
33	Georgia	243.4	10	Iowa	327.5
47	Hawaii	184.8	11	South Dakota	323.8
42	Idaho	218.1	12	Rhode Island	323.0
19	Illinois	296.8	13	Kentucky	313.8
20	Indiana	295.2	14	Alabama	311.7
10	Iowa	327.5	15	Ohio	308.7
21	Kansas	295.1	16	New Jersey	304.5
13	Kentucky	313.8	17	North Dakota	300.0
25	Louisiana	284.1	18	Tennessee	298.8
27	Maine	280.0	19	Illinois	296.8
36	Maryland	241.6	20	Indiana	295.2
24	Massachusetts	284.8	21	Kansas	295.1
23	Michigan	285.1	22	Connecticut	294.6
40	Minnesota	229.4	23	Michigan	285.1
5	Mississippi	349.1	24	Massachusetts	284.8
7	Missouri	341.9	25	Louisiana	284.1
39	Montana	231.9	26	Wisconsin	281.5
9	Nebraska	329.6	27	Maine	280.0
38	Nevada	232.1	28	North Carolina	277.8
37	New Hampshire	240.7	29	Vermont	277.4
16	New Jersey	304.5	30	South Carolina	268.0
46	New Mexico	187.5	31	Delaware	266.9
3	New York	354.0	32	Oregon	245.3
28	North Carolina	277.8	33	Georgia	243.4
17	North Dakota	300.0	34	Arizona	243.1
15	Ohio	308.7	35	Virginia	242.4
8	Oklahoma	339.1	36	Maryland	241.6
32	Oregon	245.3	37	New Hampshire	240.7
2	Pennsylvania	360.2	38	Nevada	232.1
12	Rhode Island	323.0	39	Montana	231.9
30	South Carolina	268.0	40	Minnesota	229.4
11	South Dakota	323.8	41	Texas	229.0
18	Tennessee	298.8	42	Idaho	218.1
41	Texas	229.0	43	Washington	217.5
49	Utah	151.8	44	California	217.2
29	Vermont	277.4	45	Wyoming	194.1
35	Virginia	242.4	46	New Mexico	187.5
43	Washington	217.5	47	Hawaii	184.8
1	West Virginia	382.9	48	Colorado	178.1
26	Wisconsin	281.5	49	Utah	151.8
45	Wyoming	194.1	50	Alaska	88.1
				District of Columbia	314.1

Source: U.S. Department of Health and Human Services, National Center for Health Statistics
"Monthly Vital Statistics Report" (Vol. 43, No. 6(S), March 22, 1995)
*Final data by state of residence.

Deaths by Malignant Neoplasms in 1992

National Total = 520,578 Deaths*

ALPHA ORDER					RANK ORDER			
RANK	STATE		DEATHS	% of USA	RANK	STATE	DEATHS	% of USA
20	Alabama		9,043	1.74%	1	California	50,083	9.62%
50	Alaska		518	0.10%	2	New York	38,624	7.42%
24	Arizona		7,444	1.43%	3	Florida	35,173	6.76%
30	Arkansas		5,847	1.12%	4	Pennsylvania	30,308	5.82%
1	California		50,083	9.62%	5	Texas	30,102	5.78%
33	Colorado		4,954	0.95%	6	Illinois	24,621	4.73%
25	Connecticut		7,133	1.37%	7	Ohio	24,320	4.67%
46	Delaware		1,544	0.30%	8	Michigan	19,297	3.71%
3	Florida		35,173	6.76%	9	New Jersey	17,867	3.43%
15	Georgia		11,797	2.27%	10	Massachusetts	14,182	2.72%
43	Hawaii		1,755	0.34%	11	North Carolina	13,944	2.68%
42	Idaho		1,802	0.35%	12	Indiana	12,028	2.31%
6	Illinois		24,621	4.73%	13	Virginia	12,008	2.31%
12	Indiana		12,028	2.31%	14	Missouri	11,810	2.27%
28	Iowa		6,433	1.24%	15	Georgia	11,797	2.27%
32	Kansas		5,033	0.97%	16	Tennessee	10,773	2.07%
22	Kentucky		8,549	1.64%	17	Wisconsin	10,325	1.98%
21	Louisiana		8,857	1.70%	18	Maryland	9,951	1.91%
36	Maine		2,940	0.56%	19	Washington	9,462	1.82%
18	Maryland		9,951	1.91%	20	Alabama	9,043	1.74%
10	Massachusetts		14,182	2.72%	21	Louisiana	8,857	1.70%
8	Michigan		19,297	3.71%	22	Kentucky	8,549	1.64%
23	Minnesota		8,547	1.64%	23	Minnesota	8,547	1.64%
31	Mississippi		5,560	1.07%	24	Arizona	7,444	1.43%
14	Missouri		11,810	2.27%	25	Connecticut	7,133	1.37%
44	Montana		1,707	0.33%	26	South Carolina	6,992	1.34%
35	Nebraska		3,239	0.62%	27	Oklahoma	6,773	1.30%
37	Nevada		2,678	0.51%	28	Iowa	6,433	1.24%
40	New Hampshire		2,283	0.44%	29	Oregon	6,314	1.21%
9	New Jersey		17,867	3.43%	30	Arkansas	5,847	1.12%
39	New Mexico		2,490	0.48%	31	Mississippi	5,560	1.07%
2	New York		38,624	7.42%	32	Kansas	5,033	0.97%
11	North Carolina		13,944	2.68%	33	Colorado	4,954	0.95%
47	North Dakota		1,363	0.26%	34	West Virginia	4,614	0.89%
7	Ohio		24,320	4.67%	35	Nebraska	3,239	0.62%
27	Oklahoma		6,773	1.30%	36	Maine	2,940	0.56%
29	Oregon		6,314	1.21%	37	Nevada	2,678	0.51%
4	Pennsylvania		30,308	5.82%	38	Rhode Island	2,517	0.48%
38	Rhode Island		2,517	0.48%	39	New Mexico	2,490	0.48%
26	South Carolina		6,992	1.34%	40	New Hampshire	2,283	0.44%
45	South Dakota		1,573	0.30%	41	Utah	1,961	0.38%
16	Tennessee		10,773	2.07%	42	Idaho	1,802	0.35%
5	Texas		30,102	5.78%	43	Hawaii	1,755	0.34%
41	Utah		1,961	0.38%	44	Montana	1,707	0.33%
48	Vermont		1,166	0.22%	45	South Dakota	1,573	0.30%
13	Virginia		12,008	2.31%	46	Delaware	1,544	0.30%
19	Washington		9,462	1.82%	47	North Dakota	1,363	0.26%
34	West Virginia		4,614	0.89%	48	Vermont	1,166	0.22%
17	Wisconsin		10,325	1.98%	49	Wyoming	747	0.14%
49	Wyoming		747	0.14%	50	Alaska	518	0.10%
						District of Columbia	1,527	0.29%

Source: U.S. Department of Health and Human Services, National Center for Health Statistics
  "Monthly Vital Statistics Report" (Vol. 43, No. 6(S), March 22, 1995)
*Final data by state of residence. Neoplasms are abnormal tissue, tumors. Includes many cancers.

Death Rate by Malignant Neoplasms in 1992

National Rate = 204.1 Deaths per 100,000 Population*

ALPHA ORDER			RANK ORDER		
RANK	**STATE**	**RATE**	**RANK**	**STATE**	**RATE**
15	Alabama	218.6	1	Florida	260.9
50	Alaska	88.1	2	West Virginia	255.1
36	Arizona	194.2	3	Pennsylvania	252.7
5	Arkansas	244.2	4	Rhode Island	251.4
44	California	162.1	5	Arkansas	244.2
48	Colorado	143.0	6	Maine	237.8
16	Connecticut	217.5	7	Massachusetts	236.7
12	Delaware	223.5	8	Iowa	229.5
1	Florida	260.9	9	New Jersey	228.5
41	Georgia	174.2	10	Kentucky	227.7
47	Hawaii	151.9	11	Missouri	227.5
43	Idaho	169.1	12	Delaware	223.5
23	Illinois	212.0	13	South Dakota	222.0
20	Indiana	212.6	14	Ohio	220.7
8	Iowa	229.5	15	Alabama	218.6
35	Kansas	200.1	16	Connecticut	217.5
10	Kentucky	227.7	17	North Dakota	215.0
26	Louisiana	207.0	18	Tennessee	214.4
6	Maine	237.8	19	New York	213.3
32	Maryland	202.4	20	Indiana	212.6
7	Massachusetts	236.7	20	Mississippi	212.6
29	Michigan	204.6	22	Oregon	212.5
38	Minnesota	191.3	23	Illinois	212.0
20	Mississippi	212.6	24	Oklahoma	211.3
11	Missouri	227.5	25	Montana	207.6
25	Montana	207.6	26	Louisiana	207.0
32	Nebraska	202.4	27	Wisconsin	206.8
34	Nevada	200.4	28	New Hampshire	204.7
28	New Hampshire	204.7	29	Michigan	204.6
9	New Jersey	228.5	30	Vermont	204.1
46	New Mexico	157.4	31	North Carolina	204.0
19	New York	213.3	32	Maryland	202.4
31	North Carolina	204.0	32	Nebraska	202.4
17	North Dakota	215.0	34	Nevada	200.4
14	Ohio	220.7	35	Kansas	200.1
24	Oklahoma	211.3	36	Arizona	194.2
22	Oregon	212.5	37	South Carolina	194.1
3	Pennsylvania	252.7	38	Minnesota	191.3
4	Rhode Island	251.4	39	Virginia	187.8
37	South Carolina	194.1	40	Washington	184.0
13	South Dakota	222.0	41	Georgia	174.2
18	Tennessee	214.4	42	Texas	170.2
42	Texas	170.2	43	Idaho	169.1
49	Utah	108.3	44	California	162.1
30	Vermont	204.1	45	Wyoming	160.7
39	Virginia	187.8	46	New Mexico	157.4
40	Washington	184.0	47	Hawaii	151.9
2	West Virginia	255.1	48	Colorado	143.0
27	Wisconsin	206.8	49	Utah	108.3
45	Wyoming	160.7	50	Alaska	88.1
				District of Columbia	260.9

Source: U.S. Department of Health and Human Services, National Center for Health Statistics
   "Monthly Vital Statistics Report" (Vol. 43, No. 6(S), March 22, 1995)
*Final data by state of residence. Neoplasms are abnormal tissue, tumors. Includes many cancers.

Deaths by Pneumonia and Influenza in 1992

National Total = 75,719 Deaths*

RANK	STATE	DEATHS	% of USA
22	Alabama	1,159	1.53%
50	Alaska	47	0.06%
26	Arizona	1,070	1.41%
29	Arkansas	882	1.16%
1	California	9,822	12.97%
28	Colorado	941	1.24%
24	Connecticut	1,132	1.50%
46	Delaware	231	0.31%
6	Florida	3,398	4.49%
15	Georgia	1,687	2.23%
44	Hawaii	263	0.35%
39	Idaho	323	0.43%
5	Illinois	3,549	4.69%
16	Indiana	1,676	2.21%
25	Iowa	1,117	1.48%
30	Kansas	853	1.13%
19	Kentucky	1,350	1.78%
27	Louisiana	1,000	1.32%
38	Maine	339	0.45%
23	Maryland	1,148	1.52%
9	Massachusetts	2,395	3.16%
8	Michigan	2,714	3.58%
18	Minnesota	1,392	1.84%
32	Mississippi	813	1.07%
12	Missouri	1,864	2.46%
43	Montana	274	0.36%
35	Nebraska	576	0.76%
42	Nevada	277	0.37%
40	New Hampshire	311	0.41%
10	New Jersey	2,161	2.85%
37	New Mexico	356	0.47%
2	New York	6,201	8.19%
11	North Carolina	1,918	2.53%
47	North Dakota	211	0.28%
7	Ohio	3,099	4.09%
21	Oklahoma	1,253	1.65%
31	Oregon	849	1.12%
3	Pennsylvania	4,039	5.33%
41	Rhode Island	289	0.38%
33	South Carolina	756	1.00%
45	South Dakota	262	0.35%
14	Tennessee	1,725	2.28%
4	Texas	3,712	4.90%
36	Utah	407	0.54%
48	Vermont	186	0.25%
13	Virginia	1,761	2.33%
20	Washington	1,312	1.73%
34	West Virginia	692	0.91%
17	Wisconsin	1,607	2.12%
49	Wyoming	109	0.14%

RANK	STATE	DEATHS	% of USA
1	California	9,822	12.97%
2	New York	6,201	8.19%
3	Pennsylvania	4,039	5.33%
4	Texas	3,712	4.90%
5	Illinois	3,549	4.69%
6	Florida	3,398	4.49%
7	Ohio	3,099	4.09%
8	Michigan	2,714	3.58%
9	Massachusetts	2,395	3.16%
10	New Jersey	2,161	2.85%
11	North Carolina	1,918	2.53%
12	Missouri	1,864	2.46%
13	Virginia	1,761	2.33%
14	Tennessee	1,725	2.28%
15	Georgia	1,687	2.23%
16	Indiana	1,676	2.21%
17	Wisconsin	1,607	2.12%
18	Minnesota	1,392	1.84%
19	Kentucky	1,350	1.78%
20	Washington	1,312	1.73%
21	Oklahoma	1,253	1.65%
22	Alabama	1,159	1.53%
23	Maryland	1,148	1.52%
24	Connecticut	1,132	1.50%
25	Iowa	1,117	1.48%
26	Arizona	1,070	1.41%
27	Louisiana	1,000	1.32%
28	Colorado	941	1.24%
29	Arkansas	882	1.16%
30	Kansas	853	1.13%
31	Oregon	849	1.12%
32	Mississippi	813	1.07%
33	South Carolina	756	1.00%
34	West Virginia	692	0.91%
35	Nebraska	576	0.76%
36	Utah	407	0.54%
37	New Mexico	356	0.47%
38	Maine	339	0.45%
39	Idaho	323	0.43%
40	New Hampshire	311	0.41%
41	Rhode Island	289	0.38%
42	Nevada	277	0.37%
43	Montana	274	0.36%
44	Hawaii	263	0.35%
45	South Dakota	262	0.35%
46	Delaware	231	0.31%
47	North Dakota	211	0.28%
48	Vermont	186	0.25%
49	Wyoming	109	0.14%
50	Alaska	47	0.06%
	District of Columbia	211	0.28%

Source: U.S. Department of Health and Human Services, National Center for Health Statistics
unpublished data
*By state of residence.

Death Rate by Pneumonia and Influenza in 1992

National Rate = 29.7 Deaths per 100,000 Population*

ALPHA ORDER			RANK ORDER		
RANK	**STATE**	**RATE**	**RANK**	**STATE**	**RATE**
30	Alabama	28.0	1	Massachusetts	40.0
50	Alaska	8.0	2	Iowa	39.8
32	Arizona	27.9	3	Oklahoma	39.1
6	Arkansas	36.8	4	West Virginia	38.2
20	California	31.8	5	South Dakota	37.0
37	Colorado	27.2	6	Arkansas	36.8
10	Connecticut	34.5	7	Kentucky	36.0
15	Delaware	33.4	7	Nebraska	36.0
39	Florida	25.2	9	Missouri	35.9
40	Georgia	24.9	10	Connecticut	34.5
44	Hawaii	22.8	11	Tennessee	34.3
24	Idaho	30.3	12	New York	34.2
23	Illinois	30.6	13	Kansas	33.9
25	Indiana	29.6	14	Pennsylvania	33.7
2	Iowa	39.8	15	Delaware	33.4
13	Kansas	33.9	16	Montana	33.3
7	Kentucky	36.0	16	North Dakota	33.3
42	Louisiana	23.4	18	Vermont	32.5
36	Maine	27.4	19	Wisconsin	32.2
43	Maryland	23.3	20	California	31.8
1	Massachusetts	40.0	21	Minnesota	31.1
27	Michigan	28.8	21	Mississippi	31.1
21	Minnesota	31.1	23	Illinois	30.6
21	Mississippi	31.1	24	Idaho	30.3
9	Missouri	35.9	25	Indiana	29.6
16	Montana	33.3	26	Rhode Island	28.9
7	Nebraska	36.0	27	Michigan	28.8
49	Nevada	20.7	28	Oregon	28.6
32	New Hampshire	27.9	29	Ohio	28.1
34	New Jersey	27.6	30	Alabama	28.0
45	New Mexico	22.5	30	North Carolina	28.0
12	New York	34.2	32	Arizona	27.9
30	North Carolina	28.0	32	New Hampshire	27.9
16	North Dakota	33.3	34	New Jersey	27.6
29	Ohio	28.1	35	Virginia	27.5
3	Oklahoma	39.1	36	Maine	27.4
28	Oregon	28.6	37	Colorado	27.2
14	Pennsylvania	33.7	38	Washington	25.5
26	Rhode Island	28.9	39	Florida	25.2
47	South Carolina	21.0	40	Georgia	24.9
5	South Dakota	37.0	41	Wyoming	23.5
11	Tennessee	34.3	42	Louisiana	23.4
47	Texas	21.0	43	Maryland	23.3
45	Utah	22.5	44	Hawaii	22.8
18	Vermont	32.5	45	New Mexico	22.5
35	Virginia	27.5	45	Utah	22.5
38	Washington	25.5	47	South Carolina	21.0
4	West Virginia	38.2	47	Texas	21.0
19	Wisconsin	32.2	49	Nevada	20.7
41	Wyoming	23.5	50	Alaska	8.0
				District of Columbia	35.9

Source: U.S. Department of Health and Human Services, National Center for Health Statistics unpublished data
*By state of residence.

142

Deaths by Complications of Pregnancy and Childbirth in 1992

National Total = 318 Deaths*

ALPHA ORDER

ALPHA ORDER

RANK	STATE	DEATHS	% of USA
15	Alabama	5	1.57%
41	Alaska	0	0.00%
37	Arizona	1	0.31%
22	Arkansas	3	0.94%
1	California	57	17.92%
22	Colorado	3	0.94%
37	Connecticut	1	0.31%
41	Delaware	0	0.00%
4	Florida	22	6.92%
9	Georgia	9	2.83%
29	Hawaii	2	0.63%
41	Idaho	0	0.00%
7	Illinois	11	3.46%
22	Indiana	3	0.94%
29	Iowa	2	0.63%
29	Kansas	2	0.63%
29	Kentucky	2	0.63%
29	Louisiana	2	0.63%
22	Maine	3	0.94%
29	Maryland	2	0.63%
18	Massachusetts	4	1.26%
5	Michigan	18	5.66%
22	Minnesota	3	0.94%
18	Mississippi	4	1.26%
15	Missouri	5	1.57%
41	Montana	0	0.00%
41	Nebraska	0	0.00%
18	Nevada	4	1.26%
41	New Hampshire	0	0.00%
11	New Jersey	8	2.52%
29	New Mexico	2	0.63%
2	New York	44	13.84%
6	North Carolina	13	4.09%
41	North Dakota	0	0.00%
13	Ohio	6	1.89%
18	Oklahoma	4	1.26%
37	Oregon	1	0.31%
7	Pennsylvania	11	3.46%
37	Rhode Island	1	0.31%
9	South Carolina	9	2.83%
41	South Dakota	0	0.00%
11	Tennessee	8	2.52%
3	Texas	23	7.23%
15	Utah	5	1.57%
41	Vermont	0	0.00%
13	Virginia	6	1.89%
22	Washington	3	0.94%
29	West Virginia	2	0.63%
22	Wisconsin	3	0.94%
41	Wyoming	0	0.00%

RANK ORDER

RANK	STATE	DEATHS	% of USA
1	California	57	17.92%
2	New York	44	13.84%
3	Texas	23	7.23%
4	Florida	22	6.92%
5	Michigan	18	5.66%
6	North Carolina	13	4.09%
7	Illinois	11	3.46%
7	Pennsylvania	11	3.46%
9	Georgia	9	2.83%
9	South Carolina	9	2.83%
11	New Jersey	8	2.52%
11	Tennessee	8	2.52%
13	Ohio	6	1.89%
13	Virginia	6	1.89%
15	Alabama	5	1.57%
15	Missouri	5	1.57%
15	Utah	5	1.57%
18	Massachusetts	4	1.26%
18	Mississippi	4	1.26%
18	Nevada	4	1.26%
18	Oklahoma	4	1.26%
22	Arkansas	3	0.94%
22	Colorado	3	0.94%
22	Indiana	3	0.94%
22	Maine	3	0.94%
22	Minnesota	3	0.94%
22	Washington	3	0.94%
22	Wisconsin	3	0.94%
29	Hawaii	2	0.63%
29	Iowa	2	0.63%
29	Kansas	2	0.63%
29	Kentucky	2	0.63%
29	Louisiana	2	0.63%
29	Maryland	2	0.63%
29	New Mexico	2	0.63%
29	West Virginia	2	0.63%
37	Arizona	1	0.31%
37	Connecticut	1	0.31%
37	Oregon	1	0.31%
37	Rhode Island	1	0.31%
41	Alaska	0	0.00%
41	Delaware	0	0.00%
41	Idaho	0	0.00%
41	Montana	0	0.00%
41	Nebraska	0	0.00%
41	New Hampshire	0	0.00%
41	North Dakota	0	0.00%
41	South Dakota	0	0.00%
41	Vermont	0	0.00%
41	Wyoming	0	0.00%
	District of Columbia	1	0.31%

Source: U.S. Department of Health and Human Services, National Center for Health Statistics
   unpublished data
*By state of residence.

Death Rate by Complications of Pregnancy and Childbirth in 1992

National Rate = 0.24 Deaths per 100,000 Female Population*

ALPHA ORDER				RANK ORDER		
RANK	**STATE**	**RATE**		**RANK**	**STATE**	**RATE**
18	Alabama	0.23		1	Nevada	0.61
41	Alaska	0.00		2	Utah	0.55
40	Arizona	0.05		3	South Carolina	0.49
16	Arkansas	0.24		4	Maine	0.47
6	California	0.37		4	New York	0.47
26	Colorado	0.17		6	California	0.37
39	Connecticut	0.06		6	Michigan	0.37
41	Delaware	0.00		6	North Carolina	0.37
10	Florida	0.32		9	Hawaii	0.35
13	Georgia	0.26		10	Florida	0.32
9	Hawaii	0.35		11	Tennessee	0.31
41	Idaho	0.00		12	Mississippi	0.29
23	Illinois	0.18		13	Georgia	0.26
34	Indiana	0.10		13	Texas	0.26
28	Iowa	0.14		15	New Mexico	0.25
27	Kansas	0.16		16	Arkansas	0.24
34	Kentucky	0.10		16	Oklahoma	0.24
36	Louisiana	0.09		18	Alabama	0.23
4	Maine	0.47		19	West Virginia	0.21
37	Maryland	0.08		20	New Jersey	0.20
29	Massachusetts	0.13		21	Missouri	0.19
6	Michigan	0.37		21	Rhode Island	0.19
29	Minnesota	0.13		23	Illinois	0.18
12	Mississippi	0.29		23	Pennsylvania	0.18
21	Missouri	0.19		23	Virginia	0.18
41	Montana	0.00		26	Colorado	0.17
41	Nebraska	0.00		27	Kansas	0.16
1	Nevada	0.61		28	Iowa	0.14
41	New Hampshire	0.00		29	Massachusetts	0.13
20	New Jersey	0.20		29	Minnesota	0.13
15	New Mexico	0.25		31	Washington	0.12
4	New York	0.47		31	Wisconsin	0.12
6	North Carolina	0.37		33	Ohio	0.11
41	North Dakota	0.00		34	Indiana	0.10
33	Ohio	0.11		34	Kentucky	0.10
16	Oklahoma	0.24		36	Louisiana	0.09
38	Oregon	0.07		37	Maryland	0.08
23	Pennsylvania	0.18		38	Oregon	0.07
21	Rhode Island	0.19		39	Connecticut	0.06
3	South Carolina	0.49		40	Arizona	0.05
41	South Dakota	0.00		41	Alaska	0.00
11	Tennessee	0.31		41	Delaware	0.00
13	Texas	0.26		41	Idaho	0.00
2	Utah	0.55		41	Montana	0.00
41	Vermont	0.00		41	Nebraska	0.00
23	Virginia	0.18		41	New Hampshire	0.00
31	Washington	0.12		41	North Dakota	0.00
19	West Virginia	0.21		41	South Dakota	0.00
31	Wisconsin	0.12		41	Vermont	0.00
41	Wyoming	0.00		41	Wyoming	0.00
					District of Columbia	0.32

Source: Morgan Quitno Press using data from US Dept of Health & Human Services, National Center for Health Statistics unpublished data
By state of residence.

Deaths by Syphilis in 1992

National Total = 98 Deaths*

RANK	STATE	DEATHS	% of USA
10	Alabama	3	3.06%
32	Alaska	0	0.00%
16	Arizona	2	2.04%
22	Arkansas	1	1.02%
3	California	8	8.16%
32	Colorado	0	0.00%
32	Connecticut	0	0.00%
32	Delaware	0	0.00%
1	Florida	10	10.20%
10	Georgia	3	3.06%
32	Hawaii	0	0.00%
32	Idaho	0	0.00%
6	Illinois	4	4.08%
32	Indiana	0	0.00%
32	Iowa	0	0.00%
32	Kansas	0	0.00%
32	Kentucky	0	0.00%
6	Louisiana	4	4.08%
22	Maine	1	1.02%
16	Maryland	2	2.04%
22	Massachusetts	1	1.02%
10	Michigan	3	3.06%
5	Minnesota	6	6.12%
10	Mississippi	3	3.06%
32	Missouri	0	0.00%
32	Montana	0	0.00%
32	Nebraska	0	0.00%
22	Nevada	1	1.02%
32	New Hampshire	0	0.00%
6	New Jersey	4	4.08%
22	New Mexico	1	1.02%
2	New York	9	9.18%
10	North Carolina	3	3.06%
32	North Dakota	0	0.00%
16	Ohio	2	2.04%
22	Oklahoma	1	1.02%
22	Oregon	1	1.02%
10	Pennsylvania	3	3.06%
32	Rhode Island	0	0.00%
6	South Carolina	4	4.08%
32	South Dakota	0	0.00%
16	Tennessee	2	2.04%
3	Texas	8	8.16%
32	Utah	0	0.00%
22	Vermont	1	1.02%
16	Virginia	2	2.04%
22	Washington	1	1.02%
22	West Virginia	1	1.02%
16	Wisconsin	2	2.04%
32	Wyoming	0	0.00%

RANK	STATE	DEATHS	% of USA
1	Florida	10	10.20%
2	New York	9	9.18%
3	California	8	8.16%
3	Texas	8	8.16%
5	Minnesota	6	6.12%
6	Illinois	4	4.08%
6	Louisiana	4	4.08%
6	New Jersey	4	4.08%
6	South Carolina	4	4.08%
10	Alabama	3	3.06%
10	Georgia	3	3.06%
10	Michigan	3	3.06%
10	Mississippi	3	3.06%
10	North Carolina	3	3.06%
10	Pennsylvania	3	3.06%
16	Arizona	2	2.04%
16	Maryland	2	2.04%
16	Ohio	2	2.04%
16	Tennessee	2	2.04%
16	Virginia	2	2.04%
16	Wisconsin	2	2.04%
22	Arkansas	1	1.02%
22	Maine	1	1.02%
22	Massachusetts	1	1.02%
22	Nevada	1	1.02%
22	New Mexico	1	1.02%
22	Oklahoma	1	1.02%
22	Oregon	1	1.02%
22	Vermont	1	1.02%
22	Washington	1	1.02%
22	West Virginia	1	1.02%
32	Alaska	0	0.00%
32	Colorado	0	0.00%
32	Connecticut	0	0.00%
32	Delaware	0	0.00%
32	Hawaii	0	0.00%
32	Idaho	0	0.00%
32	Indiana	0	0.00%
32	Iowa	0	0.00%
32	Kansas	0	0.00%
32	Kentucky	0	0.00%
32	Missouri	0	0.00%
32	Montana	0	0.00%
32	Nebraska	0	0.00%
32	New Hampshire	0	0.00%
32	North Dakota	0	0.00%
32	Rhode Island	0	0.00%
32	South Dakota	0	0.00%
32	Utah	0	0.00%
32	Wyoming	0	0.00%
	District of Columbia	1	1.02%

Source: U.S. Department of Health and Human Services, National Center for Health Statistics
    unpublished data

*By state of residence.

Death Rate by Syphilis in 1992

National Rate = 0.04 Deaths per 100,000 Population*

<table>
<tr><td colspan="3">ALPHA ORDER</td><td colspan="3">RANK ORDER</td></tr>
<tr><td>RANK</td><td>STATE</td><td>RATE</td><td>RANK</td><td>STATE</td><td>RATE</td></tr>
<tr><td>7</td><td>Alabama</td><td>0.07</td><td>1</td><td>Vermont</td><td>0.17</td></tr>
<tr><td>32</td><td>Alaska</td><td>0.00</td><td>2</td><td>Minnesota</td><td>0.13</td></tr>
<tr><td>12</td><td>Arizona</td><td>0.05</td><td>3</td><td>Mississippi</td><td>0.11</td></tr>
<tr><td>16</td><td>Arkansas</td><td>0.04</td><td>3</td><td>South Carolina</td><td>0.11</td></tr>
<tr><td>22</td><td>California</td><td>0.03</td><td>5</td><td>Louisiana</td><td>0.09</td></tr>
<tr><td>32</td><td>Colorado</td><td>0.00</td><td>6</td><td>Maine</td><td>0.08</td></tr>
<tr><td>32</td><td>Connecticut</td><td>0.00</td><td>7</td><td>Alabama</td><td>0.07</td></tr>
<tr><td>32</td><td>Delaware</td><td>0.00</td><td>7</td><td>Florida</td><td>0.07</td></tr>
<tr><td>7</td><td>Florida</td><td>0.07</td><td>7</td><td>Nevada</td><td>0.07</td></tr>
<tr><td>16</td><td>Georgia</td><td>0.04</td><td>10</td><td>New Mexico</td><td>0.06</td></tr>
<tr><td>32</td><td>Hawaii</td><td>0.00</td><td>10</td><td>West Virginia</td><td>0.06</td></tr>
<tr><td>32</td><td>Idaho</td><td>0.00</td><td>12</td><td>Arizona</td><td>0.05</td></tr>
<tr><td>22</td><td>Illinois</td><td>0.03</td><td>12</td><td>New Jersey</td><td>0.05</td></tr>
<tr><td>32</td><td>Indiana</td><td>0.00</td><td>12</td><td>New York</td><td>0.05</td></tr>
<tr><td>32</td><td>Iowa</td><td>0.00</td><td>12</td><td>Texas</td><td>0.05</td></tr>
<tr><td>32</td><td>Kansas</td><td>0.00</td><td>16</td><td>Arkansas</td><td>0.04</td></tr>
<tr><td>32</td><td>Kentucky</td><td>0.00</td><td>16</td><td>Georgia</td><td>0.04</td></tr>
<tr><td>5</td><td>Louisiana</td><td>0.09</td><td>16</td><td>Maryland</td><td>0.04</td></tr>
<tr><td>6</td><td>Maine</td><td>0.08</td><td>16</td><td>North Carolina</td><td>0.04</td></tr>
<tr><td>16</td><td>Maryland</td><td>0.04</td><td>16</td><td>Tennessee</td><td>0.04</td></tr>
<tr><td>29</td><td>Massachusetts</td><td>0.02</td><td>16</td><td>Wisconsin</td><td>0.04</td></tr>
<tr><td>22</td><td>Michigan</td><td>0.03</td><td>22</td><td>California</td><td>0.03</td></tr>
<tr><td>2</td><td>Minnesota</td><td>0.13</td><td>22</td><td>Illinois</td><td>0.03</td></tr>
<tr><td>3</td><td>Mississippi</td><td>0.11</td><td>22</td><td>Michigan</td><td>0.03</td></tr>
<tr><td>32</td><td>Missouri</td><td>0.00</td><td>22</td><td>Oklahoma</td><td>0.03</td></tr>
<tr><td>32</td><td>Montana</td><td>0.00</td><td>22</td><td>Oregon</td><td>0.03</td></tr>
<tr><td>32</td><td>Nebraska</td><td>0.00</td><td>22</td><td>Pennsylvania</td><td>0.03</td></tr>
<tr><td>7</td><td>Nevada</td><td>0.07</td><td>22</td><td>Virginia</td><td>0.03</td></tr>
<tr><td>32</td><td>New Hampshire</td><td>0.00</td><td>29</td><td>Massachusetts</td><td>0.02</td></tr>
<tr><td>12</td><td>New Jersey</td><td>0.05</td><td>29</td><td>Ohio</td><td>0.02</td></tr>
<tr><td>10</td><td>New Mexico</td><td>0.06</td><td>29</td><td>Washington</td><td>0.02</td></tr>
<tr><td>12</td><td>New York</td><td>0.05</td><td>32</td><td>Alaska</td><td>0.00</td></tr>
<tr><td>16</td><td>North Carolina</td><td>0.04</td><td>32</td><td>Colorado</td><td>0.00</td></tr>
<tr><td>32</td><td>North Dakota</td><td>0.00</td><td>32</td><td>Connecticut</td><td>0.00</td></tr>
<tr><td>29</td><td>Ohio</td><td>0.02</td><td>32</td><td>Delaware</td><td>0.00</td></tr>
<tr><td>22</td><td>Oklahoma</td><td>0.03</td><td>32</td><td>Hawaii</td><td>0.00</td></tr>
<tr><td>22</td><td>Oregon</td><td>0.03</td><td>32</td><td>Idaho</td><td>0.00</td></tr>
<tr><td>22</td><td>Pennsylvania</td><td>0.03</td><td>32</td><td>Indiana</td><td>0.00</td></tr>
<tr><td>32</td><td>Rhode Island</td><td>0.00</td><td>32</td><td>Iowa</td><td>0.00</td></tr>
<tr><td>3</td><td>South Carolina</td><td>0.11</td><td>32</td><td>Kansas</td><td>0.00</td></tr>
<tr><td>32</td><td>South Dakota</td><td>0.00</td><td>32</td><td>Kentucky</td><td>0.00</td></tr>
<tr><td>16</td><td>Tennessee</td><td>0.04</td><td>32</td><td>Missouri</td><td>0.00</td></tr>
<tr><td>12</td><td>Texas</td><td>0.05</td><td>32</td><td>Montana</td><td>0.00</td></tr>
<tr><td>32</td><td>Utah</td><td>0.00</td><td>32</td><td>Nebraska</td><td>0.00</td></tr>
<tr><td>1</td><td>Vermont</td><td>0.17</td><td>32</td><td>New Hampshire</td><td>0.00</td></tr>
<tr><td>22</td><td>Virginia</td><td>0.03</td><td>32</td><td>North Dakota</td><td>0.00</td></tr>
<tr><td>29</td><td>Washington</td><td>0.02</td><td>32</td><td>Rhode Island</td><td>0.00</td></tr>
<tr><td>10</td><td>West Virginia</td><td>0.06</td><td>32</td><td>South Dakota</td><td>0.00</td></tr>
<tr><td>16</td><td>Wisconsin</td><td>0.04</td><td>32</td><td>Utah</td><td>0.00</td></tr>
<tr><td>32</td><td>Wyoming</td><td>0.00</td><td>32</td><td>Wyoming</td><td>0.00</td></tr>
<tr><td></td><td></td><td></td><td></td><td>District of Columbia</td><td>0.17</td></tr>
</table>

Source: U.S. Department of Health and Human Services, National Center for Health Statistics unpublished data

*By state of residence.

146

Deaths by Tuberculosis in 1992

National Total = 1,705 Deaths*

<u>ALPHA ORDER</u>

RANK	STATE	DEATHS	% of USA
13	Alabama	45	2.64%
44	Alaska	2	0.12%
17	Arizona	33	1.94%
24	Arkansas	21	1.23%
2	California	203	11.91%
34	Colorado	7	0.41%
30	Connecticut	12	0.70%
35	Delaware	6	0.35%
3	Florida	126	7.39%
7	Georgia	55	3.23%
35	Hawaii	6	0.35%
48	Idaho	1	0.06%
5	Illinois	92	5.40%
22	Indiana	23	1.35%
35	Iowa	6	0.35%
39	Kansas	4	0.23%
22	Kentucky	23	1.35%
12	Louisiana	47	2.76%
44	Maine	2	0.12%
20	Maryland	27	1.58%
26	Massachusetts	19	1.11%
10	Michigan	49	2.87%
30	Minnesota	12	0.70%
16	Mississippi	35	2.05%
15	Missouri	37	2.17%
41	Montana	3	0.18%
44	Nebraska	2	0.12%
38	Nevada	5	0.29%
41	New Hampshire	3	0.18%
8	New Jersey	52	3.05%
32	New Mexico	9	0.53%
1	New York	251	14.72%
11	North Carolina	48	2.82%
39	North Dakota	4	0.23%
14	Ohio	38	2.23%
21	Oklahoma	25	1.47%
29	Oregon	13	0.76%
6	Pennsylvania	64	3.75%
32	Rhode Island	9	0.53%
18	South Carolina	30	1.76%
44	South Dakota	2	0.12%
8	Tennessee	52	3.05%
4	Texas	108	6.33%
41	Utah	3	0.18%
50	Vermont	0	0.00%
19	Virginia	29	1.70%
27	Washington	18	1.06%
28	West Virginia	14	0.82%
24	Wisconsin	21	1.23%
48	Wyoming	1	0.06%

<u>RANK ORDER</u>

RANK	STATE	DEATHS	% of USA
1	New York	251	14.72%
2	California	203	11.91%
3	Florida	126	7.39%
4	Texas	108	6.33%
5	Illinois	92	5.40%
6	Pennsylvania	64	3.75%
7	Georgia	55	3.23%
8	New Jersey	52	3.05%
8	Tennessee	52	3.05%
10	Michigan	49	2.87%
11	North Carolina	48	2.82%
12	Louisiana	47	2.76%
13	Alabama	45	2.64%
14	Ohio	38	2.23%
15	Missouri	37	2.17%
16	Mississippi	35	2.05%
17	Arizona	33	1.94%
18	South Carolina	30	1.76%
19	Virginia	29	1.70%
20	Maryland	27	1.58%
21	Oklahoma	25	1.47%
22	Indiana	23	1.35%
22	Kentucky	23	1.35%
24	Arkansas	21	1.23%
24	Wisconsin	21	1.23%
26	Massachusetts	19	1.11%
27	Washington	18	1.06%
28	West Virginia	14	0.82%
29	Oregon	13	0.76%
30	Connecticut	12	0.70%
30	Minnesota	12	0.70%
32	New Mexico	9	0.53%
32	Rhode Island	9	0.53%
34	Colorado	7	0.41%
35	Delaware	6	0.35%
35	Hawaii	6	0.35%
35	Iowa	6	0.35%
38	Nevada	5	0.29%
39	Kansas	4	0.23%
39	North Dakota	4	0.23%
41	Montana	3	0.18%
41	New Hampshire	3	0.18%
41	Utah	3	0.18%
44	Alaska	2	0.12%
44	Maine	2	0.12%
44	Nebraska	2	0.12%
44	South Dakota	2	0.12%
48	Idaho	1	0.06%
48	Wyoming	1	0.06%
50	Vermont	0	0.00%
	District of Columbia	8	0.47%

Source: U.S. Department of Health and Human Services, National Center for Health Statistics
     unpublished data
*By state of residence.

Death Rate by Tuberculosis in 1992

National Rate = 0.67 Deaths per 100,000 Population*

ALPHA ORDER

RANK	STATE	RATE
4	Alabama	1.09
36	Alaska	0.34
10	Arizona	0.86
8	Arkansas	0.88
18	California	0.66
44	Colorado	0.20
32	Connecticut	0.37
9	Delaware	0.87
6	Florida	0.93
12	Georgia	0.81
26	Hawaii	0.52
49	Idaho	0.09
13	Illinois	0.79
31	Indiana	0.41
43	Iowa	0.21
46	Kansas	0.16
21	Kentucky	0.61
3	Louisiana	1.10
46	Maine	0.16
24	Maryland	0.55
38	Massachusetts	0.32
26	Michigan	0.52
40	Minnesota	0.27
2	Mississippi	1.34
16	Missouri	0.71
34	Montana	0.36
48	Nebraska	0.12
32	Nevada	0.37
40	New Hampshire	0.27
18	New Jersey	0.66
23	New Mexico	0.57
1	New York	1.39
17	North Carolina	0.70
20	North Dakota	0.63
36	Ohio	0.34
14	Oklahoma	0.78
29	Oregon	0.44
25	Pennsylvania	0.53
7	Rhode Island	0.90
11	South Carolina	0.83
39	South Dakota	0.28
5	Tennessee	1.03
21	Texas	0.61
45	Utah	0.17
50	Vermont	0.00
28	Virginia	0.45
35	Washington	0.35
15	West Virginia	0.77
30	Wisconsin	0.42
42	Wyoming	0.22

RANK ORDER

RANK	STATE	RATE
1	New York	1.39
2	Mississippi	1.34
3	Louisiana	1.10
4	Alabama	1.09
5	Tennessee	1.03
6	Florida	0.93
7	Rhode Island	0.90
8	Arkansas	0.88
9	Delaware	0.87
10	Arizona	0.86
11	South Carolina	0.83
12	Georgia	0.81
13	Illinois	0.79
14	Oklahoma	0.78
15	West Virginia	0.77
16	Missouri	0.71
17	North Carolina	0.70
18	California	0.66
18	New Jersey	0.66
20	North Dakota	0.63
21	Kentucky	0.61
21	Texas	0.61
23	New Mexico	0.57
24	Maryland	0.55
25	Pennsylvania	0.53
26	Hawaii	0.52
26	Michigan	0.52
28	Virginia	0.45
29	Oregon	0.44
30	Wisconsin	0.42
31	Indiana	0.41
32	Connecticut	0.37
32	Nevada	0.37
34	Montana	0.36
35	Washington	0.35
36	Alaska	0.34
36	Ohio	0.34
38	Massachusetts	0.32
39	South Dakota	0.28
40	Minnesota	0.27
40	New Hampshire	0.27
42	Wyoming	0.22
43	Iowa	0.21
44	Colorado	0.20
45	Utah	0.17
46	Kansas	0.16
46	Maine	0.16
48	Nebraska	0.12
49	Idaho	0.09
50	Vermont	0.00
	District of Columbia	1.36

Source: U.S. Department of Health and Human Services, National Center for Health Statistics
    unpublished data
*By state of residence.

Deaths by Injury in 1992

National Total = 145,655 Deaths*

ALPHA ORDER

RANK	STATE	DEATHS	% of USA
14	Alabama	3,172	2.18%
42	Alaska	491	0.34%
19	Arizona	2,686	1.84%
30	Arkansas	1,766	1.21%
1	California	17,680	12.14%
28	Colorado	2,016	1.38%
31	Connecticut	1,401	0.96%
47	Delaware	380	0.26%
4	Florida	8,363	5.74%
10	Georgia	4,341	2.98%
43	Hawaii	481	0.33%
39	Idaho	693	0.48%
6	Illinois	6,216	4.27%
16	Indiana	3,099	2.13%
32	Iowa	1,373	0.94%
33	Kansas	1,354	0.93%
23	Kentucky	2,393	1.64%
15	Louisiana	3,139	2.16%
41	Maine	594	0.41%
20	Maryland	2,627	1.80%
25	Massachusetts	2,333	1.60%
8	Michigan	5,124	3.52%
26	Minnesota	2,180	1.50%
24	Mississippi	2,345	1.61%
12	Missouri	3,378	2.32%
40	Montana	607	0.42%
38	Nebraska	833	0.57%
36	Nevada	939	0.64%
44	New Hampshire	438	0.30%
17	New Jersey	2,984	2.05%
34	New Mexico	1,317	0.90%
3	New York	9,015	6.19%
9	North Carolina	4,422	3.04%
49	North Dakota	314	0.22%
7	Ohio	5,293	3.63%
27	Oklahoma	2,022	1.39%
29	Oregon	1,778	1.22%
5	Pennsylvania	6,441	4.42%
46	Rhode Island	384	0.26%
21	South Carolina	2,471	1.70%
45	South Dakota	407	0.28%
11	Tennessee	3,476	2.39%
2	Texas	10,872	7.46%
37	Utah	905	0.62%
50	Vermont	286	0.20%
13	Virginia	3,358	2.31%
18	Washington	2,798	1.92%
35	West Virginia	1,239	0.85%
22	Wisconsin	2,449	1.68%
48	Wyoming	346	0.24%

RANK ORDER

RANK	STATE	DEATHS	% of USA
1	California	17,680	12.14%
2	Texas	10,872	7.46%
3	New York	9,015	6.19%
4	Florida	8,363	5.74%
5	Pennsylvania	6,441	4.42%
6	Illinois	6,216	4.27%
7	Ohio	5,293	3.63%
8	Michigan	5,124	3.52%
9	North Carolina	4,422	3.04%
10	Georgia	4,341	2.98%
11	Tennessee	3,476	2.39%
12	Missouri	3,378	2.32%
13	Virginia	3,358	2.31%
14	Alabama	3,172	2.18%
15	Louisiana	3,139	2.16%
16	Indiana	3,099	2.13%
17	New Jersey	2,984	2.05%
18	Washington	2,798	1.92%
19	Arizona	2,686	1.84%
20	Maryland	2,627	1.80%
21	South Carolina	2,471	1.70%
22	Wisconsin	2,449	1.68%
23	Kentucky	2,393	1.64%
24	Mississippi	2,345	1.61%
25	Massachusetts	2,333	1.60%
26	Minnesota	2,180	1.50%
27	Oklahoma	2,022	1.39%
28	Colorado	2,016	1.38%
29	Oregon	1,778	1.22%
30	Arkansas	1,766	1.21%
31	Connecticut	1,401	0.96%
32	Iowa	1,373	0.94%
33	Kansas	1,354	0.93%
34	New Mexico	1,317	0.90%
35	West Virginia	1,239	0.85%
36	Nevada	939	0.64%
37	Utah	905	0.62%
38	Nebraska	833	0.57%
39	Idaho	693	0.48%
40	Montana	607	0.42%
41	Maine	594	0.41%
42	Alaska	491	0.34%
43	Hawaii	481	0.33%
44	New Hampshire	438	0.30%
45	South Dakota	407	0.28%
46	Rhode Island	384	0.26%
47	Delaware	380	0.26%
48	Wyoming	346	0.24%
49	North Dakota	314	0.22%
50	Vermont	286	0.20%
	District of Columbia	636	0.44%

Source: Morgan Quitno Press using data from U.S. Dept of Health & Human Services, National Center for Health Statistics "Monthly Vital Statistics Report" (Vol. 43, No. 6(S), March 22, 1995) and unpublished data
*Final data by state of residence. Injury as used here includes Accidents (including motor vehicle), Suicides, Homicides, War and Other undetermined.

Death Rate by Injury in 1992

National Rate = 57.1 Deaths by Injury per 100,000 Population*

ALPHA ORDER			RANK ORDER		
RANK	STATE	RATE	RANK	STATE	RATE
4	Alabama	76.7	1	Mississippi	89.7
2	Alaska	83.5	2	Alaska	83.5
10	Arizona	70.1	3	New Mexico	83.2
6	Arkansas	73.8	4	Alabama	76.7
25	California	57.2	5	Wyoming	74.4
23	Colorado	58.2	6	Arkansas	73.8
45	Connecticut	42.7	6	Montana	73.8
26	Delaware	55.0	8	Louisiana	73.4
20	Florida	62.0	9	Nevada	70.3
17	Georgia	64.1	10	Arizona	70.1
46	Hawaii	41.6	11	Tennessee	69.2
15	Idaho	65.0	12	South Carolina	68.6
32	Illinois	53.5	13	West Virginia	68.5
27	Indiana	54.8	14	Missouri	65.1
40	Iowa	49.0	15	Idaho	65.0
30	Kansas	53.8	16	North Carolina	64.7
18	Kentucky	63.7	17	Georgia	64.1
8	Louisiana	73.4	18	Kentucky	63.7
43	Maine	48.1	19	Oklahoma	63.1
33	Maryland	53.4	20	Florida	62.0
48	Massachusetts	38.9	21	Texas	61.5
29	Michigan	54.3	22	Oregon	59.8
42	Minnesota	48.8	23	Colorado	58.2
1	Mississippi	89.7	24	South Dakota	57.5
14	Missouri	65.1	25	California	57.2
6	Montana	73.8	26	Delaware	55.0
35	Nebraska	52.0	27	Indiana	54.8
9	Nevada	70.3	28	Washington	54.4
47	New Hampshire	39.3	29	Michigan	54.3
50	New Jersey	38.2	30	Kansas	53.8
3	New Mexico	83.2	31	Pennsylvania	53.7
38	New York	49.8	32	Illinois	53.5
16	North Carolina	64.7	33	Maryland	53.4
39	North Dakota	49.5	34	Virginia	52.5
44	Ohio	48.0	35	Nebraska	52.0
19	Oklahoma	63.1	36	Vermont	50.1
22	Oregon	59.8	37	Utah	50.0
31	Pennsylvania	53.7	38	New York	49.8
49	Rhode Island	38.4	39	North Dakota	49.5
12	South Carolina	68.6	40	Iowa	49.0
24	South Dakota	57.5	40	Wisconsin	49.0
11	Tennessee	69.2	42	Minnesota	48.8
21	Texas	61.5	43	Maine	48.1
37	Utah	50.0	44	Ohio	48.0
36	Vermont	50.1	45	Connecticut	42.7
34	Virginia	52.5	46	Hawaii	41.6
28	Washington	54.4	47	New Hampshire	39.3
13	West Virginia	68.5	48	Massachusetts	38.9
40	Wisconsin	49.0	49	Rhode Island	38.4
5	Wyoming	74.4	50	New Jersey	38.2
				District of Columbia	108.7

Source: Morgan Quitno Press using data from U.S. Dept of Health & Human Services, National Center for Health Statistics
"Monthly Vital Statistics Report" (Vol. 43, No. 6(S), March 22, 1995) and unpublished data
*Final data by state of residence. Injury as used here includes Accidents (including motor vehicle), Suicides, Homicides, War and Other undetermined.

Deaths by Accidents and Adverse Effects in 1992

National Total = 86,777 Deaths*

RANK	STATE	DEATHS	% of USA
13	Alabama	2,065	2.38%
42	Alaska	358	0.41%
20	Arizona	1,622	1.87%
29	Arkansas	1,141	1.31%
1	California	9,498	10.95%
28	Colorado	1,146	1.32%
32	Connecticut	895	1.03%
46	Delaware	247	0.28%
3	Florida	4,872	5.61%
10	Georgia	2,634	3.04%
44	Hawaii	293	0.34%
38	Idaho	476	0.55%
6	Illinois	3,511	4.05%
16	Indiana	1,932	2.23%
31	Iowa	1,020	1.18%
33	Kansas	871	1.00%
19	Kentucky	1,660	1.91%
17	Louisiana	1,775	2.05%
41	Maine	405	0.47%
26	Maryland	1,286	1.48%
25	Massachusetts	1,296	1.49%
8	Michigan	2,884	3.32%
24	Minnesota	1,487	1.71%
23	Mississippi	1,535	1.77%
12	Missouri	2,134	2.46%
40	Montana	407	0.47%
36	Nebraska	559	0.64%
39	Nevada	412	0.47%
45	New Hampshire	254	0.29%
14	New Jersey	2,021	2.33%
35	New Mexico	823	0.95%
4	New York	4,854	5.59%
9	North Carolina	2,717	3.13%
48	North Dakota	232	0.27%
7	Ohio	3,357	3.87%
27	Oklahoma	1,266	1.46%
30	Oregon	1,088	1.25%
5	Pennsylvania	4,114	4.74%
49	Rhode Island	227	0.26%
22	South Carolina	1,549	1.79%
43	South Dakota	304	0.35%
11	Tennessee	2,208	2.54%
2	Texas	6,105	7.04%
37	Utah	555	0.64%
50	Vermont	170	0.20%
15	Virginia	1,939	2.23%
18	Washington	1,718	1.98%
34	West Virginia	845	0.97%
21	Wisconsin	1,588	1.83%
47	Wyoming	237	0.27%

RANK	STATE	DEATHS	% of USA
1	California	9,498	10.95%
2	Texas	6,105	7.04%
3	Florida	4,872	5.61%
4	New York	4,854	5.59%
5	Pennsylvania	4,114	4.74%
6	Illinois	3,511	4.05%
7	Ohio	3,357	3.87%
8	Michigan	2,884	3.32%
9	North Carolina	2,717	3.13%
10	Georgia	2,634	3.04%
11	Tennessee	2,208	2.54%
12	Missouri	2,134	2.46%
13	Alabama	2,065	2.38%
14	New Jersey	2,021	2.33%
15	Virginia	1,939	2.23%
16	Indiana	1,932	2.23%
17	Louisiana	1,775	2.05%
18	Washington	1,718	1.98%
19	Kentucky	1,660	1.91%
20	Arizona	1,622	1.87%
21	Wisconsin	1,588	1.83%
22	South Carolina	1,549	1.79%
23	Mississippi	1,535	1.77%
24	Minnesota	1,487	1.71%
25	Massachusetts	1,296	1.49%
26	Maryland	1,286	1.48%
27	Oklahoma	1,266	1.46%
28	Colorado	1,146	1.32%
29	Arkansas	1,141	1.31%
30	Oregon	1,088	1.25%
31	Iowa	1,020	1.18%
32	Connecticut	895	1.03%
33	Kansas	871	1.00%
34	West Virginia	845	0.97%
35	New Mexico	823	0.95%
36	Nebraska	559	0.64%
37	Utah	555	0.64%
38	Idaho	476	0.55%
39	Nevada	412	0.47%
40	Montana	407	0.47%
41	Maine	405	0.47%
42	Alaska	358	0.41%
43	South Dakota	304	0.35%
44	Hawaii	293	0.34%
45	New Hampshire	254	0.29%
46	Delaware	247	0.28%
47	Wyoming	237	0.27%
48	North Dakota	232	0.27%
49	Rhode Island	227	0.26%
50	Vermont	170	0.20%
	District of Columbia	185	0.21%

Source: U.S. Department of Health and Human Services, National Center for Health Statistics
   "Monthly Vital Statistics Report" (Vol. 43, No. 6(S), March 22, 1995)
Final data by state of residence. Includes motor vehicle deaths, poisoning, falls, drowning and other unknown accidents.

Death Rate by Accidents and Adverse Effects in 1992

National Rate = 34.0 Deaths per 100,000 Population*

ALPHA ORDER			RANK ORDER		
RANK	STATE	RATE	RANK	STATE	RATE
5	Alabama	49.9	1	Alaska	60.9
1	Alaska	60.9	2	Mississippi	58.7
14	Arizona	42.3	3	New Mexico	52.0
7	Arkansas	47.7	4	Wyoming	51.0
36	California	30.7	5	Alabama	49.9
32	Colorado	33.1	6	Montana	49.5
43	Connecticut	27.3	7	Arkansas	47.7
24	Delaware	35.8	8	West Virginia	46.7
23	Florida	36.1	9	Idaho	44.7
19	Georgia	38.9	10	Kentucky	44.2
47	Hawaii	25.4	11	Tennessee	43.9
9	Idaho	44.7	12	South Carolina	43.0
41	Illinois	30.2	13	South Dakota	42.9
29	Indiana	34.1	14	Arizona	42.3
22	Iowa	36.4	15	Louisiana	41.5
26	Kansas	34.6	16	Missouri	41.1
10	Kentucky	44.2	17	North Carolina	39.7
15	Louisiana	41.5	18	Oklahoma	39.5
33	Maine	32.8	19	Georgia	38.9
45	Maryland	26.2	20	North Dakota	36.6
50	Massachusetts	21.6	20	Oregon	36.6
37	Michigan	30.6	22	Iowa	36.4
31	Minnesota	33.3	23	Florida	36.1
2	Mississippi	58.7	24	Delaware	35.8
16	Missouri	41.1	25	Nebraska	34.9
6	Montana	49.5	26	Kansas	34.6
25	Nebraska	34.9	27	Texas	34.5
35	Nevada	30.8	28	Pennsylvania	34.3
48	New Hampshire	22.8	29	Indiana	34.1
46	New Jersey	25.8	30	Washington	33.4
3	New Mexico	52.0	31	Minnesota	33.3
44	New York	26.8	32	Colorado	33.1
17	North Carolina	39.7	33	Maine	32.8
20	North Dakota	36.6	34	Wisconsin	31.8
39	Ohio	30.5	35	Nevada	30.8
18	Oklahoma	39.5	36	California	30.7
20	Oregon	36.6	37	Michigan	30.6
28	Pennsylvania	34.3	37	Utah	30.6
49	Rhode Island	22.7	39	Ohio	30.5
12	South Carolina	43.0	40	Virginia	30.3
13	South Dakota	42.9	41	Illinois	30.2
11	Tennessee	43.9	42	Vermont	29.8
27	Texas	34.5	43	Connecticut	27.3
37	Utah	30.6	44	New York	26.8
42	Vermont	29.8	45	Maryland	26.2
40	Virginia	30.3	46	New Jersey	25.8
30	Washington	33.4	47	Hawaii	25.4
8	West Virginia	46.7	48	New Hampshire	22.8
34	Wisconsin	31.8	49	Rhode Island	22.7
4	Wyoming	51.0	50	Massachusetts	21.6
				District of Columbia	31.6

Source: U.S. Department of Health and Human Services, National Center for Health Statistics
"Monthly Vital Statistics Report" (Vol. 43, No. 6(S), March 22, 1995)
Final data by state of residence. Includes motor vehicle deaths, poisoning, falls, drowning and other unknown accidents.

Deaths by Firearms in 1992

National Total = 37,776 Deaths by Firearms*

ALPHA ORDER

RANK ORDER

RANK	STATE	DEATHS	% of USA
14	Alabama	873	2.31%
42	Alaska	97	0.26%
18	Arizona	745	1.97%
26	Arkansas	464	1.23%
1	California	5,226	13.83%
24	Colorado	498	1.32%
35	Connecticut	271	0.72%
46	Delaware	57	0.15%
4	Florida	2,207	5.84%
8	Georgia	1,242	3.29%
48	Hawaii	55	0.15%
38	Idaho	161	0.43%
5	Illinois	1,553	4.11%
16	Indiana	772	2.04%
36	Iowa	213	0.56%
31	Kansas	334	0.88%
22	Kentucky	576	1.52%
11	Louisiana	1,079	2.86%
40	Maine	125	0.33%
17	Maryland	752	1.99%
34	Massachusetts	290	0.77%
6	Michigan	1,386	3.67%
29	Minnesota	360	0.95%
20	Mississippi	609	1.61%
15	Missouri	864	2.29%
41	Montana	124	0.33%
39	Nebraska	160	0.42%
30	Nevada	338	0.89%
43	New Hampshire	95	0.25%
28	New Jersey	416	1.10%
33	New Mexico	293	0.78%
3	New York	2,446	6.48%
10	North Carolina	1,216	3.22%
47	North Dakota	56	0.15%
9	Ohio	1,232	3.26%
23	Oklahoma	519	1.37%
27	Oregon	420	1.11%
7	Pennsylvania	1,317	3.49%
50	Rhode Island	47	0.12%
19	South Carolina	701	1.86%
49	South Dakota	54	0.14%
13	Tennessee	985	2.61%
2	Texas	3,466	9.18%
37	Utah	195	0.52%
45	Vermont	75	0.20%
12	Virginia	1,014	2.68%
21	Washington	593	1.57%
32	West Virginia	297	0.79%
25	Wisconsin	484	1.28%
44	Wyoming	83	0.22%

RANK	STATE	DEATHS	% of USA
1	California	5,226	13.83%
2	Texas	3,466	9.18%
3	New York	2,446	6.48%
4	Florida	2,207	5.84%
5	Illinois	1,553	4.11%
6	Michigan	1,386	3.67%
7	Pennsylvania	1,317	3.49%
8	Georgia	1,242	3.29%
9	Ohio	1,232	3.26%
10	North Carolina	1,216	3.22%
11	Louisiana	1,079	2.86%
12	Virginia	1,014	2.68%
13	Tennessee	985	2.61%
14	Alabama	873	2.31%
15	Missouri	864	2.29%
16	Indiana	772	2.04%
17	Maryland	752	1.99%
18	Arizona	745	1.97%
19	South Carolina	701	1.86%
20	Mississippi	609	1.61%
21	Washington	593	1.57%
22	Kentucky	576	1.52%
23	Oklahoma	519	1.37%
24	Colorado	498	1.32%
25	Wisconsin	484	1.28%
26	Arkansas	464	1.23%
27	Oregon	420	1.11%
28	New Jersey	416	1.10%
29	Minnesota	360	0.95%
30	Nevada	338	0.89%
31	Kansas	334	0.88%
32	West Virginia	297	0.79%
33	New Mexico	293	0.78%
34	Massachusetts	290	0.77%
35	Connecticut	271	0.72%
36	Iowa	213	0.56%
37	Utah	195	0.52%
38	Idaho	161	0.43%
39	Nebraska	160	0.42%
40	Maine	125	0.33%
41	Montana	124	0.33%
42	Alaska	97	0.26%
43	New Hampshire	95	0.25%
44	Wyoming	83	0.22%
45	Vermont	75	0.20%
46	Delaware	57	0.15%
47	North Dakota	56	0.15%
48	Hawaii	55	0.15%
49	South Dakota	54	0.14%
50	Rhode Island	47	0.12%
	District of Columbia	341	0.90%

Source: U.S. Department of Health and Human Services, National Center for Health Statistics
    unpublished data
*By state of residence.

Death Rate by Firearms in 1992

National Rate = 14.8 Deaths per 100,000 Population*

ALPHA ORDER				RANK ORDER		
RANK	**STATE**	**RATE**		**RANK**	**STATE**	**RATE**
4	Alabama	21.1		1	Nevada	25.3
16	Alaska	16.5		2	Louisiana	25.2
8	Arizona	19.4		3	Mississippi	23.3
8	Arkansas	19.4		4	Alabama	21.1
14	California	16.9		5	Tennessee	19.6
26	Colorado	14.4		5	Texas	19.6
42	Connecticut	8.3		7	South Carolina	19.5
42	Delaware	8.3		8	Arizona	19.4
17	Florida	16.4		8	Arkansas	19.4
11	Georgia	18.3		10	New Mexico	18.5
48	Hawaii	4.8		11	Georgia	18.3
23	Idaho	15.1		12	Wyoming	17.9
30	Illinois	13.4		13	North Carolina	17.8
28	Indiana	13.6		14	California	16.9
45	Iowa	7.6		15	Missouri	16.6
31	Kansas	13.3		16	Alaska	16.5
21	Kentucky	15.3		17	Florida	16.4
2	Louisiana	25.2		17	West Virginia	16.4
37	Maine	10.1		19	Oklahoma	16.2
21	Maryland	15.3		20	Virginia	15.9
48	Massachusetts	4.8		21	Kentucky	15.3
25	Michigan	14.7		21	Maryland	15.3
44	Minnesota	8.1		23	Idaho	15.1
3	Mississippi	23.3		23	Montana	15.1
15	Missouri	16.6		25	Michigan	14.7
23	Montana	15.1		26	Colorado	14.4
38	Nebraska	10.0		27	Oregon	14.1
1	Nevada	25.3		28	Indiana	13.6
41	New Hampshire	8.5		29	New York	13.5
47	New Jersey	5.3		30	Illinois	13.4
10	New Mexico	18.5		31	Kansas	13.3
29	New York	13.5		32	Vermont	13.1
13	North Carolina	17.8		33	Washington	11.5
40	North Dakota	8.8		34	Ohio	11.2
34	Ohio	11.2		35	Pennsylvania	11.0
19	Oklahoma	16.2		36	Utah	10.8
27	Oregon	14.1		37	Maine	10.1
35	Pennsylvania	11.0		38	Nebraska	10.0
50	Rhode Island	4.7		39	Wisconsin	9.7
7	South Carolina	19.5		40	North Dakota	8.8
45	South Dakota	7.6		41	New Hampshire	8.5
5	Tennessee	19.6		42	Connecticut	8.3
5	Texas	19.6		42	Delaware	8.3
36	Utah	10.8		44	Minnesota	8.1
32	Vermont	13.1		45	Iowa	7.6
20	Virginia	15.9		45	South Dakota	7.6
33	Washington	11.5		47	New Jersey	5.3
17	West Virginia	16.4		48	Hawaii	4.8
39	Wisconsin	9.7		48	Massachusetts	4.8
12	Wyoming	17.9		50	Rhode Island	4.7
					District of Columbia	58.0

Source: U.S. Department of Health and Human Services, National Center for Health Statistics unpublished data

*By state of residence.

Deaths by Motor Vehicle Accidents in 1992

National Total = 40,982 Deaths*

RANK	STATE	DEATHS	% of USA
12	Alabama	1,085	2.65%
47	Alaska	109	0.27%
21	Arizona	796	1.94%
27	Arkansas	603	1.47%
1	California	4,461	10.89%
29	Colorado	557	1.36%
35	Connecticut	332	0.81%
44	Delaware	132	0.32%
3	Florida	2,452	5.98%
9	Georgia	1,366	3.33%
45	Hawaii	125	0.31%
38	Idaho	236	0.58%
6	Illinois	1,514	3.69%
14	Indiana	954	2.33%
30	Iowa	470	1.15%
33	Kansas	425	1.04%
19	Kentucky	822	2.01%
15	Louisiana	896	2.19%
39	Maine	212	0.52%
26	Maryland	634	1.55%
28	Massachusetts	562	1.37%
8	Michigan	1,439	3.51%
25	Minnesota	637	1.55%
18	Mississippi	829	2.02%
13	Missouri	1,002	2.44%
41	Montana	180	0.44%
37	Nebraska	267	0.65%
39	Nevada	212	0.52%
46	New Hampshire	115	0.28%
17	New Jersey	832	2.03%
34	New Mexico	404	0.99%
4	New York	2,017	4.92%
10	North Carolina	1,314	3.21%
48	North Dakota	96	0.23%
7	Ohio	1,471	3.59%
24	Oklahoma	653	1.59%
31	Oregon	446	1.09%
5	Pennsylvania	1,637	3.99%
49	Rhode Island	93	0.23%
20	South Carolina	798	1.95%
42	South Dakota	151	0.37%
11	Tennessee	1,203	2.94%
2	Texas	3,198	7.80%
36	Utah	271	0.66%
50	Vermont	84	0.20%
16	Virginia	872	2.13%
22	Washington	722	1.76%
32	West Virginia	426	1.04%
23	Wisconsin	677	1.65%
43	Wyoming	134	0.33%

RANK	STATE	DEATHS	% of USA
1	California	4,461	10.89%
2	Texas	3,198	7.80%
3	Florida	2,452	5.98%
4	New York	2,017	4.92%
5	Pennsylvania	1,637	3.99%
6	Illinois	1,514	3.69%
7	Ohio	1,471	3.59%
8	Michigan	1,439	3.51%
9	Georgia	1,366	3.33%
10	North Carolina	1,314	3.21%
11	Tennessee	1,203	2.94%
12	Alabama	1,085	2.65%
13	Missouri	1,002	2.44%
14	Indiana	954	2.33%
15	Louisiana	896	2.19%
16	Virginia	872	2.13%
17	New Jersey	832	2.03%
18	Mississippi	829	2.02%
19	Kentucky	822	2.01%
20	South Carolina	798	1.95%
21	Arizona	796	1.94%
22	Washington	722	1.76%
23	Wisconsin	677	1.65%
24	Oklahoma	653	1.59%
25	Minnesota	637	1.55%
26	Maryland	634	1.55%
27	Arkansas	603	1.47%
28	Massachusetts	562	1.37%
29	Colorado	557	1.36%
30	Iowa	470	1.15%
31	Oregon	446	1.09%
32	West Virginia	426	1.04%
33	Kansas	425	1.04%
34	New Mexico	404	0.99%
35	Connecticut	332	0.81%
36	Utah	271	0.66%
37	Nebraska	267	0.65%
38	Idaho	236	0.58%
39	Maine	212	0.52%
39	Nevada	212	0.52%
41	Montana	180	0.44%
42	South Dakota	151	0.37%
43	Wyoming	134	0.33%
44	Delaware	132	0.32%
45	Hawaii	125	0.31%
46	New Hampshire	115	0.28%
47	Alaska	109	0.27%
48	North Dakota	96	0.23%
49	Rhode Island	93	0.23%
50	Vermont	84	0.20%
	District of Columbia	59	0.14%

Source: U.S. Department of Health and Human Services, National Center for Health Statistics
"Monthly Vital Statistics Report" (Vol. 43, No. 6(S), March 22, 1995)
*Final data by state of residence. These numbers are compiled from death certificates by the Centers for Disease Control and Prevention. They may differ from motor vehicle deaths collected by the U.S. Department of Transportation from other sources.

Death Rate by Motor Vehicle Accidents in 1992

National Rate = 16.1 Deaths per 100,000 Population*

ALPHA ORDER			RANK ORDER		
RANK	STATE	RATE	RANK	STATE	RATE
3	Alabama	26.2	1	Mississippi	31.7
20	Alaska	18.5	2	Wyoming	28.8
14	Arizona	20.8	3	Alabama	26.2
5	Arkansas	25.2	4	New Mexico	25.5
35	California	14.4	5	Arkansas	25.2
28	Colorado	16.1	6	Tennessee	23.9
48	Connecticut	10.1	7	West Virginia	23.6
19	Delaware	19.1	8	Idaho	22.1
21	Florida	18.2	8	South Carolina	22.1
16	Georgia	20.2	10	Kentucky	21.9
45	Hawaii	10.8	10	Montana	21.9
8	Idaho	22.1	12	South Dakota	21.3
42	Illinois	13.0	13	Louisiana	20.9
24	Indiana	16.9	14	Arizona	20.8
26	Iowa	16.8	15	Oklahoma	20.4
24	Kansas	16.9	16	Georgia	20.2
10	Kentucky	21.9	17	Missouri	19.3
13	Louisiana	20.9	18	North Carolina	19.2
23	Maine	17.1	19	Delaware	19.1
43	Maryland	12.9	20	Alaska	18.5
49	Massachusetts	9.4	21	Florida	18.2
30	Michigan	15.3	22	Texas	18.1
36	Minnesota	14.3	23	Maine	17.1
1	Mississippi	31.7	24	Indiana	16.9
17	Missouri	19.3	24	Kansas	16.9
10	Montana	21.9	26	Iowa	16.8
27	Nebraska	16.7	27	Nebraska	16.7
29	Nevada	15.9	28	Colorado	16.1
47	New Hampshire	10.3	29	Nevada	15.9
46	New Jersey	10.6	30	Michigan	15.3
4	New Mexico	25.5	31	North Dakota	15.1
44	New York	11.1	32	Oregon	15.0
18	North Carolina	19.2	32	Utah	15.0
31	North Dakota	15.1	34	Vermont	14.7
41	Ohio	13.3	35	California	14.4
15	Oklahoma	20.4	36	Minnesota	14.3
32	Oregon	15.0	37	Washington	14.0
38	Pennsylvania	13.6	38	Pennsylvania	13.6
50	Rhode Island	9.3	38	Virginia	13.6
8	South Carolina	22.1	38	Wisconsin	13.6
12	South Dakota	21.3	41	Ohio	13.3
6	Tennessee	23.9	42	Illinois	13.0
22	Texas	18.1	43	Maryland	12.9
32	Utah	15.0	44	New York	11.1
34	Vermont	14.7	45	Hawaii	10.8
38	Virginia	13.6	46	New Jersey	10.6
37	Washington	14.0	47	New Hampshire	10.3
7	West Virginia	23.6	48	Connecticut	10.1
38	Wisconsin	13.6	49	Massachusetts	9.4
2	Wyoming	28.8	50	Rhode Island	9.3
				District of Columbia	10.1

Source: U.S. Department of Health and Human Services, National Center for Health Statistics
    "Monthly Vital Statistics Report" (Vol. 43, No. 6(S), March 22, 1995)
*Final data by state of residence. These numbers are compiled from death certificates by the Centers for Disease Control and Prevention. They may differ from motor vehicle deaths collected by the U.S. Department of Transportation from other sources.

Ratio of Firearms Deaths to Motor Vehicle Deaths in 1992

National Ratio = 0.92 Firearms Deaths per Motor Vehicle Death*

ALPHA ORDER

RANK	STATE	RATIO
26	Alabama	0.80
15	Alaska	0.89
10	Arizona	0.94
30	Arkansas	0.77
5	California	1.17
15	Colorado	0.89
22	Connecticut	0.82
49	Delaware	0.43
14	Florida	0.90
13	Georgia	0.91
48	Hawaii	0.44
38	Idaho	0.68
8	Illinois	1.03
25	Indiana	0.81
47	Iowa	0.45
28	Kansas	0.79
35	Kentucky	0.70
3	Louisiana	1.20
41	Maine	0.59
4	Maryland	1.19
44	Massachusetts	0.52
9	Michigan	0.96
43	Minnesota	0.57
31	Mississippi	0.73
19	Missouri	0.86
37	Montana	0.69
40	Nebraska	0.60
1	Nevada	1.59
21	New Hampshire	0.83
46	New Jersey	0.50
31	New Mexico	0.73
2	New York	1.21
12	North Carolina	0.93
42	North Dakota	0.58
20	Ohio	0.84
28	Oklahoma	0.79
10	Oregon	0.94
26	Pennsylvania	0.80
45	Rhode Island	0.51
18	South Carolina	0.88
50	South Dakota	0.36
22	Tennessee	0.82
7	Texas	1.08
33	Utah	0.72
15	Vermont	0.89
6	Virginia	1.16
22	Washington	0.82
35	West Virginia	0.70
34	Wisconsin	0.71
39	Wyoming	0.62

RANK ORDER

RANK	STATE	RATIO
1	Nevada	1.59
2	New York	1.21
3	Louisiana	1.20
4	Maryland	1.19
5	California	1.17
6	Virginia	1.16
7	Texas	1.08
8	Illinois	1.03
9	Michigan	0.96
10	Arizona	0.94
10	Oregon	0.94
12	North Carolina	0.93
13	Georgia	0.91
14	Florida	0.90
15	Alaska	0.89
15	Colorado	0.89
15	Vermont	0.89
18	South Carolina	0.88
19	Missouri	0.86
20	Ohio	0.84
21	New Hampshire	0.83
22	Connecticut	0.82
22	Tennessee	0.82
22	Washington	0.82
25	Indiana	0.81
26	Alabama	0.80
26	Pennsylvania	0.80
28	Kansas	0.79
28	Oklahoma	0.79
30	Arkansas	0.77
31	Mississippi	0.73
31	New Mexico	0.73
33	Utah	0.72
34	Wisconsin	0.71
35	Kentucky	0.70
35	West Virginia	0.70
37	Montana	0.69
38	Idaho	0.68
39	Wyoming	0.62
40	Nebraska	0.60
41	Maine	0.59
42	North Dakota	0.58
43	Minnesota	0.57
44	Massachusetts	0.52
45	Rhode Island	0.51
46	New Jersey	0.50
47	Iowa	0.45
48	Hawaii	0.44
49	Delaware	0.43
50	South Dakota	0.36

| | District of Columbia | 5.78 |

Source: Morgan Quitno Press using data from US Dept of Health & Human Services, National Center for Health Statistics unpublished data
*By state of residence.

Deaths by Homicide in 1992

National Total = 25,488 Homicides*

ALPHA ORDER

RANK ORDER

RANK	STATE	HOMICIDES	% of USA		RANK	STATE	HOMICIDES	% of USA
16	Alabama	546	2.14%		1	California	4,194	16.45%
41	Alaska	41	0.16%		2	New York	2,438	9.57%
21	Arizona	368	1.44%		3	Texas	2,359	9.26%
22	Arkansas	304	1.19%		4	Illinois	1,429	5.61%
1	California	4,194	16.45%		5	Florida	1,381	5.42%
27	Colorado	218	0.86%		6	Michigan	1,059	4.15%
29	Connecticut	180	0.71%		7	Georgia	835	3.28%
43	Delaware	37	0.15%		8	North Carolina	816	3.20%
5	Florida	1,381	5.42%		9	Louisiana	791	3.10%
7	Georgia	835	3.28%		10	Pennsylvania	782	3.07%
39	Hawaii	42	0.16%		11	Ohio	676	2.65%
39	Idaho	42	0.16%		12	Maryland	647	2.54%
4	Illinois	1,429	5.61%		13	Tennessee	570	2.24%
19	Indiana	406	1.59%		14	Virginia	568	2.23%
37	Iowa	52	0.20%		15	Missouri	567	2.22%
33	Kansas	156	0.61%		16	Alabama	546	2.14%
28	Kentucky	212	0.83%		17	Mississippi	457	1.79%
9	Louisiana	791	3.10%		18	South Carolina	438	1.72%
45	Maine	30	0.12%		19	Indiana	406	1.59%
12	Maryland	647	2.54%		20	New Jersey	402	1.58%
26	Massachusetts	227	0.89%		21	Arizona	368	1.44%
6	Michigan	1,059	4.15%		22	Arkansas	304	1.19%
34	Minnesota	144	0.56%		23	Washington	301	1.18%
17	Mississippi	457	1.79%		24	Oklahoma	252	0.99%
15	Missouri	567	2.22%		25	Wisconsin	244	0.96%
42	Montana	39	0.15%		26	Massachusetts	227	0.89%
36	Nebraska	61	0.24%		27	Colorado	218	0.86%
32	Nevada	158	0.62%		28	Kentucky	212	0.83%
46	New Hampshire	22	0.09%		29	Connecticut	180	0.71%
20	New Jersey	402	1.58%		30	New Mexico	162	0.64%
30	New Mexico	162	0.64%		31	Oregon	160	0.63%
2	New York	2,438	9.57%		32	Nevada	158	0.62%
8	North Carolina	816	3.20%		33	Kansas	156	0.61%
50	North Dakota	12	0.05%		34	Minnesota	144	0.56%
11	Ohio	676	2.65%		35	West Virginia	131	0.51%
24	Oklahoma	252	0.99%		36	Nebraska	61	0.24%
31	Oregon	160	0.63%		37	Iowa	52	0.20%
10	Pennsylvania	782	3.07%		38	Utah	51	0.20%
44	Rhode Island	32	0.13%		39	Hawaii	42	0.16%
18	South Carolina	438	1.72%		39	Idaho	42	0.16%
49	South Dakota	19	0.07%		41	Alaska	41	0.16%
13	Tennessee	570	2.24%		42	Montana	39	0.15%
3	Texas	2,359	9.26%		43	Delaware	37	0.15%
38	Utah	51	0.20%		44	Rhode Island	32	0.13%
48	Vermont	20	0.08%		45	Maine	30	0.12%
14	Virginia	568	2.23%		46	New Hampshire	22	0.09%
23	Washington	301	1.18%		47	Wyoming	21	0.08%
35	West Virginia	131	0.51%		48	Vermont	20	0.08%
25	Wisconsin	244	0.96%		49	South Dakota	19	0.07%
47	Wyoming	21	0.08%		50	North Dakota	12	0.05%
						District of Columbia	389	1.53%

Source: U.S. Department of Health and Human Services, National Center for Health Statistics
    "Monthly Vital Statistics Report" (Vol. 43, No. 6(S), March 22, 1995)
Final data by state of residence. Includes legal intervention. Homicide data shown here are collected by the Centers for Disease Control and Prevention based on death certificates and differ from murder data collected by the F.B.I. from other sources.

Death Rate by Homicide in 1992

National Rate = 10.0 Deaths by Homicides per 100,000 Population*

ALPHA ORDER

RANK	STATE	RATE
6	Alabama	13.2
24	Alaska	7.0
19	Arizona	9.6
8	Arkansas	12.7
3	California	13.6
26	Colorado	6.3
31	Connecticut	5.5
32	Delaware	5.4
17	Florida	10.2
9	Georgia	12.3
41	Hawaii	3.6
38	Idaho	3.9
9	Illinois	12.3
22	Indiana	7.2
49	Iowa	1.9
27	Kansas	6.2
30	Kentucky	5.6
1	Louisiana	18.5
47	Maine	2.4
6	Maryland	13.2
39	Massachusetts	3.8
15	Michigan	11.2
43	Minnesota	3.2
2	Mississippi	17.5
16	Missouri	10.9
36	Montana	4.7
39	Nebraska	3.8
13	Nevada	11.8
48	New Hampshire	2.0
34	New Jersey	5.1
17	New Mexico	10.2
4	New York	13.5
12	North Carolina	11.9
49	North Dakota**	1.9
28	Ohio	6.1
21	Oklahoma	7.9
32	Oregon	5.4
25	Pennsylvania	6.5
43	Rhode Island	3.2
11	South Carolina	12.2
46	South Dakota**	2.7
14	Tennessee	11.3
5	Texas	13.3
45	Utah	2.8
42	Vermont	3.5
20	Virginia	8.9
29	Washington	5.9
22	West Virginia	7.2
35	Wisconsin	4.9
37	Wyoming	4.5

RANK ORDER

RANK	STATE	RATE
1	Louisiana	18.5
2	Mississippi	17.5
3	California	13.6
4	New York	13.5
5	Texas	13.3
6	Alabama	13.2
6	Maryland	13.2
8	Arkansas	12.7
9	Georgia	12.3
9	Illinois	12.3
11	South Carolina	12.2
12	North Carolina	11.9
13	Nevada	11.8
14	Tennessee	11.3
15	Michigan	11.2
16	Missouri	10.9
17	Florida	10.2
17	New Mexico	10.2
19	Arizona	9.6
20	Virginia	8.9
21	Oklahoma	7.9
22	Indiana	7.2
22	West Virginia	7.2
24	Alaska	7.0
25	Pennsylvania	6.5
26	Colorado	6.3
27	Kansas	6.2
28	Ohio	6.1
29	Washington	5.9
30	Kentucky	5.6
31	Connecticut	5.5
32	Delaware	5.4
32	Oregon	5.4
34	New Jersey	5.1
35	Wisconsin	4.9
36	Montana	4.7
37	Wyoming	4.5
38	Idaho	3.9
39	Massachusetts	3.8
39	Nebraska	3.8
41	Hawaii	3.6
42	Vermont	3.5
43	Minnesota	3.2
43	Rhode Island	3.2
45	Utah	2.8
46	South Dakota**	2.7
47	Maine	2.4
48	New Hampshire	2.0
49	Iowa	1.9
49	North Dakota**	1.9

District of Columbia	66.5

Source: U.S. Department of Health and Human Services, National Center for Health Statistics
"Monthly Vital Statistics Report" (Vol. 43, No. 6(S), March 22, 1995)
*Final data by state of residence. Includes legal intervention. Homicide data shown here are collected by the Centers for Disease Control and Prevention based on death certificates and differ from murder data collected by the F.B.I. from other sources. **Rates for South Dakota and North Dakota were calculated by the editors.

Deaths by Suicide in 1992

National Total = 30,484 Deaths by Suicide*

ALPHA ORDER				RANK ORDER			
RANK	STATE	SUICIDES	% of USA	RANK	STATE	SUICIDES	% of USA
21	Alabama	523	1.72%	1	California	3,723	12.21%
44	Alaska	90	0.30%	2	Texas	2,258	7.41%
14	Arizona	653	2.14%	3	Florida	2,027	6.65%
34	Arkansas	293	0.96%	4	New York	1,532	5.03%
1	California	3,723	12.21%	5	Pennsylvania	1,389	4.56%
17	Colorado	598	1.96%	6	Ohio	1,194	3.92%
33	Connecticut	298	0.98%	7	Illinois	1,142	3.75%
45	Delaware	88	0.29%	8	Michigan	1,068	3.50%
3	Florida	2,027	6.65%	9	North Carolina	860	2.82%
11	Georgia	811	2.66%	10	Virginia	812	2.66%
43	Hawaii	129	0.42%	11	Georgia	811	2.66%
39	Idaho	168	0.55%	12	Indiana	695	2.28%
7	Illinois	1,142	3.75%	13	Washington	694	2.28%
12	Indiana	695	2.28%	14	Arizona	653	2.14%
35	Iowa	287	0.94%	15	Tennessee	650	2.13%
31	Kansas	311	1.02%	16	Missouri	626	2.05%
24	Kentucky	493	1.62%	17	Colorado	598	1.96%
20	Louisiana	529	1.74%	18	Wisconsin	586	1.92%
40	Maine	157	0.52%	19	Massachusetts	534	1.75%
28	Maryland	461	1.51%	20	Louisiana	529	1.74%
19	Massachusetts	534	1.75%	21	Alabama	523	1.72%
8	Michigan	1,068	3.50%	22	Minnesota	513	1.68%
22	Minnesota	513	1.68%	22	New Jersey	513	1.68%
29	Mississippi	333	1.09%	24	Kentucky	493	1.62%
16	Missouri	626	2.05%	25	Oregon	488	1.60%
41	Montana	153	0.50%	26	Oklahoma	472	1.55%
38	Nebraska	188	0.62%	27	South Carolina	465	1.53%
30	Nevada	329	1.08%	28	Maryland	461	1.51%
42	New Hampshire	137	0.45%	29	Mississippi	333	1.09%
22	New Jersey	513	1.68%	30	Nevada	329	1.08%
32	New Mexico	303	0.99%	31	Kansas	311	1.02%
4	New York	1,532	5.03%	32	New Mexico	303	0.99%
9	North Carolina	860	2.82%	33	Connecticut	298	0.98%
50	North Dakota	65	0.21%	34	Arkansas	293	0.96%
6	Ohio	1,194	3.92%	35	Iowa	287	0.94%
26	Oklahoma	472	1.55%	36	Utah	256	0.84%
25	Oregon	488	1.60%	37	West Virginia	240	0.79%
5	Pennsylvania	1,389	4.56%	38	Nebraska	188	0.62%
49	Rhode Island	73	0.24%	39	Idaho	168	0.55%
27	South Carolina	465	1.53%	40	Maine	157	0.52%
48	South Dakota	79	0.26%	41	Montana	153	0.50%
15	Tennessee	650	2.13%	42	New Hampshire	137	0.45%
2	Texas	2,258	7.41%	43	Hawaii	129	0.42%
36	Utah	256	0.84%	44	Alaska	90	0.30%
47	Vermont	80	0.26%	45	Delaware	88	0.29%
10	Virginia	812	2.66%	46	Wyoming	84	0.28%
13	Washington	694	2.28%	47	Vermont	80	0.26%
37	West Virginia	240	0.79%	48	South Dakota	79	0.26%
18	Wisconsin	586	1.92%	49	Rhode Island	73	0.24%
46	Wyoming	84	0.28%	50	North Dakota	65	0.21%
					District of Columbia	34	0.11%

Source: U.S. Department of Health and Human Services, National Center for Health Statistics
   "Monthly Vital Statistics Report" (Vol. 43, No. 6(S), March 22, 1995)
Final data by state of residence.

Death Rate by Suicide in 1992

National Rate = 12.0 Suicides per 100,000 Population*

ALPHA ORDER			RANK ORDER		
RANK	STATE	RATE	RANK	STATE	RATE
24	Alabama	12.6	1	Nevada	24.6
9	Alaska	15.3	2	New Mexico	19.2
6	Arizona	17.0	3	Montana	18.6
30	Arkansas	12.2	4	Wyoming	18.1
31	California	12.1	5	Colorado	17.3
5	Colorado	17.3	6	Arizona	17.0
46	Connecticut	9.1	7	Oregon	16.4
20	Delaware	12.7	8	Idaho	15.8
10	Florida	15.0	9	Alaska	15.3
33	Georgia	12.0	10	Florida	15.0
39	Hawaii	11.2	11	Oklahoma	14.7
8	Idaho	15.8	12	Utah	14.1
44	Illinois	9.8	13	Vermont	14.0
28	Indiana	12.3	14	Washington	13.5
43	Iowa	10.2	15	West Virginia	13.3
26	Kansas	12.4	16	Kentucky	13.1
16	Kentucky	13.1	17	South Carolina	12.9
26	Louisiana	12.4	17	Tennessee	12.9
20	Maine	12.7	19	Texas	12.8
45	Maryland	9.4	20	Delaware	12.7
47	Massachusetts	8.9	20	Maine	12.7
38	Michigan	11.3	20	Mississippi	12.7
37	Minnesota	11.5	20	Virginia	12.7
20	Mississippi	12.7	24	Alabama	12.6
31	Missouri	12.1	24	North Carolina	12.6
3	Montana	18.6	26	Kansas	12.4
34	Nebraska	11.7	26	Louisiana	12.4
1	Nevada	24.6	28	Indiana	12.3
28	New Hampshire	12.3	28	New Hampshire	12.3
50	New Jersey	6.6	30	Arkansas	12.2
2	New Mexico	19.2	31	California	12.1
48	New York	8.5	31	Missouri	12.1
24	North Carolina	12.6	33	Georgia	12.0
42	North Dakota	10.3	34	Nebraska	11.7
41	Ohio	10.8	34	Wisconsin	11.7
11	Oklahoma	14.7	36	Pennsylvania	11.6
7	Oregon	16.4	37	Minnesota	11.5
36	Pennsylvania	11.6	38	Michigan	11.3
49	Rhode Island	7.3	39	Hawaii	11.2
17	South Carolina	12.9	39	South Dakota	11.2
39	South Dakota	11.2	41	Ohio	10.8
17	Tennessee	12.9	42	North Dakota	10.3
19	Texas	12.8	43	Iowa	10.2
12	Utah	14.1	44	Illinois	9.8
13	Vermont	14.0	45	Maryland	9.4
20	Virginia	12.7	46	Connecticut	9.1
14	Washington	13.5	47	Massachusetts	8.9
15	West Virginia	13.3	48	New York	8.5
34	Wisconsin	11.7	49	Rhode Island	7.3
4	Wyoming	18.1	50	New Jersey	6.6
				District of Columbia	5.8

Source: U.S. Department of Health and Human Services, National Center for Health Statistics
"Monthly Vital Statistics Report" (Vol. 43, No. 6(S), March 22, 1995)
*Final data by state of residence.

Years Lost by Premature Death in 1991

National Average = 5,501 Years Lost per 100,000 Population*

ALPHA ORDER

RANK ORDER

RANK	STATE	YEARS
3	Alabama	6,826
17	Alaska	5,675
22	Arizona	5,543
5	Arkansas	6,553
23	California	5,323
34	Colorado	4,796
37	Connecticut	4,501
24	Delaware	5,292
12	Florida	5,923
6	Georgia	6,447
46	Hawaii	4,150
35	Idaho	4,717
13	Illinois	5,852
26	Indiana	5,247
43	Iowa	4,304
32	Kansas	4,962
16	Kentucky	5,685
2	Louisiana	6,962
42	Maine	4,354
20	Maryland	5,642
44	Massachusetts	4,171
21	Michigan	5,565
49	Minnesota	3,988
1	Mississippi	7,208
14	Missouri	5,763
31	Montana	4,988
39	Nebraska	4,429
8	Nevada	6,052
50	New Hampshire	3,943
25	New Jersey	5,265
11	New Mexico	5,971
7	New York	6,232
10	North Carolina	5,994
45	North Dakota	4,158
30	Ohio	5,120
18	Oklahoma	5,654
36	Oregon	4,613
29	Pennsylvania	5,137
40	Rhode Island	4,420
4	South Carolina	6,655
33	South Dakota	4,945
9	Tennessee	6,044
19	Texas	5,650
47	Utah	4,147
48	Vermont	4,038
27	Virginia	5,174
38	Washington	4,465
15	West Virginia	5,747
41	Wisconsin	4,385
28	Wyoming	5,152

RANK	STATE	YEARS
1	Mississippi	7,208
2	Louisiana	6,962
3	Alabama	6,826
4	South Carolina	6,655
5	Arkansas	6,553
6	Georgia	6,447
7	New York	6,232
8	Nevada	6,052
9	Tennessee	6,044
10	North Carolina	5,994
11	New Mexico	5,971
12	Florida	5,923
13	Illinois	5,852
14	Missouri	5,763
15	West Virginia	5,747
16	Kentucky	5,685
17	Alaska	5,675
18	Oklahoma	5,654
19	Texas	5,650
20	Maryland	5,642
21	Michigan	5,565
22	Arizona	5,543
23	California	5,323
24	Delaware	5,292
25	New Jersey	5,265
26	Indiana	5,247
27	Virginia	5,174
28	Wyoming	5,152
29	Pennsylvania	5,137
30	Ohio	5,120
31	Montana	4,988
32	Kansas	4,962
33	South Dakota	4,945
34	Colorado	4,796
35	Idaho	4,717
36	Oregon	4,613
37	Connecticut	4,501
38	Washington	4,465
39	Nebraska	4,429
40	Rhode Island	4,420
41	Wisconsin	4,385
42	Maine	4,354
43	Iowa	4,304
44	Massachusetts	4,171
45	North Dakota	4,158
46	Hawaii	4,150
47	Utah	4,147
48	Vermont	4,038
49	Minnesota	3,988
50	New Hampshire	3,943
	District of Columbia**	NA

Source: U.S. Department of Health and Human Services, National Center for Health Statistics unpublished data

*Years of productive life lost due to death before age 65.

**Not available.

Estimated Years of Potential Life Lost Attributable to Smoking in 1990

National Estimated Total = 5,062,814 Years of Potential Life Lost*

ALPHA ORDER

RANK	STATE	YEARS	% of USA
20	Alabama	90,360	1.78%
50	Alaska	6,720	0.13%
26	Arizona	66,959	1.32%
29	Arkansas	58,742	1.16%
1	California	498,297	9.84%
33	Colorado	49,000	0.97%
27	Connecticut	60,535	1.20%
41	Delaware	15,248	0.30%
3	Florida	328,191	6.48%
11	Georgia	134,168	2.65%
42	Hawaii	15,222	0.30%
43	Idaho	14,708	0.29%
6	Illinois	235,933	4.66%
13	Indiana	123,584	2.44%
32	Iowa	50,521	1.00%
34	Kansas	42,540	0.84%
18	Kentucky	94,602	1.87%
17	Louisiana	94,886	1.87%
37	Maine	27,419	0.54%
19	Maryland	92,197	1.82%
16	Massachusetts	117,640	2.32%
8	Michigan	195,600	3.86%
25	Minnesota	67,835	1.34%
30	Mississippi	57,839	1.14%
14	Missouri	122,136	2.41%
45	Montana	14,491	0.29%
36	Nebraska	29,075	0.57%
35	Nevada	30,254	0.60%
40	New Hampshire	18,993	0.38%
9	New Jersey	151,773	3.00%
39	New Mexico	21,156	0.42%
2	New York	377,530	7.46%
10	North Carolina	147,810	2.92%
47	North Dakota	11,717	0.23%
7	Ohio	231,497	4.57%
24	Oklahoma	73,057	1.44%
28	Oregon	59,217	1.17%
5	Pennsylvania	271,839	5.37%
38	Rhode Island	21,541	0.43%
23	South Carolina	79,069	1.56%
46	South Dakota	12,684	0.25%
12	Tennessee	132,635	2.62%
4	Texas	317,631	6.27%
44	Utah	14,572	0.29%
48	Vermont	10,631	0.21%
15	Virginia	119,716	2.36%
21	Washington	89,222	1.76%
31	West Virginia	51,007	1.01%
22	Wisconsin	86,345	1.71%
49	Wyoming	7,298	0.14%

RANK ORDER

RANK	STATE	YEARS	% of USA
1	California	498,297	9.84%
2	New York	377,530	7.46%
3	Florida	328,191	6.48%
4	Texas	317,631	6.27%
5	Pennsylvania	271,839	5.37%
6	Illinois	235,933	4.66%
7	Ohio	231,497	4.57%
8	Michigan	195,600	3.86%
9	New Jersey	151,773	3.00%
10	North Carolina	147,810	2.92%
11	Georgia	134,168	2.65%
12	Tennessee	132,635	2.62%
13	Indiana	123,584	2.44%
14	Missouri	122,136	2.41%
15	Virginia	119,716	2.36%
16	Massachusetts	117,640	2.32%
17	Louisiana	94,886	1.87%
18	Kentucky	94,602	1.87%
19	Maryland	92,197	1.82%
20	Alabama	90,360	1.78%
21	Washington	89,222	1.76%
22	Wisconsin	86,345	1.71%
23	South Carolina	79,069	1.56%
24	Oklahoma	73,057	1.44%
25	Minnesota	67,835	1.34%
26	Arizona	66,959	1.32%
27	Connecticut	60,535	1.20%
28	Oregon	59,217	1.17%
29	Arkansas	58,742	1.16%
30	Mississippi	57,839	1.14%
31	West Virginia	51,007	1.01%
32	Iowa	50,521	1.00%
33	Colorado	49,000	0.97%
34	Kansas	42,540	0.84%
35	Nevada	30,254	0.60%
36	Nebraska	29,075	0.57%
37	Maine	27,419	0.54%
38	Rhode Island	21,541	0.43%
39	New Mexico	21,156	0.42%
40	New Hampshire	18,993	0.38%
41	Delaware	15,248	0.30%
42	Hawaii	15,222	0.30%
43	Idaho	14,708	0.29%
44	Utah	14,572	0.29%
45	Montana	14,491	0.29%
46	South Dakota	12,684	0.25%
47	North Dakota	11,717	0.23%
48	Vermont	10,631	0.21%
49	Wyoming	7,298	0.14%
50	Alaska	6,720	0.13%
	District of Columbia	21,172	0.42%

Source: U.S. Department of Health and Human Services, Centers for Disease Control and Prevention
"Surveillance for Smoking-Attributable Mortality, 1990" (MMWR, Vol. 43, No. SS-1, June 10, 1994)
Calculated by using life expectancy at age of death.

Estimated Deaths Attributable to Smoking in 1990

National Estimated Total = 415,226 Deaths

ALPHA ORDER				RANK ORDER			
RANK	STATE	DEATHS	% of USA	RANK	STATE	DEATHS	% of USA
22	Alabama	6,801	1.64%	1	California	42,574	10.25%
50	Alaska	402	0.10%	2	New York	30,992	7.46%
25	Arizona	5,697	1.37%	3	Florida	28,596	6.89%
30	Arkansas	4,706	1.13%	4	Texas	25,452	6.13%
1	California	42,574	10.25%	5	Pennsylvania	22,624	5.45%
33	Colorado	4,171	1.00%	6	Illinois	19,269	4.64%
27	Connecticut	5,362	1.29%	7	Ohio	18,114	4.36%
44	Delaware	1,178	0.28%	8	Michigan	15,454	3.72%
3	Florida	28,596	6.89%	9	New Jersey	12,605	3.04%
15	Georgia	9,694	2.33%	10	North Carolina	11,032	2.66%
46	Hawaii	1,174	0.28%	11	Massachusetts	10,430	2.51%
42	Idaho	1,304	0.31%	12	Indiana	10,250	2.47%
6	Illinois	19,269	4.64%	13	Tennessee	10,214	2.46%
12	Indiana	10,250	2.47%	14	Missouri	10,177	2.45%
29	Iowa	4,816	1.16%	15	Georgia	9,694	2.33%
34	Kansas	3,828	0.92%	16	Virginia	9,237	2.22%
19	Kentucky	7,449	1.79%	17	Washington	7,790	1.88%
21	Louisiana	6,887	1.66%	18	Wisconsin	7,620	1.84%
36	Maine	2,376	0.57%	19	Kentucky	7,449	1.79%
20	Maryland	7,370	1.77%	20	Maryland	7,370	1.77%
11	Massachusetts	10,430	2.51%	21	Louisiana	6,887	1.66%
8	Michigan	15,454	3.72%	22	Alabama	6,801	1.64%
24	Minnesota	6,127	1.48%	23	Oklahoma	6,138	1.48%
31	Mississippi	4,458	1.07%	24	Minnesota	6,127	1.48%
14	Missouri	10,177	2.45%	25	Arizona	5,697	1.37%
41	Montana	1,313	0.32%	26	South Carolina	5,619	1.35%
35	Nebraska	2,675	0.64%	27	Connecticut	5,362	1.29%
37	Nevada	2,234	0.54%	28	Oregon	5,226	1.26%
40	New Hampshire	1,655	0.40%	29	Iowa	4,816	1.16%
9	New Jersey	12,605	3.04%	30	Arkansas	4,706	1.13%
39	New Mexico	1,741	0.42%	31	Mississippi	4,458	1.07%
2	New York	30,992	7.46%	32	West Virginia	4,221	1.02%
10	North Carolina	11,032	2.66%	33	Colorado	4,171	1.00%
47	North Dakota	1,031	0.25%	34	Kansas	3,828	0.92%
7	Ohio	18,114	4.36%	35	Nebraska	2,675	0.64%
23	Oklahoma	6,138	1.48%	36	Maine	2,376	0.57%
28	Oregon	5,226	1.26%	37	Nevada	2,234	0.54%
5	Pennsylvania	22,624	5.45%	38	Rhode Island	1,881	0.45%
38	Rhode Island	1,881	0.45%	39	New Mexico	1,741	0.42%
26	South Carolina	5,619	1.35%	40	New Hampshire	1,655	0.40%
45	South Dakota	1,175	0.28%	41	Montana	1,313	0.32%
13	Tennessee	10,214	2.46%	42	Idaho	1,304	0.31%
4	Texas	25,452	6.13%	43	Utah	1,228	0.30%
43	Utah	1,228	0.30%	44	Delaware	1,178	0.28%
48	Vermont	913	0.22%	45	South Dakota	1,175	0.28%
16	Virginia	9,237	2.22%	46	Hawaii	1,174	0.28%
17	Washington	7,790	1.88%	47	North Dakota	1,031	0.25%
32	West Virginia	4,221	1.02%	48	Vermont	913	0.22%
18	Wisconsin	7,620	1.84%	49	Wyoming	659	0.16%
49	Wyoming	659	0.16%	50	Alaska	402	0.10%
					District of Columbia	1,287	0.31%

*Source: U.S. Department of Health and Human Services, Centers for Disease Control and Prevention
"Surveillance for Smoking-Attributable Mortality, 1990" (MMWR, Vol. 43, No. SS-1, June 10, 1994)*

Estimated Death Rate Attributable to Smoking in 1990

National Estimated Median Rate = 363.3 Deaths per 100,000 Population*

ALPHA ORDER

RANK	STATE	RATE
29	Alabama	350.4
5	Alaska	398.2
35	Arizona	339.6
16	Arkansas	376.3
24	California	366.3
38	Colorado	331.4
39	Connecticut	325.7
7	Delaware	393.1
27	Florida	357.5
13	Georgia	383.5
49	Hawaii	257.2
47	Idaho	293.2
26	Illinois	360.0
6	Indiana	394.3
44	Iowa	304.2
45	Kansas	300.8
4	Kentucky	428.7
11	Louisiana	388.2
9	Maine	389.4
15	Maryland	378.1
34	Massachusetts	345.3
18	Michigan	372.5
46	Minnesota	295.2
17	Mississippi	375.1
12	Missouri	383.8
36	Montana	334.2
40	Nebraska	321.0
1	Nevada	478.1
31	New Hampshire	349.3
37	New Jersey	334.1
48	New Mexico	287.7
28	New York	352.8
21	North Carolina	367.6
42	North Dakota	308.2
32	Ohio	347.7
8	Oklahoma	390.4
20	Oregon	369.3
33	Pennsylvania	346.8
30	Rhode Island	350.3
14	South Carolina	380.1
43	South Dakota	307.9
2	Tennessee	442.1
10	Texas	389.1
50	Utah	218.0
25	Vermont	363.3
23	Virginia	366.6
22	Washington	367.4
3	West Virginia	433.6
41	Wisconsin	313.3
19	Wyoming	371.0

RANK ORDER

RANK	STATE	RATE
1	Nevada	478.1
2	Tennessee	442.1
3	West Virginia	433.6
4	Kentucky	428.7
5	Alaska	398.2
6	Indiana	394.3
7	Delaware	393.1
8	Oklahoma	390.4
9	Maine	389.4
10	Texas	389.1
11	Louisiana	388.2
12	Missouri	383.8
13	Georgia	383.5
14	South Carolina	380.1
15	Maryland	378.1
16	Arkansas	376.3
17	Mississippi	375.1
18	Michigan	372.5
19	Wyoming	371.0
20	Oregon	369.3
21	North Carolina	367.6
22	Washington	367.4
23	Virginia	366.6
24	California	366.3
25	Vermont	363.3
26	Illinois	360.0
27	Florida	357.5
28	New York	352.8
29	Alabama	350.4
30	Rhode Island	350.3
31	New Hampshire	349.3
32	Ohio	347.7
33	Pennsylvania	346.8
34	Massachusetts	345.3
35	Arizona	339.6
36	Montana	334.2
37	New Jersey	334.1
38	Colorado	331.4
39	Connecticut	325.7
40	Nebraska	321.0
41	Wisconsin	313.3
42	North Dakota	308.2
43	South Dakota	307.9
44	Iowa	304.2
45	Kansas	300.8
46	Minnesota	295.2
47	Idaho	293.2
48	New Mexico	287.7
49	Hawaii	257.2
50	Utah	218.0

| | District of Columbia | 444.7 |

Source: U.S. Department of Health and Human Services, Centers for Disease Control and Prevention
    "Surveillance for Smoking-Attributable Mortality, 1990" (MMWR, Vol. 43, No. SS-1, June 10, 1994)
*Per 100,000 population of adults 35 years old or older in 1990. Deaths among infants and burn deaths among persons
1 to 34 years were excluded from rate calculations.

Alcohol-Induced Deaths in 1992

National Total = 19,568 Deaths*

ALPHA ORDER					RANK ORDER			
RANK	STATE		DEATHS	% of USA	RANK	STATE	DEATHS	% of USA
25	Alabama		264	1.35%	1	California	3,301	16.87%
38	Alaska		96	0.49%	2	New York	1,814	9.27%
13	Arizona		391	2.00%	3	Florida	1,192	6.09%
36	Arkansas		110	0.56%	4	Texas	1,024	5.23%
1	California		3,301	16.87%	5	Illinois	868	4.44%
13	Colorado		391	2.00%	6	North Carolina	782	4.00%
29	Connecticut		186	0.95%	7	Michigan	700	3.58%
46	Delaware		48	0.25%	8	Pennsylvania	589	3.01%
3	Florida		1,192	6.09%	9	Georgia	568	2.90%
9	Georgia		568	2.90%	10	Ohio	566	2.89%
49	Hawaii		36	0.18%	11	New Jersey	499	2.55%
45	Idaho		50	0.26%	12	South Carolina	420	2.15%
5	Illinois		868	4.44%	13	Arizona	391	2.00%
20	Indiana		305	1.56%	13	Colorado	391	2.00%
34	Iowa		128	0.65%	15	Tennessee	377	1.93%
35	Kansas		118	0.60%	16	Washington	376	1.92%
28	Kentucky		244	1.25%	17	Virginia	361	1.84%
27	Louisiana		245	1.25%	18	Massachusetts	340	1.74%
39	Maine		87	0.44%	19	Missouri	318	1.63%
24	Maryland		283	1.45%	20	Indiana	305	1.56%
18	Massachusetts		340	1.74%	21	Minnesota	294	1.50%
7	Michigan		700	3.58%	21	Wisconsin	294	1.50%
21	Minnesota		294	1.50%	23	Oregon	291	1.49%
31	Mississippi		169	0.86%	24	Maryland	283	1.45%
19	Missouri		318	1.63%	25	Alabama	264	1.35%
43	Montana		74	0.38%	26	New Mexico	259	1.32%
37	Nebraska		100	0.51%	27	Louisiana	245	1.25%
32	Nevada		156	0.80%	28	Kentucky	244	1.25%
41	New Hampshire		78	0.40%	29	Connecticut	186	0.95%
11	New Jersey		499	2.55%	29	Oklahoma	186	0.95%
26	New Mexico		259	1.32%	31	Mississippi	169	0.86%
2	New York		1,814	9.27%	32	Nevada	156	0.80%
6	North Carolina		782	4.00%	33	West Virginia	135	0.69%
47	North Dakota		40	0.20%	34	Iowa	128	0.65%
10	Ohio		566	2.89%	35	Kansas	118	0.60%
29	Oklahoma		186	0.95%	36	Arkansas	110	0.56%
23	Oregon		291	1.49%	37	Nebraska	100	0.51%
8	Pennsylvania		589	3.01%	38	Alaska	96	0.49%
43	Rhode Island		74	0.38%	39	Maine	87	0.44%
12	South Carolina		420	2.15%	40	Utah	82	0.42%
42	South Dakota		76	0.39%	41	New Hampshire	78	0.40%
15	Tennessee		377	1.93%	42	South Dakota	76	0.39%
4	Texas		1,024	5.23%	43	Montana	74	0.38%
40	Utah		82	0.42%	43	Rhode Island	74	0.38%
48	Vermont		37	0.19%	45	Idaho	50	0.26%
17	Virginia		361	1.84%	46	Delaware	48	0.25%
16	Washington		376	1.92%	47	North Dakota	40	0.20%
33	West Virginia		135	0.69%	48	Vermont	37	0.19%
21	Wisconsin		294	1.50%	49	Hawaii	36	0.18%
50	Wyoming		35	0.18%	50	Wyoming	35	0.18%
						District of Columbia	111	0.57%

Source: U.S. Department of Health and Human Services, Centers for Disease Control and Prevention
    unpublished data

*By state of residence. Includes excessive blood level of alcohol, chronic liver disease and cirrhosis, alcoholic psychoses, alcohol dependence syndrome and other alcohol related deaths. Excludes accidents, homicides and other causes indirectly related to alcohol use.

Death Rate from Alcohol–Induced Deaths in 1992

National Rate = 7.67 Deaths per 100,000 Population*

ALPHA ORDER

RANK	STATE	RATE
29	Alabama	6.38
2	Alaska	16.33
9	Arizona	10.19
47	Arkansas	4.59
8	California	10.68
6	Colorado	11.28
39	Connecticut	5.67
24	Delaware	6.95
13	Florida	8.84
14	Georgia	8.38
50	Hawaii	3.11
45	Idaho	4.69
17	Illinois	7.47
42	Indiana	5.39
48	Iowa	4.57
45	Kansas	4.69
26	Kentucky	6.50
38	Louisiana	5.73
22	Maine	7.03
37	Maryland	5.75
39	Massachusetts	5.67
19	Michigan	7.42
25	Minnesota	6.58
28	Mississippi	6.46
33	Missouri	6.12
12	Montana	9.00
32	Nebraska	6.25
3	Nevada	11.67
23	New Hampshire	6.99
29	New Jersey	6.38
1	New Mexico	16.37
10	New York	10.01
5	North Carolina	11.43
31	North Dakota	6.31
43	Ohio	5.14
35	Oklahoma	5.80
11	Oregon	9.79
44	Pennsylvania	4.91
20	Rhode Island	7.39
4	South Carolina	11.66
7	South Dakota	10.73
16	Tennessee	7.50
36	Texas	5.79
49	Utah	4.53
27	Vermont	6.47
41	Virginia	5.64
21	Washington	7.31
18	West Virginia	7.46
34	Wisconsin	5.89
15	Wyoming	7.53

RANK ORDER

RANK	STATE	RATE
1	New Mexico	16.37
2	Alaska	16.33
3	Nevada	11.67
4	South Carolina	11.66
5	North Carolina	11.43
6	Colorado	11.28
7	South Dakota	10.73
8	California	10.68
9	Arizona	10.19
10	New York	10.01
11	Oregon	9.79
12	Montana	9.00
13	Florida	8.84
14	Georgia	8.38
15	Wyoming	7.53
16	Tennessee	7.50
17	Illinois	7.47
18	West Virginia	7.46
19	Michigan	7.42
20	Rhode Island	7.39
21	Washington	7.31
22	Maine	7.03
23	New Hampshire	6.99
24	Delaware	6.95
25	Minnesota	6.58
26	Kentucky	6.50
27	Vermont	6.47
28	Mississippi	6.46
29	Alabama	6.38
29	New Jersey	6.38
31	North Dakota	6.31
32	Nebraska	6.25
33	Missouri	6.12
34	Wisconsin	5.89
35	Oklahoma	5.80
36	Texas	5.79
37	Maryland	5.75
38	Louisiana	5.73
39	Connecticut	5.67
39	Massachusetts	5.67
41	Virginia	5.64
42	Indiana	5.39
43	Ohio	5.14
44	Pennsylvania	4.91
45	Idaho	4.69
45	Kansas	4.69
47	Arkansas	4.59
48	Iowa	4.57
49	Utah	4.53
50	Hawaii	3.11

| | District of Columbia | 18.88 |

*Source: U.S. Department of Health and Human Services, Centers for Disease Control and Prevention
unpublished data*

By state of residence. Includes excessive blood level of alcohol, chronic liver disease and cirrhosis, alcoholic psychoses, alcohol dependence syndrome and other alcohol related deaths. Excludes accidents, homicides and other causes indirectly related to alcohol use.

Drug-Induced Deaths in 1992

National Total = 11,703 Deaths*

ALPHA ORDER

RANK	STATE	DEATHS	% of USA
29	Alabama	90	0.77%
47	Alaska	17	0.15%
11	Arizona	272	2.32%
33	Arkansas	69	0.59%
1	California	2,624	22.42%
18	Colorado	169	1.44%
20	Connecticut	147	1.26%
41	Delaware	37	0.32%
5	Florida	550	4.70%
16	Georgia	181	1.55%
39	Hawaii	40	0.34%
42	Idaho	31	0.26%
6	Illinois	520	4.44%
23	Indiana	131	1.12%
40	Iowa	39	0.33%
36	Kansas	56	0.48%
26	Kentucky	117	1.00%
25	Louisiana	121	1.03%
44	Maine	27	0.23%
10	Maryland	279	2.38%
8	Massachusetts	355	3.03%
7	Michigan	391	3.34%
30	Minnesota	89	0.76%
34	Mississippi	63	0.54%
17	Missouri	171	1.46%
45	Montana	22	0.19%
43	Nebraska	30	0.26%
31	Nevada	87	0.74%
38	New Hampshire	43	0.37%
13	New Jersey	266	2.27%
22	New Mexico	139	1.19%
2	New York	1,235	10.55%
14	North Carolina	189	1.61%
50	North Dakota	9	0.08%
9	Ohio	298	2.55%
28	Oklahoma	91	0.78%
19	Oregon	168	1.44%
3	Pennsylvania	739	6.31%
35	Rhode Island	62	0.53%
27	South Carolina	106	0.91%
48	South Dakota	14	0.12%
21	Tennessee	145	1.24%
4	Texas	720	6.15%
32	Utah	81	0.69%
46	Vermont	19	0.16%
14	Virginia	189	1.61%
12	Washington	271	2.32%
37	West Virginia	44	0.38%
24	Wisconsin	122	1.04%
49	Wyoming	11	0.09%

RANK ORDER

RANK	STATE	DEATHS	% of USA
1	California	2,624	22.42%
2	New York	1,235	10.55%
3	Pennsylvania	739	6.31%
4	Texas	720	6.15%
5	Florida	550	4.70%
6	Illinois	520	4.44%
7	Michigan	391	3.34%
8	Massachusetts	355	3.03%
9	Ohio	298	2.55%
10	Maryland	279	2.38%
11	Arizona	272	2.32%
12	Washington	271	2.32%
13	New Jersey	266	2.27%
14	North Carolina	189	1.61%
14	Virginia	189	1.61%
16	Georgia	181	1.55%
17	Missouri	171	1.46%
18	Colorado	169	1.44%
19	Oregon	168	1.44%
20	Connecticut	147	1.26%
21	Tennessee	145	1.24%
22	New Mexico	139	1.19%
23	Indiana	131	1.12%
24	Wisconsin	122	1.04%
25	Louisiana	121	1.03%
26	Kentucky	117	1.00%
27	South Carolina	106	0.91%
28	Oklahoma	91	0.78%
29	Alabama	90	0.77%
30	Minnesota	89	0.76%
31	Nevada	87	0.74%
32	Utah	81	0.69%
33	Arkansas	69	0.59%
34	Mississippi	63	0.54%
35	Rhode Island	62	0.53%
36	Kansas	56	0.48%
37	West Virginia	44	0.38%
38	New Hampshire	43	0.37%
39	Hawaii	40	0.34%
40	Iowa	39	0.33%
41	Delaware	37	0.32%
42	Idaho	31	0.26%
43	Nebraska	30	0.26%
44	Maine	27	0.23%
45	Montana	22	0.19%
46	Vermont	19	0.16%
47	Alaska	17	0.15%
48	South Dakota	14	0.12%
49	Wyoming	11	0.09%
50	North Dakota	9	0.08%
	District of Columbia	17	0.15%

Source: U.S. Department of Health and Human Services, Centers for Disease Control and Prevention
   unpublished data

*By state of residence. Includes drug psychoses, drug dependence, nondependent use excluding alcohol and tobacco, accidental poisoning or suicide by drugs, medicaments and biologicals. Excludes accidents, homicides and other causes indirectly related to drug use.

Death Rate from Drug–Induced Deaths in 1992

National Rate = 4.59 Deaths per 100,000 Population*

RANK	STATE	RATE
45	Alabama	2.17
29	Alaska	2.89
3	Arizona	7.09
31	Arkansas	2.88
2	California	8.49
13	Colorado	4.88
14	Connecticut	4.48
11	Delaware	5.36
18	Florida	4.08
36	Georgia	2.67
21	Hawaii	3.46
28	Idaho	2.91
14	Illinois	4.48
42	Indiana	2.31
50	Iowa	1.39
43	Kansas	2.23
25	Kentucky	3.12
33	Louisiana	2.83
44	Maine	2.18
9	Maryland	5.67
8	Massachusetts	5.92
17	Michigan	4.14
46	Minnesota	1.99
40	Mississippi	2.41
24	Missouri	3.29
36	Montana	2.67
48	Nebraska	1.87
5	Nevada	6.51
20	New Hampshire	3.85
22	New Jersey	3.40
1	New Mexico	8.79
4	New York	6.82
34	North Carolina	2.76
49	North Dakota	1.42
35	Ohio	2.70
32	Oklahoma	2.84
10	Oregon	5.65
7	Pennsylvania	6.16
6	Rhode Island	6.19
27	South Carolina	2.94
47	South Dakota	1.98
29	Tennessee	2.89
19	Texas	4.07
16	Utah	4.47
23	Vermont	3.32
26	Virginia	2.95
12	Washington	5.27
39	West Virginia	2.43
38	Wisconsin	2.44
41	Wyoming	2.37

RANK	STATE	RATE
1	New Mexico	8.79
2	California	8.49
3	Arizona	7.09
4	New York	6.82
5	Nevada	6.51
6	Rhode Island	6.19
7	Pennsylvania	6.16
8	Massachusetts	5.92
9	Maryland	5.67
10	Oregon	5.65
11	Delaware	5.36
12	Washington	5.27
13	Colorado	4.88
14	Connecticut	4.48
14	Illinois	4.48
16	Utah	4.47
17	Michigan	4.14
18	Florida	4.08
19	Texas	4.07
20	New Hampshire	3.85
21	Hawaii	3.46
22	New Jersey	3.40
23	Vermont	3.32
24	Missouri	3.29
25	Kentucky	3.12
26	Virginia	2.95
27	South Carolina	2.94
28	Idaho	2.91
29	Alaska	2.89
29	Tennessee	2.89
31	Arkansas	2.88
32	Oklahoma	2.84
33	Louisiana	2.83
34	North Carolina	2.76
35	Ohio	2.70
36	Georgia	2.67
36	Montana	2.67
38	Wisconsin	2.44
39	West Virginia	2.43
40	Mississippi	2.41
41	Wyoming	2.37
42	Indiana	2.31
43	Kansas	2.23
44	Maine	2.18
45	Alabama	2.17
46	Minnesota	1.99
47	South Dakota	1.98
48	Nebraska	1.87
49	North Dakota	1.42
50	Iowa	1.39
	District of Columbia	2.89

Source: U.S. Department of Health and Human Services, Centers for Disease Control and Prevention
    unpublished data

*By state of residence. Includes drug psychoses, drug dependence, nondependent use excluding alcohol and tobacco, accidental poisoning or suicide by drugs, medicaments and biologicals. Excludes accidents, homicides and other causes indirectly related to drug use.

III. FACILITIES

Hospitals in 1993

National Total = 6,467 Hospitals*

ALPHA ORDER

RANK	STATE	HOSPITALS	% of USA
20	Alabama	134	2.07%
46	Alaska	27	0.42%
29	Arizona	91	1.41%
28	Arkansas	99	1.53%
1	California	522	8.07%
30	Colorado	90	1.39%
35	Connecticut	62	0.96%
50	Delaware	13	0.20%
5	Florida	288	4.45%
8	Georgia	199	3.08%
47	Hawaii	26	0.40%
41	Idaho	49	0.76%
6	Illinois	243	3.76%
18	Indiana	136	2.10%
22	Iowa	130	2.01%
12	Kansas	154	2.38%
23	Kentucky	123	1.90%
10	Louisiana	167	2.58%
42	Maine	46	0.71%
32	Maryland	81	1.25%
17	Massachusetts	145	2.24%
9	Michigan	194	3.00%
11	Minnesota	158	2.44%
25	Mississippi	109	1.69%
12	Missouri	154	2.38%
37	Montana	61	0.94%
27	Nebraska	101	1.56%
44	Nevada	29	0.45%
43	New Hampshire	36	0.56%
24	New Jersey	119	1.84%
37	New Mexico	61	0.94%
3	New York	295	4.56%
12	North Carolina	154	2.38%
39	North Dakota	52	0.80%
7	Ohio	224	3.46%
18	Oklahoma	136	2.10%
33	Oregon	71	1.10%
4	Pennsylvania	292	4.52%
48	Rhode Island	18	0.28%
31	South Carolina	87	1.35%
35	South Dakota	62	0.96%
15	Tennessee	152	2.35%
2	Texas	510	7.89%
39	Utah	52	0.80%
48	Vermont	18	0.28%
21	Virginia	131	2.03%
26	Washington	107	1.65%
34	West Virginia	66	1.02%
16	Wisconsin	147	2.27%
44	Wyoming	29	0.45%

RANK ORDER

RANK	STATE	HOSPITALS	% of USA
1	California	522	8.07%
2	Texas	510	7.89%
3	New York	295	4.56%
4	Pennsylvania	292	4.52%
5	Florida	288	4.45%
6	Illinois	243	3.76%
7	Ohio	224	3.46%
8	Georgia	199	3.08%
9	Michigan	194	3.00%
10	Louisiana	167	2.58%
11	Minnesota	158	2.44%
12	Kansas	154	2.38%
12	Missouri	154	2.38%
12	North Carolina	154	2.38%
15	Tennessee	152	2.35%
16	Wisconsin	147	2.27%
17	Massachusetts	145	2.24%
18	Indiana	136	2.10%
18	Oklahoma	136	2.10%
20	Alabama	134	2.07%
21	Virginia	131	2.03%
22	Iowa	130	2.01%
23	Kentucky	123	1.90%
24	New Jersey	119	1.84%
25	Mississippi	109	1.69%
26	Washington	107	1.65%
27	Nebraska	101	1.56%
28	Arkansas	99	1.53%
29	Arizona	91	1.41%
30	Colorado	90	1.39%
31	South Carolina	87	1.35%
32	Maryland	81	1.25%
33	Oregon	71	1.10%
34	West Virginia	66	1.02%
35	Connecticut	62	0.96%
35	South Dakota	62	0.96%
37	Montana	61	0.94%
37	New Mexico	61	0.94%
39	North Dakota	52	0.80%
39	Utah	52	0.80%
41	Idaho	49	0.76%
42	Maine	46	0.71%
43	New Hampshire	36	0.56%
44	Nevada	29	0.45%
44	Wyoming	29	0.45%
46	Alaska	27	0.42%
47	Hawaii	26	0.40%
48	Rhode Island	18	0.28%
48	Vermont	18	0.28%
50	Delaware	13	0.20%
	District of Columbia	17	0.26%

Source: American Hospital Association (Chicago, IL)
   "Hospital Statistics" (1994–95 edition)
*Federal and nonfederal hospitals.

Federal Hospitals in 1993

National Total = 316 Hospitals

ALPHA ORDER

RANK	STATE	HOSPITALS	% of USA
11	Alabama	8	2.53%
11	Alaska	8	2.53%
3	Arizona	15	4.75%
36	Arkansas	3	0.95%
1	California	23	7.28%
19	Colorado	6	1.90%
36	Connecticut	3	0.95%
42	Delaware	2	0.63%
5	Florida	12	3.80%
11	Georgia	8	2.53%
48	Hawaii	1	0.32%
42	Idaho	2	0.63%
11	Illinois	8	2.53%
31	Indiana	4	1.27%
36	Iowa	3	0.95%
22	Kansas	5	1.58%
31	Kentucky	4	1.27%
22	Louisiana	5	1.58%
42	Maine	2	0.63%
11	Maryland	8	2.53%
22	Massachusetts	5	1.58%
19	Michigan	6	1.90%
31	Minnesota	4	1.27%
22	Mississippi	5	1.58%
18	Missouri	7	2.22%
22	Montana	5	1.58%
22	Nebraska	5	1.58%
36	Nevada	3	0.95%
48	New Hampshire	1	0.32%
31	New Jersey	4	1.27%
5	New Mexico	12	3.80%
3	New York	15	4.75%
9	North Carolina	9	2.85%
22	North Dakota	5	1.58%
22	Ohio	5	1.58%
7	Oklahoma	11	3.48%
42	Oregon	2	0.63%
8	Pennsylvania	10	3.16%
42	Rhode Island	2	0.63%
19	South Carolina	6	1.90%
9	South Dakota	9	2.85%
22	Tennessee	5	1.58%
2	Texas	19	6.01%
42	Utah	2	0.63%
48	Vermont	1	0.32%
11	Virginia	8	2.53%
11	Washington	8	2.53%
31	West Virginia	4	1.27%
36	Wisconsin	3	0.95%
36	Wyoming	3	0.95%

RANK ORDER

RANK	STATE	HOSPITALS	% of USA
1	California	23	7.28%
2	Texas	19	6.01%
3	Arizona	15	4.75%
3	New York	15	4.75%
5	Florida	12	3.80%
5	New Mexico	12	3.80%
7	Oklahoma	11	3.48%
8	Pennsylvania	10	3.16%
9	North Carolina	9	2.85%
9	South Dakota	9	2.85%
11	Alabama	8	2.53%
11	Alaska	8	2.53%
11	Georgia	8	2.53%
11	Illinois	8	2.53%
11	Maryland	8	2.53%
11	Virginia	8	2.53%
11	Washington	8	2.53%
18	Missouri	7	2.22%
19	Colorado	6	1.90%
19	Michigan	6	1.90%
19	South Carolina	6	1.90%
22	Kansas	5	1.58%
22	Louisiana	5	1.58%
22	Massachusetts	5	1.58%
22	Mississippi	5	1.58%
22	Montana	5	1.58%
22	Nebraska	5	1.58%
22	North Dakota	5	1.58%
22	Ohio	5	1.58%
22	Tennessee	5	1.58%
31	Indiana	4	1.27%
31	Kentucky	4	1.27%
31	Minnesota	4	1.27%
31	New Jersey	4	1.27%
31	West Virginia	4	1.27%
36	Arkansas	3	0.95%
36	Connecticut	3	0.95%
36	Iowa	3	0.95%
36	Nevada	3	0.95%
36	Wisconsin	3	0.95%
36	Wyoming	3	0.95%
42	Delaware	2	0.63%
42	Idaho	2	0.63%
42	Maine	2	0.63%
42	Oregon	2	0.63%
42	Rhode Island	2	0.63%
42	Utah	2	0.63%
48	Hawaii	1	0.32%
48	New Hampshire	1	0.32%
48	Vermont	1	0.32%
	District of Columbia	2	0.63%

Source: American Hospital Association (Chicago, IL)
"Hospital Statistics" (1994–95 edition)

Nonfederal Hospitals in 1993

National Total = 6,151 Hospitals

ALPHA ORDER

RANK	STATE	HOSPITALS	% of USA
20	Alabama	126	2.05%
47	Alaska	19	0.31%
31	Arizona	76	1.24%
27	Arkansas	96	1.56%
1	California	499	8.11%
29	Colorado	84	1.37%
35	Connecticut	59	0.96%
50	Delaware	11	0.18%
5	Florida	276	4.49%
8	Georgia	191	3.11%
46	Hawaii	25	0.41%
40	Idaho	47	0.76%
6	Illinois	235	3.82%
18	Indiana	132	2.15%
19	Iowa	127	2.06%
12	Kansas	149	2.42%
23	Kentucky	119	1.93%
10	Louisiana	162	2.63%
42	Maine	44	0.72%
32	Maryland	73	1.19%
17	Massachusetts	140	2.28%
9	Michigan	188	3.06%
11	Minnesota	154	2.50%
25	Mississippi	104	1.69%
13	Missouri	147	2.39%
36	Montana	56	0.91%
27	Nebraska	96	1.56%
44	Nevada	26	0.42%
43	New Hampshire	35	0.57%
24	New Jersey	115	1.87%
39	New Mexico	49	0.80%
4	New York	280	4.55%
15	North Carolina	145	2.36%
40	North Dakota	47	0.76%
7	Ohio	219	3.56%
21	Oklahoma	125	2.03%
33	Oregon	69	1.12%
3	Pennsylvania	282	4.58%
49	Rhode Island	16	0.26%
30	South Carolina	81	1.32%
37	South Dakota	53	0.86%
13	Tennessee	147	2.39%
2	Texas	491	7.98%
38	Utah	50	0.81%
48	Vermont	17	0.28%
22	Virginia	123	2.00%
26	Washington	99	1.61%
34	West Virginia	62	1.01%
16	Wisconsin	144	2.34%
44	Wyoming	26	0.42%

RANK ORDER

RANK	STATE	HOSPITALS	% of USA
1	California	499	8.11%
2	Texas	491	7.98%
3	Pennsylvania	282	4.58%
4	New York	280	4.55%
5	Florida	276	4.49%
6	Illinois	235	3.82%
7	Ohio	219	3.56%
8	Georgia	191	3.11%
9	Michigan	188	3.06%
10	Louisiana	162	2.63%
11	Minnesota	154	2.50%
12	Kansas	149	2.42%
13	Missouri	147	2.39%
13	Tennessee	147	2.39%
15	North Carolina	145	2.36%
16	Wisconsin	144	2.34%
17	Massachusetts	140	2.28%
18	Indiana	132	2.15%
19	Iowa	127	2.06%
20	Alabama	126	2.05%
21	Oklahoma	125	2.03%
22	Virginia	123	2.00%
23	Kentucky	119	1.93%
24	New Jersey	115	1.87%
25	Mississippi	104	1.69%
26	Washington	99	1.61%
27	Arkansas	96	1.56%
27	Nebraska	96	1.56%
29	Colorado	84	1.37%
30	South Carolina	81	1.32%
31	Arizona	76	1.24%
32	Maryland	73	1.19%
33	Oregon	69	1.12%
34	West Virginia	62	1.01%
35	Connecticut	59	0.96%
36	Montana	56	0.91%
37	South Dakota	53	0.86%
38	Utah	50	0.81%
39	New Mexico	49	0.80%
40	Idaho	47	0.76%
40	North Dakota	47	0.76%
42	Maine	44	0.72%
43	New Hampshire	35	0.57%
44	Nevada	26	0.42%
44	Wyoming	26	0.42%
46	Hawaii	25	0.41%
47	Alaska	19	0.31%
48	Vermont	17	0.28%
49	Rhode Island	16	0.26%
50	Delaware	11	0.18%
	District of Columbia	15	0.24%

Source: American Hospital Association (Chicago, IL)
"Hospital Statistics" (1994–95 edition)

Psychiatric Hospitals in 1993

National Total = 760 Hospitals*

ALPHA ORDER				RANK ORDER			
RANK	STATE	HOSPITALS	% of USA	RANK	STATE	HOSPITALS	% of USA
26	Alabama	11	1.45%	1	California	62	8.16%
43	Alaska	3	0.39%	1	Texas	62	8.16%
17	Arizona	16	2.11%	3	Florida	45	5.92%
29	Arkansas	9	1.18%	4	Pennsylvania	44	5.79%
1	California	62	8.16%	5	New York	43	5.66%
26	Colorado	11	1.45%	6	Georgia	26	3.42%
14	Connecticut	18	2.37%	6	Illinois	26	3.42%
43	Delaware	3	0.39%	6	Louisiana	26	3.42%
3	Florida	45	5.92%	6	Ohio	26	3.42%
6	Georgia	26	3.42%	10	Virginia	23	3.03%
47	Hawaii	1	0.13%	11	Massachusetts	22	2.89%
35	Idaho	6	0.79%	11	North Carolina	22	2.89%
6	Illinois	26	3.42%	13	Michigan	19	2.50%
16	Indiana	17	2.24%	14	Connecticut	18	2.37%
31	Iowa	8	1.05%	14	Wisconsin	18	2.37%
21	Kansas	14	1.84%	16	Indiana	17	2.24%
24	Kentucky	12	1.58%	17	Arizona	16	2.11%
6	Louisiana	26	3.42%	17	Maryland	16	2.11%
36	Maine	5	0.66%	19	Missouri	15	1.97%
17	Maryland	16	2.11%	19	Tennessee	15	1.97%
11	Massachusetts	22	2.89%	21	Kansas	14	1.84%
13	Michigan	19	2.50%	21	Oklahoma	14	1.84%
29	Minnesota	9	1.18%	23	New Jersey	13	1.71%
33	Mississippi	7	0.92%	24	Kentucky	12	1.58%
19	Missouri	15	1.97%	24	New Mexico	12	1.58%
47	Montana	1	0.13%	26	Alabama	11	1.45%
40	Nebraska	4	0.53%	26	Colorado	11	1.45%
36	Nevada	5	0.66%	28	South Carolina	10	1.32%
36	New Hampshire	5	0.66%	29	Arkansas	9	1.18%
23	New Jersey	13	1.71%	29	Minnesota	9	1.18%
24	New Mexico	12	1.58%	31	Iowa	8	1.05%
5	New York	43	5.66%	31	Utah	8	1.05%
11	North Carolina	22	2.89%	33	Mississippi	7	0.92%
47	North Dakota	1	0.13%	33	Washington	7	0.92%
6	Ohio	26	3.42%	35	Idaho	6	0.79%
21	Oklahoma	14	1.84%	36	Maine	5	0.66%
36	Oregon	5	0.66%	36	Nevada	5	0.66%
4	Pennsylvania	44	5.79%	36	New Hampshire	5	0.66%
40	Rhode Island	4	0.53%	36	Oregon	5	0.66%
28	South Carolina	10	1.32%	40	Nebraska	4	0.53%
47	South Dakota	1	0.13%	40	Rhode Island	4	0.53%
19	Tennessee	15	1.97%	40	West Virginia	4	0.53%
1	Texas	62	8.16%	43	Alaska	3	0.39%
31	Utah	8	1.05%	43	Delaware	3	0.39%
45	Vermont	2	0.26%	45	Vermont	2	0.26%
10	Virginia	23	3.03%	45	Wyoming	2	0.26%
33	Washington	7	0.92%	47	Hawaii	1	0.13%
40	West Virginia	4	0.53%	47	Montana	1	0.13%
14	Wisconsin	18	2.37%	47	North Dakota	1	0.13%
45	Wyoming	2	0.26%	47	South Dakota	1	0.13%

District of Columbia   2   0.26%

Source: American Hospital Association (Chicago, IL)
   "Hospital Statistics" (1994-95 edition)
*Federal and nonfederal psychiatric hospitals.

Community Hospitals in 1993

National Total = 5,261 Hospitals*

ALPHA ORDER				RANK ORDER			
RANK	STATE	HOSPITALS	% of USA	RANK	STATE	HOSPITALS	% of USA
18	Alabama	116	2.20%	1	California	429	8.15%
47	Alaska	16	0.30%	2	Texas	414	7.87%
32	Arizona	60	1.14%	3	Pennsylvania	233	4.43%
28	Arkansas	87	1.65%	4	New York	231	4.39%
1	California	429	8.15%	5	Florida	223	4.24%
29	Colorado	72	1.37%	6	Illinois	208	3.95%
42	Connecticut	35	0.67%	7	Ohio	192	3.65%
50	Delaware	8	0.15%	8	Michigan	167	3.17%
5	Florida	223	4.24%	9	Georgia	159	3.02%
9	Georgia	159	3.02%	10	Minnesota	145	2.76%
46	Hawaii	20	0.38%	11	Kansas	134	2.55%
39	Idaho	41	0.78%	12	Louisiana	132	2.51%
6	Illinois	208	3.95%	13	Missouri	130	2.47%
19	Indiana	115	2.19%	13	Tennessee	130	2.47%
16	Iowa	119	2.26%	15	Wisconsin	127	2.41%
11	Kansas	134	2.55%	16	Iowa	119	2.26%
21	Kentucky	106	2.01%	17	North Carolina	117	2.22%
12	Louisiana	132	2.51%	18	Alabama	116	2.20%
40	Maine	39	0.74%	19	Indiana	115	2.19%
36	Maryland	50	0.95%	20	Oklahoma	110	2.09%
22	Massachusetts	99	1.88%	21	Kentucky	106	2.01%
8	Michigan	167	3.17%	22	Massachusetts	99	1.88%
10	Minnesota	145	2.76%	23	Mississippi	97	1.84%
23	Mississippi	97	1.84%	23	New Jersey	97	1.84%
13	Missouri	130	2.47%	25	Virginia	96	1.82%
34	Montana	52	0.99%	26	Nebraska	90	1.71%
26	Nebraska	90	1.71%	26	Washington	90	1.71%
45	Nevada	21	0.40%	28	Arkansas	87	1.65%
43	New Hampshire	28	0.53%	29	Colorado	72	1.37%
23	New Jersey	97	1.84%	30	South Carolina	68	1.29%
41	New Mexico	37	0.70%	31	Oregon	63	1.20%
4	New York	231	4.39%	32	Arizona	60	1.14%
17	North Carolina	117	2.22%	33	West Virginia	58	1.10%
37	North Dakota	45	0.86%	34	Montana	52	0.99%
7	Ohio	192	3.65%	35	South Dakota	51	0.97%
20	Oklahoma	110	2.09%	36	Maryland	50	0.95%
31	Oregon	63	1.20%	37	North Dakota	45	0.86%
3	Pennsylvania	233	4.43%	38	Utah	42	0.80%
49	Rhode Island	11	0.21%	39	Idaho	41	0.78%
30	South Carolina	68	1.29%	40	Maine	39	0.74%
35	South Dakota	51	0.97%	41	New Mexico	37	0.70%
13	Tennessee	130	2.47%	42	Connecticut	35	0.67%
2	Texas	414	7.87%	43	New Hampshire	28	0.53%
38	Utah	42	0.80%	44	Wyoming	25	0.48%
48	Vermont	15	0.29%	45	Nevada	21	0.40%
25	Virginia	96	1.82%	46	Hawaii	20	0.38%
26	Washington	90	1.71%	47	Alaska	16	0.30%
33	West Virginia	58	1.10%	48	Vermont	15	0.29%
15	Wisconsin	127	2.41%	49	Rhode Island	11	0.21%
44	Wyoming	25	0.48%	50	Delaware	8	0.15%
					District of Columbia	11	0.21%

Source: American Hospital Association (Chicago, IL)
    "Hospital Statistics" (1994–95 edition)
*Community hospitals are a subset of nonfederal hospitals.

Community Hospitals per 100,000 Population in 1993

National Rate = 2.04 Community Hospitals per 100,000 Population*

<table>
<tr><td colspan="3"><u>ALPHA ORDER</u></td><td colspan="3"><u>RANK ORDER</u></td></tr>
<tr><td>RANK</td><td>STATE</td><td>RATE</td><td>RANK</td><td>STATE</td><td>RATE</td></tr>
<tr><td>17</td><td>Alabama</td><td>2.77</td><td>1</td><td>South Dakota</td><td>7.12</td></tr>
<tr><td>18</td><td>Alaska</td><td>2.68</td><td>2</td><td>North Dakota</td><td>7.06</td></tr>
<tr><td>41</td><td>Arizona</td><td>1.52</td><td>3</td><td>Montana</td><td>6.18</td></tr>
<tr><td>10</td><td>Arkansas</td><td>3.59</td><td>4</td><td>Nebraska</td><td>5.58</td></tr>
<tr><td>44</td><td>California</td><td>1.37</td><td>5</td><td>Wyoming</td><td>5.32</td></tr>
<tr><td>29</td><td>Colorado</td><td>2.02</td><td>6</td><td>Kansas</td><td>5.29</td></tr>
<tr><td>49</td><td>Connecticut</td><td>1.07</td><td>7</td><td>Iowa</td><td>4.22</td></tr>
<tr><td>47</td><td>Delaware</td><td>1.15</td><td>8</td><td>Idaho</td><td>3.73</td></tr>
<tr><td>40</td><td>Florida</td><td>1.62</td><td>9</td><td>Mississippi</td><td>3.67</td></tr>
<tr><td>24</td><td>Georgia</td><td>2.30</td><td>10</td><td>Arkansas</td><td>3.59</td></tr>
<tr><td>36</td><td>Hawaii</td><td>1.72</td><td>11</td><td>Oklahoma</td><td>3.40</td></tr>
<tr><td>8</td><td>Idaho</td><td>3.73</td><td>12</td><td>Minnesota</td><td>3.21</td></tr>
<tr><td>33</td><td>Illinois</td><td>1.78</td><td>13</td><td>West Virginia</td><td>3.19</td></tr>
<tr><td>29</td><td>Indiana</td><td>2.02</td><td>14</td><td>Maine</td><td>3.15</td></tr>
<tr><td>7</td><td>Iowa</td><td>4.22</td><td>15</td><td>Louisiana</td><td>3.08</td></tr>
<tr><td>6</td><td>Kansas</td><td>5.29</td><td>16</td><td>Kentucky</td><td>2.79</td></tr>
<tr><td>16</td><td>Kentucky</td><td>2.79</td><td>17</td><td>Alabama</td><td>2.77</td></tr>
<tr><td>15</td><td>Louisiana</td><td>3.08</td><td>18</td><td>Alaska</td><td>2.68</td></tr>
<tr><td>14</td><td>Maine</td><td>3.15</td><td>19</td><td>Vermont</td><td>2.60</td></tr>
<tr><td>50</td><td>Maryland</td><td>1.01</td><td>20</td><td>Tennessee</td><td>2.55</td></tr>
<tr><td>39</td><td>Massachusetts</td><td>1.65</td><td>21</td><td>Wisconsin</td><td>2.52</td></tr>
<tr><td>34</td><td>Michigan</td><td>1.77</td><td>22</td><td>New Hampshire</td><td>2.49</td></tr>
<tr><td>12</td><td>Minnesota</td><td>3.21</td><td>23</td><td>Missouri</td><td>2.48</td></tr>
<tr><td>9</td><td>Mississippi</td><td>3.67</td><td>24</td><td>Georgia</td><td>2.30</td></tr>
<tr><td>23</td><td>Missouri</td><td>2.48</td><td>24</td><td>Texas</td><td>2.30</td></tr>
<tr><td>3</td><td>Montana</td><td>6.18</td><td>26</td><td>New Mexico</td><td>2.29</td></tr>
<tr><td>4</td><td>Nebraska</td><td>5.58</td><td>27</td><td>Utah</td><td>2.26</td></tr>
<tr><td>41</td><td>Nevada</td><td>1.52</td><td>28</td><td>Oregon</td><td>2.08</td></tr>
<tr><td>22</td><td>New Hampshire</td><td>2.49</td><td>29</td><td>Colorado</td><td>2.02</td></tr>
<tr><td>46</td><td>New Jersey</td><td>1.23</td><td>29</td><td>Indiana</td><td>2.02</td></tr>
<tr><td>26</td><td>New Mexico</td><td>2.29</td><td>31</td><td>Pennsylvania</td><td>1.94</td></tr>
<tr><td>45</td><td>New York</td><td>1.27</td><td>32</td><td>South Carolina</td><td>1.87</td></tr>
<tr><td>38</td><td>North Carolina</td><td>1.68</td><td>33</td><td>Illinois</td><td>1.78</td></tr>
<tr><td>2</td><td>North Dakota</td><td>7.06</td><td>34</td><td>Michigan</td><td>1.77</td></tr>
<tr><td>35</td><td>Ohio</td><td>1.74</td><td>35</td><td>Ohio</td><td>1.74</td></tr>
<tr><td>11</td><td>Oklahoma</td><td>3.40</td><td>36</td><td>Hawaii</td><td>1.72</td></tr>
<tr><td>28</td><td>Oregon</td><td>2.08</td><td>37</td><td>Washington</td><td>1.71</td></tr>
<tr><td>31</td><td>Pennsylvania</td><td>1.94</td><td>38</td><td>North Carolina</td><td>1.68</td></tr>
<tr><td>48</td><td>Rhode Island</td><td>1.10</td><td>39</td><td>Massachusetts</td><td>1.65</td></tr>
<tr><td>32</td><td>South Carolina</td><td>1.87</td><td>40</td><td>Florida</td><td>1.62</td></tr>
<tr><td>1</td><td>South Dakota</td><td>7.12</td><td>41</td><td>Arizona</td><td>1.52</td></tr>
<tr><td>20</td><td>Tennessee</td><td>2.55</td><td>41</td><td>Nevada</td><td>1.52</td></tr>
<tr><td>24</td><td>Texas</td><td>2.30</td><td>43</td><td>Virginia</td><td>1.48</td></tr>
<tr><td>27</td><td>Utah</td><td>2.26</td><td>44</td><td>California</td><td>1.37</td></tr>
<tr><td>19</td><td>Vermont</td><td>2.60</td><td>45</td><td>New York</td><td>1.27</td></tr>
<tr><td>43</td><td>Virginia</td><td>1.48</td><td>46</td><td>New Jersey</td><td>1.23</td></tr>
<tr><td>37</td><td>Washington</td><td>1.71</td><td>47</td><td>Delaware</td><td>1.15</td></tr>
<tr><td>13</td><td>West Virginia</td><td>3.19</td><td>48</td><td>Rhode Island</td><td>1.10</td></tr>
<tr><td>21</td><td>Wisconsin</td><td>2.52</td><td>49</td><td>Connecticut</td><td>1.07</td></tr>
<tr><td>5</td><td>Wyoming</td><td>5.32</td><td>50</td><td>Maryland</td><td>1.01</td></tr>
<tr><td></td><td></td><td></td><td></td><td>District of Columbia</td><td>1.90</td></tr>
</table>

Source: Morgan Quitno Press using data from American Hospital Association (Chicago, IL)
"Hospital Statistics" (1994–95 edition)
*Community hospitals are a subset of nonfederal hospitals.

Community Hospitals per 1,000 Square Miles in 1993

National Rate = 1.39 Community Hospitals*

ALPHA ORDER			RANK ORDER		
RANK	STATE	RATE	RANK	STATE	RATE
21	Alabama	2.21	1	New Jersey	11.12
50	Alaska	0.02	2	Massachusetts	9.38
43	Arizona	0.53	3	Rhode Island	7.12
31	Arkansas	1.64	4	Connecticut	6.31
16	California	2.62	5	Pennsylvania	5.06
39	Colorado	0.69	6	Ohio	4.28
4	Connecticut	6.31	7	New York	4.23
11	Delaware	3.21	8	Maryland	4.03
10	Florida	3.39	9	Illinois	3.59
15	Georgia	2.67	10	Florida	3.39
28	Hawaii	1.83	11	Delaware	3.21
44	Idaho	0.49	12	Indiana	3.16
9	Illinois	3.59	13	Tennessee	3.08
12	Indiana	3.16	14	New Hampshire	2.99
24	Iowa	2.11	15	Georgia	2.67
32	Kansas	1.63	16	California	2.62
16	Kentucky	2.62	16	Kentucky	2.62
18	Louisiana	2.55	18	Louisiana	2.55
38	Maine	1.10	19	West Virginia	2.39
8	Maryland	4.03	20	Virginia	2.24
2	Massachusetts	9.38	21	Alabama	2.21
29	Michigan	1.73	22	North Carolina	2.17
30	Minnesota	1.67	23	South Carolina	2.12
25	Mississippi	2.00	24	Iowa	2.11
27	Missouri	1.86	25	Mississippi	2.00
46	Montana	0.35	26	Wisconsin	1.94
37	Nebraska	1.16	27	Missouri	1.86
49	Nevada	0.19	28	Hawaii	1.83
14	New Hampshire	2.99	29	Michigan	1.73
1	New Jersey	11.12	30	Minnesota	1.67
47	New Mexico	0.30	31	Arkansas	1.64
7	New York	4.23	32	Kansas	1.63
22	North Carolina	2.17	33	Oklahoma	1.57
41	North Dakota	0.64	34	Vermont	1.56
6	Ohio	4.28	35	Texas	1.54
33	Oklahoma	1.57	36	Washington	1.26
41	Oregon	0.64	37	Nebraska	1.16
5	Pennsylvania	5.06	38	Maine	1.10
3	Rhode Island	7.12	39	Colorado	0.69
23	South Carolina	2.12	40	South Dakota	0.66
40	South Dakota	0.66	41	North Dakota	0.64
13	Tennessee	3.08	41	Oregon	0.64
35	Texas	1.54	43	Arizona	0.53
44	Utah	0.49	44	Idaho	0.49
34	Vermont	1.56	44	Utah	0.49
20	Virginia	2.24	46	Montana	0.35
36	Washington	1.26	47	New Mexico	0.30
19	West Virginia	2.39	48	Wyoming	0.26
26	Wisconsin	1.94	49	Nevada	0.19
48	Wyoming	0.26	50	Alaska	0.02

District of Columbia**   NA

Source: Morgan Quitno Corporation using data from American Hospital Association
   "Hospital Statistics" (1994-95 edition)
*Based on 1990 Census land and water area figures. Community hospitals are a subset of nonfederal hospitals.
**The District of Columbia has 11 community hospitals for its 68 square miles.

176

Nongovernment Not-For-Profit Hospitals in 1993

National Total = 3,154 Hospitals*

ALPHA ORDER

RANK	STATE	HOSPITALS	% of USA
33	Alabama	35	1.11%
48	Alaska	7	0.22%
21	Arizona	48	1.52%
25	Arkansas	44	1.40%
1	California	238	7.55%
31	Colorado	38	1.20%
35	Connecticut	34	1.08%
47	Delaware	8	0.25%
9	Florida	98	3.11%
25	Georgia	44	1.40%
44	Hawaii	12	0.38%
45	Idaho	11	0.35%
5	Illinois	159	5.04%
17	Indiana	59	1.87%
20	Iowa	54	1.71%
17	Kansas	59	1.87%
16	Kentucky	69	2.19%
38	Louisiana	32	1.01%
33	Maine	35	1.11%
21	Maryland	48	1.52%
11	Massachusetts	86	2.73%
6	Michigan	135	4.28%
12	Minnesota	83	2.63%
36	Mississippi	33	1.05%
12	Missouri	83	2.63%
30	Montana	41	1.30%
24	Nebraska	46	1.46%
50	Nevada	6	0.19%
40	New Hampshire	24	0.76%
10	New Jersey	92	2.92%
42	New Mexico	22	0.70%
3	New York	191	6.06%
15	North Carolina	71	2.25%
28	North Dakota	43	1.36%
4	Ohio	166	5.26%
31	Oklahoma	38	1.20%
29	Oregon	42	1.33%
2	Pennsylvania	223	7.07%
45	Rhode Island	11	0.35%
39	South Carolina	28	0.89%
25	South Dakota	44	1.40%
19	Tennessee	56	1.78%
7	Texas	126	3.99%
40	Utah	24	0.76%
43	Vermont	15	0.48%
14	Virginia	78	2.47%
23	Washington	47	1.49%
36	West Virginia	33	1.05%
8	Wisconsin	119	3.77%
48	Wyoming	7	0.22%

RANK ORDER

RANK	STATE	HOSPITALS	% of USA
1	California	238	7.55%
2	Pennsylvania	223	7.07%
3	New York	191	6.06%
4	Ohio	166	5.26%
5	Illinois	159	5.04%
6	Michigan	135	4.28%
7	Texas	126	3.99%
8	Wisconsin	119	3.77%
9	Florida	98	3.11%
10	New Jersey	92	2.92%
11	Massachusetts	86	2.73%
12	Minnesota	83	2.63%
12	Missouri	83	2.63%
14	Virginia	78	2.47%
15	North Carolina	71	2.25%
16	Kentucky	69	2.19%
17	Indiana	59	1.87%
17	Kansas	59	1.87%
19	Tennessee	56	1.78%
20	Iowa	54	1.71%
21	Arizona	48	1.52%
21	Maryland	48	1.52%
23	Washington	47	1.49%
24	Nebraska	46	1.46%
25	Arkansas	44	1.40%
25	Georgia	44	1.40%
25	South Dakota	44	1.40%
28	North Dakota	43	1.36%
29	Oregon	42	1.33%
30	Montana	41	1.30%
31	Colorado	38	1.20%
31	Oklahoma	38	1.20%
33	Alabama	35	1.11%
33	Maine	35	1.11%
35	Connecticut	34	1.08%
36	Mississippi	33	1.05%
36	West Virginia	33	1.05%
38	Louisiana	32	1.01%
39	South Carolina	28	0.89%
40	New Hampshire	24	0.76%
40	Utah	24	0.76%
42	New Mexico	22	0.70%
43	Vermont	15	0.48%
44	Hawaii	12	0.38%
45	Idaho	11	0.35%
45	Rhode Island	11	0.35%
47	Delaware	8	0.25%
48	Alaska	7	0.22%
48	Wyoming	7	0.22%
50	Nevada	6	0.19%
	District of Columbia	9	0.29%

Source: American Hospital Association (Chicago, IL)
"Hospital Statistics" (1994-95 edition)
*Nongovernment not-for-profit hospitals are a subset of community hospitals.

Investor-Owned (For-Profit) Hospitals in 1993

National Total = 717 Hospitals*

ALPHA ORDER

RANK	STATE	HOSPITALS	% of USA
7	Alabama	28	3.91%
36	Alaska	1	0.14%
21	Arizona	8	1.12%
9	Arkansas	16	2.23%
2	California	102	14.23%
27	Colorado	4	0.56%
44	Connecticut	0	0.00%
44	Delaware	0	0.00%
3	Florida	96	13.39%
6	Georgia	33	4.60%
36	Hawaii	1	0.14%
31	Idaho	3	0.42%
15	Illinois	12	1.67%
23	Indiana	7	0.98%
33	Iowa	2	0.28%
18	Kansas	10	1.39%
8	Kentucky	22	3.07%
5	Louisiana	38	5.30%
36	Maine	1	0.14%
33	Maryland	2	0.28%
27	Massachusetts	4	0.56%
36	Michigan	1	0.14%
44	Minnesota	0	0.00%
15	Mississippi	12	1.67%
18	Missouri	10	1.39%
44	Montana	0	0.00%
36	Nebraska	1	0.14%
24	Nevada	6	0.84%
27	New Hampshire	4	0.56%
36	New Jersey	1	0.14%
25	New Mexico	5	0.70%
11	New York	13	1.81%
11	North Carolina	13	1.81%
36	North Dakota	1	0.14%
31	Ohio	3	0.42%
11	Oklahoma	13	1.81%
25	Oregon	5	0.70%
21	Pennsylvania	8	1.12%
44	Rhode Island	0	0.00%
17	South Carolina	11	1.53%
44	South Dakota	0	0.00%
4	Tennessee	44	6.14%
1	Texas	132	18.41%
20	Utah	9	1.26%
44	Vermont	0	0.00%
11	Virginia	13	1.81%
27	Washington	4	0.56%
10	West Virginia	14	1.95%
36	Wisconsin	1	0.14%
33	Wyoming	2	0.28%

RANK ORDER

RANK	STATE	HOSPITALS	% of USA
1	Texas	132	18.41%
2	California	102	14.23%
3	Florida	96	13.39%
4	Tennessee	44	6.14%
5	Louisiana	38	5.30%
6	Georgia	33	4.60%
7	Alabama	28	3.91%
8	Kentucky	22	3.07%
9	Arkansas	16	2.23%
10	West Virginia	14	1.95%
11	New York	13	1.81%
11	North Carolina	13	1.81%
11	Oklahoma	13	1.81%
11	Virginia	13	1.81%
15	Illinois	12	1.67%
15	Mississippi	12	1.67%
17	South Carolina	11	1.53%
18	Kansas	10	1.39%
18	Missouri	10	1.39%
20	Utah	9	1.26%
21	Arizona	8	1.12%
21	Pennsylvania	8	1.12%
23	Indiana	7	0.98%
24	Nevada	6	0.84%
25	New Mexico	5	0.70%
25	Oregon	5	0.70%
27	Colorado	4	0.56%
27	Massachusetts	4	0.56%
27	New Hampshire	4	0.56%
27	Washington	4	0.56%
31	Idaho	3	0.42%
31	Ohio	3	0.42%
33	Iowa	2	0.28%
33	Maryland	2	0.28%
33	Wyoming	2	0.28%
36	Alaska	1	0.14%
36	Hawaii	1	0.14%
36	Maine	1	0.14%
36	Michigan	1	0.14%
36	Nebraska	1	0.14%
36	New Jersey	1	0.14%
36	North Dakota	1	0.14%
36	Wisconsin	1	0.14%
44	Connecticut	0	0.00%
44	Delaware	0	0.00%
44	Minnesota	0	0.00%
44	Montana	0	0.00%
44	Rhode Island	0	0.00%
44	South Dakota	0	0.00%
44	Vermont	0	0.00%
	District of Columbia	1	0.14%

Source: American Hospital Association (Chicago, IL)
    "Hospital Statistics" (1994-95 edition)
*Investor-owned (for-profit) hospitals are a subset of community hospitals.

State and Local Government-Owned Hospitals in 1993

National Total = 1,390 Hospitals*

ALPHA ORDER

RANK	STATE	HOSPITALS	% of USA
9	Alabama	53	3.81%
35	Alaska	8	0.58%
40	Arizona	4	0.29%
22	Arkansas	27	1.94%
2	California	89	6.40%
18	Colorado	30	2.16%
44	Connecticut	1	0.07%
46	Delaware	0	0.00%
20	Florida	29	2.09%
3	Georgia	82	5.90%
36	Hawaii	7	0.50%
22	Idaho	27	1.94%
14	Illinois	37	2.66%
11	Indiana	49	3.53%
5	Iowa	63	4.53%
4	Kansas	65	4.68%
28	Kentucky	15	1.08%
6	Louisiana	62	4.46%
42	Maine	3	0.22%
46	Maryland	0	0.00%
32	Massachusetts	9	0.65%
17	Michigan	31	2.23%
6	Minnesota	62	4.46%
10	Mississippi	52	3.74%
14	Missouri	37	2.66%
29	Montana	11	0.79%
12	Nebraska	43	3.09%
32	Nevada	9	0.65%
46	New Hampshire	0	0.00%
40	New Jersey	4	0.29%
31	New Mexico	10	0.72%
22	New York	27	1.94%
16	North Carolina	33	2.37%
44	North Dakota	1	0.07%
25	Ohio	23	1.65%
8	Oklahoma	59	4.24%
26	Oregon	16	1.15%
43	Pennsylvania	2	0.14%
46	Rhode Island	0	0.00%
20	South Carolina	29	2.09%
36	South Dakota	7	0.50%
18	Tennessee	30	2.16%
1	Texas	156	11.22%
32	Utah	9	0.65%
46	Vermont	0	0.00%
39	Virginia	5	0.36%
13	Washington	39	2.81%
29	West Virginia	11	0.79%
36	Wisconsin	7	0.50%
26	Wyoming	16	1.15%

RANK ORDER

RANK	STATE	HOSPITALS	% of USA
1	Texas	156	11.22%
2	California	89	6.40%
3	Georgia	82	5.90%
4	Kansas	65	4.68%
5	Iowa	63	4.53%
6	Louisiana	62	4.46%
6	Minnesota	62	4.46%
8	Oklahoma	59	4.24%
9	Alabama	53	3.81%
10	Mississippi	52	3.74%
11	Indiana	49	3.53%
12	Nebraska	43	3.09%
13	Washington	39	2.81%
14	Illinois	37	2.66%
14	Missouri	37	2.66%
16	North Carolina	33	2.37%
17	Michigan	31	2.23%
18	Colorado	30	2.16%
18	Tennessee	30	2.16%
20	Florida	29	2.09%
20	South Carolina	29	2.09%
22	Arkansas	27	1.94%
22	Idaho	27	1.94%
22	New York	27	1.94%
25	Ohio	23	1.65%
26	Oregon	16	1.15%
26	Wyoming	16	1.15%
28	Kentucky	15	1.08%
29	Montana	11	0.79%
29	West Virginia	11	0.79%
31	New Mexico	10	0.72%
32	Massachusetts	9	0.65%
32	Nevada	9	0.65%
32	Utah	9	0.65%
35	Alaska	8	0.58%
36	Hawaii	7	0.50%
36	South Dakota	7	0.50%
36	Wisconsin	7	0.50%
39	Virginia	5	0.36%
40	Arizona	4	0.29%
40	New Jersey	4	0.29%
42	Maine	3	0.22%
43	Pennsylvania	2	0.14%
44	Connecticut	1	0.07%
44	North Dakota	1	0.07%
46	Delaware	0	0.00%
46	Maryland	0	0.00%
46	New Hampshire	0	0.00%
46	Rhode Island	0	0.00%
46	Vermont	0	0.00%
	District of Columbia	1	0.07%

Source: American Hospital Association (Chicago, IL)
"Hospital Statistics" (1994-95 edition)
*State and local government-owned hospitals are a subset of community hospitals.

Hospital Beds in 1993

National Total = 1,163,460 Beds*

ALPHA ORDER				RANK ORDER			
RANK	STATE	BEDS	% of USA	RANK	STATE	BEDS	% of USA
18	Alabama	23,071	1.98%	1	New York	101,461	8.72%
50	Alaska	1,937	0.17%	2	California	100,218	8.61%
30	Arizona	13,198	1.13%	3	Texas	74,641	6.42%
32	Arkansas	12,985	1.12%	4	Pennsylvania	67,456	5.80%
2	California	100,218	8.61%	5	Florida	62,805	5.40%
29	Colorado	13,218	1.14%	6	Illinois	54,820	4.71%
31	Connecticut	13,066	1.12%	7	Ohio	48,541	4.17%
47	Delaware	2,842	0.24%	8	New Jersey	37,408	3.22%
5	Florida	62,805	5.40%	9	Michigan	36,919	3.17%
10	Georgia	35,224	3.03%	10	Georgia	35,224	3.03%
46	Hawaii	3,934	0.34%	11	North Carolina	30,069	2.58%
45	Idaho	4,078	0.35%	12	Massachusetts	29,800	2.56%
6	Illinois	54,820	4.71%	13	Missouri	28,431	2.44%
16	Indiana	25,275	2.17%	14	Tennessee	28,101	2.42%
24	Iowa	15,992	1.37%	15	Virginia	27,788	2.39%
26	Kansas	15,251	1.31%	16	Indiana	25,275	2.17%
22	Kentucky	18,929	1.63%	17	Louisiana	23,463	2.02%
17	Louisiana	23,463	2.02%	18	Alabama	23,071	1.98%
37	Maine	5,489	0.47%	19	Minnesota	22,754	1.96%
21	Maryland	19,314	1.66%	20	Wisconsin	21,996	1.89%
12	Massachusetts	29,800	2.56%	21	Maryland	19,314	1.66%
9	Michigan	36,919	3.17%	22	Kentucky	18,929	1.63%
19	Minnesota	22,754	1.96%	23	Mississippi	16,244	1.40%
23	Mississippi	16,244	1.40%	24	Iowa	15,992	1.37%
13	Missouri	28,431	2.44%	25	Washington	15,413	1.32%
41	Montana	4,664	0.40%	26	Kansas	15,251	1.31%
34	Nebraska	10,321	0.89%	27	South Carolina	14,292	1.23%
43	Nevada	4,345	0.37%	28	Oklahoma	14,002	1.20%
42	New Hampshire	4,542	0.39%	29	Colorado	13,218	1.14%
8	New Jersey	37,408	3.22%	30	Arizona	13,198	1.13%
36	New Mexico	6,621	0.57%	31	Connecticut	13,066	1.12%
1	New York	101,461	8.72%	32	Arkansas	12,985	1.12%
11	North Carolina	30,069	2.58%	33	West Virginia	10,344	0.89%
40	North Dakota	5,043	0.43%	34	Nebraska	10,321	0.89%
7	Ohio	48,541	4.17%	35	Oregon	9,663	0.83%
28	Oklahoma	14,002	1.20%	36	New Mexico	6,621	0.57%
35	Oregon	9,663	0.83%	37	Maine	5,489	0.47%
4	Pennsylvania	67,456	5.80%	38	Utah	5,475	0.47%
44	Rhode Island	4,244	0.36%	39	South Dakota	5,286	0.45%
27	South Carolina	14,292	1.23%	40	North Dakota	5,043	0.43%
39	South Dakota	5,286	0.45%	41	Montana	4,664	0.40%
14	Tennessee	28,101	2.42%	42	New Hampshire	4,542	0.39%
3	Texas	74,641	6.42%	43	Nevada	4,345	0.37%
38	Utah	5,475	0.47%	44	Rhode Island	4,244	0.36%
49	Vermont	2,363	0.20%	45	Idaho	4,078	0.35%
15	Virginia	27,788	2.39%	46	Hawaii	3,934	0.34%
25	Washington	15,413	1.32%	47	Delaware	2,842	0.24%
33	West Virginia	10,344	0.89%	48	Wyoming	2,776	0.24%
20	Wisconsin	21,996	1.89%	49	Vermont	2,363	0.20%
48	Wyoming	2,776	0.24%	50	Alaska	1,937	0.17%
					District of Columbia	7,348	0.63%

Source: American Hospital Association (Chicago, IL)
  "Hospital Statistics" (1994-95 edition)
*In federal and nonfederal hospitals.

Hospital Beds per 100,000 Population in 1993

National Rate = 451 Beds per 100,000 Population*

ALPHA ORDER			RANK ORDER		
RANK	STATE	RATE	RANK	STATE	RATE
12	Alabama	552	1	North Dakota	792
45	Alaska	324	2	South Dakota	738
44	Arizona	335	3	Nebraska	640
16	Arkansas	535	4	Mississippi	615
46	California	321	5	Kansas	602
41	Colorado	371	6	Wyoming	591
37	Connecticut	399	7	West Virginia	569
35	Delaware	407	8	Iowa	567
23	Florida	458	9	Pennsylvania	561
17	Georgia	510	10	New York	559
43	Hawaii	337	11	Montana	555
41	Idaho	371	12	Alabama	552
22	Illinois	469	12	Tennessee	552
24	Indiana	443	14	Louisiana	547
8	Iowa	567	15	Missouri	543
5	Kansas	602	16	Arkansas	535
19	Kentucky	499	17	Georgia	510
14	Louisiana	547	18	Minnesota	503
24	Maine	443	19	Kentucky	499
39	Maryland	390	20	Massachusetts	495
20	Massachusetts	495	21	New Jersey	476
39	Michigan	390	22	Illinois	469
18	Minnesota	503	23	Florida	458
4	Mississippi	615	24	Indiana	443
15	Missouri	543	24	Maine	443
11	Montana	555	26	Ohio	439
3	Nebraska	640	27	Wisconsin	436
48	Nevada	314	28	North Carolina	433
36	New Hampshire	404	28	Oklahoma	433
21	New Jersey	476	30	Virginia	429
33	New Mexico	410	31	Rhode Island	424
10	New York	559	32	Texas	414
28	North Carolina	433	33	New Mexico	410
1	North Dakota	792	33	Vermont	410
26	Ohio	439	35	Delaware	407
28	Oklahoma	433	36	New Hampshire	404
47	Oregon	318	37	Connecticut	399
9	Pennsylvania	561	38	South Carolina	394
31	Rhode Island	424	39	Maryland	390
38	South Carolina	394	39	Michigan	390
2	South Dakota	738	41	Colorado	371
12	Tennessee	552	41	Idaho	371
32	Texas	414	43	Hawaii	337
49	Utah	294	44	Arizona	335
33	Vermont	410	45	Alaska	324
30	Virginia	429	46	California	321
50	Washington	293	47	Oregon	318
7	West Virginia	569	48	Nevada	314
27	Wisconsin	436	49	Utah	294
6	Wyoming	591	50	Washington	293
				District of Columbia	1,269

Source: Morgan Quitno Press using data from American Hospital Association (Chicago, IL)
"Hospital Statistics" (1994–95 edition)
*In federal and nonfederal hospitals.

Average Number of Beds per Hospital in 1993

National Average = 180 Beds per Hospital*

ALPHA ORDER			RANK ORDER		
RANK	**STATE**	**BEDS**	**RANK**	**STATE**	**BEDS**
20	Alabama	172	1	New York	344
50	Alaska	72	2	New Jersey	314
30	Arizona	145	3	Maryland	238
35	Arkansas	131	4	Rhode Island	236
14	California	192	5	Pennsylvania	231
28	Colorado	147	6	Illinois	226
11	Connecticut	211	7	Delaware	219
7	Delaware	219	8	Florida	218
8	Florida	218	9	Ohio	217
19	Georgia	177	10	Virginia	212
24	Hawaii	151	11	Connecticut	211
48	Idaho	83	12	Massachusetts	206
6	Illinois	226	13	North Carolina	195
16	Indiana	186	14	California	192
38	Iowa	123	15	Michigan	190
44	Kansas	99	16	Indiana	186
23	Kentucky	154	17	Missouri	185
33	Louisiana	140	17	Tennessee	185
39	Maine	119	19	Georgia	177
3	Maryland	238	20	Alabama	172
12	Massachusetts	206	21	South Carolina	164
15	Michigan	190	22	West Virginia	157
31	Minnesota	144	23	Kentucky	154
27	Mississippi	149	24	Hawaii	151
17	Missouri	185	25	Nevada	150
49	Montana	76	25	Wisconsin	150
43	Nebraska	102	27	Mississippi	149
25	Nevada	150	28	Colorado	147
37	New Hampshire	126	29	Texas	146
2	New Jersey	314	30	Arizona	145
40	New Mexico	109	31	Minnesota	144
1	New York	344	31	Washington	144
13	North Carolina	195	33	Louisiana	140
45	North Dakota	97	34	Oregon	136
9	Ohio	217	35	Arkansas	131
42	Oklahoma	103	35	Vermont	131
34	Oregon	136	37	New Hampshire	126
5	Pennsylvania	231	38	Iowa	123
4	Rhode Island	236	39	Maine	119
21	South Carolina	164	40	New Mexico	109
47	South Dakota	85	41	Utah	105
17	Tennessee	185	42	Oklahoma	103
29	Texas	146	43	Nebraska	102
41	Utah	105	44	Kansas	99
35	Vermont	131	45	North Dakota	97
10	Virginia	212	46	Wyoming	96
31	Washington	144	47	South Dakota	85
22	West Virginia	157	48	Idaho	83
25	Wisconsin	150	49	Montana	76
46	Wyoming	96	50	Alaska	72
				District of Columbia	432

Source: Morgan Quitno Press using data from American Hospital Association (Chicago, IL)
   "Hospital Statistics" (1994–95 edition)
*In federal and nonfederal hospitals.

Beds in Federal Hospitals in 1993

National Total = 87,847 Beds

RANK	STATE	BEDS	% of USA
15	Alabama	2,049	2.33%
38	Alaska	434	0.49%
17	Arizona	1,815	2.07%
26	Arkansas	1,205	1.37%
3	California	6,791	7.73%
25	Colorado	1,242	1.41%
36	Connecticut	700	0.80%
45	Delaware	241	0.27%
5	Florida	4,118	4.69%
8	Georgia	2,891	3.29%
39	Hawaii	421	0.48%
49	Idaho	201	0.23%
6	Illinois	3,960	4.51%
30	Indiana	1,100	1.25%
31	Iowa	985	1.12%
24	Kansas	1,274	1.45%
22	Kentucky	1,310	1.49%
28	Louisiana	1,143	1.30%
41	Maine	353	0.40%
14	Maryland	2,192	2.50%
9	Massachusetts	2,473	2.82%
16	Michigan	1,948	2.22%
27	Minnesota	1,159	1.32%
23	Mississippi	1,283	1.46%
11	Missouri	2,280	2.60%
44	Montana	255	0.29%
37	Nebraska	634	0.72%
47	Nevada	229	0.26%
48	New Hampshire	228	0.26%
18	New Jersey	1,732	1.97%
32	New Mexico	918	1.04%
2	New York	7,014	7.98%
13	North Carolina	2,200	2.50%
43	North Dakota	292	0.33%
7	Ohio	3,331	3.79%
35	Oklahoma	869	0.99%
33	Oregon	904	1.03%
4	Pennsylvania	4,478	5.10%
45	Rhode Island	241	0.27%
29	South Carolina	1,134	1.29%
34	South Dakota	876	1.00%
12	Tennessee	2,269	2.58%
1	Texas	7,401	8.42%
42	Utah	332	0.38%
50	Vermont	150	0.17%
10	Virginia	2,335	2.66%
19	Washington	1,643	1.87%
20	West Virginia	1,514	1.72%
21	Wisconsin	1,408	1.60%
40	Wyoming	383	0.44%

RANK	STATE	BEDS	% of USA
1	Texas	7,401	8.42%
2	New York	7,014	7.98%
3	California	6,791	7.73%
4	Pennsylvania	4,478	5.10%
5	Florida	4,118	4.69%
6	Illinois	3,960	4.51%
7	Ohio	3,331	3.79%
8	Georgia	2,891	3.29%
9	Massachusetts	2,473	2.82%
10	Virginia	2,335	2.66%
11	Missouri	2,280	2.60%
12	Tennessee	2,269	2.58%
13	North Carolina	2,200	2.50%
14	Maryland	2,192	2.50%
15	Alabama	2,049	2.33%
16	Michigan	1,948	2.22%
17	Arizona	1,815	2.07%
18	New Jersey	1,732	1.97%
19	Washington	1,643	1.87%
20	West Virginia	1,514	1.72%
21	Wisconsin	1,408	1.60%
22	Kentucky	1,310	1.49%
23	Mississippi	1,283	1.46%
24	Kansas	1,274	1.45%
25	Colorado	1,242	1.41%
26	Arkansas	1,205	1.37%
27	Minnesota	1,159	1.32%
28	Louisiana	1,143	1.30%
29	South Carolina	1,134	1.29%
30	Indiana	1,100	1.25%
31	Iowa	985	1.12%
32	New Mexico	918	1.04%
33	Oregon	904	1.03%
34	South Dakota	876	1.00%
35	Oklahoma	869	0.99%
36	Connecticut	700	0.80%
37	Nebraska	634	0.72%
38	Alaska	434	0.49%
39	Hawaii	421	0.48%
40	Wyoming	383	0.44%
41	Maine	353	0.40%
42	Utah	332	0.38%
43	North Dakota	292	0.33%
44	Montana	255	0.29%
45	Delaware	241	0.27%
45	Rhode Island	241	0.27%
47	Nevada	229	0.26%
48	New Hampshire	228	0.26%
49	Idaho	201	0.23%
50	Vermont	150	0.17%
	District of Columbia	1,509	1.72%

Source: American Hospital Association (Chicago, IL)
"Hospital Statistics" (1994–95 edition)

Beds in Nonfederal Hospitals in 1993

National Total = 1,075,613 Beds

ALPHA ORDER					RANK ORDER			
RANK	STATE		BEDS	% of USA	RANK	STATE	BEDS	% of USA
19	Alabama		21,022	1.95%	1	New York	94,447	8.78%
50	Alaska		1,503	0.14%	2	California	93,427	8.69%
32	Arizona		11,383	1.06%	3	Texas	67,240	6.25%
31	Arkansas		11,780	1.10%	4	Pennsylvania	62,978	5.86%
2	California		93,427	8.69%	5	Florida	58,687	5.46%
30	Colorado		11,976	1.11%	6	Illinois	50,860	4.73%
29	Connecticut		12,366	1.15%	7	Ohio	45,210	4.20%
47	Delaware		2,601	0.24%	8	New Jersey	35,676	3.32%
5	Florida		58,687	5.46%	9	Michigan	34,971	3.25%
10	Georgia		32,333	3.01%	10	Georgia	32,333	3.01%
46	Hawaii		3,513	0.33%	11	North Carolina	27,869	2.59%
45	Idaho		3,877	0.36%	12	Massachusetts	27,327	2.54%
6	Illinois		50,860	4.73%	13	Missouri	26,151	2.43%
16	Indiana		24,175	2.25%	14	Tennessee	25,832	2.40%
23	Iowa		15,007	1.40%	15	Virginia	25,453	2.37%
25	Kansas		13,977	1.30%	16	Indiana	24,175	2.25%
21	Kentucky		17,619	1.64%	17	Louisiana	22,320	2.08%
17	Louisiana		22,320	2.08%	18	Minnesota	21,595	2.01%
38	Maine		5,136	0.48%	19	Alabama	21,022	1.95%
22	Maryland		17,122	1.59%	20	Wisconsin	20,588	1.91%
12	Massachusetts		27,327	2.54%	21	Kentucky	17,619	1.64%
9	Michigan		34,971	3.25%	22	Maryland	17,122	1.59%
18	Minnesota		21,595	2.01%	23	Iowa	15,007	1.40%
24	Mississippi		14,961	1.39%	24	Mississippi	14,961	1.39%
13	Missouri		26,151	2.43%	25	Kansas	13,977	1.30%
41	Montana		4,409	0.41%	26	Washington	13,770	1.28%
33	Nebraska		9,687	0.90%	27	South Carolina	13,158	1.22%
43	Nevada		4,116	0.38%	28	Oklahoma	13,133	1.22%
42	New Hampshire		4,314	0.40%	29	Connecticut	12,366	1.15%
8	New Jersey		35,676	3.32%	30	Colorado	11,976	1.11%
36	New Mexico		5,703	0.53%	31	Arkansas	11,780	1.10%
1	New York		94,447	8.78%	32	Arizona	11,383	1.06%
11	North Carolina		27,869	2.59%	33	Nebraska	9,687	0.90%
39	North Dakota		4,751	0.44%	34	West Virginia	8,830	0.82%
7	Ohio		45,210	4.20%	35	Oregon	8,759	0.81%
28	Oklahoma		13,133	1.22%	36	New Mexico	5,703	0.53%
35	Oregon		8,759	0.81%	37	Utah	5,143	0.48%
4	Pennsylvania		62,978	5.86%	38	Maine	5,136	0.48%
44	Rhode Island		4,003	0.37%	39	North Dakota	4,751	0.44%
27	South Carolina		13,158	1.22%	40	South Dakota	4,410	0.41%
40	South Dakota		4,410	0.41%	41	Montana	4,409	0.41%
14	Tennessee		25,832	2.40%	42	New Hampshire	4,314	0.40%
3	Texas		67,240	6.25%	43	Nevada	4,116	0.38%
37	Utah		5,143	0.48%	44	Rhode Island	4,003	0.37%
49	Vermont		2,213	0.21%	45	Idaho	3,877	0.36%
15	Virginia		25,453	2.37%	46	Hawaii	3,513	0.33%
26	Washington		13,770	1.28%	47	Delaware	2,601	0.24%
34	West Virginia		8,830	0.82%	48	Wyoming	2,393	0.22%
20	Wisconsin		20,588	1.91%	49	Vermont	2,213	0.21%
48	Wyoming		2,393	0.22%	50	Alaska	1,503	0.14%
						District of Columbia	5,839	0.54%

Source: American Hospital Association (Chicago, IL)
"Hospital Statistics" (1994–95 edition)

Beds in Psychiatric Hospitals in 1993

National Total = 145,385 Beds*

ALPHA ORDER				RANK ORDER			
RANK	STATE	BEDS	% of USA	RANK	STATE	BEDS	% of USA
17	Alabama	3,140	2.16%	1	New York	15,128	10.41%
47	Alaska	228	0.16%	2	California	13,145	9.04%
30	Arizona	1,587	1.09%	3	Pennsylvania	10,158	6.99%
36	Arkansas	741	0.51%	4	Texas	7,978	5.49%
2	California	13,145	9.04%	5	Florida	6,665	4.58%
26	Colorado	1,860	1.28%	6	Illinois	6,556	4.51%
25	Connecticut	1,892	1.30%	7	North Carolina	5,409	3.72%
42	Delaware	448	0.31%	8	Virginia	5,155	3.55%
5	Florida	6,665	4.58%	9	New Jersey	5,139	3.53%
13	Georgia	3,527	2.43%	10	Michigan	4,560	3.14%
48	Hawaii	195	0.13%	11	Ohio	4,111	2.83%
39	Idaho	502	0.35%	12	Massachusetts	3,604	2.48%
6	Illinois	6,556	4.51%	13	Georgia	3,527	2.43%
15	Indiana	3,289	2.26%	14	Minnesota	3,478	2.39%
24	Iowa	2,236	1.54%	15	Indiana	3,289	2.26%
20	Kansas	2,643	1.82%	16	Maryland	3,264	2.25%
29	Kentucky	1,630	1.12%	17	Alabama	3,140	2.16%
19	Louisiana	2,859	1.97%	17	Wisconsin	3,140	2.16%
38	Maine	666	0.46%	19	Louisiana	2,859	1.97%
16	Maryland	3,264	2.25%	20	Kansas	2,643	1.82%
12	Massachusetts	3,604	2.48%	21	Mississippi	2,374	1.63%
10	Michigan	4,560	3.14%	22	Missouri	2,272	1.56%
14	Minnesota	3,478	2.39%	23	Tennessee	2,238	1.54%
21	Mississippi	2,374	1.63%	24	Iowa	2,236	1.54%
22	Missouri	2,272	1.56%	25	Connecticut	1,892	1.30%
50	Montana	37	0.03%	26	Colorado	1,860	1.28%
34	Nebraska	785	0.54%	27	Washington	1,742	1.20%
43	Nevada	397	0.27%	28	South Carolina	1,645	1.13%
37	New Hampshire	727	0.50%	29	Kentucky	1,630	1.12%
9	New Jersey	5,139	3.53%	30	Arizona	1,587	1.09%
31	New Mexico	1,583	1.09%	31	New Mexico	1,583	1.09%
1	New York	15,128	10.41%	32	Oklahoma	1,327	0.91%
7	North Carolina	5,409	3.72%	33	Oregon	1,251	0.86%
45	North Dakota	327	0.22%	34	Nebraska	785	0.54%
11	Ohio	4,111	2.83%	35	Utah	773	0.53%
32	Oklahoma	1,327	0.91%	36	Arkansas	741	0.51%
33	Oregon	1,251	0.86%	37	New Hampshire	727	0.50%
3	Pennsylvania	10,158	6.99%	38	Maine	666	0.46%
44	Rhode Island	390	0.27%	39	Idaho	502	0.35%
28	South Carolina	1,645	1.13%	40	West Virginia	492	0.34%
49	South Dakota	60	0.04%	41	Wyoming	456	0.31%
23	Tennessee	2,238	1.54%	42	Delaware	448	0.31%
4	Texas	7,978	5.49%	43	Nevada	397	0.27%
35	Utah	773	0.53%	44	Rhode Island	390	0.27%
46	Vermont	289	0.20%	45	North Dakota	327	0.22%
8	Virginia	5,155	3.55%	46	Vermont	289	0.20%
27	Washington	1,742	1.20%	47	Alaska	228	0.16%
40	West Virginia	492	0.34%	48	Hawaii	195	0.13%
17	Wisconsin	3,140	2.16%	49	South Dakota	60	0.04%
41	Wyoming	456	0.31%	50	Montana	37	0.03%
					District of Columbia	1,287	0.89%

Source: American Hospital Association (Chicago, IL)
"Hospital Statistics" (1994-95 edition)
*In federal and nonfederal psychiatric hospitals.

Beds in Community Hospitals in 1993

National Total = 918,786 Beds*

ALPHA ORDER				RANK ORDER			
RANK	STATE	BEDS	% of USA	RANK	STATE	BEDS	% of USA
18	Alabama	18,545	2.02%	1	California	78,023	8.49%
50	Alaska	1,275	0.14%	2	New York	77,445	8.43%
31	Arizona	9,796	1.07%	3	Texas	58,157	6.33%
29	Arkansas	11,039	1.20%	4	Pennsylvania	53,751	5.85%
1	California	78,023	8.49%	5	Florida	51,302	5.58%
30	Colorado	10,272	1.12%	6	Illinois	44,322	4.82%
32	Connecticut	9,290	1.01%	7	Ohio	41,510	4.52%
48	Delaware	2,153	0.23%	8	Michigan	31,034	3.38%
5	Florida	51,302	5.58%	9	New Jersey	31,033	3.38%
10	Georgia	26,493	2.88%	10	Georgia	26,493	2.88%
46	Hawaii	2,924	0.32%	11	Missouri	23,599	2.57%
44	Idaho	3,375	0.37%	12	Tennessee	22,965	2.50%
6	Illinois	44,322	4.82%	13	North Carolina	22,675	2.47%
14	Indiana	21,444	2.33%	14	Indiana	21,444	2.33%
22	Iowa	13,371	1.46%	15	Massachusetts	21,142	2.30%
28	Kansas	11,288	1.23%	16	Virginia	19,645	2.14%
21	Kentucky	15,963	1.74%	17	Louisiana	18,909	2.06%
17	Louisiana	18,909	2.06%	18	Alabama	18,545	2.02%
36	Maine	4,470	0.49%	19	Minnesota	18,459	2.01%
23	Maryland	13,133	1.43%	20	Wisconsin	18,044	1.96%
15	Massachusetts	21,142	2.30%	21	Kentucky	15,963	1.74%
8	Michigan	31,034	3.38%	22	Iowa	13,371	1.46%
19	Minnesota	18,459	2.01%	23	Maryland	13,133	1.43%
24	Mississippi	12,587	1.37%	24	Mississippi	12,587	1.37%
11	Missouri	23,599	2.57%	25	Washington	11,943	1.30%
39	Montana	4,299	0.47%	26	Oklahoma	11,770	1.28%
33	Nebraska	8,418	0.92%	27	South Carolina	11,374	1.24%
42	Nevada	3,719	0.40%	28	Kansas	11,288	1.23%
43	New Hampshire	3,437	0.37%	29	Arkansas	11,039	1.20%
9	New Jersey	31,033	3.38%	30	Colorado	10,272	1.12%
41	New Mexico	4,120	0.45%	31	Arizona	9,796	1.07%
2	New York	77,445	8.43%	32	Connecticut	9,290	1.01%
13	North Carolina	22,675	2.47%	33	Nebraska	8,418	0.92%
37	North Dakota	4,398	0.48%	34	West Virginia	8,338	0.91%
7	Ohio	41,510	4.52%	35	Oregon	7,476	0.81%
26	Oklahoma	11,770	1.28%	36	Maine	4,470	0.49%
35	Oregon	7,476	0.81%	37	North Dakota	4,398	0.48%
4	Pennsylvania	53,751	5.85%	38	Utah	4,370	0.48%
45	Rhode Island	3,050	0.33%	39	Montana	4,299	0.47%
27	South Carolina	11,374	1.24%	40	South Dakota	4,267	0.46%
40	South Dakota	4,267	0.46%	41	New Mexico	4,120	0.45%
12	Tennessee	22,965	2.50%	42	Nevada	3,719	0.40%
3	Texas	58,157	6.33%	43	New Hampshire	3,437	0.37%
38	Utah	4,370	0.48%	44	Idaho	3,375	0.37%
49	Vermont	1,924	0.21%	45	Rhode Island	3,050	0.33%
16	Virginia	19,645	2.14%	46	Hawaii	2,924	0.32%
25	Washington	11,943	1.30%	47	Wyoming	2,167	0.24%
34	West Virginia	8,338	0.91%	48	Delaware	2,153	0.23%
20	Wisconsin	18,044	1.96%	49	Vermont	1,924	0.21%
47	Wyoming	2,167	0.24%	50	Alaska	1,275	0.14%
					District of Columbia	4,283	0.47%

Source: American Hospital Association (Chicago, IL)
   "Hospital Statistics" (1994–95 edition)
*Community hospital beds are a subset of nonfederal hospital beds.

Beds in Community Hospitals per 100,000 Population in 1993

National Rate = 356 Beds per 100,000 Population*

RANK	STATE	RATE
14	Alabama	444
50	Alaska	213
46	Arizona	248
9	Arkansas	455
45	California	250
39	Colorado	288
40	Connecticut	283
34	Delaware	308
24	Florida	374
20	Georgia	384
44	Hawaii	251
35	Idaho	307
21	Illinois	379
22	Indiana	376
6	Iowa	474
13	Kansas	445
17	Kentucky	421
15	Louisiana	441
26	Maine	360
42	Maryland	265
28	Massachusetts	351
30	Michigan	328
18	Minnesota	408
5	Mississippi	477
10	Missouri	451
4	Montana	511
3	Nebraska	522
41	Nevada	269
36	New Hampshire	306
19	New Jersey	395
43	New Mexico	255
16	New York	427
31	North Carolina	326
1	North Dakota	690
23	Ohio	375
25	Oklahoma	364
47	Oregon	246
12	Pennsylvania	447
37	Rhode Island	305
33	South Carolina	313
2	South Dakota	596
10	Tennessee	451
32	Texas	323
48	Utah	235
29	Vermont	334
38	Virginia	303
49	Washington	227
8	West Virginia	459
27	Wisconsin	358
7	Wyoming	461

RANK	STATE	RATE
1	North Dakota	690
2	South Dakota	596
3	Nebraska	522
4	Montana	511
5	Mississippi	477
6	Iowa	474
7	Wyoming	461
8	West Virginia	459
9	Arkansas	455
10	Missouri	451
10	Tennessee	451
12	Pennsylvania	447
13	Kansas	445
14	Alabama	444
15	Louisiana	441
16	New York	427
17	Kentucky	421
18	Minnesota	408
19	New Jersey	395
20	Georgia	384
21	Illinois	379
22	Indiana	376
23	Ohio	375
24	Florida	374
25	Oklahoma	364
26	Maine	360
27	Wisconsin	358
28	Massachusetts	351
29	Vermont	334
30	Michigan	328
31	North Carolina	326
32	Texas	323
33	South Carolina	313
34	Delaware	308
35	Idaho	307
36	New Hampshire	306
37	Rhode Island	305
38	Virginia	303
39	Colorado	288
40	Connecticut	283
41	Nevada	269
42	Maryland	265
43	New Mexico	255
44	Hawaii	251
45	California	250
46	Arizona	248
47	Oregon	246
48	Utah	235
49	Washington	227
50	Alaska	213
	District of Columbia	740

Source: Morgan Quitno Press using data from American Hospital Association (Chicago, IL)
"Hospital Statistics" (1994-95 edition)
*Community hospital beds are a subset of nonfederal hospital beds.

Average Number of Beds per Community Hospital in 1993

National Average = 175 Beds per Community Hospital*

ALPHA ORDER				RANK ORDER		
RANK	STATE	BEDS		RANK	STATE	BEDS
23	Alabama	160		1	New York	335
50	Alaska	80		2	New Jersey	320
22	Arizona	163		3	Rhode Island	277
34	Arkansas	127		4	Delaware	269
16	California	182		5	Connecticut	265
27	Colorado	143		6	Maryland	263
5	Connecticut	265		7	Pennsylvania	231
4	Delaware	269		8	Florida	230
8	Florida	230		9	Ohio	216
20	Georgia	167		10	Massachusetts	214
25	Hawaii	146		11	Illinois	213
49	Idaho	82		12	Virginia	205
11	Illinois	213		13	North Carolina	194
14	Indiana	186		14	Indiana	186
39	Iowa	112		14	Michigan	186
46	Kansas	84		16	California	182
24	Kentucky	151		16	Missouri	182
27	Louisiana	143		18	Nevada	177
38	Maine	115		18	Tennessee	177
6	Maryland	263		20	Georgia	167
10	Massachusetts	214		20	South Carolina	167
14	Michigan	186		22	Arizona	163
34	Minnesota	127		23	Alabama	160
32	Mississippi	130		24	Kentucky	151
16	Missouri	182		25	Hawaii	146
48	Montana	83		26	West Virginia	144
44	Nebraska	94		27	Colorado	143
18	Nevada	177		27	Louisiana	143
36	New Hampshire	123		29	Wisconsin	142
2	New Jersey	320		30	Texas	140
40	New Mexico	111		31	Washington	133
1	New York	335		32	Mississippi	130
13	North Carolina	194		33	Vermont	128
43	North Dakota	98		34	Arkansas	127
9	Ohio	216		34	Minnesota	127
41	Oklahoma	107		36	New Hampshire	123
37	Oregon	119		37	Oregon	119
7	Pennsylvania	231		38	Maine	115
3	Rhode Island	277		39	Iowa	112
20	South Carolina	167		40	New Mexico	111
46	South Dakota	84		41	Oklahoma	107
18	Tennessee	177		42	Utah	104
30	Texas	140		43	North Dakota	98
42	Utah	104		44	Nebraska	94
33	Vermont	128		45	Wyoming	87
12	Virginia	205		46	Kansas	84
31	Washington	133		46	South Dakota	84
26	West Virginia	144		48	Montana	83
29	Wisconsin	142		49	Idaho	82
45	Wyoming	87		50	Alaska	80
					District of Columbia	389

Source: Morgan Quitno Press using data from American Hospital Association (Chicago, IL)
"Hospital Statistics" (1994–95 edition)
*Community hospital beds are a subset of nonfederal hospital beds.

Beds in Nongovernment Not-For-Profit Hospitals in 1993

National Total = 651,272 Beds*

ALPHA ORDER

RANK	STATE	BEDS	% of USA
28	Alabama	6,599	1.01%
49	Alaska	800	0.12%
24	Arizona	8,054	1.24%
27	Arkansas	7,095	1.09%
3	California	50,770	7.80%
26	Colorado	7,434	1.14%
21	Connecticut	9,058	1.39%
45	Delaware	2,153	0.33%
9	Florida	25,705	3.95%
20	Georgia	10,455	1.61%
44	Hawaii	2,175	0.33%
47	Idaho	1,281	0.20%
4	Illinois	38,259	5.87%
13	Indiana	14,827	2.28%
22	Iowa	8,761	1.35%
29	Kansas	6,394	0.98%
19	Kentucky	10,606	1.63%
25	Louisiana	7,564	1.16%
37	Maine	4,222	0.65%
17	Maryland	12,755	1.96%
11	Massachusetts	18,706	2.87%
7	Michigan	27,670	4.25%
18	Minnesota	12,695	1.95%
35	Mississippi	5,370	0.82%
10	Missouri	18,927	2.91%
39	Montana	3,829	0.59%
34	Nebraska	5,405	0.83%
48	Nevada	1,178	0.18%
40	New Hampshire	3,082	0.47%
6	New Jersey	28,433	4.37%
43	New Mexico	2,241	0.34%
1	New York	60,310	9.26%
15	North Carolina	14,203	2.18%
36	North Dakota	4,246	0.65%
5	Ohio	36,967	5.68%
31	Oklahoma	6,260	0.96%
32	Oregon	5,930	0.91%
2	Pennsylvania	52,955	8.13%
41	Rhode Island	3,050	0.47%
33	South Carolina	5,709	0.88%
38	South Dakota	3,944	0.61%
16	Tennessee	13,421	2.06%
8	Texas	26,591	4.08%
42	Utah	2,676	0.41%
46	Vermont	1,924	0.30%
14	Virginia	14,658	2.25%
23	Washington	8,512	1.31%
30	West Virginia	6,363	0.98%
12	Wisconsin	16,726	2.57%
50	Wyoming	572	0.09%

RANK ORDER

RANK	STATE	BEDS	% of USA
1	New York	60,310	9.26%
2	Pennsylvania	52,955	8.13%
3	California	50,770	7.80%
4	Illinois	38,259	5.87%
5	Ohio	36,967	5.68%
6	New Jersey	28,433	4.37%
7	Michigan	27,670	4.25%
8	Texas	26,591	4.08%
9	Florida	25,705	3.95%
10	Missouri	18,927	2.91%
11	Massachusetts	18,706	2.87%
12	Wisconsin	16,726	2.57%
13	Indiana	14,827	2.28%
14	Virginia	14,658	2.25%
15	North Carolina	14,203	2.18%
16	Tennessee	13,421	2.06%
17	Maryland	12,755	1.96%
18	Minnesota	12,695	1.95%
19	Kentucky	10,606	1.63%
20	Georgia	10,455	1.61%
21	Connecticut	9,058	1.39%
22	Iowa	8,761	1.35%
23	Washington	8,512	1.31%
24	Arizona	8,054	1.24%
25	Louisiana	7,564	1.16%
26	Colorado	7,434	1.14%
27	Arkansas	7,095	1.09%
28	Alabama	6,599	1.01%
29	Kansas	6,394	0.98%
30	West Virginia	6,363	0.98%
31	Oklahoma	6,260	0.96%
32	Oregon	5,930	0.91%
33	South Carolina	5,709	0.88%
34	Nebraska	5,405	0.83%
35	Mississippi	5,370	0.82%
36	North Dakota	4,246	0.65%
37	Maine	4,222	0.65%
38	South Dakota	3,944	0.61%
39	Montana	3,829	0.59%
40	New Hampshire	3,082	0.47%
41	Rhode Island	3,050	0.47%
42	Utah	2,676	0.41%
43	New Mexico	2,241	0.34%
44	Hawaii	2,175	0.33%
45	Delaware	2,153	0.33%
46	Vermont	1,924	0.30%
47	Idaho	1,281	0.20%
48	Nevada	1,178	0.18%
49	Alaska	800	0.12%
50	Wyoming	572	0.09%
	District of Columbia	3,752	0.58%

Source: American Hospital Association (Chicago, IL)
"Hospital Statistics" (1994-95 edition)
*Nongovernment not-for-profit hospital beds are a subset of community hospital beds.

Beds in Investor-Owned (For-Profit) Hospitals in 1993

National Total = 98,964 Beds*

ALPHA ORDER

RANK ORDER

RANK	STATE	BEDS	% of USA
7	Alabama	3,668	3.71%
35	Alaska	238	0.24%
20	Arizona	1,058	1.07%
12	Arkansas	1,715	1.73%
3	California	12,661	12.79%
27	Colorado	456	0.46%
44	Connecticut	0	0.00%
44	Delaware	0	0.00%
2	Florida	17,303	17.48%
5	Georgia	4,249	4.29%
39	Hawaii	143	0.14%
28	Idaho	448	0.45%
11	Illinois	1,751	1.77%
22	Indiana	997	1.01%
36	Iowa	216	0.22%
19	Kansas	1,314	1.33%
8	Kentucky	3,474	3.51%
6	Louisiana	4,197	4.24%
42	Maine	80	0.08%
31	Maryland	378	0.38%
26	Massachusetts	552	0.56%
41	Michigan	101	0.10%
44	Minnesota	0	0.00%
18	Mississippi	1,344	1.36%
15	Missouri	1,506	1.52%
44	Montana	0	0.00%
34	Nebraska	297	0.30%
13	Nevada	1,672	1.69%
32	New Hampshire	355	0.36%
38	New Jersey	151	0.15%
24	New Mexico	768	0.78%
9	New York	3,051	3.08%
16	North Carolina	1,469	1.48%
40	North Dakota	110	0.11%
33	Ohio	308	0.31%
17	Oklahoma	1,463	1.48%
29	Oregon	412	0.42%
25	Pennsylvania	727	0.73%
44	Rhode Island	0	0.00%
14	South Carolina	1,602	1.62%
44	South Dakota	0	0.00%
4	Tennessee	4,853	4.90%
1	Texas	18,344	18.54%
23	Utah	963	0.97%
44	Vermont	0	0.00%
10	Virginia	2,755	2.78%
30	Washington	411	0.42%
21	West Virginia	1,055	1.07%
43	Wisconsin	74	0.07%
37	Wyoming	172	0.17%

RANK	STATE	BEDS	% of USA
1	Texas	18,344	18.54%
2	Florida	17,303	17.48%
3	California	12,661	12.79%
4	Tennessee	4,853	4.90%
5	Georgia	4,249	4.29%
6	Louisiana	4,197	4.24%
7	Alabama	3,668	3.71%
8	Kentucky	3,474	3.51%
9	New York	3,051	3.08%
10	Virginia	2,755	2.78%
11	Illinois	1,751	1.77%
12	Arkansas	1,715	1.73%
13	Nevada	1,672	1.69%
14	South Carolina	1,602	1.62%
15	Missouri	1,506	1.52%
16	North Carolina	1,469	1.48%
17	Oklahoma	1,463	1.48%
18	Mississippi	1,344	1.36%
19	Kansas	1,314	1.33%
20	Arizona	1,058	1.07%
21	West Virginia	1,055	1.07%
22	Indiana	997	1.01%
23	Utah	963	0.97%
24	New Mexico	768	0.78%
25	Pennsylvania	727	0.73%
26	Massachusetts	552	0.56%
27	Colorado	456	0.46%
28	Idaho	448	0.45%
29	Oregon	412	0.42%
30	Washington	411	0.42%
31	Maryland	378	0.38%
32	New Hampshire	355	0.36%
33	Ohio	308	0.31%
34	Nebraska	297	0.30%
35	Alaska	238	0.24%
36	Iowa	216	0.22%
37	Wyoming	172	0.17%
38	New Jersey	151	0.15%
39	Hawaii	143	0.14%
40	North Dakota	110	0.11%
41	Michigan	101	0.10%
42	Maine	80	0.08%
43	Wisconsin	74	0.07%
44	Connecticut	0	0.00%
44	Delaware	0	0.00%
44	Minnesota	0	0.00%
44	Montana	0	0.00%
44	Rhode Island	0	0.00%
44	South Dakota	0	0.00%
44	Vermont	0	0.00%
	District of Columbia	103	0.10%

Source: American Hospital Association (Chicago, IL)
  "Hospital Statistics" (1994-95 edition)
*Investor-owned (for-profit) hospital beds are a subset of community hospital beds.

Beds in State and Local Government–Owned Hospitals in 1993

National Total = 168,550 Beds*

ALPHA ORDER					RANK ORDER			

RANK	STATE	BEDS	% of USA
6	Alabama	8,278	4.91%
41	Alaska	237	0.14%
37	Arizona	684	0.41%
26	Arkansas	2,229	1.32%
1	California	14,592	8.66%
24	Colorado	2,382	1.41%
42	Connecticut	232	0.14%
46	Delaware	0	0.00%
5	Florida	8,294	4.92%
4	Georgia	11,789	6.99%
38	Hawaii	606	0.36%
29	Idaho	1,646	0.98%
14	Illinois	4,312	2.56%
11	Indiana	5,620	3.33%
13	Iowa	4,394	2.61%
18	Kansas	3,580	2.12%
28	Kentucky	1,883	1.12%
7	Louisiana	7,148	4.24%
43	Maine	168	0.10%
46	Maryland	0	0.00%
27	Massachusetts	1,884	1.12%
19	Michigan	3,263	1.94%
10	Minnesota	5,764	3.42%
9	Mississippi	5,873	3.48%
20	Missouri	3,166	1.88%
39	Montana	470	0.28%
22	Nebraska	2,716	1.61%
35	Nevada	869	0.52%
46	New Hampshire	0	0.00%
23	New Jersey	2,449	1.45%
33	New Mexico	1,111	0.66%
2	New York	14,084	8.36%
8	North Carolina	7,003	4.15%
45	North Dakota	42	0.02%
15	Ohio	4,235	2.51%
17	Oklahoma	4,047	2.40%
32	Oregon	1,134	0.67%
44	Pennsylvania	69	0.04%
46	Rhode Island	0	0.00%
16	South Carolina	4,063	2.41%
40	South Dakota	323	0.19%
12	Tennessee	4,691	2.78%
3	Texas	13,222	7.84%
36	Utah	731	0.43%
46	Vermont	0	0.00%
25	Virginia	2,232	1.32%
21	Washington	3,020	1.79%
34	West Virginia	920	0.55%
31	Wisconsin	1,244	0.74%
30	Wyoming	1,423	0.84%

RANK	STATE	BEDS	% of USA
1	California	14,592	8.66%
2	New York	14,084	8.36%
3	Texas	13,222	7.84%
4	Georgia	11,789	6.99%
5	Florida	8,294	4.92%
6	Alabama	8,278	4.91%
7	Louisiana	7,148	4.24%
8	North Carolina	7,003	4.15%
9	Mississippi	5,873	3.48%
10	Minnesota	5,764	3.42%
11	Indiana	5,620	3.33%
12	Tennessee	4,691	2.78%
13	Iowa	4,394	2.61%
14	Illinois	4,312	2.56%
15	Ohio	4,235	2.51%
16	South Carolina	4,063	2.41%
17	Oklahoma	4,047	2.40%
18	Kansas	3,580	2.12%
19	Michigan	3,263	1.94%
20	Missouri	3,166	1.88%
21	Washington	3,020	1.79%
22	Nebraska	2,716	1.61%
23	New Jersey	2,449	1.45%
24	Colorado	2,382	1.41%
25	Virginia	2,232	1.32%
26	Arkansas	2,229	1.32%
27	Massachusetts	1,884	1.12%
28	Kentucky	1,883	1.12%
29	Idaho	1,646	0.98%
30	Wyoming	1,423	0.84%
31	Wisconsin	1,244	0.74%
32	Oregon	1,134	0.67%
33	New Mexico	1,111	0.66%
34	West Virginia	920	0.55%
35	Nevada	869	0.52%
36	Utah	731	0.43%
37	Arizona	684	0.41%
38	Hawaii	606	0.36%
39	Montana	470	0.28%
40	South Dakota	323	0.19%
41	Alaska	237	0.14%
42	Connecticut	232	0.14%
43	Maine	168	0.10%
44	Pennsylvania	69	0.04%
45	North Dakota	42	0.02%
46	Delaware	0	0.00%
46	Maryland	0	0.00%
46	New Hampshire	0	0.00%
46	Rhode Island	0	0.00%
46	Vermont	0	0.00%
	District of Columbia	428	0.25%

Source: American Hospital Association (Chicago, IL)
"Hospital Statistics" (1994–95 edition)
*State and local government–owned hospital beds are a subset of community hospital beds.

Hospital Admissions in 1993

National Total = 33,200,500 Admissions*

ALPHA ORDER			
RANK	STATE	ADMISSIONS	% of USA
18	Alabama	643,979	1.94%
49	Alaska	59,590	0.18%
24	Arizona	468,397	1.41%
30	Arkansas	371,941	1.12%
1	California	3,280,402	9.88%
28	Colorado	389,596	1.17%
29	Connecticut	371,990	1.12%
47	Delaware	87,564	0.26%
5	Florida	1,834,814	5.53%
10	Georgia	958,467	2.89%
42	Hawaii	117,024	0.35%
44	Idaho	107,136	0.32%
6	Illinois	1,560,537	4.70%
16	Indiana	738,974	2.23%
31	Iowa	365,341	1.10%
32	Kansas	318,743	0.96%
21	Kentucky	576,842	1.74%
17	Louisiana	650,598	1.96%
38	Maine	154,827	0.47%
19	Maryland	621,218	1.87%
12	Massachusetts	868,936	2.62%
9	Michigan	1,109,428	3.34%
23	Minnesota	522,393	1.57%
27	Mississippi	407,717	1.23%
15	Missouri	764,198	2.30%
45	Montana	105,383	0.32%
35	Nebraska	198,040	0.60%
39	Nevada	134,376	0.40%
41	New Hampshire	119,858	0.36%
8	New Jersey	1,134,732	3.42%
36	New Mexico	190,262	0.57%
2	New York	2,479,495	7.47%
11	North Carolina	872,053	2.63%
46	North Dakota	102,513	0.31%
7	Ohio	1,475,942	4.45%
26	Oklahoma	408,099	1.23%
33	Oregon	312,343	0.94%
4	Pennsylvania	1,912,079	5.76%
40	Rhode Island	133,702	0.40%
25	South Carolina	439,260	1.32%
43	South Dakota	116,521	0.35%
13	Tennessee	797,925	2.40%
3	Texas	2,184,239	6.58%
37	Utah	189,635	0.57%
48	Vermont	62,549	0.19%
14	Virginia	786,064	2.37%
22	Washington	550,015	1.66%
34	West Virginia	297,758	0.90%
20	Wisconsin	602,028	1.81%
50	Wyoming	47,989	0.14%

RANK ORDER			
RANK	STATE	ADMISSIONS	% of USA
1	California	3,280,402	9.88%
2	New York	2,479,495	7.47%
3	Texas	2,184,239	6.58%
4	Pennsylvania	1,912,079	5.76%
5	Florida	1,834,814	5.53%
6	Illinois	1,560,537	4.70%
7	Ohio	1,475,942	4.45%
8	New Jersey	1,134,732	3.42%
9	Michigan	1,109,428	3.34%
10	Georgia	958,467	2.89%
11	North Carolina	872,053	2.63%
12	Massachusetts	868,936	2.62%
13	Tennessee	797,925	2.40%
14	Virginia	786,064	2.37%
15	Missouri	764,198	2.30%
16	Indiana	738,974	2.23%
17	Louisiana	650,598	1.96%
18	Alabama	643,979	1.94%
19	Maryland	621,218	1.87%
20	Wisconsin	602,028	1.81%
21	Kentucky	576,842	1.74%
22	Washington	550,015	1.66%
23	Minnesota	522,393	1.57%
24	Arizona	468,397	1.41%
25	South Carolina	439,260	1.32%
26	Oklahoma	408,099	1.23%
27	Mississippi	407,717	1.23%
28	Colorado	389,596	1.17%
29	Connecticut	371,990	1.12%
30	Arkansas	371,941	1.12%
31	Iowa	365,341	1.10%
32	Kansas	318,743	0.96%
33	Oregon	312,343	0.94%
34	West Virginia	297,758	0.90%
35	Nebraska	198,040	0.60%
36	New Mexico	190,262	0.57%
37	Utah	189,635	0.57%
38	Maine	154,827	0.47%
39	Nevada	134,376	0.40%
40	Rhode Island	133,702	0.40%
41	New Hampshire	119,858	0.36%
42	Hawaii	117,024	0.35%
43	South Dakota	116,521	0.35%
44	Idaho	107,136	0.32%
45	Montana	105,383	0.32%
46	North Dakota	102,513	0.31%
47	Delaware	87,564	0.26%
48	Vermont	62,549	0.19%
49	Alaska	59,590	0.18%
50	Wyoming	47,989	0.14%
	District of Columbia	196,988	0.59%

Source: American Hospital Association (Chicago, IL)
"Hospital Statistics" (1994–95 edition)
*Admissions to federal and nonfederal hospitals.

Admissions to Federal Hospitals in 1993

National Total = 1,625,600 Admissions

ALPHA ORDER

RANK	STATE	ADMISSIONS	% of USA
20	Alabama	29,338	1.80%
28	Alaska	19,911	1.22%
9	Arizona	49,261	3.03%
26	Arkansas	22,257	1.37%
2	California	147,278	9.06%
14	Colorado	39,066	2.40%
39	Connecticut	12,063	0.74%
46	Delaware	5,235	0.32%
3	Florida	84,003	5.17%
7	Georgia	57,267	3.52%
30	Hawaii	19,375	1.19%
45	Idaho	5,438	0.33%
6	Illinois	58,709	3.61%
38	Indiana	13,075	0.80%
37	Iowa	13,233	0.81%
29	Kansas	19,717	1.21%
19	Kentucky	29,725	1.83%
23	Louisiana	27,261	1.68%
44	Maine	5,450	0.34%
11	Maryland	45,978	2.83%
25	Massachusetts	25,318	1.56%
24	Michigan	25,864	1.59%
31	Minnesota	19,372	1.19%
21	Mississippi	28,466	1.75%
12	Missouri	40,135	2.47%
42	Montana	7,588	0.47%
33	Nebraska	15,439	0.95%
43	Nevada	7,183	0.44%
50	New Hampshire	2,967	0.18%
32	New Jersey	18,519	1.14%
22	New Mexico	28,437	1.75%
4	New York	69,436	4.27%
8	North Carolina	54,900	3.38%
41	North Dakota	10,013	0.62%
13	Ohio	40,067	2.46%
17	Oklahoma	33,410	2.06%
36	Oregon	14,214	0.87%
15	Pennsylvania	38,227	2.35%
48	Rhode Island	4,548	0.28%
16	South Carolina	34,613	2.13%
27	South Dakota	20,832	1.28%
18	Tennessee	31,257	1.92%
1	Texas	155,942	9.59%
40	Utah	10,322	0.63%
49	Vermont	3,459	0.21%
5	Virginia	64,408	3.96%
10	Washington	47,011	2.89%
34	West Virginia	15,072	0.93%
35	Wisconsin	14,332	0.88%
47	Wyoming	4,694	0.29%

RANK ORDER

RANK	STATE	ADMISSIONS	% of USA
1	Texas	155,942	9.59%
2	California	147,278	9.06%
3	Florida	84,003	5.17%
4	New York	69,436	4.27%
5	Virginia	64,408	3.96%
6	Illinois	58,709	3.61%
7	Georgia	57,267	3.52%
8	North Carolina	54,900	3.38%
9	Arizona	49,261	3.03%
10	Washington	47,011	2.89%
11	Maryland	45,978	2.83%
12	Missouri	40,135	2.47%
13	Ohio	40,067	2.46%
14	Colorado	39,066	2.40%
15	Pennsylvania	38,227	2.35%
16	South Carolina	34,613	2.13%
17	Oklahoma	33,410	2.06%
18	Tennessee	31,257	1.92%
19	Kentucky	29,725	1.83%
20	Alabama	29,338	1.80%
21	Mississippi	28,466	1.75%
22	New Mexico	28,437	1.75%
23	Louisiana	27,261	1.68%
24	Michigan	25,864	1.59%
25	Massachusetts	25,318	1.56%
26	Arkansas	22,257	1.37%
27	South Dakota	20,832	1.28%
28	Alaska	19,911	1.22%
29	Kansas	19,717	1.21%
30	Hawaii	19,375	1.19%
31	Minnesota	19,372	1.19%
32	New Jersey	18,519	1.14%
33	Nebraska	15,439	0.95%
34	West Virginia	15,072	0.93%
35	Wisconsin	14,332	0.88%
36	Oregon	14,214	0.87%
37	Iowa	13,233	0.81%
38	Indiana	13,075	0.80%
39	Connecticut	12,063	0.74%
40	Utah	10,322	0.63%
41	North Dakota	10,013	0.62%
42	Montana	7,588	0.47%
43	Nevada	7,183	0.44%
44	Maine	5,450	0.34%
45	Idaho	5,438	0.33%
46	Delaware	5,235	0.32%
47	Wyoming	4,694	0.29%
48	Rhode Island	4,548	0.28%
49	Vermont	3,459	0.21%
50	New Hampshire	2,967	0.18%
	District of Columbia	35,915	2.21%

Source: American Hospital Association (Chicago, IL)
   "Hospital Statistics" (1994-95 edition)

Admissions to Nonfederal Hospitals in 1993

National Total = 31,574,900 Admissions

<table>
<tr><td colspan="4"><u>ALPHA ORDER</u></td><td colspan="4"><u>RANK ORDER</u></td></tr>
<tr><th>RANK</th><th>STATE</th><th>ADMISSIONS</th><th>% of USA</th><th>RANK</th><th>STATE</th><th>ADMISSIONS</th><th>% of USA</th></tr>
<tr><td>18</td><td>Alabama</td><td>614,641</td><td>1.95%</td><td>1</td><td>California</td><td>3,133,124</td><td>9.92%</td></tr>
<tr><td>50</td><td>Alaska</td><td>39,679</td><td>0.13%</td><td>2</td><td>New York</td><td>2,410,059</td><td>7.63%</td></tr>
<tr><td>24</td><td>Arizona</td><td>419,136</td><td>1.33%</td><td>3</td><td>Texas</td><td>2,028,297</td><td>6.42%</td></tr>
<tr><td>31</td><td>Arkansas</td><td>349,684</td><td>1.11%</td><td>4</td><td>Pennsylvania</td><td>1,873,852</td><td>5.93%</td></tr>
<tr><td>1</td><td>California</td><td>3,133,124</td><td>9.92%</td><td>5</td><td>Florida</td><td>1,750,811</td><td>5.54%</td></tr>
<tr><td>30</td><td>Colorado</td><td>350,530</td><td>1.11%</td><td>6</td><td>Illinois</td><td>1,501,828</td><td>4.76%</td></tr>
<tr><td>28</td><td>Connecticut</td><td>359,927</td><td>1.14%</td><td>7</td><td>Ohio</td><td>1,435,875</td><td>4.55%</td></tr>
<tr><td>47</td><td>Delaware</td><td>82,329</td><td>0.26%</td><td>8</td><td>New Jersey</td><td>1,116,213</td><td>3.54%</td></tr>
<tr><td>5</td><td>Florida</td><td>1,750,811</td><td>5.54%</td><td>9</td><td>Michigan</td><td>1,083,564</td><td>3.43%</td></tr>
<tr><td>10</td><td>Georgia</td><td>901,200</td><td>2.85%</td><td>10</td><td>Georgia</td><td>901,200</td><td>2.85%</td></tr>
<tr><td>44</td><td>Hawaii</td><td>97,649</td><td>0.31%</td><td>11</td><td>Massachusetts</td><td>843,618</td><td>2.67%</td></tr>
<tr><td>42</td><td>Idaho</td><td>101,698</td><td>0.32%</td><td>12</td><td>North Carolina</td><td>817,153</td><td>2.59%</td></tr>
<tr><td>6</td><td>Illinois</td><td>1,501,828</td><td>4.76%</td><td>13</td><td>Tennessee</td><td>766,668</td><td>2.43%</td></tr>
<tr><td>14</td><td>Indiana</td><td>725,899</td><td>2.30%</td><td>14</td><td>Indiana</td><td>725,899</td><td>2.30%</td></tr>
<tr><td>29</td><td>Iowa</td><td>352,108</td><td>1.12%</td><td>15</td><td>Missouri</td><td>724,063</td><td>2.29%</td></tr>
<tr><td>32</td><td>Kansas</td><td>299,026</td><td>0.95%</td><td>16</td><td>Virginia</td><td>721,656</td><td>2.29%</td></tr>
<tr><td>21</td><td>Kentucky</td><td>547,117</td><td>1.73%</td><td>17</td><td>Louisiana</td><td>623,337</td><td>1.97%</td></tr>
<tr><td>17</td><td>Louisiana</td><td>623,337</td><td>1.97%</td><td>18</td><td>Alabama</td><td>614,641</td><td>1.95%</td></tr>
<tr><td>38</td><td>Maine</td><td>149,377</td><td>0.47%</td><td>19</td><td>Wisconsin</td><td>587,696</td><td>1.86%</td></tr>
<tr><td>20</td><td>Maryland</td><td>575,240</td><td>1.82%</td><td>20</td><td>Maryland</td><td>575,240</td><td>1.82%</td></tr>
<tr><td>11</td><td>Massachusetts</td><td>843,618</td><td>2.67%</td><td>21</td><td>Kentucky</td><td>547,117</td><td>1.73%</td></tr>
<tr><td>9</td><td>Michigan</td><td>1,083,564</td><td>3.43%</td><td>22</td><td>Minnesota</td><td>503,021</td><td>1.59%</td></tr>
<tr><td>22</td><td>Minnesota</td><td>503,021</td><td>1.59%</td><td>23</td><td>Washington</td><td>503,004</td><td>1.59%</td></tr>
<tr><td>26</td><td>Mississippi</td><td>379,251</td><td>1.20%</td><td>24</td><td>Arizona</td><td>419,136</td><td>1.33%</td></tr>
<tr><td>15</td><td>Missouri</td><td>724,063</td><td>2.29%</td><td>25</td><td>South Carolina</td><td>404,647</td><td>1.28%</td></tr>
<tr><td>43</td><td>Montana</td><td>97,795</td><td>0.31%</td><td>26</td><td>Mississippi</td><td>379,251</td><td>1.20%</td></tr>
<tr><td>35</td><td>Nebraska</td><td>182,601</td><td>0.58%</td><td>27</td><td>Oklahoma</td><td>374,689</td><td>1.19%</td></tr>
<tr><td>40</td><td>Nevada</td><td>127,193</td><td>0.40%</td><td>28</td><td>Connecticut</td><td>359,927</td><td>1.14%</td></tr>
<tr><td>41</td><td>New Hampshire</td><td>116,891</td><td>0.37%</td><td>29</td><td>Iowa</td><td>352,108</td><td>1.12%</td></tr>
<tr><td>8</td><td>New Jersey</td><td>1,116,213</td><td>3.54%</td><td>30</td><td>Colorado</td><td>350,530</td><td>1.11%</td></tr>
<tr><td>37</td><td>New Mexico</td><td>161,825</td><td>0.51%</td><td>31</td><td>Arkansas</td><td>349,684</td><td>1.11%</td></tr>
<tr><td>2</td><td>New York</td><td>2,410,059</td><td>7.63%</td><td>32</td><td>Kansas</td><td>299,026</td><td>0.95%</td></tr>
<tr><td>12</td><td>North Carolina</td><td>817,153</td><td>2.59%</td><td>33</td><td>Oregon</td><td>298,129</td><td>0.94%</td></tr>
<tr><td>46</td><td>North Dakota</td><td>92,500</td><td>0.29%</td><td>34</td><td>West Virginia</td><td>282,686</td><td>0.90%</td></tr>
<tr><td>7</td><td>Ohio</td><td>1,435,875</td><td>4.55%</td><td>35</td><td>Nebraska</td><td>182,601</td><td>0.58%</td></tr>
<tr><td>27</td><td>Oklahoma</td><td>374,689</td><td>1.19%</td><td>36</td><td>Utah</td><td>179,313</td><td>0.57%</td></tr>
<tr><td>33</td><td>Oregon</td><td>298,129</td><td>0.94%</td><td>37</td><td>New Mexico</td><td>161,825</td><td>0.51%</td></tr>
<tr><td>4</td><td>Pennsylvania</td><td>1,873,852</td><td>5.93%</td><td>38</td><td>Maine</td><td>149,377</td><td>0.47%</td></tr>
<tr><td>39</td><td>Rhode Island</td><td>129,154</td><td>0.41%</td><td>39</td><td>Rhode Island</td><td>129,154</td><td>0.41%</td></tr>
<tr><td>25</td><td>South Carolina</td><td>404,647</td><td>1.28%</td><td>40</td><td>Nevada</td><td>127,193</td><td>0.40%</td></tr>
<tr><td>45</td><td>South Dakota</td><td>95,689</td><td>0.30%</td><td>41</td><td>New Hampshire</td><td>116,891</td><td>0.37%</td></tr>
<tr><td>13</td><td>Tennessee</td><td>766,668</td><td>2.43%</td><td>42</td><td>Idaho</td><td>101,698</td><td>0.32%</td></tr>
<tr><td>3</td><td>Texas</td><td>2,028,297</td><td>6.42%</td><td>43</td><td>Montana</td><td>97,795</td><td>0.31%</td></tr>
<tr><td>36</td><td>Utah</td><td>179,313</td><td>0.57%</td><td>44</td><td>Hawaii</td><td>97,649</td><td>0.31%</td></tr>
<tr><td>48</td><td>Vermont</td><td>59,090</td><td>0.19%</td><td>45</td><td>South Dakota</td><td>95,689</td><td>0.30%</td></tr>
<tr><td>16</td><td>Virginia</td><td>721,656</td><td>2.29%</td><td>46</td><td>North Dakota</td><td>92,500</td><td>0.29%</td></tr>
<tr><td>23</td><td>Washington</td><td>503,004</td><td>1.59%</td><td>47</td><td>Delaware</td><td>82,329</td><td>0.26%</td></tr>
<tr><td>34</td><td>West Virginia</td><td>282,686</td><td>0.90%</td><td>48</td><td>Vermont</td><td>59,090</td><td>0.19%</td></tr>
<tr><td>19</td><td>Wisconsin</td><td>587,696</td><td>1.86%</td><td>49</td><td>Wyoming</td><td>43,295</td><td>0.14%</td></tr>
<tr><td>49</td><td>Wyoming</td><td>43,295</td><td>0.14%</td><td>50</td><td>Alaska</td><td>39,679</td><td>0.13%</td></tr>
<tr><td></td><td></td><td></td><td></td><td></td><td>District of Columbia</td><td>161,073</td><td>0.51%</td></tr>
</table>

Source: American Hospital Association (Chicago, IL)
  "Hospital Statistics" (1994–95 edition)

Admissions to Psychiatric Hospitals in 1993

National Total = 798,216 Admissions*

ALPHA ORDER

ALPHA ORDER

RANK	STATE	ADMISSIONS	% of USA
22	Alabama	12,994	1.63%
43	Alaska	2,408	0.30%
17	Arizona	15,525	1.94%
32	Arkansas	7,624	0.96%
1	California	66,077	8.28%
26	Colorado	9,856	1.23%
25	Connecticut	9,953	1.25%
41	Delaware	2,984	0.37%
5	Florida	42,342	5.30%
6	Georgia	42,325	5.30%
49	Hawaii	447	0.06%
42	Idaho	2,657	0.33%
7	Illinois	35,426	4.44%
19	Indiana	15,397	1.93%
34	Iowa	6,344	0.79%
28	Kansas	8,992	1.13%
21	Kentucky	14,441	1.81%
12	Louisiana	23,931	3.00%
39	Maine	4,258	0.53%
18	Maryland	15,433	1.93%
13	Massachusetts	21,699	2.72%
11	Michigan	26,228	3.29%
30	Minnesota	8,132	1.02%
29	Mississippi	8,476	1.06%
16	Missouri	17,787	2.23%
50	Montana	147	0.02%
36	Nebraska	5,724	0.72%
40	Nevada	4,159	0.52%
33	New Hampshire	6,813	0.85%
20	New Jersey	14,455	1.81%
24	New Mexico	10,722	1.34%
4	New York	46,090	5.77%
8	North Carolina	30,228	3.79%
46	North Dakota	1,614	0.20%
10	Ohio	28,305	3.55%
23	Oklahoma	11,308	1.42%
37	Oregon	4,893	0.61%
3	Pennsylvania	46,742	5.86%
44	Rhode Island	2,215	0.28%
27	South Carolina	9,835	1.23%
48	South Dakota	761	0.10%
15	Tennessee	18,404	2.31%
2	Texas	57,802	7.24%
35	Utah	5,791	0.73%
47	Vermont	1,586	0.20%
9	Virginia	29,808	3.73%
31	Washington	7,978	1.00%
38	West Virginia	4,378	0.55%
14	Wisconsin	21,659	2.71%
45	Wyoming	2,039	0.26%

RANK ORDER

RANK	STATE	ADMISSIONS	% of USA
1	California	66,077	8.28%
2	Texas	57,802	7.24%
3	Pennsylvania	46,742	5.86%
4	New York	46,090	5.77%
5	Florida	42,342	5.30%
6	Georgia	42,325	5.30%
7	Illinois	35,426	4.44%
8	North Carolina	30,228	3.79%
9	Virginia	29,808	3.73%
10	Ohio	28,305	3.55%
11	Michigan	26,228	3.29%
12	Louisiana	23,931	3.00%
13	Massachusetts	21,699	2.72%
14	Wisconsin	21,659	2.71%
15	Tennessee	18,404	2.31%
16	Missouri	17,787	2.23%
17	Arizona	15,525	1.94%
18	Maryland	15,433	1.93%
19	Indiana	15,397	1.93%
20	New Jersey	14,455	1.81%
21	Kentucky	14,441	1.81%
22	Alabama	12,994	1.63%
23	Oklahoma	11,308	1.42%
24	New Mexico	10,722	1.34%
25	Connecticut	9,953	1.25%
26	Colorado	9,856	1.23%
27	South Carolina	9,835	1.23%
28	Kansas	8,992	1.13%
29	Mississippi	8,476	1.06%
30	Minnesota	8,132	1.02%
31	Washington	7,978	1.00%
32	Arkansas	7,624	0.96%
33	New Hampshire	6,813	0.85%
34	Iowa	6,344	0.79%
35	Utah	5,791	0.73%
36	Nebraska	5,724	0.72%
37	Oregon	4,893	0.61%
38	West Virginia	4,378	0.55%
39	Maine	4,258	0.53%
40	Nevada	4,159	0.52%
41	Delaware	2,984	0.37%
42	Idaho	2,657	0.33%
43	Alaska	2,408	0.30%
44	Rhode Island	2,215	0.28%
45	Wyoming	2,039	0.26%
46	North Dakota	1,614	0.20%
47	Vermont	1,586	0.20%
48	South Dakota	761	0.10%
49	Hawaii	447	0.06%
50	Montana	147	0.02%
	District of Columbia	3,024	0.38%

Source: American Hospital Association (Chicago, IL)
   "Hospital Statistics" (1994–95 edition)
*Admissions to federal and nonfederal psychiatric hospitals.

Admissions to Community Hospitals in 1993

National Total = 30,784,051 Admissions*

<table>
<tr><td colspan="4"><u>ALPHA ORDER</u></td><td colspan="4"><u>RANK ORDER</u></td></tr>
<tr><td>RANK</td><td>STATE</td><td>ADMISSIONS</td><td>% of USA</td><td>RANK</td><td>STATE</td><td>ADMISSIONS</td><td>% of USA</td></tr>
<tr><td>17</td><td>Alabama</td><td>604,896</td><td>1.97%</td><td>1</td><td>California</td><td>3,052,158</td><td>9.93%</td></tr>
<tr><td>50</td><td>Alaska</td><td>37,271</td><td>0.12%</td><td>2</td><td>New York</td><td>2,359,947</td><td>7.68%</td></tr>
<tr><td>24</td><td>Arizona</td><td>403,611</td><td>1.31%</td><td>3</td><td>Texas</td><td>1,963,869</td><td>6.39%</td></tr>
<tr><td>30</td><td>Arkansas</td><td>342,060</td><td>1.11%</td><td>4</td><td>Pennsylvania</td><td>1,830,705</td><td>5.95%</td></tr>
<tr><td>1</td><td>California</td><td>3,052,158</td><td>9.93%</td><td>5</td><td>Florida</td><td>1,705,636</td><td>5.55%</td></tr>
<tr><td>31</td><td>Colorado</td><td>340,015</td><td>1.11%</td><td>6</td><td>Illinois</td><td>1,467,767</td><td>4.77%</td></tr>
<tr><td>29</td><td>Connecticut</td><td>346,315</td><td>1.13%</td><td>7</td><td>Ohio</td><td>1,413,700</td><td>4.60%</td></tr>
<tr><td>47</td><td>Delaware</td><td>79,345</td><td>0.26%</td><td>8</td><td>New Jersey</td><td>1,103,244</td><td>3.59%</td></tr>
<tr><td>5</td><td>Florida</td><td>1,705,636</td><td>5.55%</td><td>9</td><td>Michigan</td><td>1,059,423</td><td>3.45%</td></tr>
<tr><td>10</td><td>Georgia</td><td>853,149</td><td>2.77%</td><td>10</td><td>Georgia</td><td>853,149</td><td>2.77%</td></tr>
<tr><td>44</td><td>Hawaii</td><td>96,859</td><td>0.32%</td><td>11</td><td>Massachusetts</td><td>817,255</td><td>2.66%</td></tr>
<tr><td>42</td><td>Idaho</td><td>99,041</td><td>0.32%</td><td>12</td><td>North Carolina</td><td>785,519</td><td>2.55%</td></tr>
<tr><td>6</td><td>Illinois</td><td>1,467,767</td><td>4.77%</td><td>13</td><td>Tennessee</td><td>747,256</td><td>2.43%</td></tr>
<tr><td>14</td><td>Indiana</td><td>712,260</td><td>2.32%</td><td>14</td><td>Indiana</td><td>712,260</td><td>2.32%</td></tr>
<tr><td>28</td><td>Iowa</td><td>348,442</td><td>1.13%</td><td>15</td><td>Missouri</td><td>705,086</td><td>2.29%</td></tr>
<tr><td>33</td><td>Kansas</td><td>289,830</td><td>0.94%</td><td>16</td><td>Virginia</td><td>690,737</td><td>2.25%</td></tr>
<tr><td>21</td><td>Kentucky</td><td>532,615</td><td>1.73%</td><td>17</td><td>Alabama</td><td>604,896</td><td>1.97%</td></tr>
<tr><td>18</td><td>Louisiana</td><td>598,048</td><td>1.94%</td><td>18</td><td>Louisiana</td><td>598,048</td><td>1.94%</td></tr>
<tr><td>38</td><td>Maine</td><td>145,119</td><td>0.47%</td><td>19</td><td>Wisconsin</td><td>568,412</td><td>1.85%</td></tr>
<tr><td>20</td><td>Maryland</td><td>559,278</td><td>1.82%</td><td>20</td><td>Maryland</td><td>559,278</td><td>1.82%</td></tr>
<tr><td>11</td><td>Massachusetts</td><td>817,255</td><td>2.66%</td><td>21</td><td>Kentucky</td><td>532,615</td><td>1.73%</td></tr>
<tr><td>9</td><td>Michigan</td><td>1,059,423</td><td>3.45%</td><td>22</td><td>Minnesota</td><td>496,129</td><td>1.61%</td></tr>
<tr><td>22</td><td>Minnesota</td><td>496,129</td><td>1.61%</td><td>23</td><td>Washington</td><td>494,242</td><td>1.61%</td></tr>
<tr><td>26</td><td>Mississippi</td><td>370,775</td><td>1.21%</td><td>24</td><td>Arizona</td><td>403,611</td><td>1.31%</td></tr>
<tr><td>15</td><td>Missouri</td><td>705,086</td><td>2.29%</td><td>25</td><td>South Carolina</td><td>394,225</td><td>1.28%</td></tr>
<tr><td>43</td><td>Montana</td><td>97,502</td><td>0.32%</td><td>26</td><td>Mississippi</td><td>370,775</td><td>1.21%</td></tr>
<tr><td>35</td><td>Nebraska</td><td>175,133</td><td>0.57%</td><td>27</td><td>Oklahoma</td><td>363,163</td><td>1.18%</td></tr>
<tr><td>40</td><td>Nevada</td><td>123,034</td><td>0.40%</td><td>28</td><td>Iowa</td><td>348,442</td><td>1.13%</td></tr>
<tr><td>41</td><td>New Hampshire</td><td>109,708</td><td>0.36%</td><td>29</td><td>Connecticut</td><td>346,315</td><td>1.13%</td></tr>
<tr><td>8</td><td>New Jersey</td><td>1,103,244</td><td>3.59%</td><td>30</td><td>Arkansas</td><td>342,060</td><td>1.11%</td></tr>
<tr><td>37</td><td>New Mexico</td><td>151,103</td><td>0.49%</td><td>31</td><td>Colorado</td><td>340,015</td><td>1.11%</td></tr>
<tr><td>2</td><td>New York</td><td>2,359,947</td><td>7.68%</td><td>32</td><td>Oregon</td><td>293,172</td><td>0.95%</td></tr>
<tr><td>12</td><td>North Carolina</td><td>785,519</td><td>2.55%</td><td>33</td><td>Kansas</td><td>289,830</td><td>0.94%</td></tr>
<tr><td>46</td><td>North Dakota</td><td>90,762</td><td>0.30%</td><td>34</td><td>West Virginia</td><td>278,308</td><td>0.91%</td></tr>
<tr><td>7</td><td>Ohio</td><td>1,413,700</td><td>4.60%</td><td>35</td><td>Nebraska</td><td>175,133</td><td>0.57%</td></tr>
<tr><td>27</td><td>Oklahoma</td><td>363,163</td><td>1.18%</td><td>36</td><td>Utah</td><td>173,522</td><td>0.56%</td></tr>
<tr><td>32</td><td>Oregon</td><td>293,172</td><td>0.95%</td><td>37</td><td>New Mexico</td><td>151,103</td><td>0.49%</td></tr>
<tr><td>4</td><td>Pennsylvania</td><td>1,830,705</td><td>5.95%</td><td>38</td><td>Maine</td><td>145,119</td><td>0.47%</td></tr>
<tr><td>39</td><td>Rhode Island</td><td>126,781</td><td>0.41%</td><td>39</td><td>Rhode Island</td><td>126,781</td><td>0.41%</td></tr>
<tr><td>25</td><td>South Carolina</td><td>394,225</td><td>1.28%</td><td>40</td><td>Nevada</td><td>123,034</td><td>0.40%</td></tr>
<tr><td>45</td><td>South Dakota</td><td>94,877</td><td>0.31%</td><td>41</td><td>New Hampshire</td><td>109,708</td><td>0.36%</td></tr>
<tr><td>13</td><td>Tennessee</td><td>747,256</td><td>2.43%</td><td>42</td><td>Idaho</td><td>99,041</td><td>0.32%</td></tr>
<tr><td>3</td><td>Texas</td><td>1,963,869</td><td>6.39%</td><td>43</td><td>Montana</td><td>97,502</td><td>0.32%</td></tr>
<tr><td>36</td><td>Utah</td><td>173,522</td><td>0.56%</td><td>44</td><td>Hawaii</td><td>96,859</td><td>0.32%</td></tr>
<tr><td>48</td><td>Vermont</td><td>57,504</td><td>0.19%</td><td>45</td><td>South Dakota</td><td>94,877</td><td>0.31%</td></tr>
<tr><td>16</td><td>Virginia</td><td>690,737</td><td>2.25%</td><td>46</td><td>North Dakota</td><td>90,762</td><td>0.30%</td></tr>
<tr><td>23</td><td>Washington</td><td>494,242</td><td>1.61%</td><td>47</td><td>Delaware</td><td>79,345</td><td>0.26%</td></tr>
<tr><td>34</td><td>West Virginia</td><td>278,308</td><td>0.91%</td><td>48</td><td>Vermont</td><td>57,504</td><td>0.19%</td></tr>
<tr><td>19</td><td>Wisconsin</td><td>568,412</td><td>1.85%</td><td>49</td><td>Wyoming</td><td>42,833</td><td>0.14%</td></tr>
<tr><td>49</td><td>Wyoming</td><td>42,833</td><td>0.14%</td><td>50</td><td>Alaska</td><td>37,271</td><td>0.12%</td></tr>
<tr><td></td><td></td><td></td><td></td><td></td><td>District of Columbia</td><td>156,410</td><td>0.51%</td></tr>
</table>

Source: American Hospital Association (Chicago, IL)
"Hospital Statistics" (1994-95 edition)
Community hospital admissions are a subset of nonfederal hospital admissions.

Admissions to Nongovernment Not–For–Profit Hospitals in 1993

National Total = 22,748,731 Admissions*

ALPHA ORDER

RANK	STATE	ADMISSIONS	% of USA
29	Alabama	223,432	0.98%
49	Alaska	26,339	0.12%
23	Arizona	336,858	1.48%
28	Arkansas	236,076	1.04%
1	California	2,055,893	9.04%
25	Colorado	250,758	1.10%
22	Connecticut	339,767	1.49%
44	Delaware	79,345	0.35%
9	Florida	896,539	3.94%
20	Georgia	374,195	1.64%
45	Hawaii	69,946	0.31%
47	Idaho	47,717	0.21%
4	Illinois	1,300,377	5.72%
15	Indiana	509,343	2.24%
27	Iowa	242,461	1.07%
33	Kansas	178,707	0.79%
21	Kentucky	370,027	1.63%
24	Louisiana	251,845	1.11%
35	Maine	138,860	0.61%
12	Maryland	546,182	2.40%
10	Massachusetts	747,820	3.29%
7	Michigan	985,127	4.33%
18	Minnesota	390,975	1.72%
34	Mississippi	165,652	0.73%
11	Missouri	587,040	2.58%
40	Montana	91,793	0.40%
37	Nebraska	125,117	0.55%
48	Nevada	38,824	0.17%
39	New Hampshire	99,941	0.44%
6	New Jersey	1,072,540	4.71%
43	New Mexico	85,048	0.37%
2	New York	1,925,749	8.47%
16	North Carolina	486,738	2.14%
42	North Dakota	85,997	0.38%
5	Ohio	1,271,279	5.59%
32	Oklahoma	205,543	0.90%
26	Oregon	245,643	1.08%
3	Pennsylvania	1,817,744	7.99%
36	Rhode Island	126,781	0.56%
31	South Carolina	207,735	0.91%
41	South Dakota	90,790	0.40%
17	Tennessee	474,272	2.08%
8	Texas	985,051	4.33%
38	Utah	118,935	0.52%
46	Vermont	57,504	0.25%
14	Virginia	511,425	2.25%
19	Washington	374,446	1.65%
30	West Virginia	217,077	0.95%
13	Wisconsin	530,065	2.33%
50	Wyoming	12,134	0.05%

RANK ORDER

RANK	STATE	ADMISSIONS	% of USA
1	California	2,055,893	9.04%
2	New York	1,925,749	8.47%
3	Pennsylvania	1,817,744	7.99%
4	Illinois	1,300,377	5.72%
5	Ohio	1,271,279	5.59%
6	New Jersey	1,072,540	4.71%
7	Michigan	985,127	4.33%
8	Texas	985,051	4.33%
9	Florida	896,539	3.94%
10	Massachusetts	747,820	3.29%
11	Missouri	587,040	2.58%
12	Maryland	546,182	2.40%
13	Wisconsin	530,065	2.33%
14	Virginia	511,425	2.25%
15	Indiana	509,343	2.24%
16	North Carolina	486,738	2.14%
17	Tennessee	474,272	2.08%
18	Minnesota	390,975	1.72%
19	Washington	374,446	1.65%
20	Georgia	374,195	1.64%
21	Kentucky	370,027	1.63%
22	Connecticut	339,767	1.49%
23	Arizona	336,858	1.48%
24	Louisiana	251,845	1.11%
25	Colorado	250,758	1.10%
26	Oregon	245,643	1.08%
27	Iowa	242,461	1.07%
28	Arkansas	236,076	1.04%
29	Alabama	223,432	0.98%
30	West Virginia	217,077	0.95%
31	South Carolina	207,735	0.91%
32	Oklahoma	205,543	0.90%
33	Kansas	178,707	0.79%
34	Mississippi	165,652	0.73%
35	Maine	138,860	0.61%
36	Rhode Island	126,781	0.56%
37	Nebraska	125,117	0.55%
38	Utah	118,935	0.52%
39	New Hampshire	99,941	0.44%
40	Montana	91,793	0.40%
41	South Dakota	90,790	0.40%
42	North Dakota	85,997	0.38%
43	New Mexico	85,048	0.37%
44	Delaware	79,345	0.35%
45	Hawaii	69,946	0.31%
46	Vermont	57,504	0.25%
47	Idaho	47,717	0.21%
48	Nevada	38,824	0.17%
49	Alaska	26,339	0.12%
50	Wyoming	12,134	0.05%
	District of Columbia	139,279	0.61%

Source: American Hospital Association (Chicago, IL)
"Hospital Statistics" (1994–95 edition)
*Nongovernment not–for–profit hospital admissions are a subset of community hospital admissions.

197

Admissions to Investor-Owned (For-Profit) Hospitals in 1993

National Total = 2,945,807 Admissions*

ALPHA ORDER					RANK ORDER			
RANK	STATE	ADMISSIONS	% of USA		RANK	STATE	ADMISSIONS	% of USA
6	Alabama	115,470	3.92%		1	Texas	534,118	18.13%
36	Alaska	5,934	0.20%		2	Florida	514,598	17.47%
20	Arizona	35,834	1.22%		3	California	417,845	14.18%
14	Arkansas	43,840	1.49%		4	Georgia	133,233	4.52%
3	California	417,845	14.18%		5	Tennessee	128,771	4.37%
26	Colorado	14,049	0.48%		6	Alabama	115,470	3.92%
44	Connecticut	0	0.00%		7	Kentucky	109,746	3.73%
44	Delaware	0	0.00%		8	Louisiana	106,111	3.60%
2	Florida	514,598	17.47%		9	Virginia	90,556	3.07%
4	Georgia	133,233	4.52%		10	New York	84,744	2.88%
35	Hawaii	6,468	0.22%		11	Illinois	57,957	1.97%
25	Idaho	14,847	0.50%		12	Nevada	56,611	1.92%
11	Illinois	57,957	1.97%		13	South Carolina	56,468	1.92%
24	Indiana	22,160	0.75%		14	Arkansas	43,840	1.49%
39	Iowa	3,105	0.11%		15	North Carolina	43,566	1.48%
16	Kansas	43,022	1.46%		16	Kansas	43,022	1.46%
7	Kentucky	109,746	3.73%		17	Oklahoma	40,966	1.39%
8	Louisiana	106,111	3.60%		18	Mississippi	37,665	1.28%
42	Maine	790	0.03%		19	Missouri	36,723	1.25%
28	Maryland	13,096	0.44%		20	Arizona	35,834	1.22%
32	Massachusetts	10,349	0.35%		21	Utah	33,425	1.13%
43	Michigan	669	0.02%		22	West Virginia	31,277	1.06%
44	Minnesota	0	0.00%		23	New Mexico	23,175	0.79%
18	Mississippi	37,665	1.28%		24	Indiana	22,160	0.75%
19	Missouri	36,723	1.25%		25	Idaho	14,847	0.50%
44	Montana	0	0.00%		26	Colorado	14,049	0.48%
34	Nebraska	9,667	0.33%		27	Washington	13,185	0.45%
12	Nevada	56,611	1.92%		28	Maryland	13,096	0.44%
33	New Hampshire	9,767	0.33%		29	Oregon	11,733	0.40%
40	New Jersey	1,517	0.05%		30	Pennsylvania	11,100	0.38%
23	New Mexico	23,175	0.79%		31	Ohio	10,543	0.36%
10	New York	84,744	2.88%		32	Massachusetts	10,349	0.35%
15	North Carolina	43,566	1.48%		33	New Hampshire	9,767	0.33%
37	North Dakota	4,060	0.14%		34	Nebraska	9,667	0.33%
31	Ohio	10,543	0.36%		35	Hawaii	6,468	0.22%
17	Oklahoma	40,966	1.39%		36	Alaska	5,934	0.20%
29	Oregon	11,733	0.40%		37	North Dakota	4,060	0.14%
30	Pennsylvania	11,100	0.38%		38	Wyoming	3,732	0.13%
44	Rhode Island	0	0.00%		39	Iowa	3,105	0.11%
13	South Carolina	56,468	1.92%		40	New Jersey	1,517	0.05%
44	South Dakota	0	0.00%		41	Wisconsin	939	0.03%
5	Tennessee	128,771	4.37%		42	Maine	790	0.03%
1	Texas	534,118	18.13%		43	Michigan	669	0.02%
21	Utah	33,425	1.13%		44	Connecticut	0	0.00%
44	Vermont	0	0.00%		44	Delaware	0	0.00%
9	Virginia	90,556	3.07%		44	Minnesota	0	0.00%
27	Washington	13,185	0.45%		44	Montana	0	0.00%
22	West Virginia	31,277	1.06%		44	Rhode Island	0	0.00%
41	Wisconsin	939	0.03%		44	South Dakota	0	0.00%
38	Wyoming	3,732	0.13%		44	Vermont	0	0.00%
					District of Columbia		2,376	0.08%

Source: American Hospital Association (Chicago, IL)
  "Hospital Statistics" (1994-95 edition)
*Investor-owned (for-profit) hospital admissions are a subset of community hospital admissions.

Admissions to State and Local Government-Owned Hospitals in 1993

National Total = 5,053,513 Admissions*

ALPHA ORDER

RANK	STATE	ADMISSIONS	% of USA
6	Alabama	265,994	5.26%
42	Alaska	4,998	0.10%
32	Arizona	30,919	0.61%
24	Arkansas	62,144	1.23%
1	California	578,420	11.45%
21	Colorado	75,208	1.49%
39	Connecticut	6,548	0.13%
46	Delaware	0	0.00%
5	Florida	294,499	5.83%
4	Georgia	345,721	6.84%
38	Hawaii	20,445	0.40%
30	Idaho	36,477	0.72%
15	Illinois	109,433	2.17%
9	Indiana	180,757	3.58%
18	Iowa	102,876	2.04%
23	Kansas	68,101	1.35%
26	Kentucky	52,842	1.05%
8	Louisiana	240,092	4.75%
41	Maine	5,469	0.11%
46	Maryland	0	0.00%
25	Massachusetts	59,086	1.17%
22	Michigan	73,627	1.46%
17	Minnesota	105,154	2.08%
10	Mississippi	167,458	3.31%
20	Missouri	81,323	1.61%
40	Montana	5,709	0.11%
28	Nebraska	40,349	0.80%
35	Nevada	27,599	0.55%
46	New Hampshire	0	0.00%
34	New Jersey	29,187	0.58%
27	New Mexico	42,880	0.85%
3	New York	349,454	6.92%
7	North Carolina	255,215	5.05%
45	North Dakota	705	0.01%
12	Ohio	131,878	2.61%
14	Oklahoma	116,654	2.31%
31	Oregon	35,796	0.71%
44	Pennsylvania	1,861	0.04%
46	Rhode Island	0	0.00%
13	South Carolina	130,022	2.57%
43	South Dakota	4,087	0.08%
11	Tennessee	144,213	2.85%
2	Texas	444,700	8.80%
37	Utah	21,162	0.42%
46	Vermont	0	0.00%
19	Virginia	88,756	1.76%
16	Washington	106,611	2.11%
33	West Virginia	29,954	0.59%
29	Wisconsin	37,408	0.74%
36	Wyoming	26,967	0.53%

RANK ORDER

RANK	STATE	ADMISSIONS	% of USA
1	California	578,420	11.45%
2	Texas	444,700	8.80%
3	New York	349,454	6.92%
4	Georgia	345,721	6.84%
5	Florida	294,499	5.83%
6	Alabama	265,994	5.26%
7	North Carolina	255,215	5.05%
8	Louisiana	240,092	4.75%
9	Indiana	180,757	3.58%
10	Mississippi	167,458	3.31%
11	Tennessee	144,213	2.85%
12	Ohio	131,878	2.61%
13	South Carolina	130,022	2.57%
14	Oklahoma	116,654	2.31%
15	Illinois	109,433	2.17%
16	Washington	106,611	2.11%
17	Minnesota	105,154	2.08%
18	Iowa	102,876	2.04%
19	Virginia	88,756	1.76%
20	Missouri	81,323	1.61%
21	Colorado	75,208	1.49%
22	Michigan	73,627	1.46%
23	Kansas	68,101	1.35%
24	Arkansas	62,144	1.23%
25	Massachusetts	59,086	1.17%
26	Kentucky	52,842	1.05%
27	New Mexico	42,880	0.85%
28	Nebraska	40,349	0.80%
29	Wisconsin	37,408	0.74%
30	Idaho	36,477	0.72%
31	Oregon	35,796	0.71%
32	Arizona	30,919	0.61%
33	West Virginia	29,954	0.59%
34	New Jersey	29,187	0.58%
35	Nevada	27,599	0.55%
36	Wyoming	26,967	0.53%
37	Utah	21,162	0.42%
38	Hawaii	20,445	0.40%
39	Connecticut	6,548	0.13%
40	Montana	5,709	0.11%
41	Maine	5,469	0.11%
42	Alaska	4,998	0.10%
43	South Dakota	4,087	0.08%
44	Pennsylvania	1,861	0.04%
45	North Dakota	705	0.01%
46	Delaware	0	0.00%
46	Maryland	0	0.00%
46	New Hampshire	0	0.00%
46	Rhode Island	0	0.00%
46	Vermont	0	0.00%
	District of Columbia	14,755	0.29%

Source: American Hospital Association (Chicago, IL)
  "Hospital Statistics" (1994-95 edition)
*State and local government-owned hospital admissions are a subset of community hospital admissions.

Inpatient Days in Community Hospitals in 1993

National Total = 215,888,741 Inpatient Days*

ALPHA ORDER

RANK ORDER

RANK	STATE	DAYS	% of USA	RANK	STATE	DAYS	% of USA
18	Alabama	4,108,104	1.90%	1	New York	23,402,454	10.84%
50	Alaska	245,818	0.11%	2	California	17,365,463	8.04%
32	Arizona	2,052,605	0.95%	3	Pennsylvania	14,139,233	6.55%
28	Arkansas	2,335,646	1.08%	4	Texas	11,811,104	5.47%
2	California	17,365,463	8.04%	5	Florida	11,273,286	5.22%
31	Colorado	2,196,090	1.02%	6	Illinois	10,211,839	4.73%
27	Connecticut	2,502,350	1.16%	7	Ohio	9,082,749	4.21%
47	Delaware	561,190	0.26%	8	New Jersey	8,732,017	4.04%
5	Florida	11,273,286	5.22%	9	Michigan	7,308,050	3.39%
10	Georgia	6,120,063	2.83%	10	Georgia	6,120,063	2.83%
41	Hawaii	887,575	0.41%	11	North Carolina	5,756,125	2.67%
46	Idaho	683,071	0.32%	12	Massachusetts	5,502,284	2.55%
6	Illinois	10,211,839	4.73%	13	Missouri	5,073,434	2.35%
16	Indiana	4,560,893	2.11%	14	Tennessee	5,062,785	2.35%
23	Iowa	2,827,700	1.31%	15	Virginia	4,579,844	2.12%
30	Kansas	2,233,372	1.03%	16	Indiana	4,560,893	2.11%
21	Kentucky	3,608,607	1.67%	17	Minnesota	4,430,314	2.05%
20	Louisiana	3,965,313	1.84%	18	Alabama	4,108,104	1.90%
36	Maine	1,100,319	0.51%	19	Wisconsin	4,090,257	1.89%
22	Maryland	3,569,632	1.65%	20	Louisiana	3,965,313	1.84%
12	Massachusetts	5,502,284	2.55%	21	Kentucky	3,608,607	1.67%
9	Michigan	7,308,050	3.39%	22	Maryland	3,569,632	1.65%
17	Minnesota	4,430,314	2.05%	23	Iowa	2,827,700	1.31%
25	Mississippi	2,710,871	1.26%	24	South Carolina	2,798,795	1.30%
13	Missouri	5,073,434	2.35%	25	Mississippi	2,710,871	1.26%
38	Montana	989,324	0.46%	26	Washington	2,519,676	1.17%
34	Nebraska	1,685,237	0.78%	27	Connecticut	2,502,350	1.16%
40	Nevada	919,175	0.43%	28	Arkansas	2,335,646	1.08%
45	New Hampshire	783,161	0.36%	29	Oklahoma	2,330,892	1.08%
8	New Jersey	8,732,017	4.04%	30	Kansas	2,233,372	1.03%
43	New Mexico	812,333	0.38%	31	Colorado	2,196,090	1.02%
1	New York	23,402,454	10.84%	32	Arizona	2,052,605	0.95%
11	North Carolina	5,756,125	2.67%	33	West Virginia	1,882,320	0.87%
37	North Dakota	1,025,437	0.47%	34	Nebraska	1,685,237	0.78%
7	Ohio	9,082,749	4.21%	35	Oregon	1,483,377	0.69%
29	Oklahoma	2,330,892	1.08%	36	Maine	1,100,319	0.51%
35	Oregon	1,483,377	0.69%	37	North Dakota	1,025,437	0.47%
3	Pennsylvania	14,139,233	6.55%	38	Montana	989,324	0.46%
44	Rhode Island	810,515	0.38%	39	South Dakota	943,666	0.44%
24	South Carolina	2,798,795	1.30%	40	Nevada	919,175	0.43%
39	South Dakota	943,666	0.44%	41	Hawaii	887,575	0.41%
14	Tennessee	5,062,785	2.35%	42	Utah	856,010	0.40%
4	Texas	11,811,104	5.47%	43	New Mexico	812,333	0.38%
42	Utah	856,010	0.40%	44	Rhode Island	810,515	0.38%
48	Vermont	453,141	0.21%	45	New Hampshire	783,161	0.36%
15	Virginia	4,579,844	2.12%	46	Idaho	683,071	0.32%
26	Washington	2,519,676	1.17%	47	Delaware	561,190	0.26%
33	West Virginia	1,882,320	0.87%	48	Vermont	453,141	0.21%
19	Wisconsin	4,090,257	1.89%	49	Wyoming	386,378	0.18%
49	Wyoming	386,378	0.18%	50	Alaska	245,818	0.11%
					District of Columbia	1,118,847	0.52%

Source: American Hospital Association (Chicago, IL)
    "Hospital Statistics" (1994–95 edition)
Community hospital inpatient days are a subset of nonfederal hospital inpatient days.

Average Daily Census in Community Hospitals in 1993

National Average = 591,702 Daily Census*

ALPHA ORDER

RANK	STATE	PATIENTS	% of USA
18	Alabama	11,259	1.90%
50	Alaska	674	0.11%
32	Arizona	5,626	0.95%
28	Arkansas	6,401	1.08%
2	California	47,579	8.04%
31	Colorado	6,018	1.02%
27	Connecticut	6,854	1.16%
47	Delaware	1,537	0.26%
5	Florida	30,977	5.24%
10	Georgia	16,786	2.84%
41	Hawaii	2,435	0.41%
46	Idaho	1,869	0.32%
6	Illinois	28,006	4.73%
16	Indiana	12,497	2.11%
23	Iowa	7,744	1.31%
30	Kansas	6,116	1.03%
21	Kentucky	9,887	1.67%
20	Louisiana	10,864	1.84%
36	Maine	3,017	0.51%
22	Maryland	9,791	1.65%
12	Massachusetts	15,078	2.55%
9	Michigan	20,023	3.38%
17	Minnesota	12,140	2.05%
25	Mississippi	7,429	1.26%
13	Missouri	13,899	2.35%
38	Montana	2,713	0.46%
34	Nebraska	4,613	0.78%
40	Nevada	2,517	0.43%
45	New Hampshire	2,146	0.36%
8	New Jersey	23,919	4.04%
43	New Mexico	2,224	0.38%
1	New York	64,086	10.83%
11	North Carolina	15,772	2.67%
37	North Dakota	2,809	0.47%
7	Ohio	24,877	4.20%
29	Oklahoma	6,391	1.08%
35	Oregon	4,067	0.69%
3	Pennsylvania	38,740	6.55%
44	Rhode Island	2,221	0.38%
24	South Carolina	7,668	1.30%
39	South Dakota	2,584	0.44%
14	Tennessee	13,867	2.34%
4	Texas	32,465	5.49%
42	Utah	2,348	0.40%
48	Vermont	1,241	0.21%
15	Virginia	12,549	2.12%
26	Washington	6,904	1.17%
33	West Virginia	5,157	0.87%
19	Wisconsin	11,195	1.89%
49	Wyoming	1,058	0.18%

RANK ORDER

RANK	STATE	PATIENTS	% of USA
1	New York	64,086	10.83%
2	California	47,579	8.04%
3	Pennsylvania	38,740	6.55%
4	Texas	32,465	5.49%
5	Florida	30,977	5.24%
6	Illinois	28,006	4.73%
7	Ohio	24,877	4.20%
8	New Jersey	23,919	4.04%
9	Michigan	20,023	3.38%
10	Georgia	16,786	2.84%
11	North Carolina	15,772	2.67%
12	Massachusetts	15,078	2.55%
13	Missouri	13,899	2.35%
14	Tennessee	13,867	2.34%
15	Virginia	12,549	2.12%
16	Indiana	12,497	2.11%
17	Minnesota	12,140	2.05%
18	Alabama	11,259	1.90%
19	Wisconsin	11,195	1.89%
20	Louisiana	10,864	1.84%
21	Kentucky	9,887	1.67%
22	Maryland	9,791	1.65%
23	Iowa	7,744	1.31%
24	South Carolina	7,668	1.30%
25	Mississippi	7,429	1.26%
26	Washington	6,904	1.17%
27	Connecticut	6,854	1.16%
28	Arkansas	6,401	1.08%
29	Oklahoma	6,391	1.08%
30	Kansas	6,116	1.03%
31	Colorado	6,018	1.02%
32	Arizona	5,626	0.95%
33	West Virginia	5,157	0.87%
34	Nebraska	4,613	0.78%
35	Oregon	4,067	0.69%
36	Maine	3,017	0.51%
37	North Dakota	2,809	0.47%
38	Montana	2,713	0.46%
39	South Dakota	2,584	0.44%
40	Nevada	2,517	0.43%
41	Hawaii	2,435	0.41%
42	Utah	2,348	0.40%
43	New Mexico	2,224	0.38%
44	Rhode Island	2,221	0.38%
45	New Hampshire	2,146	0.36%
46	Idaho	1,869	0.32%
47	Delaware	1,537	0.26%
48	Vermont	1,241	0.21%
49	Wyoming	1,058	0.18%
50	Alaska	674	0.11%
	District of Columbia	3,065	0.52%

Source: American Hospital Association (Chicago, IL)
    "Hospital Statistics" (1994-95 edition)
*Average total of inpatients receiving care. Excludes newborns.

Average Stay in Community Hospitals in 1993

National Average = 7.0 Days*

ALPHA ORDER			RANK ORDER		
RANK	STATE	DAYS	RANK	STATE	DAYS
28	Alabama	6.8	1	North Dakota	11.3
34	Alaska	6.6	2	Montana	10.1
47	Arizona	5.1	3	New York	9.9
28	Arkansas	6.8	3	South Dakota	9.9
45	California	5.7	5	Nebraska	9.6
38	Colorado	6.5	6	Hawaii	9.2
18	Connecticut	7.2	7	Wyoming	9.0
22	Delaware	7.1	8	Minnesota	8.9
34	Florida	6.6	9	Iowa	8.1
18	Georgia	7.2	10	New Jersey	7.9
6	Hawaii	9.2	10	Vermont	7.9
26	Idaho	6.9	12	Kansas	7.7
25	Illinois	7.0	12	Pennsylvania	7.7
39	Indiana	6.4	14	Maine	7.6
9	Iowa	8.1	15	Nevada	7.5
12	Kansas	7.7	16	Mississippi	7.3
28	Kentucky	6.8	16	North Carolina	7.3
34	Louisiana	6.6	18	Connecticut	7.2
14	Maine	7.6	18	Georgia	7.2
39	Maryland	6.4	18	Missouri	7.2
33	Massachusetts	6.7	18	Wisconsin	7.2
26	Michigan	6.9	22	Delaware	7.1
8	Minnesota	8.9	22	New Hampshire	7.1
16	Mississippi	7.3	22	South Carolina	7.1
18	Missouri	7.2	25	Illinois	7.0
2	Montana	10.1	26	Idaho	6.9
5	Nebraska	9.6	26	Michigan	6.9
15	Nevada	7.5	28	Alabama	6.8
22	New Hampshire	7.1	28	Arkansas	6.8
10	New Jersey	7.9	28	Kentucky	6.8
46	New Mexico	5.4	28	Tennessee	6.8
3	New York	9.9	28	West Virginia	6.8
16	North Carolina	7.3	33	Massachusetts	6.7
1	North Dakota	11.3	34	Alaska	6.6
39	Ohio	6.4	34	Florida	6.6
39	Oklahoma	6.4	34	Louisiana	6.6
47	Oregon	5.1	34	Virginia	6.6
12	Pennsylvania	7.7	38	Colorado	6.5
39	Rhode Island	6.4	39	Indiana	6.4
22	South Carolina	7.1	39	Maryland	6.4
3	South Dakota	9.9	39	Ohio	6.4
28	Tennessee	6.8	39	Oklahoma	6.4
44	Texas	6.0	39	Rhode Island	6.4
50	Utah	4.9	44	Texas	6.0
10	Vermont	7.9	45	California	5.7
34	Virginia	6.6	46	New Mexico	5.4
47	Washington	5.1	47	Arizona	5.1
28	West Virginia	6.8	47	Oregon	5.1
18	Wisconsin	7.2	47	Washington	5.1
7	Wyoming	9.0	50	Utah	4.9

District of Columbia   7.2

Source: American Hospital Association (Chicago, IL)
"Hospital Statistics" (1994–95 edition)
Community hospitals are a subset of nonfederal hospitals.

Occupancy Rates in Community Hospitals in 1993

National Rate = 64.4% of Community Hospital Beds Occupied*

ALPHA ORDER

RANK	STATE	RATE
27	Alabama	60.7
49	Alaska	52.9
40	Arizona	57.4
36	Arkansas	58.0
26	California	61.0
34	Colorado	58.6
5	Connecticut	73.8
8	Delaware	71.4
29	Florida	60.4
19	Georgia	63.4
1	Hawaii	83.3
42	Idaho	55.4
20	Illinois	63.2
35	Indiana	58.3
37	Iowa	57.9
46	Kansas	54.2
24	Kentucky	61.9
39	Louisiana	57.5
12	Maine	67.5
4	Maryland	74.6
9	Massachusetts	71.3
15	Michigan	64.5
14	Minnesota	65.8
32	Mississippi	59.0
33	Missouri	58.9
21	Montana	63.1
43	Nebraska	54.8
11	Nevada	67.7
22	New Hampshire	62.4
3	New Jersey	77.1
47	New Mexico	54.0
2	New York	82.8
10	North Carolina	69.6
17	North Dakota	63.9
31	Ohio	59.9
45	Oklahoma	54.3
44	Oregon	54.4
7	Pennsylvania	72.1
6	Rhode Island	72.8
13	South Carolina	67.4
28	South Dakota	60.6
29	Tennessee	60.4
41	Texas	55.8
48	Utah	53.7
15	Vermont	64.5
17	Virginia	63.9
38	Washington	57.8
25	West Virginia	61.8
23	Wisconsin	62.0
50	Wyoming	48.8

RANK ORDER

RANK	STATE	RATE
1	Hawaii	83.3
2	New York	82.8
3	New Jersey	77.1
4	Maryland	74.6
5	Connecticut	73.8
6	Rhode Island	72.8
7	Pennsylvania	72.1
8	Delaware	71.4
9	Massachusetts	71.3
10	North Carolina	69.6
11	Nevada	67.7
12	Maine	67.5
13	South Carolina	67.4
14	Minnesota	65.8
15	Michigan	64.5
15	Vermont	64.5
17	North Dakota	63.9
17	Virginia	63.9
19	Georgia	63.4
20	Illinois	63.2
21	Montana	63.1
22	New Hampshire	62.4
23	Wisconsin	62.0
24	Kentucky	61.9
25	West Virginia	61.8
26	California	61.0
27	Alabama	60.7
28	South Dakota	60.6
29	Florida	60.4
29	Tennessee	60.4
31	Ohio	59.9
32	Mississippi	59.0
33	Missouri	58.9
34	Colorado	58.6
35	Indiana	58.3
36	Arkansas	58.0
37	Iowa	57.9
38	Washington	57.8
39	Louisiana	57.5
40	Arizona	57.4
41	Texas	55.8
42	Idaho	55.4
43	Nebraska	54.8
44	Oregon	54.4
45	Oklahoma	54.3
46	Kansas	54.2
47	New Mexico	54.0
48	Utah	53.7
49	Alaska	52.9
50	Wyoming	48.8

	District of Columbia	71.6

Source: Morgan Quitno Press using data from American Hospital Association (Chicago, IL)
"Hospital Statistics" (1994-95 edition)
*Average daily census compared to number of community hospitals beds.

Outpatient Visits to Hospitals in 1993

National Total = 435,619,234 Visits*

ALPHA ORDER

ALPHA ORDER

RANK	STATE	VISITS	% of USA
23	Alabama	6,349,147	1.46%
47	Alaska	1,315,427	0.30%
27	Arizona	5,386,035	1.24%
35	Arkansas	3,478,478	0.80%
1	California	44,015,994	10.10%
22	Colorado	6,509,642	1.49%
25	Connecticut	5,721,401	1.31%
46	Delaware	1,449,760	0.33%
7	Florida	19,136,273	4.39%
12	Georgia	11,144,486	2.56%
37	Hawaii	2,819,588	0.65%
41	Idaho	1,792,327	0.41%
5	Illinois	21,598,440	4.96%
11	Indiana	11,253,721	2.58%
28	Iowa	5,355,826	1.23%
31	Kansas	4,537,105	1.04%
20	Kentucky	7,077,125	1.62%
19	Louisiana	8,161,303	1.87%
39	Maine	2,419,242	0.56%
21	Maryland	6,592,705	1.51%
9	Massachusetts	13,699,136	3.14%
8	Michigan	17,720,237	4.07%
24	Minnesota	5,818,520	1.34%
34	Mississippi	3,680,029	0.84%
15	Missouri	9,671,838	2.22%
44	Montana	1,515,588	0.35%
38	Nebraska	2,654,465	0.61%
42	Nevada	1,638,332	0.38%
40	New Hampshire	1,869,837	0.43%
10	New Jersey	12,206,095	2.80%
32	New Mexico	4,038,228	0.93%
2	New York	37,813,921	8.68%
13	North Carolina	9,979,402	2.29%
48	North Dakota	1,234,130	0.28%
6	Ohio	20,813,797	4.78%
30	Oklahoma	4,618,265	1.06%
29	Oregon	4,884,789	1.12%
3	Pennsylvania	25,898,389	5.95%
43	Rhode Island	1,618,259	0.37%
26	South Carolina	5,420,432	1.24%
45	South Dakota	1,477,182	0.34%
17	Tennessee	8,417,393	1.93%
4	Texas	23,909,603	5.49%
36	Utah	3,331,132	0.76%
49	Vermont	953,176	0.22%
14	Virginia	9,895,408	2.27%
16	Washington	9,177,300	2.11%
33	West Virginia	3,849,625	0.88%
18	Wisconsin	8,258,431	1.90%
50	Wyoming	831,723	0.19%

RANK ORDER

RANK	STATE	VISITS	% of USA
1	California	44,015,994	10.10%
2	New York	37,813,921	8.68%
3	Pennsylvania	25,898,389	5.95%
4	Texas	23,909,603	5.49%
5	Illinois	21,598,440	4.96%
6	Ohio	20,813,797	4.78%
7	Florida	19,136,273	4.39%
8	Michigan	17,720,237	4.07%
9	Massachusetts	13,699,136	3.14%
10	New Jersey	12,206,095	2.80%
11	Indiana	11,253,721	2.58%
12	Georgia	11,144,486	2.56%
13	North Carolina	9,979,402	2.29%
14	Virginia	9,895,408	2.27%
15	Missouri	9,671,838	2.22%
16	Washington	9,177,300	2.11%
17	Tennessee	8,417,393	1.93%
18	Wisconsin	8,258,431	1.90%
19	Louisiana	8,161,303	1.87%
20	Kentucky	7,077,125	1.62%
21	Maryland	6,592,705	1.51%
22	Colorado	6,509,642	1.49%
23	Alabama	6,349,147	1.46%
24	Minnesota	5,818,520	1.34%
25	Connecticut	5,721,401	1.31%
26	South Carolina	5,420,432	1.24%
27	Arizona	5,386,035	1.24%
28	Iowa	5,355,826	1.23%
29	Oregon	4,884,789	1.12%
30	Oklahoma	4,618,265	1.06%
31	Kansas	4,537,105	1.04%
32	New Mexico	4,038,228	0.93%
33	West Virginia	3,849,625	0.88%
34	Mississippi	3,680,029	0.84%
35	Arkansas	3,478,478	0.80%
36	Utah	3,331,132	0.76%
37	Hawaii	2,819,588	0.65%
38	Nebraska	2,654,465	0.61%
39	Maine	2,419,242	0.56%
40	New Hampshire	1,869,837	0.43%
41	Idaho	1,792,327	0.41%
42	Nevada	1,638,332	0.38%
43	Rhode Island	1,618,259	0.37%
44	Montana	1,515,588	0.35%
45	South Dakota	1,477,182	0.34%
46	Delaware	1,449,760	0.33%
47	Alaska	1,315,427	0.30%
48	North Dakota	1,234,130	0.28%
49	Vermont	953,176	0.22%
50	Wyoming	831,723	0.19%
	District of Columbia	2,610,547	0.60%

Source: American Hospital Association (Chicago, IL)
"Hospital Statistics" (1994–95 edition)
*To federal and nonfederal hospitals. Includes emergency and other visits.

Emergency Outpatient Visits to Hospitals in 1993

National Total = 97,379,119 Visits*

ALPHA ORDER

RANK	STATE	VISITS	% of USA
18	Alabama	2,035,095	2.09%
46	Alaska	253,504	0.26%
25	Arizona	1,324,045	1.36%
30	Arkansas	1,090,812	1.12%
1	California	9,311,601	9.56%
27	Colorado	1,186,847	1.22%
26	Connecticut	1,307,531	1.34%
45	Delaware	273,633	0.28%
4	Florida	5,338,364	5.48%
9	Georgia	3,333,476	3.42%
43	Hawaii	290,876	0.30%
42	Idaho	372,328	0.38%
7	Illinois	4,240,904	4.36%
15	Indiana	2,205,897	2.27%
33	Iowa	975,536	1.00%
34	Kansas	824,328	0.85%
20	Kentucky	1,825,036	1.87%
17	Louisiana	2,039,850	2.09%
35	Maine	614,171	0.63%
22	Maryland	1,518,310	1.56%
11	Massachusetts	2,811,412	2.89%
8	Michigan	3,428,738	3.52%
29	Minnesota	1,147,366	1.18%
24	Mississippi	1,339,665	1.38%
16	Missouri	2,128,675	2.19%
44	Montana	285,266	0.29%
40	Nebraska	431,138	0.44%
41	Nevada	420,217	0.43%
39	New Hampshire	445,681	0.46%
13	New Jersey	2,579,580	2.65%
37	New Mexico	579,318	0.59%
2	New York	6,743,867	6.93%
10	North Carolina	2,879,133	2.96%
48	North Dakota	244,270	0.25%
6	Ohio	4,818,874	4.95%
28	Oklahoma	1,152,386	1.18%
31	Oregon	1,065,693	1.09%
5	Pennsylvania	5,119,070	5.26%
38	Rhode Island	468,802	0.48%
23	South Carolina	1,492,830	1.53%
47	South Dakota	246,392	0.25%
12	Tennessee	2,592,534	2.66%
3	Texas	6,047,177	6.21%
36	Utah	601,264	0.62%
49	Vermont	205,417	0.21%
14	Virginia	2,424,106	2.49%
19	Washington	2,013,278	2.07%
32	West Virginia	1,045,937	1.07%
21	Wisconsin	1,638,080	1.68%
50	Wyoming	193,151	0.20%

RANK ORDER

RANK	STATE	VISITS	% of USA
1	California	9,311,601	9.56%
2	New York	6,743,867	6.93%
3	Texas	6,047,177	6.21%
4	Florida	5,338,364	5.48%
5	Pennsylvania	5,119,070	5.26%
6	Ohio	4,818,874	4.95%
7	Illinois	4,240,904	4.36%
8	Michigan	3,428,738	3.52%
9	Georgia	3,333,476	3.42%
10	North Carolina	2,879,133	2.96%
11	Massachusetts	2,811,412	2.89%
12	Tennessee	2,592,534	2.66%
13	New Jersey	2,579,580	2.65%
14	Virginia	2,424,106	2.49%
15	Indiana	2,205,897	2.27%
16	Missouri	2,128,675	2.19%
17	Louisiana	2,039,850	2.09%
18	Alabama	2,035,095	2.09%
19	Washington	2,013,278	2.07%
20	Kentucky	1,825,036	1.87%
21	Wisconsin	1,638,080	1.68%
22	Maryland	1,518,310	1.56%
23	South Carolina	1,492,830	1.53%
24	Mississippi	1,339,665	1.38%
25	Arizona	1,324,045	1.36%
26	Connecticut	1,307,531	1.34%
27	Colorado	1,186,847	1.22%
28	Oklahoma	1,152,386	1.18%
29	Minnesota	1,147,366	1.18%
30	Arkansas	1,090,812	1.12%
31	Oregon	1,065,693	1.09%
32	West Virginia	1,045,937	1.07%
33	Iowa	975,536	1.00%
34	Kansas	824,328	0.85%
35	Maine	614,171	0.63%
36	Utah	601,264	0.62%
37	New Mexico	579,318	0.59%
38	Rhode Island	468,802	0.48%
39	New Hampshire	445,681	0.46%
40	Nebraska	431,138	0.44%
41	Nevada	420,217	0.43%
42	Idaho	372,328	0.38%
43	Hawaii	290,876	0.30%
44	Montana	285,266	0.29%
45	Delaware	273,633	0.28%
46	Alaska	253,504	0.26%
47	South Dakota	246,392	0.25%
48	North Dakota	244,270	0.25%
49	Vermont	205,417	0.21%
50	Wyoming	193,151	0.20%
	District of Columbia	427,658	0.44%

Source: American Hospital Association (Chicago, IL)
   "Hospital Statistics" (1994–95 edition)
*To federal and nonfederal hospitals.

Surgical Operations in Hospitals in 1993

National Total = 23,842,543 Surgical Operations*

ALPHA ORDER

RANK	STATE	OPERATIONS	% of USA
22	Alabama	404,801	1.70%
50	Alaska	38,699	0.16%
25	Arizona	307,004	1.29%
31	Arkansas	246,882	1.04%
1	California	2,070,306	8.68%
27	Colorado	294,463	1.24%
30	Connecticut	267,654	1.12%
42	Delaware	86,158	0.36%
5	Florida	1,318,805	5.53%
11	Georgia	620,294	2.60%
46	Hawaii	72,464	0.30%
44	Idaho	80,033	0.34%
7	Illinois	1,046,272	4.39%
13	Indiana	586,898	2.46%
24	Iowa	389,943	1.64%
33	Kansas	238,402	1.00%
20	Kentucky	426,691	1.79%
21	Louisiana	415,969	1.74%
38	Maine	120,740	0.51%
15	Maryland	556,594	2.33%
10	Massachusetts	673,416	2.82%
8	Michigan	904,800	3.79%
23	Minnesota	392,538	1.65%
34	Mississippi	235,299	0.99%
14	Missouri	569,347	2.39%
47	Montana	68,952	0.29%
35	Nebraska	179,492	0.75%
40	Nevada	110,340	0.46%
41	New Hampshire	88,652	0.37%
9	New Jersey	681,158	2.86%
36	New Mexico	147,842	0.62%
2	New York	1,666,765	6.99%
12	North Carolina	598,990	2.51%
43	North Dakota	80,162	0.34%
6	Ohio	1,164,691	4.88%
28	Oklahoma	287,222	1.20%
29	Oregon	268,179	1.12%
4	Pennsylvania	1,497,009	6.28%
39	Rhode Island	112,587	0.47%
26	South Carolina	306,835	1.29%
45	South Dakota	74,818	0.31%
16	Tennessee	555,390	2.33%
3	Texas	1,519,720	6.37%
37	Utah	142,007	0.60%
48	Vermont	44,319	0.19%
17	Virginia	528,202	2.22%
18	Washington	509,228	2.14%
32	West Virginia	238,513	1.00%
19	Wisconsin	449,549	1.89%
49	Wyoming	39,853	0.17%

RANK ORDER

RANK	STATE	OPERATIONS	% of USA
1	California	2,070,306	8.68%
2	New York	1,666,765	6.99%
3	Texas	1,519,720	6.37%
4	Pennsylvania	1,497,009	6.28%
5	Florida	1,318,805	5.53%
6	Ohio	1,164,691	4.88%
7	Illinois	1,046,272	4.39%
8	Michigan	904,800	3.79%
9	New Jersey	681,158	2.86%
10	Massachusetts	673,416	2.82%
11	Georgia	620,294	2.60%
12	North Carolina	598,990	2.51%
13	Indiana	586,898	2.46%
14	Missouri	569,347	2.39%
15	Maryland	556,594	2.33%
16	Tennessee	555,390	2.33%
17	Virginia	528,202	2.22%
18	Washington	509,228	2.14%
19	Wisconsin	449,549	1.89%
20	Kentucky	426,691	1.79%
21	Louisiana	415,969	1.74%
22	Alabama	404,801	1.70%
23	Minnesota	392,538	1.65%
24	Iowa	389,943	1.64%
25	Arizona	307,004	1.29%
26	South Carolina	306,835	1.29%
27	Colorado	294,463	1.24%
28	Oklahoma	287,222	1.20%
29	Oregon	268,179	1.12%
30	Connecticut	267,654	1.12%
31	Arkansas	246,882	1.04%
32	West Virginia	238,513	1.00%
33	Kansas	238,402	1.00%
34	Mississippi	235,299	0.99%
35	Nebraska	179,492	0.75%
36	New Mexico	147,842	0.62%
37	Utah	142,007	0.60%
38	Maine	120,740	0.51%
39	Rhode Island	112,587	0.47%
40	Nevada	110,340	0.46%
41	New Hampshire	88,652	0.37%
42	Delaware	86,158	0.36%
43	North Dakota	80,162	0.34%
44	Idaho	80,033	0.34%
45	South Dakota	74,818	0.31%
46	Hawaii	72,464	0.30%
47	Montana	68,952	0.29%
48	Vermont	44,319	0.19%
49	Wyoming	39,853	0.17%
50	Alaska	38,699	0.16%
	District of Columbia	117,596	0.49%

Source: American Hospital Association (Chicago, IL)
"Hospital Statistics" (1994–95 edition)
In federal and nonfederal hospital operating rooms.

Medicare and Medicaid Certified Hospitals in 1995

National Total = 6,357 Hospitals*

ALPHA ORDER					RANK ORDER			
RANK	STATE		HOSPITALS	% of USA	RANK	STATE	HOSPITALS	% of USA
20	Alabama		129	2.03%	1	California	535	8.42%
47	Alaska		25	0.39%	2	Texas	520	8.18%
29	Arizona		87	1.37%	3	Florida	281	4.42%
28	Arkansas		97	1.53%	4	New York	274	4.31%
1	California		535	8.42%	5	Pennsylvania	266	4.18%
29	Colorado		87	1.37%	6	Illinois	227	3.57%
40	Connecticut		51	0.80%	7	Ohio	219	3.45%
50	Delaware		12	0.19%	8	Louisiana	198	3.11%
3	Florida		281	4.42%	9	Georgia	196	3.08%
9	Georgia		196	3.08%	10	Michigan	193	3.04%
46	Hawaii		26	0.41%	11	Indiana	160	2.52%
41	Idaho		49	0.77%	12	Tennessee	154	2.42%
6	Illinois		227	3.57%	13	Minnesota	153	2.41%
11	Indiana		160	2.52%	14	Missouri	151	2.38%
22	Iowa		123	1.93%	15	Oklahoma	149	2.34%
16	Kansas		148	2.33%	16	Kansas	148	2.33%
22	Kentucky		123	1.93%	17	Wisconsin	147	2.31%
8	Louisiana		198	3.11%	18	North Carolina	145	2.28%
42	Maine		44	0.69%	19	Massachusetts	137	2.16%
32	Maryland		74	1.16%	20	Alabama	129	2.03%
19	Massachusetts		137	2.16%	21	Virginia	126	1.98%
10	Michigan		193	3.04%	22	Iowa	123	1.93%
13	Minnesota		153	2.41%	22	Kentucky	123	1.93%
25	Mississippi		109	1.71%	24	New Jersey	112	1.76%
14	Missouri		151	2.38%	25	Mississippi	109	1.71%
37	Montana		55	0.87%	26	Nebraska	100	1.57%
26	Nebraska		100	1.57%	27	Washington	99	1.56%
43	Nevada		34	0.53%	28	Arkansas	97	1.53%
44	New Hampshire		31	0.49%	29	Arizona	87	1.37%
24	New Jersey		112	1.76%	29	Colorado	87	1.37%
36	New Mexico		58	0.91%	31	South Carolina	76	1.20%
4	New York		274	4.31%	32	Maryland	74	1.16%
18	North Carolina		145	2.28%	33	West Virginia	68	1.07%
38	North Dakota		52	0.82%	34	Oregon	67	1.05%
7	Ohio		219	3.45%	35	South Dakota	60	0.94%
15	Oklahoma		149	2.34%	36	New Mexico	58	0.91%
34	Oregon		67	1.05%	37	Montana	55	0.87%
5	Pennsylvania		266	4.18%	38	North Dakota	52	0.82%
48	Rhode Island		18	0.28%	38	Utah	52	0.82%
31	South Carolina		76	1.20%	40	Connecticut	51	0.80%
35	South Dakota		60	0.94%	41	Idaho	49	0.77%
12	Tennessee		154	2.42%	42	Maine	44	0.69%
2	Texas		520	8.18%	43	Nevada	34	0.53%
38	Utah		52	0.82%	44	New Hampshire	31	0.49%
49	Vermont		17	0.27%	45	Wyoming	29	0.46%
21	Virginia		126	1.98%	46	Hawaii	26	0.41%
27	Washington		99	1.56%	47	Alaska	25	0.39%
33	West Virginia		68	1.07%	48	Rhode Island	18	0.28%
17	Wisconsin		147	2.31%	49	Vermont	17	0.27%
45	Wyoming		29	0.46%	50	Delaware	12	0.19%
						District of Columbia	14	0.22%

Source: U.S. Department of Health and Human Services, Health Care Financing Administration unpublished data (February 27, 1995)

*Certified by HCFA to participate in the Medicare/Medicaid programs. National total does not include 61 certified hospitals in U.S. territories.

Medicare and Medicaid Certified Hospices in 1995

National Total = 1,685 Hospices*

<u>ALPHA ORDER</u>

RANK	STATE	HOSPICES	% of USA
15	Alabama	38	2.26%
50	Alaska	2	0.12%
27	Arizona	25	1.48%
12	Arkansas	42	2.49%
1	California	129	7.66%
24	Colorado	30	1.78%
27	Connecticut	25	1.48%
48	Delaware	4	0.24%
17	Florida	37	2.20%
15	Georgia	38	2.26%
45	Hawaii	7	0.42%
37	Idaho	18	1.07%
5	Illinois	72	4.27%
21	Indiana	32	1.90%
17	Iowa	37	2.20%
30	Kansas	24	1.42%
25	Kentucky	29	1.72%
31	Louisiana	23	1.36%
39	Maine	12	0.71%
23	Maryland	31	1.84%
14	Massachusetts	41	2.43%
7	Michigan	62	3.68%
12	Minnesota	42	2.49%
32	Mississippi	22	1.31%
8	Missouri	55	3.26%
40	Montana	11	0.65%
38	Nebraska	14	0.83%
48	Nevada	4	0.24%
35	New Hampshire	20	1.19%
17	New Jersey	37	2.20%
32	New Mexico	22	1.31%
9	New York	52	3.09%
6	North Carolina	67	3.98%
41	North Dakota	10	0.59%
4	Ohio	76	4.51%
20	Oklahoma	34	2.02%
21	Oregon	32	1.90%
3	Pennsylvania	92	5.46%
45	Rhode Island	7	0.42%
26	South Carolina	27	1.60%
42	South Dakota	8	0.47%
10	Tennessee	51	3.03%
2	Texas	103	6.11%
47	Utah	6	0.36%
42	Vermont	8	0.47%
32	Virginia	22	1.31%
27	Washington	25	1.48%
36	West Virginia	19	1.13%
11	Wisconsin	50	2.97%
42	Wyoming	8	0.47%

<u>RANK ORDER</u>

RANK	STATE	HOSPICES	% of USA
1	California	129	7.66%
2	Texas	103	6.11%
3	Pennsylvania	92	5.46%
4	Ohio	76	4.51%
5	Illinois	72	4.27%
6	North Carolina	67	3.98%
7	Michigan	62	3.68%
8	Missouri	55	3.26%
9	New York	52	3.09%
10	Tennessee	51	3.03%
11	Wisconsin	50	2.97%
12	Arkansas	42	2.49%
12	Minnesota	42	2.49%
14	Massachusetts	41	2.43%
15	Alabama	38	2.26%
15	Georgia	38	2.26%
17	Florida	37	2.20%
17	Iowa	37	2.20%
17	New Jersey	37	2.20%
20	Oklahoma	34	2.02%
21	Indiana	32	1.90%
21	Oregon	32	1.90%
23	Maryland	31	1.84%
24	Colorado	30	1.78%
25	Kentucky	29	1.72%
26	South Carolina	27	1.60%
27	Arizona	25	1.48%
27	Connecticut	25	1.48%
27	Washington	25	1.48%
30	Kansas	24	1.42%
31	Louisiana	23	1.36%
32	Mississippi	22	1.31%
32	New Mexico	22	1.31%
32	Virginia	22	1.31%
35	New Hampshire	20	1.19%
36	West Virginia	19	1.13%
37	Idaho	18	1.07%
38	Nebraska	14	0.83%
39	Maine	12	0.71%
40	Montana	11	0.65%
41	North Dakota	10	0.59%
42	South Dakota	8	0.47%
42	Vermont	8	0.47%
42	Wyoming	8	0.47%
45	Hawaii	7	0.42%
45	Rhode Island	7	0.42%
47	Utah	6	0.36%
48	Delaware	4	0.24%
48	Nevada	4	0.24%
50	Alaska	2	0.12%
	District of Columbia	3	0.18%

Source: U.S. Department of Health and Human Services, Health Care Financing Administration unpublished data (February 27, 1995)

*Certified by HCFA to participate in the Medicare/Medicaid programs. National total does not include 44 certified hospices in U.S. territories.

Medicare and Medicaid Certified Rural Health Clinics in 1995

National Total = 2,148 Rural Health Clinics*

ALPHA ORDER

RANK	STATE	CLINICS	% of USA
16	Alabama	52	2.42%
40	Alaska	8	0.37%
41	Arizona	5	0.23%
11	Arkansas	71	3.31%
2	California	138	6.42%
28	Colorado	23	1.07%
46	Connecticut	0	0.00%
46	Delaware	0	0.00%
8	Florida	83	3.86%
12	Georgia	70	3.26%
43	Hawaii	2	0.09%
30	Idaho	20	0.93%
5	Illinois	94	4.38%
37	Indiana	10	0.47%
8	Iowa	83	3.86%
4	Kansas	123	5.73%
22	Kentucky	28	1.30%
24	Louisiana	25	1.16%
31	Maine	18	0.84%
46	Maryland	0	0.00%
46	Massachusetts	0	0.00%
15	Michigan	53	2.47%
27	Minnesota	24	1.12%
3	Mississippi	128	5.96%
7	Missouri	87	4.05%
24	Montana	25	1.16%
17	Nebraska	49	2.28%
44	Nevada	1	0.05%
35	New Hampshire	12	0.56%
46	New Jersey	0	0.00%
37	New Mexico	10	0.47%
36	New York	11	0.51%
6	North Carolina	92	4.28%
14	North Dakota	63	2.93%
42	Ohio	4	0.19%
13	Oklahoma	67	3.12%
29	Oregon	22	1.02%
23	Pennsylvania	27	1.26%
44	Rhode Island	1	0.05%
19	South Carolina	40	1.86%
18	South Dakota	44	2.05%
10	Tennessee	72	3.35%
1	Texas	314	14.62%
34	Utah	14	0.65%
32	Vermont	16	0.74%
32	Virginia	16	0.74%
21	Washington	29	1.35%
20	West Virginia	39	1.82%
24	Wisconsin	25	1.16%
37	Wyoming	10	0.47%

RANK ORDER

RANK	STATE	CLINICS	% of USA
1	Texas	314	14.62%
2	California	138	6.42%
3	Mississippi	128	5.96%
4	Kansas	123	5.73%
5	Illinois	94	4.38%
6	North Carolina	92	4.28%
7	Missouri	87	4.05%
8	Florida	83	3.86%
8	Iowa	83	3.86%
10	Tennessee	72	3.35%
11	Arkansas	71	3.31%
12	Georgia	70	3.26%
13	Oklahoma	67	3.12%
14	North Dakota	63	2.93%
15	Michigan	53	2.47%
16	Alabama	52	2.42%
17	Nebraska	49	2.28%
18	South Dakota	44	2.05%
19	South Carolina	40	1.86%
20	West Virginia	39	1.82%
21	Washington	29	1.35%
22	Kentucky	28	1.30%
23	Pennsylvania	27	1.26%
24	Louisiana	25	1.16%
24	Montana	25	1.16%
24	Wisconsin	25	1.16%
27	Minnesota	24	1.12%
28	Colorado	23	1.07%
29	Oregon	22	1.02%
30	Idaho	20	0.93%
31	Maine	18	0.84%
32	Vermont	16	0.74%
32	Virginia	16	0.74%
34	Utah	14	0.65%
35	New Hampshire	12	0.56%
36	New York	11	0.51%
37	Indiana	10	0.47%
37	New Mexico	10	0.47%
37	Wyoming	10	0.47%
40	Alaska	8	0.37%
41	Arizona	5	0.23%
42	Ohio	4	0.19%
43	Hawaii	2	0.09%
44	Nevada	1	0.05%
44	Rhode Island	1	0.05%
46	Connecticut	0	0.00%
46	Delaware	0	0.00%
46	Maryland	0	0.00%
46	Massachusetts	0	0.00%
46	New Jersey	0	0.00%
	District of Columbia	0	0.00%

Source: U.S. Department of Health and Human Services, Health Care Financing Administration
    unpublished data (February 27, 1995)
*Certified by HCFA to participate in the Medicare/Medicaid programs. There are no certified rural health clinics in U.S. territories.

Medicare and Medicaid Certified Home Health Agencies in 1995

National Total = 8,222 Home Health Agencies*

ALPHA ORDER

RANK	STATE	AGENCIES	% of USA
18	Alabama	176	2.14%
47	Alaska	21	0.26%
26	Arizona	99	1.20%
15	Arkansas	204	2.48%
2	California	652	7.93%
22	Colorado	160	1.95%
24	Connecticut	116	1.41%
49	Delaware	19	0.23%
7	Florida	314	3.82%
28	Georgia	82	1.00%
46	Hawaii	26	0.32%
37	Idaho	57	0.69%
6	Illinois	325	3.95%
12	Indiana	219	2.66%
17	Iowa	178	2.16%
21	Kansas	168	2.04%
25	Kentucky	107	1.30%
3	Louisiana	430	5.23%
45	Maine	30	0.36%
31	Maryland	74	0.90%
19	Massachusetts	174	2.12%
16	Michigan	181	2.20%
9	Minnesota	241	2.93%
30	Mississippi	75	0.91%
11	Missouri	237	2.88%
39	Montana	53	0.64%
32	Nebraska	68	0.83%
41	Nevada	45	0.55%
43	New Hampshire	39	0.47%
39	New Jersey	53	0.64%
27	New Mexico	83	1.01%
13	New York	213	2.59%
23	North Carolina	150	1.82%
44	North Dakota	33	0.40%
4	Ohio	367	4.46%
8	Oklahoma	253	3.08%
29	Oregon	81	0.99%
5	Pennsylvania	329	4.00%
47	Rhode Island	21	0.26%
35	South Carolina	66	0.80%
42	South Dakota	40	0.49%
10	Tennessee	238	2.89%
1	Texas	1,061	12.90%
32	Utah	68	0.83%
50	Vermont	13	0.16%
14	Virginia	207	2.52%
36	Washington	62	0.75%
34	West Virginia	67	0.81%
20	Wisconsin	171	2.08%
37	Wyoming	57	0.69%

RANK ORDER

RANK	STATE	AGENCIES	% of USA
1	Texas	1,061	12.90%
2	California	652	7.93%
3	Louisiana	430	5.23%
4	Ohio	367	4.46%
5	Pennsylvania	329	4.00%
6	Illinois	325	3.95%
7	Florida	314	3.82%
8	Oklahoma	253	3.08%
9	Minnesota	241	2.93%
10	Tennessee	238	2.89%
11	Missouri	237	2.88%
12	Indiana	219	2.66%
13	New York	213	2.59%
14	Virginia	207	2.52%
15	Arkansas	204	2.48%
16	Michigan	181	2.20%
17	Iowa	178	2.16%
18	Alabama	176	2.14%
19	Massachusetts	174	2.12%
20	Wisconsin	171	2.08%
21	Kansas	168	2.04%
22	Colorado	160	1.95%
23	North Carolina	150	1.82%
24	Connecticut	116	1.41%
25	Kentucky	107	1.30%
26	Arizona	99	1.20%
27	New Mexico	83	1.01%
28	Georgia	82	1.00%
29	Oregon	81	0.99%
30	Mississippi	75	0.91%
31	Maryland	74	0.90%
32	Nebraska	68	0.83%
32	Utah	68	0.83%
34	West Virginia	67	0.81%
35	South Carolina	66	0.80%
36	Washington	62	0.75%
37	Idaho	57	0.69%
37	Wyoming	57	0.69%
39	Montana	53	0.64%
39	New Jersey	53	0.64%
41	Nevada	45	0.55%
42	South Dakota	40	0.49%
43	New Hampshire	39	0.47%
44	North Dakota	33	0.40%
45	Maine	30	0.36%
46	Hawaii	26	0.32%
47	Alaska	21	0.26%
47	Rhode Island	21	0.26%
49	Delaware	19	0.23%
50	Vermont	13	0.16%
	District of Columbia	19	0.23%

Source: U.S. Department of Health and Human Services, Health Care Financing Administration unpublished data (February 27, 1995)
Certified by HCFA to participate in the Medicare/Medicaid programs. National total does not include 46 certified home health agencies in U.S. territories.

Medicare and Medicaid Certified Nursing Care Facilities in 1995

National Total = 16,869 Nursing Care Facilities*

ALPHA ORDER					RANK ORDER			
RANK	STATE	FACILITIES	% of USA		RANK	STATE	FACILITIES	% of USA
29	Alabama	220	1.30%		1	California	1,381	8.19%
50	Alaska	16	0.09%		2	Texas	1,313	7.78%
34	Arizona	149	0.88%		3	Ohio	992	5.88%
25	Arkansas	276	1.64%		4	Illinois	846	5.02%
1	California	1,381	8.19%		5	Pennsylvania	727	4.31%
30	Colorado	218	1.29%		6	Florida	650	3.85%
26	Connecticut	267	1.58%		7	New York	640	3.79%
46	Delaware	43	0.25%		8	Indiana	597	3.54%
6	Florida	650	3.85%		9	Massachusetts	558	3.31%
19	Georgia	357	2.12%		10	Missouri	541	3.21%
47	Hawaii	42	0.25%		11	Iowa	470	2.79%
43	Idaho	78	0.46%		12	Minnesota	461	2.73%
4	Illinois	846	5.02%		13	Oklahoma	446	2.64%
8	Indiana	597	3.54%		14	Michigan	442	2.62%
11	Iowa	470	2.79%		15	Kansas	437	2.59%
15	Kansas	437	2.59%		16	Wisconsin	413	2.45%
22	Kentucky	293	1.74%		17	North Carolina	390	2.31%
18	Louisiana	362	2.15%		18	Louisiana	362	2.15%
35	Maine	139	0.82%		19	Georgia	357	2.12%
28	Maryland	232	1.38%		20	Tennessee	320	1.90%
9	Massachusetts	558	3.31%		21	New Jersey	317	1.88%
14	Michigan	442	2.62%		22	Kentucky	293	1.74%
12	Minnesota	461	2.73%		23	Washington	283	1.68%
31	Mississippi	182	1.08%		24	Virginia	279	1.65%
10	Missouri	541	3.21%		25	Arkansas	276	1.64%
38	Montana	100	0.59%		26	Connecticut	267	1.58%
27	Nebraska	233	1.38%		27	Nebraska	233	1.38%
47	Nevada	42	0.25%		28	Maryland	232	1.38%
44	New Hampshire	77	0.46%		29	Alabama	220	1.30%
21	New Jersey	317	1.88%		30	Colorado	218	1.29%
42	New Mexico	82	0.49%		31	Mississippi	182	1.08%
7	New York	640	3.79%		32	South Carolina	167	0.99%
17	North Carolina	390	2.31%		33	Oregon	162	0.96%
41	North Dakota	86	0.51%		34	Arizona	149	0.88%
3	Ohio	992	5.88%		35	Maine	139	0.82%
13	Oklahoma	446	2.64%		36	West Virginia	131	0.78%
33	Oregon	162	0.96%		37	South Dakota	116	0.69%
5	Pennsylvania	727	4.31%		38	Montana	100	0.59%
39	Rhode Island	95	0.56%		39	Rhode Island	95	0.56%
32	South Carolina	167	0.99%		39	Utah	95	0.56%
37	South Dakota	116	0.69%		41	North Dakota	86	0.51%
20	Tennessee	320	1.90%		42	New Mexico	82	0.49%
2	Texas	1,313	7.78%		43	Idaho	78	0.46%
39	Utah	95	0.56%		44	New Hampshire	77	0.46%
45	Vermont	48	0.28%		45	Vermont	48	0.28%
24	Virginia	279	1.65%		46	Delaware	43	0.25%
23	Washington	283	1.68%		47	Hawaii	42	0.25%
36	West Virginia	131	0.78%		47	Nevada	42	0.25%
16	Wisconsin	413	2.45%		49	Wyoming	38	0.23%
49	Wyoming	38	0.23%		50	Alaska	16	0.09%
						District of Columbia	20	0.12%

Source: U.S. Department of Health and Human Services, Health Care Financing Administration
     unpublished data (February 27, 1995)

*Certified by HCFA to participate in the Medicare/Medicaid programs. National total does not include 8 certified nursing care facilities in U.S. territories.

Nursing Home Beds in 1991

National Total = 1,559,394 Nursing Home Beds

RANK	STATE	BEDS	% of USA		RANK	STATE	BEDS	% of USA
28	Alabama	21,323	1.37%		1	Texas	108,285	6.94%
50	Alaska	780	0.05%		2	California	105,781	6.78%
33	Arizona	13,265	0.85%		3	Illinois	95,465	6.12%
27	Arkansas	21,706	1.39%		4	New York	94,884	6.08%
2	California	105,781	6.78%		5	Pennsylvania	85,387	5.48%
30	Colorado	17,609	1.13%		6	Ohio	82,516	5.29%
21	Connecticut	27,983	1.79%		7	Florida	63,752	4.09%
45	Delaware	4,101	0.26%		8	Indiana	55,701	3.57%
7	Florida	63,752	4.09%		9	Missouri	51,652	3.31%
16	Georgia	35,011	2.25%		10	Massachusetts	50,133	3.21%
49	Hawaii	1,958	0.13%		11	Michigan	48,886	3.13%
44	Idaho	4,887	0.31%		12	Wisconsin	48,710	3.12%
3	Illinois	95,465	6.12%		13	Minnesota	42,001	2.69%
8	Indiana	55,701	3.57%		14	New Jersey	39,970	2.56%
17	Iowa	34,521	2.21%		15	Louisiana	36,644	2.35%
23	Kansas	27,115	1.74%		16	Georgia	35,011	2.25%
26	Kentucky	25,685	1.65%		17	Iowa	34,521	2.21%
15	Louisiana	36,644	2.35%		18	Tennessee	32,493	2.08%
37	Maine	9,192	0.59%		19	Oklahoma	32,421	2.08%
22	Maryland	27,163	1.74%		20	North Carolina	28,259	1.81%
10	Massachusetts	50,133	3.21%		21	Connecticut	27,983	1.79%
11	Michigan	48,886	3.13%		22	Maryland	27,163	1.74%
13	Minnesota	42,001	2.69%		23	Kansas	27,115	1.74%
31	Mississippi	14,431	0.93%		24	Washington	26,506	1.70%
9	Missouri	51,652	3.31%		25	Virginia	26,324	1.69%
43	Montana	5,713	0.37%		26	Kentucky	25,685	1.65%
29	Nebraska	17,846	1.14%		27	Arkansas	21,706	1.39%
47	Nevada	3,171	0.20%		28	Alabama	21,323	1.37%
39	New Hampshire	7,493	0.48%		29	Nebraska	17,846	1.14%
14	New Jersey	39,970	2.56%		30	Colorado	17,609	1.13%
42	New Mexico	5,933	0.38%		31	Mississippi	14,431	0.93%
4	New York	94,884	6.08%		32	Oregon	14,382	0.92%
20	North Carolina	28,259	1.81%		33	Arizona	13,265	0.85%
41	North Dakota	6,056	0.39%		34	South Carolina	13,122	0.84%
6	Ohio	82,516	5.29%		35	Rhode Island	9,915	0.64%
19	Oklahoma	32,421	2.08%		36	West Virginia	9,792	0.63%
32	Oregon	14,382	0.92%		37	Maine	9,192	0.59%
5	Pennsylvania	85,387	5.48%		38	South Dakota	8,448	0.54%
35	Rhode Island	9,915	0.64%		39	New Hampshire	7,493	0.48%
34	South Carolina	13,122	0.84%		40	Utah	6,292	0.40%
38	South Dakota	8,448	0.54%		41	North Dakota	6,056	0.39%
18	Tennessee	32,493	2.08%		42	New Mexico	5,933	0.38%
1	Texas	108,285	6.94%		43	Montana	5,713	0.37%
40	Utah	6,292	0.40%		44	Idaho	4,887	0.31%
46	Vermont	3,478	0.22%		45	Delaware	4,101	0.26%
25	Virginia	26,324	1.69%		46	Vermont	3,478	0.22%
24	Washington	26,506	1.70%		47	Nevada	3,171	0.20%
36	West Virginia	9,792	0.63%		48	Wyoming	2,243	0.14%
12	Wisconsin	48,710	3.12%		49	Hawaii	1,958	0.13%
48	Wyoming	2,243	0.14%		50	Alaska	780	0.05%
						District of Columbia	3,010	0.19%

ALPHA ORDER

RANK ORDER

Source: U.S. Department of Health and Human Services, National Center for Health Statistics unpublished data

Rate of Nursing Home Beds in 1991

National Rate = 49.1 Nursing Home Beds per 1,000 Population Age 65 and Older

<table>
<tr><td colspan="3">ALPHA ORDER</td><td colspan="3">RANK ORDER</td></tr>
<tr><th>RANK</th><th>STATE</th><th>RATE</th><th>RANK</th><th>STATE</th><th>RATE</th></tr>
<tr><td>35</td><td>Alabama</td><td>40.2</td><td>1</td><td>South Dakota</td><td>82.0</td></tr>
<tr><td>45</td><td>Alaska</td><td>32.5</td><td>2</td><td>Iowa</td><td>80.1</td></tr>
<tr><td>47</td><td>Arizona</td><td>26.7</td><td>3</td><td>Nebraska</td><td>79.0</td></tr>
<tr><td>16</td><td>Arkansas</td><td>61.3</td><td>4</td><td>Indiana</td><td>78.7</td></tr>
<tr><td>44</td><td>California</td><td>33.2</td><td>5</td><td>Kansas</td><td>78.4</td></tr>
<tr><td>24</td><td>Colorado</td><td>51.8</td><td>6</td><td>Louisiana</td><td>77.3</td></tr>
<tr><td>14</td><td>Connecticut</td><td>61.9</td><td>7</td><td>Minnesota</td><td>75.5</td></tr>
<tr><td>28</td><td>Delaware</td><td>50.0</td><td>8</td><td>Oklahoma</td><td>75.4</td></tr>
<tr><td>48</td><td>Florida</td><td>26.2</td><td>9</td><td>Wisconsin</td><td>73.7</td></tr>
<tr><td>23</td><td>Georgia</td><td>52.3</td><td>10</td><td>Missouri</td><td>71.2</td></tr>
<tr><td>50</td><td>Hawaii</td><td>15.1</td><td>11</td><td>Illinois</td><td>65.8</td></tr>
<tr><td>37</td><td>Idaho</td><td>39.1</td><td>12</td><td>Rhode Island</td><td>65.7</td></tr>
<tr><td>11</td><td>Illinois</td><td>65.8</td><td>13</td><td>North Dakota</td><td>65.1</td></tr>
<tr><td>4</td><td>Indiana</td><td>78.7</td><td>14</td><td>Connecticut</td><td>61.9</td></tr>
<tr><td>2</td><td>Iowa</td><td>80.1</td><td>15</td><td>Texas</td><td>61.6</td></tr>
<tr><td>5</td><td>Kansas</td><td>78.4</td><td>16</td><td>Arkansas</td><td>61.3</td></tr>
<tr><td>21</td><td>Kentucky</td><td>54.4</td><td>17</td><td>Massachusetts</td><td>60.7</td></tr>
<tr><td>6</td><td>Louisiana</td><td>77.3</td><td>18</td><td>New Hampshire</td><td>58.1</td></tr>
<tr><td>20</td><td>Maine</td><td>55.7</td><td>19</td><td>Ohio</td><td>57.5</td></tr>
<tr><td>26</td><td>Maryland</td><td>51.3</td><td>20</td><td>Maine</td><td>55.7</td></tr>
<tr><td>17</td><td>Massachusetts</td><td>60.7</td><td>21</td><td>Kentucky</td><td>54.4</td></tr>
<tr><td>33</td><td>Michigan</td><td>43.3</td><td>22</td><td>Montana</td><td>52.9</td></tr>
<tr><td>7</td><td>Minnesota</td><td>75.5</td><td>23</td><td>Georgia</td><td>52.3</td></tr>
<tr><td>32</td><td>Mississippi</td><td>44.8</td><td>24</td><td>Colorado</td><td>51.8</td></tr>
<tr><td>10</td><td>Missouri</td><td>71.2</td><td>25</td><td>Tennessee</td><td>51.6</td></tr>
<tr><td>22</td><td>Montana</td><td>52.9</td><td>26</td><td>Maryland</td><td>51.3</td></tr>
<tr><td>3</td><td>Nebraska</td><td>79.0</td><td>27</td><td>Vermont</td><td>51.1</td></tr>
<tr><td>49</td><td>Nevada</td><td>23.1</td><td>28</td><td>Delaware</td><td>50.0</td></tr>
<tr><td>18</td><td>New Hampshire</td><td>58.1</td><td>29</td><td>Pennsylvania</td><td>46.0</td></tr>
<tr><td>39</td><td>New Jersey</td><td>38.3</td><td>30</td><td>Wyoming</td><td>45.8</td></tr>
<tr><td>42</td><td>New Mexico</td><td>35.3</td><td>31</td><td>Washington</td><td>45.0</td></tr>
<tr><td>35</td><td>New York</td><td>40.2</td><td>32</td><td>Mississippi</td><td>44.8</td></tr>
<tr><td>43</td><td>North Carolina</td><td>34.2</td><td>33</td><td>Michigan</td><td>43.3</td></tr>
<tr><td>13</td><td>North Dakota</td><td>65.1</td><td>34</td><td>Utah</td><td>40.6</td></tr>
<tr><td>19</td><td>Ohio</td><td>57.5</td><td>35</td><td>Alabama</td><td>40.2</td></tr>
<tr><td>8</td><td>Oklahoma</td><td>75.4</td><td>35</td><td>New York</td><td>40.2</td></tr>
<tr><td>41</td><td>Oregon</td><td>35.9</td><td>37</td><td>Idaho</td><td>39.1</td></tr>
<tr><td>29</td><td>Pennsylvania</td><td>46.0</td><td>38</td><td>Virginia</td><td>38.6</td></tr>
<tr><td>12</td><td>Rhode Island</td><td>65.7</td><td>39</td><td>New Jersey</td><td>38.3</td></tr>
<tr><td>46</td><td>South Carolina</td><td>32.3</td><td>40</td><td>West Virginia</td><td>36.0</td></tr>
<tr><td>1</td><td>South Dakota</td><td>82.0</td><td>41</td><td>Oregon</td><td>35.9</td></tr>
<tr><td>25</td><td>Tennessee</td><td>51.6</td><td>42</td><td>New Mexico</td><td>35.3</td></tr>
<tr><td>15</td><td>Texas</td><td>61.6</td><td>43</td><td>North Carolina</td><td>34.2</td></tr>
<tr><td>34</td><td>Utah</td><td>40.6</td><td>44</td><td>California</td><td>33.2</td></tr>
<tr><td>27</td><td>Vermont</td><td>51.1</td><td>45</td><td>Alaska</td><td>32.5</td></tr>
<tr><td>38</td><td>Virginia</td><td>38.6</td><td>46</td><td>South Carolina</td><td>32.3</td></tr>
<tr><td>31</td><td>Washington</td><td>45.0</td><td>47</td><td>Arizona</td><td>26.7</td></tr>
<tr><td>40</td><td>West Virginia</td><td>36.0</td><td>48</td><td>Florida</td><td>26.2</td></tr>
<tr><td>9</td><td>Wisconsin</td><td>73.7</td><td>49</td><td>Nevada</td><td>23.1</td></tr>
<tr><td>30</td><td>Wyoming</td><td>45.8</td><td>50</td><td>Hawaii</td><td>15.1</td></tr>
<tr><td></td><td></td><td></td><td></td><td>District of Columbia</td><td>38.6</td></tr>
</table>

Source: U.S. Department of Health and Human Services, National Center for Health Statistics
unpublished data

Nursing Home Population in 1990

National Total = 1,772,032 Persons in Nursing Homes*

ALPHA ORDER					RANK ORDER			
RANK	STATE	POPULATION	% of USA		RANK	STATE	POPULATION	% of USA
27	Alabama	24,031	1.36%		1	California	148,362	8.37%
50	Alaska	1,202	0.07%		2	New York	126,175	7.12%
34	Arizona	14,472	0.82%		3	Pennsylvania	106,454	6.01%
28	Arkansas	21,809	1.23%		4	Texas	101,005	5.70%
1	California	148,362	8.37%		5	Ohio	93,769	5.29%
30	Colorado	18,506	1.04%		6	Illinois	93,662	5.29%
22	Connecticut	30,962	1.75%		7	Florida	80,298	4.53%
46	Delaware	4,596	0.26%		8	Michigan	57,622	3.25%
7	Florida	80,298	4.53%		9	Massachusetts	55,662	3.14%
17	Georgia	36,549	2.06%		10	Missouri	52,060	2.94%
48	Hawaii	3,225	0.18%		11	Indiana	50,845	2.87%
42	Idaho	6,318	0.36%		12	Wisconsin	50,345	2.84%
6	Illinois	93,662	5.29%		13	New Jersey	47,054	2.66%
11	Indiana	50,845	2.87%		14	Minnesota	47,051	2.66%
18	Iowa	36,455	2.06%		15	North Carolina	47,014	2.65%
26	Kansas	26,155	1.48%		16	Virginia	37,762	2.13%
24	Kentucky	27,874	1.57%		17	Georgia	36,549	2.06%
21	Louisiana	32,072	1.81%		18	Iowa	36,455	2.06%
37	Maine	9,855	0.56%		19	Tennessee	35,192	1.99%
25	Maryland	26,884	1.52%		20	Washington	32,840	1.85%
9	Massachusetts	55,662	3.14%		21	Louisiana	32,072	1.81%
8	Michigan	57,622	3.25%		22	Connecticut	30,962	1.75%
14	Minnesota	47,051	2.66%		23	Oklahoma	29,666	1.67%
33	Mississippi	15,803	0.89%		24	Kentucky	27,874	1.57%
10	Missouri	52,060	2.94%		25	Maryland	26,884	1.52%
41	Montana	7,764	0.44%		26	Kansas	26,155	1.48%
29	Nebraska	19,171	1.08%		27	Alabama	24,031	1.36%
47	Nevada	3,605	0.20%		28	Arkansas	21,809	1.23%
39	New Hampshire	8,202	0.46%		29	Nebraska	19,171	1.08%
13	New Jersey	47,054	2.66%		30	Colorado	18,506	1.04%
43	New Mexico	6,276	0.35%		31	South Carolina	18,228	1.03%
2	New York	126,175	7.12%		32	Oregon	18,200	1.03%
15	North Carolina	47,014	2.65%		33	Mississippi	15,803	0.89%
40	North Dakota	8,159	0.46%		34	Arizona	14,472	0.82%
5	Ohio	93,769	5.29%		35	West Virginia	12,591	0.71%
23	Oklahoma	29,666	1.67%		36	Rhode Island	10,156	0.57%
32	Oregon	18,200	1.03%		37	Maine	9,855	0.56%
3	Pennsylvania	106,454	6.01%		38	South Dakota	9,356	0.53%
36	Rhode Island	10,156	0.57%		39	New Hampshire	8,202	0.46%
31	South Carolina	18,228	1.03%		40	North Dakota	8,159	0.46%
38	South Dakota	9,356	0.53%		41	Montana	7,764	0.44%
19	Tennessee	35,192	1.99%		42	Idaho	6,318	0.36%
4	Texas	101,005	5.70%		43	New Mexico	6,276	0.35%
44	Utah	6,222	0.35%		44	Utah	6,222	0.35%
45	Vermont	4,809	0.27%		45	Vermont	4,809	0.27%
16	Virginia	37,762	2.13%		46	Delaware	4,596	0.26%
20	Washington	32,840	1.85%		47	Nevada	3,605	0.20%
35	West Virginia	12,591	0.71%		48	Hawaii	3,225	0.18%
12	Wisconsin	50,345	2.84%		49	Wyoming	2,679	0.15%
49	Wyoming	2,679	0.15%		50	Alaska	1,202	0.07%
						District of Columbia	7,008	0.40%

Source: U.S. Bureau of the Census
"Nursing Home Population 1990" (CPH-L-137)
Census uses a broader definition of "Nursing Home" than does HHS. Caution should be used in comparing data from the two sources.

Percent of Population in Nursing Homes in 1990

National Percent = 0.71% of Population in Nursing Homes*

ALPHA ORDER			RANK ORDER		
RANK	**STATE**	**PERCENT**	**RANK**	**STATE**	**PERCENT**
37	Alabama	0.59	1	South Dakota	1.34
50	Alaska	0.22	2	Iowa	1.31
46	Arizona	0.39	3	North Dakota	1.28
13	Arkansas	0.93	4	Nebraska	1.21
44	California	0.50	5	Minnesota	1.08
40	Colorado	0.56	6	Kansas	1.06
11	Connecticut	0.94	7	Wisconsin	1.03
28	Delaware	0.69	8	Missouri	1.02
32	Florida	0.62	9	Rhode Island	1.01
40	Georgia	0.56	10	Montana	0.97
49	Hawaii	0.29	11	Connecticut	0.94
31	Idaho	0.63	11	Oklahoma	0.94
19	Illinois	0.82	13	Arkansas	0.93
15	Indiana	0.92	13	Massachusetts	0.93
2	Iowa	1.31	15	Indiana	0.92
6	Kansas	1.06	16	Pennsylvania	0.90
21	Kentucky	0.76	17	Ohio	0.86
21	Louisiana	0.76	18	Vermont	0.85
20	Maine	0.80	19	Illinois	0.82
40	Maryland	0.56	20	Maine	0.80
13	Massachusetts	0.93	21	Kentucky	0.76
32	Michigan	0.62	21	Louisiana	0.76
5	Minnesota	1.08	23	New Hampshire	0.74
34	Mississippi	0.61	24	Tennessee	0.72
8	Missouri	1.02	25	North Carolina	0.71
10	Montana	0.97	26	New York	0.70
4	Nebraska	1.21	26	West Virginia	0.70
48	Nevada	0.30	28	Delaware	0.69
23	New Hampshire	0.74	29	Washington	0.67
34	New Jersey	0.61	30	Oregon	0.64
45	New Mexico	0.41	31	Idaho	0.63
26	New York	0.70	32	Florida	0.62
25	North Carolina	0.71	32	Michigan	0.62
3	North Dakota	1.28	34	Mississippi	0.61
17	Ohio	0.86	34	New Jersey	0.61
11	Oklahoma	0.94	34	Virginia	0.61
30	Oregon	0.64	37	Alabama	0.59
16	Pennsylvania	0.90	37	Texas	0.59
9	Rhode Island	1.01	37	Wyoming	0.59
43	South Carolina	0.52	40	Colorado	0.56
1	South Dakota	1.34	40	Georgia	0.56
24	Tennessee	0.72	40	Maryland	0.56
37	Texas	0.59	43	South Carolina	0.52
47	Utah	0.36	44	California	0.50
18	Vermont	0.85	45	New Mexico	0.41
34	Virginia	0.61	46	Arizona	0.39
29	Washington	0.67	47	Utah	0.36
26	West Virginia	0.70	48	Nevada	0.30
7	Wisconsin	1.03	49	Hawaii	0.29
37	Wyoming	0.59	50	Alaska	0.22
				District of Columbia	1.15

Source: Morgan Quitno Press using data from U.S. Bureau of the Census
"Nursing Home Population 1990" (CPH-L-137)
*Census uses a broader definition of "Nursing Home" than does HHS. Caution should be used in comparing data from the two sources.

Nursing Home Population in 1980

National Total = 1,426,371 Persons in Nursing Homes

ALPHA ORDER					RANK ORDER			

RANK	STATE	POPULATION	% of USA
27	Alabama	18,702	1.31%
50	Alaska	854	0.06%
35	Arizona	8,424	0.59%
28	Arkansas	18,631	1.31%
1	California	134,756	9.45%
30	Colorado	16,109	1.13%
19	Connecticut	27,873	1.95%
46	Delaware	2,771	0.19%
13	Florida	36,306	2.55%
17	Georgia	29,376	2.06%
45	Hawaii	3,159	0.22%
42	Idaho	5,084	0.36%
4	Illinois	80,410	5.64%
11	Indiana	40,112	2.81%
14	Iowa	36,217	2.54%
21	Kansas	24,545	1.72%
23	Kentucky	23,591	1.65%
24	Louisiana	22,776	1.60%
34	Maine	9,570	0.67%
26	Maryland	19,821	1.39%
8	Massachusetts	49,728	3.49%
7	Michigan	55,805	3.91%
10	Minnesota	44,553	3.12%
32	Mississippi	12,753	0.89%
12	Missouri	37,942	2.66%
41	Montana	5,479	0.38%
29	Nebraska	17,650	1.24%
48	Nevada	2,339	0.16%
39	New Hampshire	6,673	0.47%
15	New Jersey	34,414	2.41%
47	New Mexico	2,585	0.18%
2	New York	114,276	8.01%
16	North Carolina	29,596	2.07%
38	North Dakota	7,486	0.52%
6	Ohio	71,479	5.01%
20	Oklahoma	25,732	1.80%
31	Oregon	16,052	1.13%
5	Pennsylvania	72,285	5.07%
36	Rhode Island	8,146	0.57%
33	South Carolina	11,666	0.82%
37	South Dakota	8,087	0.57%
25	Tennessee	22,014	1.54%
3	Texas	89,275	6.26%
43	Utah	4,921	0.35%
44	Vermont	4,354	0.31%
22	Virginia	24,323	1.71%
18	Washington	27,970	1.96%
40	West Virginia	6,355	0.45%
9	Wisconsin	48,282	3.38%
49	Wyoming	2,198	0.15%

RANK	STATE	POPULATION	% of USA
1	California	134,756	9.45%
2	New York	114,276	8.01%
3	Texas	89,275	6.26%
4	Illinois	80,410	5.64%
5	Pennsylvania	72,285	5.07%
6	Ohio	71,479	5.01%
7	Michigan	55,805	3.91%
8	Massachusetts	49,728	3.49%
9	Wisconsin	48,282	3.38%
10	Minnesota	44,553	3.12%
11	Indiana	40,112	2.81%
12	Missouri	37,942	2.66%
13	Florida	36,306	2.55%
14	Iowa	36,217	2.54%
15	New Jersey	34,414	2.41%
16	North Carolina	29,596	2.07%
17	Georgia	29,376	2.06%
18	Washington	27,970	1.96%
19	Connecticut	27,873	1.95%
20	Oklahoma	25,732	1.80%
21	Kansas	24,545	1.72%
22	Virginia	24,323	1.71%
23	Kentucky	23,591	1.65%
24	Louisiana	22,776	1.60%
25	Tennessee	22,014	1.54%
26	Maryland	19,821	1.39%
27	Alabama	18,702	1.31%
28	Arkansas	18,631	1.31%
29	Nebraska	17,650	1.24%
30	Colorado	16,109	1.13%
31	Oregon	16,052	1.13%
32	Mississippi	12,753	0.89%
33	South Carolina	11,666	0.82%
34	Maine	9,570	0.67%
35	Arizona	8,424	0.59%
36	Rhode Island	8,146	0.57%
37	South Dakota	8,087	0.57%
38	North Dakota	7,486	0.52%
39	New Hampshire	6,673	0.47%
40	West Virginia	6,355	0.45%
41	Montana	5,479	0.38%
42	Idaho	5,084	0.36%
43	Utah	4,921	0.35%
44	Vermont	4,354	0.31%
45	Hawaii	3,159	0.22%
46	Delaware	2,771	0.19%
47	New Mexico	2,585	0.18%
48	Nevada	2,339	0.16%
49	Wyoming	2,198	0.15%
50	Alaska	854	0.06%
	District of Columbia	2,866	0.20%

Source: U.S. Bureau of the Census
"Nursing Homes Persons in Institutions and Other Group Quarters" (PC80-2-4D)

Percent of Population in Nursing Homes in 1980

National Percent = 0.63% of Population in Nursing Homes

ALPHA ORDER

RANK ORDER

RANK	STATE	PERCENT
35	Alabama	0.48
49	Alaska	0.21
47	Arizona	0.31
14	Arkansas	0.81
28	California	0.57
29	Colorado	0.56
8	Connecticut	0.90
37	Delaware	0.47
42	Florida	0.37
30	Georgia	0.54
45	Hawaii	0.33
30	Idaho	0.54
18	Illinois	0.70
16	Indiana	0.73
1	Iowa	1.24
6	Kansas	1.04
23	Kentucky	0.64
30	Louisiana	0.54
11	Maine	0.85
37	Maryland	0.47
9	Massachusetts	0.87
27	Michigan	0.60
5	Minnesota	1.09
33	Mississippi	0.51
15	Missouri	0.77
18	Montana	0.70
4	Nebraska	1.12
48	Nevada	0.29
17	New Hampshire	0.72
37	New Jersey	0.47
50	New Mexico	0.20
22	New York	0.65
34	North Carolina	0.50
3	North Dakota	1.15
21	Ohio	0.66
11	Oklahoma	0.85
25	Oregon	0.61
25	Pennsylvania	0.61
10	Rhode Island	0.86
42	South Carolina	0.37
2	South Dakota	1.17
35	Tennessee	0.48
24	Texas	0.63
44	Utah	0.34
11	Vermont	0.85
41	Virginia	0.45
20	Washington	0.68
45	West Virginia	0.33
7	Wisconsin	1.03
37	Wyoming	0.47

RANK	STATE	PERCENT
1	Iowa	1.24
2	South Dakota	1.17
3	North Dakota	1.15
4	Nebraska	1.12
5	Minnesota	1.09
6	Kansas	1.04
7	Wisconsin	1.03
8	Connecticut	0.90
9	Massachusetts	0.87
10	Rhode Island	0.86
11	Maine	0.85
11	Oklahoma	0.85
11	Vermont	0.85
14	Arkansas	0.81
15	Missouri	0.77
16	Indiana	0.73
17	New Hampshire	0.72
18	Illinois	0.70
18	Montana	0.70
20	Washington	0.68
21	Ohio	0.66
22	New York	0.65
23	Kentucky	0.64
24	Texas	0.63
25	Oregon	0.61
25	Pennsylvania	0.61
27	Michigan	0.60
28	California	0.57
29	Colorado	0.56
30	Georgia	0.54
30	Idaho	0.54
30	Louisiana	0.54
33	Mississippi	0.51
34	North Carolina	0.50
35	Alabama	0.48
35	Tennessee	0.48
37	Delaware	0.47
37	Maryland	0.47
37	New Jersey	0.47
37	Wyoming	0.47
41	Virginia	0.45
42	Florida	0.37
42	South Carolina	0.37
44	Utah	0.34
45	Hawaii	0.33
45	West Virginia	0.33
47	Arizona	0.31
48	Nevada	0.29
49	Alaska	0.21
50	New Mexico	0.20
	District of Columbia	0.45

Source: Morgan Quitno Press using data from U.S. Bureau of the Census
"Nursing Homes Persons in Institutions and Other Group Quarters" (PC80-2-4D)

Change in Nursing Home Population: 1980 to 1990

National Change = 345,661 Increase in Nursing Home Population

ALPHA ORDER				RANK ORDER			
RANK	STATE	INCREASE	% of USA	RANK	STATE	INCREASE	% of USA
21	Alabama	5,329	1.54%	1	Florida	43,992	12.73%
47	Alaska	348	0.10%	2	Pennsylvania	34,169	9.89%
19	Arizona	6,048	1.75%	3	Ohio	22,290	6.45%
26	Arkansas	3,178	0.92%	4	North Carolina	17,418	5.04%
6	California	13,606	3.94%	5	Missouri	14,118	4.08%
30	Colorado	2,397	0.69%	6	California	13,606	3.94%
27	Connecticut	3,089	0.89%	7	Virginia	13,439	3.89%
35	Delaware	1,825	0.53%	8	Illinois	13,252	3.83%
1	Florida	43,992	12.73%	9	Tennessee	13,178	3.81%
15	Georgia	7,173	2.08%	10	New Jersey	12,640	3.66%
50	Hawaii	66	0.02%	11	New York	11,899	3.44%
43	Idaho	1,234	0.36%	12	Texas	11,730	3.39%
8	Illinois	13,252	3.83%	13	Indiana	10,733	3.11%
13	Indiana	10,733	3.11%	14	Louisiana	9,296	2.69%
49	Iowa	238	0.07%	15	Georgia	7,173	2.08%
37	Kansas	1,610	0.47%	16	Maryland	7,063	2.04%
23	Kentucky	4,283	1.24%	17	South Carolina	6,562	1.90%
14	Louisiana	9,296	2.69%	18	West Virginia	6,236	1.80%
48	Maine	285	0.08%	19	Arizona	6,048	1.75%
16	Maryland	7,063	2.04%	20	Massachusetts	5,934	1.72%
20	Massachusetts	5,934	1.72%	21	Alabama	5,329	1.54%
36	Michigan	1,817	0.53%	22	Washington	4,870	1.41%
29	Minnesota	2,498	0.72%	23	Kentucky	4,283	1.24%
28	Mississippi	3,050	0.88%	24	Oklahoma	3,934	1.14%
5	Missouri	14,118	4.08%	25	New Mexico	3,691	1.07%
31	Montana	2,285	0.66%	26	Arkansas	3,178	0.92%
39	Nebraska	1,521	0.44%	27	Connecticut	3,089	0.89%
42	Nevada	1,266	0.37%	28	Mississippi	3,050	0.88%
38	New Hampshire	1,529	0.44%	29	Minnesota	2,498	0.72%
10	New Jersey	12,640	3.66%	30	Colorado	2,397	0.69%
25	New Mexico	3,691	1.07%	31	Montana	2,285	0.66%
11	New York	11,899	3.44%	32	Oregon	2,148	0.62%
4	North Carolina	17,418	5.04%	33	Wisconsin	2,063	0.60%
44	North Dakota	673	0.19%	34	Rhode Island	2,010	0.58%
3	Ohio	22,290	6.45%	35	Delaware	1,825	0.53%
24	Oklahoma	3,934	1.14%	36	Michigan	1,817	0.53%
32	Oregon	2,148	0.62%	37	Kansas	1,610	0.47%
2	Pennsylvania	34,169	9.89%	38	New Hampshire	1,529	0.44%
34	Rhode Island	2,010	0.58%	39	Nebraska	1,521	0.44%
17	South Carolina	6,562	1.90%	40	Utah	1,301	0.38%
41	South Dakota	1,269	0.37%	41	South Dakota	1,269	0.37%
9	Tennessee	13,178	3.81%	42	Nevada	1,266	0.37%
12	Texas	11,730	3.39%	43	Idaho	1,234	0.36%
40	Utah	1,301	0.38%	44	North Dakota	673	0.19%
46	Vermont	455	0.13%	45	Wyoming	481	0.14%
7	Virginia	13,439	3.89%	46	Vermont	455	0.13%
22	Washington	4,870	1.41%	47	Alaska	348	0.10%
18	West Virginia	6,236	1.80%	48	Maine	285	0.08%
33	Wisconsin	2,063	0.60%	49	Iowa	238	0.07%
45	Wyoming	481	0.14%	50	Hawaii	66	0.02%
					District of Columbia	4,142	1.20%

Source: Morgan Quitno Press using data from U.S. Bureau of the Census
"Nursing Homes Persons in Institutions and Other Group Quarters" (PC80-2-4D) and
"Nursing Home Population 1990" (CPH-L-137)

Percent Change in Nursing Home Population: 1980 to 1990

National Percent Change = 24.2% Increase*

ALPHA ORDER

RANK	STATE	PERCENT
19	Alabama	28.5
14	Alaska	40.7
4	Arizona	71.8
30	Arkansas	17.1
41	California	10.1
34	Colorado	14.9
38	Connecticut	11.1
5	Delaware	65.9
2	Florida	121.2
23	Georgia	24.4
49	Hawaii	2.1
24	Idaho	24.3
31	Illinois	16.5
20	Indiana	26.8
50	Iowa	0.7
44	Kansas	6.6
28	Kentucky	18.2
13	Louisiana	40.8
48	Maine	3.0
17	Maryland	35.6
37	Massachusetts	11.9
47	Michigan	3.3
45	Minnesota	5.6
25	Mississippi	23.9
15	Missouri	37.2
12	Montana	41.7
43	Nebraska	8.6
10	Nevada	54.1
26	New Hampshire	22.9
16	New Jersey	36.7
1	New Mexico	142.8
40	New York	10.4
7	North Carolina	58.9
42	North Dakota	9.0
18	Ohio	31.2
33	Oklahoma	15.3
35	Oregon	13.4
11	Pennsylvania	47.3
22	Rhode Island	24.7
8	South Carolina	56.2
32	South Dakota	15.7
6	Tennessee	59.9
36	Texas	13.1
21	Utah	26.4
39	Vermont	10.5
9	Virginia	55.3
29	Washington	17.4
3	West Virginia	98.1
46	Wisconsin	4.3
27	Wyoming	21.9

RANK ORDER

RANK	STATE	PERCENT
1	New Mexico	142.8
2	Florida	121.2
3	West Virginia	98.1
4	Arizona	71.8
5	Delaware	65.9
6	Tennessee	59.9
7	North Carolina	58.9
8	South Carolina	56.2
9	Virginia	55.3
10	Nevada	54.1
11	Pennsylvania	47.3
12	Montana	41.7
13	Louisiana	40.8
14	Alaska	40.7
15	Missouri	37.2
16	New Jersey	36.7
17	Maryland	35.6
18	Ohio	31.2
19	Alabama	28.5
20	Indiana	26.8
21	Utah	26.4
22	Rhode Island	24.7
23	Georgia	24.4
24	Idaho	24.3
25	Mississippi	23.9
26	New Hampshire	22.9
27	Wyoming	21.9
28	Kentucky	18.2
29	Washington	17.4
30	Arkansas	17.1
31	Illinois	16.5
32	South Dakota	15.7
33	Oklahoma	15.3
34	Colorado	14.9
35	Oregon	13.4
36	Texas	13.1
37	Massachusetts	11.9
38	Connecticut	11.1
39	Vermont	10.5
40	New York	10.4
41	California	10.1
42	North Dakota	9.0
43	Nebraska	8.6
44	Kansas	6.6
45	Minnesota	5.6
46	Wisconsin	4.3
47	Michigan	3.3
48	Maine	3.0
49	Hawaii	2.1
50	Iowa	0.7

| | District of Columbia | 144.5 |

Source: Morgan Quitno Press using data from U.S. Bureau of the Census
"Nursing Homes Persons in Institutions and Other Group Quarters" (PC80-2-4D) and
"Nursing Home Population 1990" (CPH-L-137)

Health Services Establishments in 1992

National Total = 465,356 Establishments*

ALPHA ORDER					RANK ORDER			

RANK	STATE	ESTABLISHMENTS	% of USA
27	Alabama	5,852	1.26%
49	Alaska	939	0.20%
20	Arizona	7,464	1.60%
32	Arkansas	3,799	0.82%
1	California	63,219	13.59%
21	Colorado	7,400	1.59%
23	Connecticut	6,941	1.49%
45	Delaware	1,254	0.27%
4	Florida	30,511	6.56%
10	Georgia	11,468	2.46%
40	Hawaii	2,330	0.50%
43	Idaho	1,837	0.39%
7	Illinois	19,757	4.25%
16	Indiana	9,342	2.01%
30	Iowa	4,671	1.00%
31	Kansas	4,238	0.91%
25	Kentucky	5,991	1.29%
22	Louisiana	7,132	1.53%
38	Maine	2,393	0.51%
14	Maryland	9,504	2.04%
11	Massachusetts	11,346	2.44%
9	Michigan	16,745	3.60%
24	Minnesota	6,680	1.44%
33	Mississippi	3,309	0.71%
17	Missouri	8,892	1.91%
44	Montana	1,683	0.36%
37	Nebraska	2,583	0.56%
39	Nevada	2,367	0.51%
42	New Hampshire	2,013	0.43%
8	New Jersey	17,020	3.66%
36	New Mexico	2,598	0.56%
2	New York	34,254	7.36%
15	North Carolina	9,355	2.01%
48	North Dakota	951	0.20%
6	Ohio	19,795	4.25%
28	Oklahoma	5,617	1.21%
26	Oregon	5,894	1.27%
5	Pennsylvania	23,341	5.02%
41	Rhode Island	2,068	0.44%
29	South Carolina	4,870	1.05%
46	South Dakota	1,145	0.25%
18	Tennessee	8,665	1.86%
3	Texas	31,024	6.67%
34	Utah	3,147	0.68%
47	Vermont	1,078	0.23%
12	Virginia	10,119	2.17%
13	Washington	9,719	2.09%
35	West Virginia	2,932	0.63%
19	Wisconsin	7,848	1.69%
50	Wyoming	789	0.17%

RANK	STATE	ESTABLISHMENTS	% of USA
1	California	63,219	13.59%
2	New York	34,254	7.36%
3	Texas	31,024	6.67%
4	Florida	30,511	6.56%
5	Pennsylvania	23,341	5.02%
6	Ohio	19,795	4.25%
7	Illinois	19,757	4.25%
8	New Jersey	17,020	3.66%
9	Michigan	16,745	3.60%
10	Georgia	11,468	2.46%
11	Massachusetts	11,346	2.44%
12	Virginia	10,119	2.17%
13	Washington	9,719	2.09%
14	Maryland	9,504	2.04%
15	North Carolina	9,355	2.01%
16	Indiana	9,342	2.01%
17	Missouri	8,892	1.91%
18	Tennessee	8,665	1.86%
19	Wisconsin	7,848	1.69%
20	Arizona	7,464	1.60%
21	Colorado	7,400	1.59%
22	Louisiana	7,132	1.53%
23	Connecticut	6,941	1.49%
24	Minnesota	6,680	1.44%
25	Kentucky	5,991	1.29%
26	Oregon	5,894	1.27%
27	Alabama	5,852	1.26%
28	Oklahoma	5,617	1.21%
29	South Carolina	4,870	1.05%
30	Iowa	4,671	1.00%
31	Kansas	4,238	0.91%
32	Arkansas	3,799	0.82%
33	Mississippi	3,309	0.71%
34	Utah	3,147	0.68%
35	West Virginia	2,932	0.63%
36	New Mexico	2,598	0.56%
37	Nebraska	2,583	0.56%
38	Maine	2,393	0.51%
39	Nevada	2,367	0.51%
40	Hawaii	2,330	0.50%
41	Rhode Island	2,068	0.44%
42	New Hampshire	2,013	0.43%
43	Idaho	1,837	0.39%
44	Montana	1,683	0.36%
45	Delaware	1,254	0.27%
46	South Dakota	1,145	0.25%
47	Vermont	1,078	0.23%
48	North Dakota	951	0.20%
49	Alaska	939	0.20%
50	Wyoming	789	0.17%
	District of Columbia	1,467	0.32%

Source: Morgan Quitno Press using data from U.S. Bureau of the Census
  "1992 Census of Service Industries, Geographic Area Series, United States" (SC92-A-52)
*Includes establishments exempt from as well as subject to the federal income tax. Includes those establishments within the Standard Industry Classification (SIC) 80. These include those primarily engaged in furnishing medical, surgical and other health services to persons.

220

Offices and Clinics of Doctors of Medicine in 1992

National Total = 197,701 Establishments*

ALPHA ORDER

RANK	STATE	ESTABLISHMENTS	% of USA
23	Alabama	2,611	1.32%
47	Alaska	349	0.18%
20	Arizona	3,150	1.59%
29	Arkansas	1,664	0.84%
1	California	28,494	14.41%
22	Colorado	2,698	1.36%
21	Connecticut	3,039	1.54%
45	Delaware	587	0.30%
3	Florida	14,487	7.33%
10	Georgia	5,214	2.64%
37	Hawaii	1,066	0.54%
43	Idaho	728	0.37%
6	Illinois	8,424	4.26%
16	Indiana	3,744	1.89%
33	Iowa	1,349	0.68%
32	Kansas	1,382	0.70%
24	Kentucky	2,565	1.30%
18	Louisiana	3,293	1.67%
39	Maine	914	0.46%
11	Maryland	4,760	2.41%
13	Massachusetts	4,524	2.29%
9	Michigan	5,935	3.00%
30	Minnesota	1,480	0.75%
31	Mississippi	1,458	0.74%
19	Missouri	3,280	1.66%
44	Montana	599	0.30%
41	Nebraska	886	0.45%
36	Nevada	1,096	0.55%
42	New Hampshire	754	0.38%
8	New Jersey	7,718	3.90%
38	New Mexico	1,033	0.52%
2	New York	16,226	8.21%
15	North Carolina	3,826	1.94%
50	North Dakota	243	0.12%
7	Ohio	8,004	4.05%
28	Oklahoma	2,052	1.04%
26	Oregon	2,263	1.14%
5	Pennsylvania	9,347	4.73%
40	Rhode Island	889	0.45%
27	South Carolina	2,219	1.12%
47	South Dakota	349	0.18%
14	Tennessee	3,840	1.94%
4	Texas	14,367	7.27%
35	Utah	1,261	0.64%
46	Vermont	393	0.20%
12	Virginia	4,724	2.39%
17	Washington	3,464	1.75%
34	West Virginia	1,340	0.68%
25	Wisconsin	2,546	1.29%
49	Wyoming	294	0.15%

RANK ORDER

RANK	STATE	ESTABLISHMENTS	% of USA
1	California	28,494	14.41%
2	New York	16,226	8.21%
3	Florida	14,487	7.33%
4	Texas	14,367	7.27%
5	Pennsylvania	9,347	4.73%
6	Illinois	8,424	4.26%
7	Ohio	8,004	4.05%
8	New Jersey	7,718	3.90%
9	Michigan	5,935	3.00%
10	Georgia	5,214	2.64%
11	Maryland	4,760	2.41%
12	Virginia	4,724	2.39%
13	Massachusetts	4,524	2.29%
14	Tennessee	3,840	1.94%
15	North Carolina	3,826	1.94%
16	Indiana	3,744	1.89%
17	Washington	3,464	1.75%
18	Louisiana	3,293	1.67%
19	Missouri	3,280	1.66%
20	Arizona	3,150	1.59%
21	Connecticut	3,039	1.54%
22	Colorado	2,698	1.36%
23	Alabama	2,611	1.32%
24	Kentucky	2,565	1.30%
25	Wisconsin	2,546	1.29%
26	Oregon	2,263	1.14%
27	South Carolina	2,219	1.12%
28	Oklahoma	2,052	1.04%
29	Arkansas	1,664	0.84%
30	Minnesota	1,480	0.75%
31	Mississippi	1,458	0.74%
32	Kansas	1,382	0.70%
33	Iowa	1,349	0.68%
34	West Virginia	1,340	0.68%
35	Utah	1,261	0.64%
36	Nevada	1,096	0.55%
37	Hawaii	1,066	0.54%
38	New Mexico	1,033	0.52%
39	Maine	914	0.46%
40	Rhode Island	889	0.45%
41	Nebraska	886	0.45%
42	New Hampshire	754	0.38%
43	Idaho	728	0.37%
44	Montana	599	0.30%
45	Delaware	587	0.30%
46	Vermont	393	0.20%
47	Alaska	349	0.18%
47	South Dakota	349	0.18%
49	Wyoming	294	0.15%
50	North Dakota	243	0.12%
	District of Columbia	773	0.39%

Source: U.S. Bureau of the Census
"1992 Census of Service Industries, Geographic Area Series, United States" (SC92-A-52)
*Includes only establishments subject to the federal income tax.

Offices and Clinics of Dentists in 1992

National Total = 108,804 Establishments*

ALPHA ORDER

RANK	STATE	ESTABLISHMENTS	% of USA
27	Alabama	1,331	1.22%
45	Alaska	262	0.24%
25	Arizona	1,522	1.40%
33	Arkansas	822	0.76%
1	California	14,806	13.61%
21	Colorado	1,911	1.76%
22	Connecticut	1,740	1.60%
49	Delaware	215	0.20%
4	Florida	5,374	4.94%
13	Georgia	2,346	2.16%
36	Hawaii	640	0.59%
42	Idaho	455	0.42%
6	Illinois	5,156	4.74%
16	Indiana	2,177	2.00%
30	Iowa	1,149	1.06%
31	Kansas	1,003	0.92%
26	Kentucky	1,462	1.34%
24	Louisiana	1,548	1.42%
41	Maine	458	0.42%
15	Maryland	2,195	2.02%
10	Massachusetts	2,941	2.70%
8	Michigan	4,348	4.00%
19	Minnesota	2,010	1.85%
34	Mississippi	784	0.72%
18	Missouri	2,047	1.88%
44	Montana	397	0.36%
35	Nebraska	747	0.69%
40	Nevada	478	0.44%
39	New Hampshire	514	0.47%
9	New Jersey	4,033	3.71%
38	New Mexico	532	0.49%
2	New York	8,560	7.87%
17	North Carolina	2,162	1.99%
47	North Dakota	250	0.23%
7	Ohio	4,497	4.13%
28	Oklahoma	1,229	1.13%
23	Oregon	1,587	1.46%
5	Pennsylvania	5,316	4.89%
43	Rhode Island	406	0.37%
29	South Carolina	1,153	1.06%
46	South Dakota	260	0.24%
20	Tennessee	1,984	1.82%
3	Texas	6,233	5.73%
32	Utah	974	0.90%
48	Vermont	245	0.23%
12	Virginia	2,524	2.32%
11	Washington	2,674	2.46%
37	West Virginia	563	0.52%
14	Wisconsin	2,235	2.05%
50	Wyoming	202	0.19%

RANK ORDER

RANK	STATE	ESTABLISHMENTS	% of USA
1	California	14,806	13.61%
2	New York	8,560	7.87%
3	Texas	6,233	5.73%
4	Florida	5,374	4.94%
5	Pennsylvania	5,316	4.89%
6	Illinois	5,156	4.74%
7	Ohio	4,497	4.13%
8	Michigan	4,348	4.00%
9	New Jersey	4,033	3.71%
10	Massachusetts	2,941	2.70%
11	Washington	2,674	2.46%
12	Virginia	2,524	2.32%
13	Georgia	2,346	2.16%
14	Wisconsin	2,235	2.05%
15	Maryland	2,195	2.02%
16	Indiana	2,177	2.00%
17	North Carolina	2,162	1.99%
18	Missouri	2,047	1.88%
19	Minnesota	2,010	1.85%
20	Tennessee	1,984	1.82%
21	Colorado	1,911	1.76%
22	Connecticut	1,740	1.60%
23	Oregon	1,587	1.46%
24	Louisiana	1,548	1.42%
25	Arizona	1,522	1.40%
26	Kentucky	1,462	1.34%
27	Alabama	1,331	1.22%
28	Oklahoma	1,229	1.13%
29	South Carolina	1,153	1.06%
30	Iowa	1,149	1.06%
31	Kansas	1,003	0.92%
32	Utah	974	0.90%
33	Arkansas	822	0.76%
34	Mississippi	784	0.72%
35	Nebraska	747	0.69%
36	Hawaii	640	0.59%
37	West Virginia	563	0.52%
38	New Mexico	532	0.49%
39	New Hampshire	514	0.47%
40	Nevada	478	0.44%
41	Maine	458	0.42%
42	Idaho	455	0.42%
43	Rhode Island	406	0.37%
44	Montana	397	0.36%
45	Alaska	262	0.24%
46	South Dakota	260	0.24%
47	North Dakota	250	0.23%
48	Vermont	245	0.23%
49	Delaware	215	0.20%
50	Wyoming	202	0.19%
	District of Columbia	347	0.32%

Source: U.S. Bureau of the Census
   "1992 Census of Service Industries, Geographic Area Series, United States" (SC92-A-52)
Includes only establishments subject to the federal income tax.

Offices and Clinics of Doctors of Osteopathy in 1992

National Total = 8,708 Establishments*

ALPHA ORDER

RANK	STATE	ESTABLISHMENT	% of USA
31	Alabama	32	0.37%
41	Alaska	11	0.13%
10	Arizona	317	3.64%
32	Arkansas	26	0.30%
9	California	322	3.70%
11	Colorado	207	2.38%
38	Connecticut	14	0.16%
26	Delaware	50	0.57%
4	Florida	762	8.75%
17	Georgia	124	1.42%
41	Hawaii	11	0.13%
39	Idaho	13	0.15%
14	Illinois	173	1.99%
16	Indiana	142	1.63%
13	Iowa	193	2.22%
20	Kansas	97	1.11%
30	Kentucky	38	0.44%
47	Louisiana	6	0.07%
18	Maine	120	1.38%
36	Maryland	16	0.18%
28	Massachusetts	40	0.46%
1	Michigan	1,201	13.79%
36	Minnesota	16	0.18%
34	Mississippi	20	0.23%
6	Missouri	446	5.12%
40	Montana	12	0.14%
49	Nebraska	2	0.02%
27	Nevada	41	0.47%
45	New Hampshire	9	0.10%
7	New Jersey	399	4.58%
23	New Mexico	57	0.65%
12	New York	201	2.31%
35	North Carolina	19	0.22%
49	North Dakota	2	0.02%
3	Ohio	821	9.43%
8	Oklahoma	328	3.77%
19	Oregon	112	1.29%
2	Pennsylvania	1,062	12.20%
24	Rhode Island	55	0.63%
33	South Carolina	21	0.24%
45	South Dakota	9	0.10%
25	Tennessee	52	0.60%
5	Texas	707	8.12%
43	Utah	10	0.11%
47	Vermont	6	0.07%
29	Virginia	39	0.45%
15	Washington	149	1.71%
22	West Virginia	90	1.03%
21	Wisconsin	96	1.10%
43	Wyoming	10	0.11%

RANK ORDER

RANK	STATE	ESTABLISHMENT	% of USA
1	Michigan	1,201	13.79%
2	Pennsylvania	1,062	12.20%
3	Ohio	821	9.43%
4	Florida	762	8.75%
5	Texas	707	8.12%
6	Missouri	446	5.12%
7	New Jersey	399	4.58%
8	Oklahoma	328	3.77%
9	California	322	3.70%
10	Arizona	317	3.64%
11	Colorado	207	2.38%
12	New York	201	2.31%
13	Iowa	193	2.22%
14	Illinois	173	1.99%
15	Washington	149	1.71%
16	Indiana	142	1.63%
17	Georgia	124	1.42%
18	Maine	120	1.38%
19	Oregon	112	1.29%
20	Kansas	97	1.11%
21	Wisconsin	96	1.10%
22	West Virginia	90	1.03%
23	New Mexico	57	0.65%
24	Rhode Island	55	0.63%
25	Tennessee	52	0.60%
26	Delaware	50	0.57%
27	Nevada	41	0.47%
28	Massachusetts	40	0.46%
29	Virginia	39	0.45%
30	Kentucky	38	0.44%
31	Alabama	32	0.37%
32	Arkansas	26	0.30%
33	South Carolina	21	0.24%
34	Mississippi	20	0.23%
35	North Carolina	19	0.22%
36	Maryland	16	0.18%
36	Minnesota	16	0.18%
38	Connecticut	14	0.16%
39	Idaho	13	0.15%
40	Montana	12	0.14%
41	Alaska	11	0.13%
41	Hawaii	11	0.13%
43	Utah	10	0.11%
43	Wyoming	10	0.11%
45	New Hampshire	9	0.10%
45	South Dakota	9	0.10%
47	Louisiana	6	0.07%
47	Vermont	6	0.07%
49	Nebraska	2	0.02%
49	North Dakota	2	0.02%
	District of Columbia	2	0.02%

Source: U.S. Bureau of the Census

"1992 Census of Service Industries, Geographic Area Series, United States" (SC92-A-52)

*Includes only establishments subject to the federal income tax.

Offices and Clinics of Chiropractors in 1992

National Total = 27,329 Establishments*

ALPHA ORDER

RANK	STATE	ESTABLISHMENTS	% of USA
29	Alabama	282	1.03%
47	Alaska	71	0.26%
14	Arizona	622	2.28%
31	Arkansas	237	0.87%
1	California	4,364	15.97%
16	Colorado	589	2.16%
24	Connecticut	347	1.27%
49	Delaware	50	0.18%
2	Florida	1,847	6.76%
12	Georgia	760	2.78%
39	Hawaii	119	0.44%
37	Idaho	134	0.49%
7	Illinois	1,068	3.91%
20	Indiana	436	1.60%
18	Iowa	446	1.63%
25	Kansas	321	1.17%
30	Kentucky	269	0.98%
28	Louisiana	284	1.04%
38	Maine	126	0.46%
32	Maryland	231	0.85%
17	Massachusetts	575	2.10%
8	Michigan	938	3.43%
10	Minnesota	824	3.02%
42	Mississippi	113	0.41%
15	Missouri	598	2.19%
41	Montana	117	0.43%
35	Nebraska	163	0.60%
34	Nevada	166	0.61%
43	New Hampshire	108	0.40%
6	New Jersey	1,245	4.56%
33	New Mexico	185	0.68%
3	New York	1,741	6.37%
19	North Carolina	439	1.61%
45	North Dakota	90	0.33%
9	Ohio	871	3.19%
27	Oklahoma	316	1.16%
21	Oregon	428	1.57%
5	Pennsylvania	1,310	4.79%
46	Rhode Island	79	0.29%
26	South Carolina	319	1.17%
40	South Dakota	118	0.43%
22	Tennessee	356	1.30%
4	Texas	1,426	5.22%
36	Utah	153	0.56%
48	Vermont	65	0.24%
23	Virginia	355	1.30%
11	Washington	804	2.94%
44	West Virginia	105	0.38%
13	Wisconsin	665	2.43%
50	Wyoming	41	0.15%

RANK ORDER

RANK	STATE	ESTABLISHMENTS	% of USA
1	California	4,364	15.97%
2	Florida	1,847	6.76%
3	New York	1,741	6.37%
4	Texas	1,426	5.22%
5	Pennsylvania	1,310	4.79%
6	New Jersey	1,245	4.56%
7	Illinois	1,068	3.91%
8	Michigan	938	3.43%
9	Ohio	871	3.19%
10	Minnesota	824	3.02%
11	Washington	804	2.94%
12	Georgia	760	2.78%
13	Wisconsin	665	2.43%
14	Arizona	622	2.28%
15	Missouri	598	2.19%
16	Colorado	589	2.16%
17	Massachusetts	575	2.10%
18	Iowa	446	1.63%
19	North Carolina	439	1.61%
20	Indiana	436	1.60%
21	Oregon	428	1.57%
22	Tennessee	356	1.30%
23	Virginia	355	1.30%
24	Connecticut	347	1.27%
25	Kansas	321	1.17%
26	South Carolina	319	1.17%
27	Oklahoma	316	1.16%
28	Louisiana	284	1.04%
29	Alabama	282	1.03%
30	Kentucky	269	0.98%
31	Arkansas	237	0.87%
32	Maryland	231	0.85%
33	New Mexico	185	0.68%
34	Nevada	166	0.61%
35	Nebraska	163	0.60%
36	Utah	153	0.56%
37	Idaho	134	0.49%
38	Maine	126	0.46%
39	Hawaii	119	0.44%
40	South Dakota	118	0.43%
41	Montana	117	0.43%
42	Mississippi	113	0.41%
43	New Hampshire	108	0.40%
44	West Virginia	105	0.38%
45	North Dakota	90	0.33%
46	Rhode Island	79	0.29%
47	Alaska	71	0.26%
48	Vermont	65	0.24%
49	Delaware	50	0.18%
50	Wyoming	41	0.15%
	District of Columbia	13	0.05%

Source: U.S. Bureau of the Census
"1992 Census of Service Industries, Geographic Area Series, United States" (SC92-A-52)
*Includes only establishments subject to the federal income tax.

Offices and Clinics of Optometrists in 1992

National Total = 17,135 Establishments*

ALPHA ORDER

RANK	STATE	ESTABLISHMENTS	% of USA
26	Alabama	229	1.34%
49	Alaska	44	0.26%
32	Arizona	189	1.10%
29	Arkansas	202	1.18%
1	California	2,382	13.90%
22	Colorado	257	1.50%
27	Connecticut	228	1.33%
50	Delaware	40	0.23%
4	Florida	854	4.98%
13	Georgia	373	2.18%
40	Hawaii	99	0.58%
41	Idaho	94	0.55%
7	Illinois	698	4.07%
11	Indiana	463	2.70%
21	Iowa	270	1.58%
24	Kansas	247	1.44%
23	Kentucky	248	1.45%
31	Louisiana	196	1.14%
35	Maine	123	0.72%
25	Maryland	235	1.37%
14	Massachusetts	370	2.16%
8	Michigan	607	3.54%
20	Minnesota	281	1.64%
34	Mississippi	148	0.86%
19	Missouri	301	1.76%
39	Montana	103	0.60%
36	Nebraska	121	0.71%
37	Nevada	110	0.64%
44	New Hampshire	74	0.43%
9	New Jersey	550	3.21%
38	New Mexico	104	0.61%
6	New York	791	4.62%
10	North Carolina	498	2.91%
46	North Dakota	64	0.37%
5	Ohio	836	4.88%
18	Oklahoma	317	1.85%
28	Oregon	222	1.30%
3	Pennsylvania	869	5.07%
45	Rhode Island	72	0.42%
30	South Carolina	198	1.16%
43	South Dakota	80	0.47%
15	Tennessee	364	2.12%
2	Texas	1,100	6.42%
42	Utah	81	0.47%
48	Vermont	50	0.29%
12	Virginia	436	2.54%
17	Washington	341	1.99%
33	West Virginia	151	0.88%
16	Wisconsin	347	2.03%
47	Wyoming	54	0.32%

RANK ORDER

RANK	STATE	ESTABLISHMENTS	% of USA
1	California	2,382	13.90%
2	Texas	1,100	6.42%
3	Pennsylvania	869	5.07%
4	Florida	854	4.98%
5	Ohio	836	4.88%
6	New York	791	4.62%
7	Illinois	698	4.07%
8	Michigan	607	3.54%
9	New Jersey	550	3.21%
10	North Carolina	498	2.91%
11	Indiana	463	2.70%
12	Virginia	436	2.54%
13	Georgia	373	2.18%
14	Massachusetts	370	2.16%
15	Tennessee	364	2.12%
16	Wisconsin	347	2.03%
17	Washington	341	1.99%
18	Oklahoma	317	1.85%
19	Missouri	301	1.76%
20	Minnesota	281	1.64%
21	Iowa	270	1.58%
22	Colorado	257	1.50%
23	Kentucky	248	1.45%
24	Kansas	247	1.44%
25	Maryland	235	1.37%
26	Alabama	229	1.34%
27	Connecticut	228	1.33%
28	Oregon	222	1.30%
29	Arkansas	202	1.18%
30	South Carolina	198	1.16%
31	Louisiana	196	1.14%
32	Arizona	189	1.10%
33	West Virginia	151	0.88%
34	Mississippi	148	0.86%
35	Maine	123	0.72%
36	Nebraska	121	0.71%
37	Nevada	110	0.64%
38	New Mexico	104	0.61%
39	Montana	103	0.60%
40	Hawaii	99	0.58%
41	Idaho	94	0.55%
42	Utah	81	0.47%
43	South Dakota	80	0.47%
44	New Hampshire	74	0.43%
45	Rhode Island	72	0.42%
46	North Dakota	64	0.37%
47	Wyoming	54	0.32%
48	Vermont	50	0.29%
49	Alaska	44	0.26%
50	Delaware	40	0.23%
	District of Columbia	24	0.14%

Source: U.S. Bureau of the Census
"1992 Census of Service Industries, Geographic Area Series, United States" (SC92-A-52)
*Includes only establishments subject to the federal income tax.

Offices and Clinics of Podiatrists in 1992

National Total = 7,948 Establishments*

ALPHA ORDER

RANK	STATE	ESTABLISHMENTS	% of USA
29	Alabama	49	0.62%
49	Alaska	5	0.06%
18	Arizona	121	1.52%
41	Arkansas	20	0.25%
2	California	930	11.70%
22	Colorado	88	1.11%
14	Connecticut	152	1.91%
39	Delaware	25	0.31%
4	Florida	564	7.10%
17	Georgia	139	1.75%
44	Hawaii	16	0.20%
43	Idaho	17	0.21%
7	Illinois	419	5.27%
12	Indiana	166	2.09%
23	Iowa	75	0.94%
26	Kansas	55	0.69%
31	Kentucky	46	0.58%
30	Louisiana	48	0.60%
34	Maine	36	0.45%
10	Maryland	211	2.65%
11	Massachusetts	208	2.62%
8	Michigan	400	5.03%
25	Minnesota	60	0.75%
42	Mississippi	18	0.23%
20	Missouri	98	1.23%
44	Montana	16	0.20%
35	Nebraska	34	0.43%
37	Nevada	28	0.35%
40	New Hampshire	24	0.30%
6	New Jersey	449	5.65%
36	New Mexico	33	0.42%
1	New York	938	11.80%
16	North Carolina	140	1.76%
48	North Dakota	7	0.09%
5	Ohio	490	6.17%
27	Oklahoma	52	0.65%
24	Oregon	61	0.77%
3	Pennsylvania	589	7.41%
28	Rhode Island	50	0.63%
33	South Carolina	40	0.50%
46	South Dakota	14	0.18%
21	Tennessee	90	1.13%
9	Texas	382	4.81%
32	Utah	44	0.55%
47	Vermont	9	0.11%
13	Virginia	164	2.06%
15	Washington	146	1.84%
38	West Virginia	26	0.33%
19	Wisconsin	119	1.50%
49	Wyoming	5	0.06%

RANK ORDER

RANK	STATE	ESTABLISHMENTS	% of USA
1	New York	938	11.80%
2	California	930	11.70%
3	Pennsylvania	589	7.41%
4	Florida	564	7.10%
5	Ohio	490	6.17%
6	New Jersey	449	5.65%
7	Illinois	419	5.27%
8	Michigan	400	5.03%
9	Texas	382	4.81%
10	Maryland	211	2.65%
11	Massachusetts	208	2.62%
12	Indiana	166	2.09%
13	Virginia	164	2.06%
14	Connecticut	152	1.91%
15	Washington	146	1.84%
16	North Carolina	140	1.76%
17	Georgia	139	1.75%
18	Arizona	121	1.52%
19	Wisconsin	119	1.50%
20	Missouri	98	1.23%
21	Tennessee	90	1.13%
22	Colorado	88	1.11%
23	Iowa	75	0.94%
24	Oregon	61	0.77%
25	Minnesota	60	0.75%
26	Kansas	55	0.69%
27	Oklahoma	52	0.65%
28	Rhode Island	50	0.63%
29	Alabama	49	0.62%
30	Louisiana	48	0.60%
31	Kentucky	46	0.58%
32	Utah	44	0.55%
33	South Carolina	40	0.50%
34	Maine	36	0.45%
35	Nebraska	34	0.43%
36	New Mexico	33	0.42%
37	Nevada	28	0.35%
38	West Virginia	26	0.33%
39	Delaware	25	0.31%
40	New Hampshire	24	0.30%
41	Arkansas	20	0.25%
42	Mississippi	18	0.23%
43	Idaho	17	0.21%
44	Hawaii	16	0.20%
44	Montana	16	0.20%
46	South Dakota	14	0.18%
47	Vermont	9	0.11%
48	North Dakota	7	0.09%
49	Alaska	5	0.06%
49	Wyoming	5	0.06%
	District of Columbia	32	0.40%

Source: U.S. Bureau of the Census
  "1992 Census of Service Industries, Geographic Area Series, United States" (SC92-A-52)
*Includes only establishments subject to the federal income tax.

Offices and Clinics of Other Health Practitioners in 1992

National Total = 22,260 Establishments*

ALPHA ORDER

RANK	STATE	ESTABLISHMENTS	% of USA
28	Alabama	174	0.78%
47	Alaska	60	0.27%
17	Arizona	447	2.01%
33	Arkansas	156	0.70%
1	California	3,954	17.76%
14	Colorado	515	2.31%
24	Connecticut	312	1.40%
43	Delaware	76	0.34%
2	Florida	1,644	7.39%
12	Georgia	544	2.44%
37	Hawaii	120	0.54%
42	Idaho	79	0.35%
7	Illinois	722	3.24%
25	Indiana	275	1.24%
33	Iowa	156	0.70%
32	Kansas	158	0.71%
27	Kentucky	212	0.95%
23	Louisiana	324	1.46%
38	Maine	112	0.50%
11	Maryland	592	2.66%
13	Massachusetts	526	2.36%
8	Michigan	669	3.01%
19	Minnesota	361	1.62%
40	Mississippi	102	0.46%
18	Missouri	374	1.68%
41	Montana	86	0.39%
39	Nebraska	107	0.48%
35	Nevada	130	0.58%
36	New Hampshire	128	0.58%
9	New Jersey	666	2.99%
30	New Mexico	167	0.75%
4	New York	1,344	6.04%
15	North Carolina	497	2.23%
50	North Dakota	31	0.14%
6	Ohio	860	3.86%
26	Oklahoma	228	1.02%
19	Oregon	361	1.62%
5	Pennsylvania	899	4.04%
46	Rhode Island	66	0.30%
29	South Carolina	169	0.76%
48	South Dakota	37	0.17%
22	Tennessee	330	1.48%
3	Texas	1,636	7.35%
31	Utah	166	0.75%
44	Vermont	69	0.31%
16	Virginia	485	2.18%
10	Washington	620	2.79%
44	West Virginia	69	0.31%
21	Wisconsin	340	1.53%
48	Wyoming	37	0.17%

RANK ORDER

RANK	STATE	ESTABLISHMENTS	% of USA
1	California	3,954	17.76%
2	Florida	1,644	7.39%
3	Texas	1,636	7.35%
4	New York	1,344	6.04%
5	Pennsylvania	899	4.04%
6	Ohio	860	3.86%
7	Illinois	722	3.24%
8	Michigan	669	3.01%
9	New Jersey	666	2.99%
10	Washington	620	2.79%
11	Maryland	592	2.66%
12	Georgia	544	2.44%
13	Massachusetts	526	2.36%
14	Colorado	515	2.31%
15	North Carolina	497	2.23%
16	Virginia	485	2.18%
17	Arizona	447	2.01%
18	Missouri	374	1.68%
19	Minnesota	361	1.62%
19	Oregon	361	1.62%
21	Wisconsin	340	1.53%
22	Tennessee	330	1.48%
23	Louisiana	324	1.46%
24	Connecticut	312	1.40%
25	Indiana	275	1.24%
26	Oklahoma	228	1.02%
27	Kentucky	212	0.95%
28	Alabama	174	0.78%
29	South Carolina	169	0.76%
30	New Mexico	167	0.75%
31	Utah	166	0.75%
32	Kansas	158	0.71%
33	Arkansas	156	0.70%
33	Iowa	156	0.70%
35	Nevada	130	0.58%
36	New Hampshire	128	0.58%
37	Hawaii	120	0.54%
38	Maine	112	0.50%
39	Nebraska	107	0.48%
40	Mississippi	102	0.46%
41	Montana	86	0.39%
42	Idaho	79	0.35%
43	Delaware	76	0.34%
44	Vermont	69	0.31%
44	West Virginia	69	0.31%
46	Rhode Island	66	0.30%
47	Alaska	60	0.27%
48	South Dakota	37	0.17%
48	Wyoming	37	0.17%
50	North Dakota	31	0.14%
	District of Columbia	68	0.31%

Source: U.S. Bureau of the Census
    "1992 Census of Service Industries, Geographic Area Series, United States" (SC92-A-52)
*Includes only establishments subject to the federal income tax. Includes health practitioners not otherwise classified such as acupuncturists, midwives, nutritionists, physical and occupational therapists and psychologists.

IV. FINANCE

IV. FINANCE (Continued)

DEFINITIONS

The following definitions are from Lewin VHI for their report for Families USA Foundation and pertain to tables 247-259:

"Families" are groups of one or more persons related by birth, marriage or adoption and who are residing together.

"Health Care Payments" cover expenditures for the delivery of all health services and supplies and the purchase of medical products, including prescription drugs and vision products in retail outlets. It also includes government public health expenditures, the administrative costs of public health programs and the net cost of private insurance.

"Expenditures" represent the amount actually spent on health care in each state.

"Payments" are health care payments made by residents of a given state whether the funds were spent in that state or not.

Persons Not Covered by Health Insurance in 1993

National Total = 39,440,799 Uninsured*

ALPHA ORDER

RANK ORDER

RANK	STATE	UNINSURED	% of USA
16	Alabama	719,132	1.82%
48	Alaska	79,534	0.20%
14	Arizona	796,890	2.02%
24	Arkansas	477,922	1.21%
1	California	6,149,749	15.59%
28	Colorado	449,064	1.14%
33	Connecticut	327,800	0.83%
45	Delaware	93,532	0.24%
3	Florida	2,690,296	6.82%
7	Georgia	1,269,968	3.22%
42	Hawaii	129,426	0.33%
39	Idaho	162,800	0.41%
5	Illinois	1,472,436	3.73%
18	Indiana	679,014	1.72%
35	Iowa	259,532	0.66%
34	Kansas	321,945	0.82%
25	Kentucky	474,250	1.20%
11	Louisiana	1,025,310	2.60%
41	Maine	137,640	0.35%
20	Maryland	669,330	1.70%
17	Massachusetts	704,106	1.79%
10	Michigan	1,059,520	2.69%
27	Minnesota	456,924	1.16%
26	Mississippi	469,920	1.19%
22	Missouri	638,670	1.62%
43	Montana	128,673	0.33%
38	Nebraska	191,947	0.49%
36	Nevada	250,142	0.63%
40	New Hampshire	140,500	0.36%
9	New Jersey	1,076,683	2.73%
31	New Mexico	355,520	0.90%
4	New York	2,523,267	6.40%
12	North Carolina	973,280	2.47%
47	North Dakota	85,358	0.22%
8	Ohio	1,227,771	3.11%
15	Oklahoma	762,988	1.93%
29	Oregon	446,145	1.13%
6	Pennsylvania	1,299,240	3.29%
44	Rhode Island	103,000	0.26%
23	South Carolina	613,470	1.56%
46	South Dakota	93,080	0.24%
19	Tennessee	672,408	1.70%
2	Texas	3,928,796	9.96%
37	Utah	210,180	0.53%
50	Vermont	68,544	0.17%
13	Virginia	841,490	2.13%
21	Washington	662,634	1.68%
32	West Virginia	332,694	0.84%
30	Wisconsin	438,828	1.11%
49	Wyoming	70,500	0.18%

RANK	STATE	UNINSURED	% of USA
1	California	6,149,749	15.59%
2	Texas	3,928,796	9.96%
3	Florida	2,690,296	6.82%
4	New York	2,523,267	6.40%
5	Illinois	1,472,436	3.73%
6	Pennsylvania	1,299,240	3.29%
7	Georgia	1,269,968	3.22%
8	Ohio	1,227,771	3.11%
9	New Jersey	1,076,683	2.73%
10	Michigan	1,059,520	2.69%
11	Louisiana	1,025,310	2.60%
12	North Carolina	973,280	2.47%
13	Virginia	841,490	2.13%
14	Arizona	796,890	2.02%
15	Oklahoma	762,988	1.93%
16	Alabama	719,132	1.82%
17	Massachusetts	704,106	1.79%
18	Indiana	679,014	1.72%
19	Tennessee	672,408	1.70%
20	Maryland	669,330	1.70%
21	Washington	662,634	1.68%
22	Missouri	638,670	1.62%
23	South Carolina	613,470	1.56%
24	Arkansas	477,922	1.21%
25	Kentucky	474,250	1.20%
26	Mississippi	469,920	1.19%
27	Minnesota	456,924	1.16%
28	Colorado	449,064	1.14%
29	Oregon	446,145	1.13%
30	Wisconsin	438,828	1.11%
31	New Mexico	355,520	0.90%
32	West Virginia	332,694	0.84%
33	Connecticut	327,800	0.83%
34	Kansas	321,945	0.82%
35	Iowa	259,532	0.66%
36	Nevada	250,142	0.63%
37	Utah	210,180	0.53%
38	Nebraska	191,947	0.49%
39	Idaho	162,800	0.41%
40	New Hampshire	140,500	0.36%
41	Maine	137,640	0.35%
42	Hawaii	129,426	0.33%
43	Montana	128,673	0.33%
44	Rhode Island	103,000	0.26%
45	Delaware	93,532	0.24%
46	South Dakota	93,080	0.24%
47	North Dakota	85,358	0.22%
48	Alaska	79,534	0.20%
49	Wyoming	70,500	0.18%
50	Vermont	68,544	0.17%
	District of Columbia	119,853	0.30%

Source: Morgan Quitno Press using data from U.S. Bureau of the Census
"Health Insurance Coverage - 1993" (Statistical Brief, SB/94-28, October 1994)
*Based on percent of uninsured in each state issued by Census and updated 1993 state population estimates. National total calculated using 1993 national population estimate multiplied by Census national uninsured figure of 15.3%.

Percent of Population Not Covered by Health Insurance in 1993

National Percent = 15.3% Not Covered by Health Insurance

ALPHA ORDER

RANK	STATE	PERCENT
13	Alabama	17.2
25	Alaska	13.3
5	Arizona	20.2
6	Arkansas	19.7
6	California	19.7
30	Colorado	12.6
48	Connecticut	10.0
23	Delaware	13.4
8	Florida	19.6
9	Georgia	18.4
42	Hawaii	11.1
17	Idaho	14.8
30	Illinois	12.6
36	Indiana	11.9
49	Iowa	9.2
29	Kansas	12.7
33	Kentucky	12.5
1	Louisiana	23.9
42	Maine	11.1
22	Maryland	13.5
39	Massachusetts	11.7
41	Michigan	11.2
47	Minnesota	10.1
12	Mississippi	17.8
35	Missouri	12.2
15	Montana	15.3
36	Nebraska	11.9
11	Nevada	18.1
33	New Hampshire	12.5
21	New Jersey	13.7
3	New Mexico	22.0
20	New York	13.9
19	North Carolina	14.0
23	North Dakota	13.4
42	Ohio	11.1
2	Oklahoma	23.6
18	Oregon	14.7
45	Pennsylvania	10.8
46	Rhode Island	10.3
14	South Carolina	16.9
27	South Dakota	13.0
26	Tennessee	13.2
4	Texas	21.8
40	Utah	11.3
36	Vermont	11.9
27	Virginia	13.0
30	Washington	12.6
10	West Virginia	18.3
50	Wisconsin	8.7
16	Wyoming	15.0

RANK ORDER

RANK	STATE	PERCENT
1	Louisiana	23.9
2	Oklahoma	23.6
3	New Mexico	22.0
4	Texas	21.8
5	Arizona	20.2
6	Arkansas	19.7
6	California	19.7
8	Florida	19.6
9	Georgia	18.4
10	West Virginia	18.3
11	Nevada	18.1
12	Mississippi	17.8
13	Alabama	17.2
14	South Carolina	16.9
15	Montana	15.3
16	Wyoming	15.0
17	Idaho	14.8
18	Oregon	14.7
19	North Carolina	14.0
20	New York	13.9
21	New Jersey	13.7
22	Maryland	13.5
23	Delaware	13.4
23	North Dakota	13.4
25	Alaska	13.3
26	Tennessee	13.2
27	South Dakota	13.0
27	Virginia	13.0
29	Kansas	12.7
30	Colorado	12.6
30	Illinois	12.6
30	Washington	12.6
33	Kentucky	12.5
33	New Hampshire	12.5
35	Missouri	12.2
36	Indiana	11.9
36	Nebraska	11.9
36	Vermont	11.9
39	Massachusetts	11.7
40	Utah	11.3
41	Michigan	11.2
42	Hawaii	11.1
42	Maine	11.1
42	Ohio	11.1
45	Pennsylvania	10.8
46	Rhode Island	10.3
47	Minnesota	10.1
48	Connecticut	10.0
49	Iowa	9.2
50	Wisconsin	8.7

District of Columbia 20.7

Source: U.S. Bureau of the Census
"Health Insurance Coverage - 1993" (Statistical Brief, SB/94-28, October 1994)

Persons Covered by Health Insurance in 1993

National Total = 218,342,201 Insured*

ALPHA ORDER

RANK	STATE	INSURED	% of USA
21	Alabama	3,461,868	1.59%
48	Alaska	518,466	0.24%
24	Arizona	3,148,110	1.44%
33	Arkansas	1,948,078	0.89%
1	California	25,067,251	11.48%
25	Colorado	3,114,936	1.43%
27	Connecticut	2,950,200	1.35%
46	Delaware	604,468	0.28%
4	Florida	11,035,704	5.05%
11	Georgia	5,632,032	2.58%
40	Hawaii	1,036,574	0.47%
42	Idaho	937,200	0.43%
6	Illinois	10,213,564	4.68%
14	Indiana	5,026,986	2.30%
29	Iowa	2,561,468	1.17%
31	Kansas	2,213,055	1.01%
22	Kentucky	3,319,750	1.52%
23	Louisiana	3,264,690	1.50%
39	Maine	1,102,360	0.50%
19	Maryland	4,288,670	1.96%
13	Massachusetts	5,313,894	2.43%
8	Michigan	8,400,480	3.85%
20	Minnesota	4,067,076	1.86%
32	Mississippi	2,170,080	0.99%
17	Missouri	4,596,330	2.11%
44	Montana	712,327	0.33%
36	Nebraska	1,421,053	0.65%
38	Nevada	1,131,858	0.52%
41	New Hampshire	983,500	0.45%
9	New Jersey	6,782,317	3.11%
37	New Mexico	1,260,480	0.58%
2	New York	15,629,733	7.16%
10	North Carolina	5,978,720	2.74%
47	North Dakota	551,642	0.25%
7	Ohio	9,833,229	4.50%
30	Oklahoma	2,470,012	1.13%
28	Oregon	2,588,855	1.19%
5	Pennsylvania	10,730,760	4.91%
43	Rhode Island	897,000	0.41%
26	South Carolina	3,016,530	1.38%
45	South Dakota	622,920	0.29%
18	Tennessee	4,421,592	2.03%
3	Texas	14,093,204	6.45%
34	Utah	1,649,820	0.76%
49	Vermont	507,456	0.23%
12	Virginia	5,631,510	2.58%
16	Washington	4,596,366	2.11%
35	West Virginia	1,485,306	0.68%
15	Wisconsin	4,605,172	2.11%
50	Wyoming	399,500	0.18%

RANK ORDER

RANK	STATE	INSURED	% of USA
1	California	25,067,251	11.48%
2	New York	15,629,733	7.16%
3	Texas	14,093,204	6.45%
4	Florida	11,035,704	5.05%
5	Pennsylvania	10,730,760	4.91%
6	Illinois	10,213,564	4.68%
7	Ohio	9,833,229	4.50%
8	Michigan	8,400,480	3.85%
9	New Jersey	6,782,317	3.11%
10	North Carolina	5,978,720	2.74%
11	Georgia	5,632,032	2.58%
12	Virginia	5,631,510	2.58%
13	Massachusetts	5,313,894	2.43%
14	Indiana	5,026,986	2.30%
15	Wisconsin	4,605,172	2.11%
16	Washington	4,596,366	2.11%
17	Missouri	4,596,330	2.11%
18	Tennessee	4,421,592	2.03%
19	Maryland	4,288,670	1.96%
20	Minnesota	4,067,076	1.86%
21	Alabama	3,461,868	1.59%
22	Kentucky	3,319,750	1.52%
23	Louisiana	3,264,690	1.50%
24	Arizona	3,148,110	1.44%
25	Colorado	3,114,936	1.43%
26	South Carolina	3,016,530	1.38%
27	Connecticut	2,950,200	1.35%
28	Oregon	2,588,855	1.19%
29	Iowa	2,561,468	1.17%
30	Oklahoma	2,470,012	1.13%
31	Kansas	2,213,055	1.01%
32	Mississippi	2,170,080	0.99%
33	Arkansas	1,948,078	0.89%
34	Utah	1,649,820	0.76%
35	West Virginia	1,485,306	0.68%
36	Nebraska	1,421,053	0.65%
37	New Mexico	1,260,480	0.58%
38	Nevada	1,131,858	0.52%
39	Maine	1,102,360	0.50%
40	Hawaii	1,036,574	0.47%
41	New Hampshire	983,500	0.45%
42	Idaho	937,200	0.43%
43	Rhode Island	897,000	0.41%
44	Montana	712,327	0.33%
45	South Dakota	622,920	0.29%
46	Delaware	604,468	0.28%
47	North Dakota	551,642	0.25%
48	Alaska	518,466	0.24%
49	Vermont	507,456	0.23%
50	Wyoming	399,500	0.18%
	District of Columbia	459,147	0.21%

Source: Morgan Quitno Press using data from U.S. Bureau of the Census
"Health Insurance Coverage - 1993" (Statistical Brief, SB/94-28, October 1994)
This is the reverse of persons not covered which is based on percent of uninsured in each state issued by Census and latest 1993 resident state population estimates.

Percent of Population Covered by Health Insurance in 1993

National Percent = 84.7% of Covered by Health Insurance*

ALPHA ORDER				RANK ORDER		
RANK	**STATE**	**PERCENT**		**RANK**	**STATE**	**PERCENT**
38	Alabama	82.8		1	Wisconsin	91.3
26	Alaska	86.7		2	Iowa	90.8
46	Arizona	79.8		3	Connecticut	90.0
44	Arkansas	80.3		4	Minnesota	89.9
44	California	80.3		5	Rhode Island	89.7
19	Colorado	87.4		6	Pennsylvania	89.2
3	Connecticut	90.0		7	Hawaii	88.9
27	Delaware	86.6		7	Maine	88.9
43	Florida	80.4		7	Ohio	88.9
42	Georgia	81.6		10	Michigan	88.8
7	Hawaii	88.9		11	Utah	88.7
34	Idaho	85.2		12	Massachusetts	88.3
19	Illinois	87.4		13	Indiana	88.1
13	Indiana	88.1		13	Nebraska	88.1
2	Iowa	90.8		13	Vermont	88.1
22	Kansas	87.3		16	Missouri	87.8
17	Kentucky	87.5		17	Kentucky	87.5
50	Louisiana	76.1		17	New Hampshire	87.5
7	Maine	88.9		19	Colorado	87.4
29	Maryland	86.5		19	Illinois	87.4
12	Massachusetts	88.3		19	Washington	87.4
10	Michigan	88.8		22	Kansas	87.3
4	Minnesota	89.9		23	South Dakota	87.0
39	Mississippi	82.2		23	Virginia	87.0
16	Missouri	87.8		25	Tennessee	86.8
36	Montana	84.7		26	Alaska	86.7
13	Nebraska	88.1		27	Delaware	86.6
40	Nevada	81.9		27	North Dakota	86.6
17	New Hampshire	87.5		29	Maryland	86.5
30	New Jersey	86.3		30	New Jersey	86.3
48	New Mexico	78.0		31	New York	86.1
31	New York	86.1		32	North Carolina	86.0
32	North Carolina	86.0		33	Oregon	85.3
27	North Dakota	86.6		34	Idaho	85.2
7	Ohio	88.9		35	Wyoming	85.0
49	Oklahoma	76.4		36	Montana	84.7
33	Oregon	85.3		37	South Carolina	83.1
6	Pennsylvania	89.2		38	Alabama	82.8
5	Rhode Island	89.7		39	Mississippi	82.2
37	South Carolina	83.1		40	Nevada	81.9
23	South Dakota	87.0		41	West Virginia	81.7
25	Tennessee	86.8		42	Georgia	81.6
47	Texas	78.2		43	Florida	80.4
11	Utah	88.7		44	Arkansas	80.3
13	Vermont	88.1		44	California	80.3
23	Virginia	87.0		46	Arizona	79.8
19	Washington	87.4		47	Texas	78.2
41	West Virginia	81.7		48	New Mexico	78.0
1	Wisconsin	91.3		49	Oklahoma	76.4
35	Wyoming	85.0		50	Louisiana	76.1

District of Columbia   79.3

Source: Morgan Quitno Press using data from U.S. Bureau of the Census
"Health Insurance Coverage - 1993" (Statistical Brief, SB/94-28, October 1994)
This is the reverse of percent of population not covered which is based on percent of uninsured in each state issued by Census.

Persons Not Covered by Health Insurance in 1991

National Total = 36,306,864 Uninsured*

ALPHA ORDER					RANK ORDER			
RANK	STATE	UNINSURED	% of USA		RANK	STATE	UNINSURED	% of USA
14	Alabama	739,747	2.04%		1	California	5,900,704	16.25%
46	Alaska	77,953	0.21%		2	Texas	3,954,432	10.89%
18	Arizona	659,472	1.82%		3	Florida	2,511,432	6.92%
29	Arkansas	374,618	1.03%		4	New York	2,291,207	6.31%
1	California	5,900,704	16.25%		5	Illinois	1,359,950	3.75%
30	Colorado	347,110	0.96%		6	Ohio	1,125,996	3.10%
35	Connecticut	250,116	0.69%		7	Virginia	1,031,068	2.84%
44	Delaware	92,480	0.25%		8	North Carolina	1,012,800	2.79%
3	Florida	2,511,432	6.92%		9	Pennsylvania	955,760	2.63%
10	Georgia	940,608	2.59%		10	Georgia	940,608	2.59%
45	Hawaii	80,514	0.22%		11	Louisiana	886,369	2.44%
38	Idaho	187,020	0.52%		12	New Jersey	854,370	2.35%
5	Illinois	1,359,950	3.75%		13	Michigan	852,670	2.35%
15	Indiana	733,993	2.02%		14	Alabama	739,747	2.04%
34	Iowa	251,280	0.69%		15	Indiana	733,993	2.02%
32	Kansas	286,580	0.79%		16	Massachusetts	666,222	1.83%
24	Kentucky	486,665	1.34%		17	Tennessee	663,300	1.83%
11	Louisiana	886,369	2.44%		18	Arizona	659,472	1.82%
39	Maine	137,307	0.38%		19	Maryland	641,388	1.77%
19	Maryland	641,388	1.77%		20	Missouri	634,434	1.75%
16	Massachusetts	666,222	1.83%		21	Oklahoma	586,080	1.61%
13	Michigan	852,670	2.35%		22	Washington	531,908	1.47%
27	Minnesota	411,897	1.13%		23	Mississippi	495,454	1.36%
23	Mississippi	495,454	1.36%		24	Kentucky	486,665	1.34%
20	Missouri	634,434	1.75%		25	South Carolina	473,081	1.30%
42	Montana	103,424	0.28%		26	Oregon	426,320	1.17%
40	Nebraska	132,136	0.36%		27	Minnesota	411,897	1.13%
37	Nevada	242,865	0.67%		28	Wisconsin	400,869	1.10%
41	New Hampshire	111,908	0.31%		29	Arkansas	374,618	1.03%
12	New Jersey	854,370	2.35%		30	Colorado	347,110	0.96%
31	New Mexico	341,887	0.94%		31	New Mexico	341,887	0.94%
4	New York	2,291,207	6.31%		32	Kansas	286,580	0.79%
8	North Carolina	1,012,800	2.79%		33	West Virginia	282,443	0.78%
50	North Dakota	47,550	0.13%		34	Iowa	251,280	0.69%
6	Ohio	1,125,996	3.10%		35	Connecticut	250,116	0.69%
21	Oklahoma	586,080	1.61%		36	Utah	247,380	0.68%
26	Oregon	426,320	1.17%		37	Nevada	242,865	0.67%
9	Pennsylvania	955,760	2.63%		38	Idaho	187,020	0.52%
43	Rhode Island	103,412	0.28%		39	Maine	137,307	0.38%
25	South Carolina	473,081	1.30%		40	Nebraska	132,136	0.36%
48	South Dakota	70,200	0.19%		41	New Hampshire	111,908	0.31%
17	Tennessee	663,300	1.83%		42	Montana	103,424	0.28%
2	Texas	3,954,432	10.89%		43	Rhode Island	103,412	0.28%
36	Utah	247,380	0.68%		44	Delaware	92,480	0.25%
47	Vermont	72,704	0.20%		45	Hawaii	80,514	0.22%
7	Virginia	1,031,068	2.84%		46	Alaska	77,953	0.21%
22	Washington	531,908	1.47%		47	Vermont	72,704	0.20%
33	West Virginia	282,443	0.78%		48	South Dakota	70,200	0.19%
28	Wisconsin	400,869	1.10%		49	Wyoming	51,296	0.14%
49	Wyoming	51,296	0.14%		50	North Dakota	47,550	0.13%
						District of Columbia	155,628	0.43%

Source: Morgan Quitno Press using data from U.S. Bureau of the Census
"Health Insurance Coverage - 1993" (Statistical Brief, SB/94-28, October 1994)
*Based on percent of uninsured in each state issued by Census and updated 1991 state population estimates. National total calculated using 1991 national population estimate multiplied by Census national uninsured figure of 14.4%.

Percent of Persons Not Covered by Health Insurance in 1991

National Percent = 14.4% Uninsured

ALPHA ORDER

RANK	STATE	PERCENT		RANK	STATE	PERCENT
9	Alabama	18.1		1	Texas	22.8
19	Alaska	13.7		2	New Mexico	22.1
11	Arizona	17.6		3	Louisiana	20.9
13	Arkansas	15.8		4	California	19.4
4	California	19.4		5	Mississippi	19.1
37	Colorado	10.3		6	Florida	18.9
48	Connecticut	7.6		6	Nevada	18.9
20	Delaware	13.6		8	Oklahoma	18.5
6	Florida	18.9		9	Alabama	18.1
17	Georgia	14.2		10	Idaho	18.0
50	Hawaii	7.1		11	Arizona	17.6
10	Idaho	18.0		12	Virginia	16.4
30	Illinois	11.8		13	Arkansas	15.8
24	Indiana	13.1		14	West Virginia	15.7
44	Iowa	9.0		15	North Carolina	15.0
31	Kansas	11.5		16	Oregon	14.6
24	Kentucky	13.1		17	Georgia	14.2
3	Louisiana	20.9		18	Utah	14.0
33	Maine	11.1		19	Alaska	13.7
23	Maryland	13.2		20	Delaware	13.6
33	Massachusetts	11.1		21	Tennessee	13.4
43	Michigan	9.1		22	South Carolina	13.3
42	Minnesota	9.3		23	Maryland	13.2
5	Mississippi	19.1		24	Indiana	13.1
29	Missouri	12.3		24	Kentucky	13.1
26	Montana	12.8		26	Montana	12.8
45	Nebraska	8.3		26	Vermont	12.8
6	Nevada	18.9		28	New York	12.7
40	New Hampshire	10.1		29	Missouri	12.3
35	New Jersey	11.0		30	Illinois	11.8
2	New Mexico	22.1		31	Kansas	11.5
28	New York	12.7		32	Wyoming	11.2
15	North Carolina	15.0		33	Maine	11.1
49	North Dakota	7.5		33	Massachusetts	11.1
37	Ohio	10.3		35	New Jersey	11.0
8	Oklahoma	18.5		36	Washington	10.6
16	Oregon	14.6		37	Colorado	10.3
47	Pennsylvania	8.0		37	Ohio	10.3
37	Rhode Island	10.3		37	Rhode Island	10.3
22	South Carolina	13.3		40	New Hampshire	10.1
41	South Dakota	10.0		41	South Dakota	10.0
21	Tennessee	13.4		42	Minnesota	9.3
1	Texas	22.8		43	Michigan	9.1
18	Utah	14.0		44	Iowa	9.0
26	Vermont	12.8		45	Nebraska	8.3
12	Virginia	16.4		46	Wisconsin	8.1
36	Washington	10.6		47	Pennsylvania	8.0
14	West Virginia	15.7		48	Connecticut	7.6
46	Wisconsin	8.1		49	North Dakota	7.5
32	Wyoming	11.2		50	Hawaii	7.1

District of Columbia   26.2

Source: U.S. Bureau of the Census
"Health Insurance Coverage – 1993" (Statistical Brief, SB/94-28, October 1994)

Change in Number of Uninsured Persons: 1991 to 1993

National Change = 3,133,935 Increase*

ALPHA ORDER				RANK ORDER		
RANK	STATE	CHANGE		RANK	STATE	CHANGE
43	Alabama	(20,615)		1	Pennsylvania	343,480
37	Alaska	1,581		2	Georgia	329,360
11	Arizona	137,418		3	California	249,045
14	Arkansas	103,304		4	New York	232,060
3	California	249,045		5	New Jersey	222,313
15	Colorado	101,954		6	Michigan	206,850
17	Connecticut	77,684		7	Florida	178,864
38	Delaware	1,052		8	Oklahoma	176,908
7	Florida	178,864		9	South Carolina	140,389
2	Georgia	329,360		10	Louisiana	138,941
20	Hawaii	48,912		11	Arizona	137,418
44	Idaho	(24,220)		12	Washington	130,726
13	Illinois	112,486		13	Illinois	112,486
49	Indiana	(54,979)		14	Arkansas	103,304
34	Iowa	8,252		15	Colorado	101,954
25	Kansas	35,365		16	Ohio	101,775
42	Kentucky	(12,415)		17	Connecticut	77,684
10	Louisiana	138,941		18	Nebraska	59,811
39	Maine	333		19	West Virginia	50,251
27	Maryland	27,942		20	Hawaii	48,912
23	Massachusetts	37,884		21	Minnesota	45,027
6	Michigan	206,850		22	Wisconsin	37,959
21	Minnesota	45,027		23	Massachusetts	37,884
45	Mississippi	(25,534)		24	North Dakota	37,808
36	Missouri	4,236		25	Kansas	35,365
28	Montana	25,249		26	New Hampshire	28,592
18	Nebraska	59,811		27	Maryland	27,942
35	Nevada	7,277		28	Montana	25,249
26	New Hampshire	28,592		29	South Dakota	22,880
5	New Jersey	222,313		30	Oregon	19,825
32	New Mexico	13,633		31	Wyoming	19,204
4	New York	232,060		32	New Mexico	13,633
48	North Carolina	(39,520)		33	Tennessee	9,108
24	North Dakota	37,808		34	Iowa	8,252
16	Ohio	101,775		35	Nevada	7,277
8	Oklahoma	176,908		36	Missouri	4,236
30	Oregon	19,825		37	Alaska	1,581
1	Pennsylvania	343,480		38	Delaware	1,052
40	Rhode Island	(412)		39	Maine	333
9	South Carolina	140,389		40	Rhode Island	(412)
29	South Dakota	22,880		41	Vermont	(4,160)
33	Tennessee	9,108		42	Kentucky	(12,415)
46	Texas	(25,636)		43	Alabama	(20,615)
47	Utah	(37,200)		44	Idaho	(24,220)
41	Vermont	(4,160)		45	Mississippi	(25,534)
50	Virginia	(189,578)		46	Texas	(25,636)
12	Washington	130,726		47	Utah	(37,200)
19	West Virginia	50,251		48	North Carolina	(39,520)
22	Wisconsin	37,959		49	Indiana	(54,979)
31	Wyoming	19,204		50	Virginia	(189,578)
					District of Columbia	(35,775)

Source: Morgan Quitno Press using data from U.S. Bureau of the Census
    "Health Insurance Coverage - 1993" (Statistical Brief, SB/94-28, October 1994)
*Based on percent of uninsured in each state issued by Census and updated 1993 and 1991 state population estimates.

234

Percent Change in Number of Uninsured: 1991 to 1993

National Percent Change = 8.63% Increase*

ALPHA ORDER

RANK	STATE	PERCENT CHANGE
43	Alabama	(2.79)
35	Alaska	2.03
18	Arizona	20.84
12	Arkansas	27.58
31	California	4.22
11	Colorado	29.37
8	Connecticut	31.06
37	Delaware	1.14
27	Florida	7.12
6	Georgia	35.02
2	Hawaii	60.75
48	Idaho	(12.95)
26	Illinois	8.27
47	Indiana	(7.49)
33	Iowa	3.28
21	Kansas	12.34
42	Kentucky	(2.55)
20	Louisiana	15.68
39	Maine	0.24
30	Maryland	4.36
28	Massachusetts	5.69
17	Michigan	24.26
22	Minnesota	10.93
45	Mississippi	(5.15)
38	Missouri	0.67
16	Montana	24.41
3	Nebraska	45.26
34	Nevada	3.00
14	New Hampshire	25.55
13	New Jersey	26.02
32	New Mexico	3.99
23	New York	10.13
44	North Carolina	(3.90)
1	North Dakota	79.51
25	Ohio	9.04
9	Oklahoma	30.18
29	Oregon	4.65
5	Pennsylvania	35.94
40	Rhode Island	(0.40)
10	South Carolina	29.68
7	South Dakota	32.59
36	Tennessee	1.37
41	Texas	(0.65)
49	Utah	(15.04)
46	Vermont	(5.72)
50	Virginia	(18.39)
15	Washington	24.58
19	West Virginia	17.79
24	Wisconsin	9.47
4	Wyoming	37.44

RANK ORDER

RANK	STATE	PERCENT CHANGE
1	North Dakota	79.51
2	Hawaii	60.75
3	Nebraska	45.26
4	Wyoming	37.44
5	Pennsylvania	35.94
6	Georgia	35.02
7	South Dakota	32.59
8	Connecticut	31.06
9	Oklahoma	30.18
10	South Carolina	29.68
11	Colorado	29.37
12	Arkansas	27.58
13	New Jersey	26.02
14	New Hampshire	25.55
15	Washington	24.58
16	Montana	24.41
17	Michigan	24.26
18	Arizona	20.84
19	West Virginia	17.79
20	Louisiana	15.68
21	Kansas	12.34
22	Minnesota	10.93
23	New York	10.13
24	Wisconsin	9.47
25	Ohio	9.04
26	Illinois	8.27
27	Florida	7.12
28	Massachusetts	5.69
29	Oregon	4.65
30	Maryland	4.36
31	California	4.22
32	New Mexico	3.99
33	Iowa	3.28
34	Nevada	3.00
35	Alaska	2.03
36	Tennessee	1.37
37	Delaware	1.14
38	Missouri	0.67
39	Maine	0.24
40	Rhode Island	(0.40)
41	Texas	(0.65)
42	Kentucky	(2.55)
43	Alabama	(2.79)
44	North Carolina	(3.90)
45	Mississippi	(5.15)
46	Vermont	(5.72)
47	Indiana	(7.49)
48	Idaho	(12.95)
49	Utah	(15.04)
50	Virginia	(18.39)
	District of Columbia	(22.99)

Source: Morgan Quitno Press using data from U.S. Bureau of the Census
 "Health Insurance Coverage - 1993" (Statistical Brief, SB/94-28, October 1994)
*Based on percent of uninsured in each state issued by Census and updated 1993 and 1991 state population estimates.

Percent Change in Percent of Population Uninsured: 1991 to 1993

National Percent Change = 6.25% Increase*

ALPHA ORDER			RANK ORDER		
RANK	STATE	PERCENT CHANGE	RANK	STATE	PERCENT CHANGE
43	Alabama	(5.0)	1	North Dakota	78.7
39	Alaska	(2.9)	2	Hawaii	56.3
19	Arizona	14.8	3	Nebraska	43.4
11	Arkansas	24.7	4	Pennsylvania	35.0
31	California	1.6	5	Wyoming	33.9
15	Colorado	22.3	6	Connecticut	31.6
6	Connecticut	31.6	7	South Dakota	30.0
37	Delaware	(1.5)	8	Georgia	29.6
28	Florida	3.7	9	Oklahoma	27.6
8	Georgia	29.6	10	South Carolina	27.1
2	Hawaii	56.3	11	Arkansas	24.7
48	Idaho	(17.8)	12	New Jersey	24.6
26	Illinois	6.8	13	New Hampshire	23.8
47	Indiana	(9.2)	14	Michigan	23.1
30	Iowa	2.2	15	Colorado	22.3
21	Kansas	10.4	16	Montana	19.5
42	Kentucky	(4.6)	17	Washington	18.9
20	Louisiana	14.4	18	West Virginia	16.6
33	Maine	0.0	19	Arizona	14.8
29	Maryland	2.3	20	Louisiana	14.4
27	Massachusetts	5.4	21	Kansas	10.4
14	Michigan	23.1	22	New York	9.5
23	Minnesota	8.6	23	Minnesota	8.6
45	Mississippi	(6.8)	24	Ohio	7.8
36	Missouri	(0.8)	25	Wisconsin	7.4
16	Montana	19.5	26	Illinois	6.8
3	Nebraska	43.4	27	Massachusetts	5.4
40	Nevada	(4.2)	28	Florida	3.7
13	New Hampshire	23.8	29	Maryland	2.3
12	New Jersey	24.6	30	Iowa	2.2
35	New Mexico	(0.5)	31	California	1.6
22	New York	9.5	32	Oregon	0.7
44	North Carolina	(6.7)	33	Maine	0.0
1	North Dakota	78.7	33	Rhode Island	0.0
24	Ohio	7.8	35	New Mexico	(0.5)
9	Oklahoma	27.6	36	Missouri	(0.8)
32	Oregon	0.7	37	Delaware	(1.5)
4	Pennsylvania	35.0	38	Tennessee	(1.5)
33	Rhode Island	0.0	39	Alaska	(2.9)
10	South Carolina	27.1	40	Nevada	(4.2)
7	South Dakota	30.0	41	Texas	(4.4)
38	Tennessee	(1.5)	42	Kentucky	(4.6)
41	Texas	(4.4)	43	Alabama	(5.0)
49	Utah	(19.3)	44	North Carolina	(6.7)
46	Vermont	(7.0)	45	Mississippi	(6.8)
50	Virginia	(20.7)	46	Vermont	(7.0)
17	Washington	18.9	47	Indiana	(9.2)
18	West Virginia	16.6	48	Idaho	(17.8)
25	Wisconsin	7.4	49	Utah	(19.3)
5	Wyoming	33.9	50	Virginia	(20.7)
				District of Columbia	(21.0)

Source: Morgan Quitno Press using data from U.S. Bureau of the Census
   "Health Insurance Coverage - 1993" (Statistical Brief, SB/94-28, October 1994)
*Based on percent of uninsured in each state issued by Census.

Number of Health Maintenance Organizations (HMOs) in 1993

National Total = 543 HMOs*

ALPHA ORDER

RANK	STATE	HMOs	% of USA
22	Alabama	9	1.66%
48	Alaska	0	0.00%
9	Arizona	19	3.50%
33	Arkansas	5	0.92%
1	California	40	7.37%
13	Colorado	14	2.58%
13	Connecticut	14	2.58%
36	Delaware	4	0.74%
2	Florida	35	6.45%
22	Georgia	9	1.66%
29	Hawaii	6	1.10%
42	Idaho	1	0.18%
5	Illinois	26	4.79%
16	Indiana	12	2.21%
38	Iowa	3	0.55%
22	Kansas	9	1.66%
29	Kentucky	6	1.10%
22	Louisiana	9	1.66%
40	Maine	2	0.37%
13	Maryland	14	2.58%
12	Massachusetts	16	2.95%
11	Michigan	17	3.13%
22	Minnesota	9	1.66%
42	Mississippi	1	0.18%
10	Missouri	18	3.31%
42	Montana	1	0.18%
33	Nebraska	5	0.92%
29	Nevada	6	1.10%
40	New Hampshire	2	0.37%
20	New Jersey	10	1.84%
29	New Mexico	6	1.10%
3	New York	34	6.26%
20	North Carolina	10	1.84%
42	North Dakota	1	0.18%
4	Ohio	32	5.89%
33	Oklahoma	5	0.92%
28	Oregon	7	1.29%
8	Pennsylvania	20	3.68%
38	Rhode Island	3	0.55%
36	South Carolina	4	0.74%
42	South Dakota	1	0.18%
18	Tennessee	11	2.03%
5	Texas	26	4.79%
27	Utah	8	1.47%
42	Vermont	1	0.18%
16	Virginia	12	2.21%
18	Washington	11	2.03%
48	West Virginia	0	0.00%
5	Wisconsin	26	4.79%
48	Wyoming	0	0.00%

RANK ORDER

RANK	STATE	HMOs	% of USA
1	California	40	7.37%
2	Florida	35	6.45%
3	New York	34	6.26%
4	Ohio	32	5.89%
5	Illinois	26	4.79%
5	Texas	26	4.79%
5	Wisconsin	26	4.79%
8	Pennsylvania	20	3.68%
9	Arizona	19	3.50%
10	Missouri	18	3.31%
11	Michigan	17	3.13%
12	Massachusetts	16	2.95%
13	Colorado	14	2.58%
13	Connecticut	14	2.58%
13	Maryland	14	2.58%
16	Indiana	12	2.21%
16	Virginia	12	2.21%
18	Tennessee	11	2.03%
18	Washington	11	2.03%
20	New Jersey	10	1.84%
20	North Carolina	10	1.84%
22	Alabama	9	1.66%
22	Georgia	9	1.66%
22	Kansas	9	1.66%
22	Louisiana	9	1.66%
22	Minnesota	9	1.66%
27	Utah	8	1.47%
28	Oregon	7	1.29%
29	Hawaii	6	1.10%
29	Kentucky	6	1.10%
29	Nevada	6	1.10%
29	New Mexico	6	1.10%
33	Arkansas	5	0.92%
33	Nebraska	5	0.92%
33	Oklahoma	5	0.92%
36	Delaware	4	0.74%
36	South Carolina	4	0.74%
38	Iowa	3	0.55%
38	Rhode Island	3	0.55%
40	Maine	2	0.37%
40	New Hampshire	2	0.37%
42	Idaho	1	0.18%
42	Mississippi	1	0.18%
42	Montana	1	0.18%
42	North Dakota	1	0.18%
42	South Dakota	1	0.18%
42	Vermont	1	0.18%
48	Alaska	0	0.00%
48	West Virginia	0	0.00%
48	Wyoming	0	0.00%
	District of Columbia	3	0.55%

Source: Group Health Association of America

"Patterns in HMO Enrollment" (4th Edition, June 1994, Reprinted with permission of GHAA, 1129 20th Street, NW, Washington, DC 20036)

*As of December 31, 1993. Total does not include two HMOs in Guam.

Enrollees in Health Maintenance Organizations (HMOs) in 1993

National Total = 45,126,556 Enrollees*

<u>ALPHA ORDER</u>

RANK	STATE	ENROLLEES	% of USA
27	Alabama	267,361	0.59%
48	Alaska	0	0.00%
12	Arizona	1,302,851	2.89%
40	Arkansas	67,281	0.15%
1	California	10,999,128	24.37%
16	Colorado	834,967	1.85%
17	Connecticut	805,928	1.79%
36	Delaware	120,753	0.27%
3	Florida	2,414,714	5.35%
20	Georgia	495,949	1.10%
28	Hawaii	263,172	0.58%
44	Idaho	11,926	0.03%
6	Illinois	1,890,512	4.19%
23	Indiana	384,205	0.85%
39	Iowa	106,194	0.24%
33	Kansas	191,997	0.43%
31	Kentucky	250,223	0.55%
25	Louisiana	305,392	0.68%
42	Maine	53,637	0.12%
10	Maryland	1,598,083	3.54%
5	Massachusetts	2,063,481	4.57%
8	Michigan	1,753,593	3.89%
11	Minnesota	1,366,552	3.03%
46	Mississippi	3,200	0.01%
19	Missouri	752,900	1.67%
45	Montana	11,390	0.03%
38	Nebraska	108,975	0.24%
34	Nevada	176,883	0.39%
35	New Hampshire	153,356	0.34%
14	New Jersey	1,026,143	2.27%
30	New Mexico	254,664	0.56%
2	New York	3,919,013	8.68%
22	North Carolina	459,392	1.02%
47	North Dakota	3,008	0.01%
9	Ohio	1,698,013	3.76%
32	Oklahoma	235,841	0.52%
15	Oregon	959,573	2.13%
4	Pennsylvania	2,293,233	5.08%
29	Rhode Island	260,552	0.58%
37	South Carolina	119,892	0.27%
43	South Dakota	20,890	0.05%
26	Tennessee	291,286	0.65%
7	Texas	1,757,713	3.90%
24	Utah	345,612	0.77%
41	Vermont	64,489	0.14%
21	Virginia	468,605	1.04%
18	Washington	803,847	1.78%
48	West Virginia	0	0.00%
13	Wisconsin	1,171,819	2.60%
48	Wyoming	0	0.00%

<u>RANK ORDER</u>

RANK	STATE	ENROLLEES	% of USA
1	California	10,999,128	24.37%
2	New York	3,919,013	8.68%
3	Florida	2,414,714	5.35%
4	Pennsylvania	2,293,233	5.08%
5	Massachusetts	2,063,481	4.57%
6	Illinois	1,890,512	4.19%
7	Texas	1,757,713	3.90%
8	Michigan	1,753,593	3.89%
9	Ohio	1,698,013	3.76%
10	Maryland	1,598,083	3.54%
11	Minnesota	1,366,552	3.03%
12	Arizona	1,302,851	2.89%
13	Wisconsin	1,171,819	2.60%
14	New Jersey	1,026,143	2.27%
15	Oregon	959,573	2.13%
16	Colorado	834,967	1.85%
17	Connecticut	805,928	1.79%
18	Washington	803,847	1.78%
19	Missouri	752,900	1.67%
20	Georgia	495,949	1.10%
21	Virginia	468,605	1.04%
22	North Carolina	459,392	1.02%
23	Indiana	384,205	0.85%
24	Utah	345,612	0.77%
25	Louisiana	305,392	0.68%
26	Tennessee	291,286	0.65%
27	Alabama	267,361	0.59%
28	Hawaii	263,172	0.58%
29	Rhode Island	260,552	0.58%
30	New Mexico	254,664	0.56%
31	Kentucky	250,223	0.55%
32	Oklahoma	235,841	0.52%
33	Kansas	191,997	0.43%
34	Nevada	176,883	0.39%
35	New Hampshire	153,356	0.34%
36	Delaware	120,753	0.27%
37	South Carolina	119,892	0.27%
38	Nebraska	108,975	0.24%
39	Iowa	106,194	0.24%
40	Arkansas	67,281	0.15%
41	Vermont	64,489	0.14%
42	Maine	53,637	0.12%
43	South Dakota	20,890	0.05%
44	Idaho	11,926	0.03%
45	Montana	11,390	0.03%
46	Mississippi	3,200	0.01%
47	North Dakota	3,008	0.01%
48	Alaska	0	0.00%
48	West Virginia	0	0.00%
48	Wyoming	0	0.00%
	District of Columbia	218,368	0.48%

Source: Group Health Association of America
   "Patterns in HMO Enrollment" (4th Edition, June 1994, Reprinted with permission of GHAA, 1129 20th Street, NW, Washington, DC 20036)
*As of December 31, 1993. Total does not include 78,791 enrollees in Guam.

Percent of Population Enrolled in Health Maintenance Organizations (HMOs) in 1993

National Percent = 17.51% Enrolled in HMOs*

<u>ALPHA ORDER</u>

RANK	STATE	PERCENT
37	Alabama	6.39
48	Alaska	0.00
3	Arizona	33.03
43	Arkansas	2.77
1	California	35.23
9	Colorado	23.43
8	Connecticut	24.59
17	Delaware	17.30
16	Florida	17.59
31	Georgia	7.19
11	Hawaii	22.57
45	Idaho	1.08
18	Illinois	16.18
34	Indiana	6.73
40	Iowa	3.76
28	Kansas	7.57
36	Kentucky	6.60
32	Louisiana	7.12
39	Maine	4.33
4	Maryland	32.23
2	Massachusetts	34.29
15	Michigan	18.54
6	Minnesota	30.21
47	Mississippi	0.12
22	Missouri	14.38
44	Montana	1.35
33	Nebraska	6.76
25	Nevada	12.80
23	New Hampshire	13.64
24	New Jersey	13.06
19	New Mexico	15.76
12	New York	21.59
35	North Carolina	6.61
46	North Dakota	0.47
20	Ohio	15.35
29	Oklahoma	7.29
5	Oregon	31.62
13	Pennsylvania	19.06
7	Rhode Island	26.06
41	South Carolina	3.30
42	South Dakota	2.92
38	Tennessee	5.72
27	Texas	9.75
14	Utah	18.58
26	Vermont	11.20
30	Virginia	7.24
21	Washington	15.29
48	West Virginia	0.00
10	Wisconsin	23.23
48	Wyoming	0.00

<u>RANK ORDER</u>

RANK	STATE	PERCENT
1	California	35.23
2	Massachusetts	34.29
3	Arizona	33.03
4	Maryland	32.23
5	Oregon	31.62
6	Minnesota	30.21
7	Rhode Island	26.06
8	Connecticut	24.59
9	Colorado	23.43
10	Wisconsin	23.23
11	Hawaii	22.57
12	New York	21.59
13	Pennsylvania	19.06
14	Utah	18.58
15	Michigan	18.54
16	Florida	17.59
17	Delaware	17.30
18	Illinois	16.18
19	New Mexico	15.76
20	Ohio	15.35
21	Washington	15.29
22	Missouri	14.38
23	New Hampshire	13.64
24	New Jersey	13.06
25	Nevada	12.80
26	Vermont	11.20
27	Texas	9.75
28	Kansas	7.57
29	Oklahoma	7.29
30	Virginia	7.24
31	Georgia	7.19
32	Louisiana	7.12
33	Nebraska	6.76
34	Indiana	6.73
35	North Carolina	6.61
36	Kentucky	6.60
37	Alabama	6.39
38	Tennessee	5.72
39	Maine	4.33
40	Iowa	3.76
41	South Carolina	3.30
42	South Dakota	2.92
43	Arkansas	2.77
44	Montana	1.35
45	Idaho	1.08
46	North Dakota	0.47
47	Mississippi	0.12
48	Alaska	0.00
48	West Virginia	0.00
48	Wyoming	0.00

District of Columbia**   NA

Source: Morgan Quitno Press using data from Group Health Association of America
   "Patterns in HMO Enrollment" (4th Edition, June 1994, Reprinted with permission of GHAA, 1129 20th Street, NW, Washington, DC 20036)
*As of December 31, 1993. Based on updated 1993 Census population estimates. National percent does not include enrollees in Guam.
**Not available.

239

Percent of Insured Population
Enrolled in Health Maintenance Organizations (HMOs) in 1993
National Percent = 20.67% of Insured are Enrolled in HMOs*

RANK	STATE	PERCENT	RANK	STATE	PERCENT
33	Alabama	7.72	1	California	43.88
48	Alaska	0.00	2	Arizona	41.39
2	Arizona	41.39	3	Massachusetts	38.83
42	Arkansas	3.45	4	Maryland	37.26
1	California	43.88	5	Oregon	37.07
9	Colorado	26.81	6	Minnesota	33.60
8	Connecticut	27.32	7	Rhode Island	29.05
18	Delaware	19.98	8	Connecticut	27.32
13	Florida	21.88	9	Colorado	26.81
30	Georgia	8.81	10	Wisconsin	25.45
11	Hawaii	25.39	11	Hawaii	25.39
45	Idaho	1.27	12	New York	25.07
19	Illinois	18.51	13	Florida	21.88
36	Indiana	7.64	14	Pennsylvania	21.37
40	Iowa	4.15	15	Utah	20.95
31	Kansas	8.68	16	Michigan	20.87
37	Kentucky	7.54	17	New Mexico	20.20
29	Louisiana	9.35	18	Delaware	19.98
39	Maine	4.87	19	Illinois	18.51
4	Maryland	37.26	20	Washington	17.49
3	Massachusetts	38.83	21	Ohio	17.27
16	Michigan	20.87	22	Missouri	16.38
6	Minnesota	33.60	23	Nevada	15.63
47	Mississippi	0.15	24	New Hampshire	15.59
22	Missouri	16.38	25	New Jersey	15.13
44	Montana	1.60	26	Vermont	12.71
35	Nebraska	7.67	27	Texas	12.47
23	Nevada	15.63	28	Oklahoma	9.55
24	New Hampshire	15.59	29	Louisiana	9.35
25	New Jersey	15.13	30	Georgia	8.81
17	New Mexico	20.20	31	Kansas	8.68
12	New York	25.07	32	Virginia	8.32
34	North Carolina	7.68	33	Alabama	7.72
46	North Dakota	0.55	34	North Carolina	7.68
21	Ohio	17.27	35	Nebraska	7.67
28	Oklahoma	9.55	36	Indiana	7.64
5	Oregon	37.07	37	Kentucky	7.54
14	Pennsylvania	21.37	38	Tennessee	6.59
7	Rhode Island	29.05	39	Maine	4.87
41	South Carolina	3.97	40	Iowa	4.15
43	South Dakota	3.35	41	South Carolina	3.97
38	Tennessee	6.59	42	Arkansas	3.45
27	Texas	12.47	43	South Dakota	3.35
15	Utah	20.95	44	Montana	1.60
26	Vermont	12.71	45	Idaho	1.27
32	Virginia	8.32	46	North Dakota	0.55
20	Washington	17.49	47	Mississippi	0.15
48	West Virginia	0.00	48	Alaska	0.00
10	Wisconsin	25.45	48	West Virginia	0.00
48	Wyoming	0.00	48	Wyoming	0.00
				District of Columbia**	NA

Source: Morgan Quitno Press using data from Group Health Association of America
 "Patterns in HMO Enrollment" (4th Edition, June 1994, Reprinted with permission of GHAA, 1129 20th Street, NW,
  Washington, DC 20036)
*As of December 31, 1993. Based on updated 1993 Census population estimates. National percent does not include
enrollees in Guam.
**Not available.

Preferred Provider Organizations (PPOs) in 1994

National Total = 1,105 PPOs*

ALPHA ORDER					RANK ORDER			
RANK	STATE		PPOs	% of USA	RANK	STATE		PPOs	% of USA

RANK	STATE	PPOs	% of USA
14	Alabama	29	2.62%
43	Alaska	3	0.27%
12	Arizona	30	2.71%
36	Arkansas	9	0.81%
1	California	84	7.60%
10	Colorado	33	2.99%
28	Connecticut	16	1.45%
39	Delaware	6	0.54%
2	Florida	78	7.06%
7	Georgia	39	3.53%
39	Hawaii	6	0.54%
46	Idaho	2	0.18%
5	Illinois	50	4.52%
8	Indiana	37	3.35%
31	Iowa	13	1.18%
21	Kansas	21	1.90%
28	Kentucky	16	1.45%
12	Louisiana	30	2.71%
39	Maine	6	0.54%
21	Maryland	21	1.90%
18	Massachusetts	23	2.08%
15	Michigan	28	2.53%
30	Minnesota	14	1.27%
35	Mississippi	10	0.90%
11	Missouri	31	2.81%
47	Montana	1	0.09%
33	Nebraska	11	1.00%
24	Nevada	20	1.81%
42	New Hampshire	5	0.45%
18	New Jersey	23	2.08%
37	New Mexico	7	0.63%
18	New York	23	2.08%
17	North Carolina	24	2.17%
49	North Dakota	0	0.00%
6	Ohio	47	4.25%
24	Oklahoma	20	1.81%
31	Oregon	13	1.18%
4	Pennsylvania	56	5.07%
43	Rhode Island	3	0.27%
27	South Carolina	18	1.63%
43	South Dakota	3	0.27%
8	Tennessee	37	3.35%
3	Texas	67	6.06%
33	Utah	11	1.00%
47	Vermont	1	0.09%
26	Virginia	19	1.72%
21	Washington	21	1.90%
37	West Virginia	7	0.63%
16	Wisconsin	26	2.35%
49	Wyoming	0	0.00%

RANK	STATE	PPOs	% of USA
1	California	84	7.60%
2	Florida	78	7.06%
3	Texas	67	6.06%
4	Pennsylvania	56	5.07%
5	Illinois	50	4.52%
6	Ohio	47	4.25%
7	Georgia	39	3.53%
8	Indiana	37	3.35%
8	Tennessee	37	3.35%
10	Colorado	33	2.99%
11	Missouri	31	2.81%
12	Arizona	30	2.71%
12	Louisiana	30	2.71%
14	Alabama	29	2.62%
15	Michigan	28	2.53%
16	Wisconsin	26	2.35%
17	North Carolina	24	2.17%
18	Massachusetts	23	2.08%
18	New Jersey	23	2.08%
18	New York	23	2.08%
21	Kansas	21	1.90%
21	Maryland	21	1.90%
21	Washington	21	1.90%
24	Nevada	20	1.81%
24	Oklahoma	20	1.81%
26	Virginia	19	1.72%
27	South Carolina	18	1.63%
28	Connecticut	16	1.45%
28	Kentucky	16	1.45%
30	Minnesota	14	1.27%
31	Iowa	13	1.18%
31	Oregon	13	1.18%
33	Nebraska	11	1.00%
33	Utah	11	1.00%
35	Mississippi	10	0.90%
36	Arkansas	9	0.81%
37	New Mexico	7	0.63%
37	West Virginia	7	0.63%
39	Delaware	6	0.54%
39	Hawaii	6	0.54%
39	Maine	6	0.54%
42	New Hampshire	5	0.45%
43	Alaska	3	0.27%
43	Rhode Island	3	0.27%
43	South Dakota	3	0.27%
46	Idaho	2	0.18%
47	Montana	1	0.09%
47	Vermont	1	0.09%
49	North Dakota	0	0.00%
49	Wyoming	0	0.00%
	District of Columbia	7	0.63%

Source: American Managed Care and Review Association, Washington, D.C. (reprinted with permission)
"AMCRA Foundation Managed Health Care Database"
*As of October 1994. Total does not include two PPOs in Puerto Rico.

Enrollment in Preferred Provider Organizations (PPOs) in 1993

National Total = 60,037,800 Enrollees*

ALPHA ORDER

RANK ORDER

RANK	STATE	ENROLLEES	% of USA	RANK	STATE	ENROLLEES	% of USA
10	Alabama	1,447,382	2.41%	1	California	7,309,847	12.18%
42	Alaska	17,977	0.03%	2	Texas	5,180,493	8.63%
21	Arizona	650,372	1.08%	3	Florida	3,039,137	5.06%
38	Arkansas	62,092	0.10%	4	Illinois	2,852,985	4.75%
1	California	7,309,847	12.18%	5	Ohio	2,190,132	3.65%
6	Colorado	1,816,605	3.03%	6	Colorado	1,816,605	3.03%
35	Connecticut	151,790	0.25%	7	Pennsylvania	1,671,562	2.78%
45	Delaware	8,754	0.01%	8	Tennessee	1,625,072	2.71%
3	Florida	3,039,137	5.06%	9	Minnesota	1,490,398	2.48%
15	Georgia	923,543	1.54%	10	Alabama	1,447,382	2.41%
25	Hawaii	476,921	0.79%	11	Washington	1,263,936	2.11%
46	Idaho	2,735	0.00%	12	Missouri	1,177,764	1.96%
4	Illinois	2,852,985	4.75%	13	Maryland	1,043,793	1.74%
16	Indiana	911,003	1.52%	14	New Jersey	1,033,625	1.72%
33	Iowa	251,762	0.42%	15	Georgia	923,543	1.54%
31	Kansas	381,090	0.63%	16	Indiana	911,003	1.52%
28	Kentucky	441,403	0.74%	17	North Carolina	784,023	1.31%
20	Louisiana	665,660	1.11%	18	Michigan	736,796	1.23%
44	Maine	9,374	0.02%	19	New York	707,893	1.18%
13	Maryland	1,043,793	1.74%	20	Louisiana	665,660	1.11%
27	Massachusetts	456,712	0.76%	21	Arizona	650,372	1.08%
18	Michigan	736,796	1.23%	22	Wisconsin	568,195	0.95%
9	Minnesota	1,490,398	2.48%	23	Nebraska	533,509	0.89%
39	Mississippi	60,407	0.10%	24	Virginia	514,958	0.86%
12	Missouri	1,177,764	1.96%	25	Hawaii	476,921	0.79%
48	Montana	1,778	0.00%	26	Oregon	474,455	0.79%
23	Nebraska	533,509	0.89%	27	Massachusetts	456,712	0.76%
32	Nevada	256,919	0.43%	28	Kentucky	441,403	0.74%
41	New Hampshire	36,899	0.06%	29	South Carolina	422,353	0.70%
14	New Jersey	1,033,625	1.72%	30	Oklahoma	416,815	0.69%
40	New Mexico	38,436	0.06%	31	Kansas	381,090	0.63%
19	New York	707,893	1.18%	32	Nevada	256,919	0.43%
17	North Carolina	784,023	1.31%	33	Iowa	251,762	0.42%
49	North Dakota	0	0.00%	34	Utah	160,948	0.27%
5	Ohio	2,190,132	3.65%	35	Connecticut	151,790	0.25%
30	Oklahoma	416,815	0.69%	36	Rhode Island	96,269	0.16%
26	Oregon	474,455	0.79%	37	West Virginia	78,011	0.13%
7	Pennsylvania	1,671,562	2.78%	38	Arkansas	62,092	0.10%
36	Rhode Island	96,269	0.16%	39	Mississippi	60,407	0.10%
29	South Carolina	422,353	0.70%	40	New Mexico	38,436	0.06%
43	South Dakota	11,281	0.02%	41	New Hampshire	36,899	0.06%
8	Tennessee	1,625,072	2.71%	42	Alaska	17,977	0.03%
2	Texas	5,180,493	8.63%	43	South Dakota	11,281	0.02%
34	Utah	160,948	0.27%	44	Maine	9,374	0.02%
47	Vermont	1,832	0.00%	45	Delaware	8,754	0.01%
24	Virginia	514,958	0.86%	46	Idaho	2,735	0.00%
11	Washington	1,263,936	2.11%	47	Vermont	1,832	0.00%
37	West Virginia	78,011	0.13%	48	Montana	1,778	0.00%
22	Wisconsin	568,195	0.95%	49	North Dakota	0	0.00%
49	Wyoming	0	0.00%	49	Wyoming	0	0.00%
					District of Columbia	57,771	0.10%

Source: American Managed Care and Review Association, Washington, D.C. (reprinted with permission)
 "AMCRA Foundation Managed Health Care Database"
As of December 31, 1993. Total includes 15,450,707 enrollees for whom state of resident is not known and 73,636 enrollees in Puerto Rico.

Percent of Population Enrolled in a Preferred Provider Organization (PPO) in 1993

National Percent = 23.3% of Population*

ALPHA ORDER

RANK	STATE	PERCENT
3	Alabama	34.5
40	Alaska	3.1
17	Arizona	16.5
41	Arkansas	2.5
10	California	23.4
1	Colorado	50.9
36	Connecticut	4.6
44	Delaware	1.2
13	Florida	22.2
23	Georgia	13.3
2	Hawaii	40.7
47	Idaho	0.2
8	Illinois	24.4
18	Indiana	15.9
31	Iowa	8.9
21	Kansas	15.1
26	Kentucky	11.6
20	Louisiana	15.5
45	Maine	0.8
14	Maryland	21.1
35	Massachusetts	7.6
34	Michigan	7.7
5	Minnesota	32.9
11	Mississippi	22.8
12	Missouri	22.5
47	Montana	0.2
4	Nebraska	33.2
16	Nevada	18.5
39	New Hampshire	3.3
24	New Jersey	13.1
42	New Mexico	2.4
38	New York	3.8
28	North Carolina	11.2
49	North Dakota	0.0
15	Ohio	19.7
25	Oklahoma	12.9
19	Oregon	15.6
22	Pennsylvania	13.8
30	Rhode Island	9.6
26	South Carolina	11.6
43	South Dakota	1.6
6	Tennessee	31.8
7	Texas	28.7
32	Utah	8.6
46	Vermont	0.3
33	Virginia	7.9
9	Washington	24.1
37	West Virginia	4.2
28	Wisconsin	11.2
49	Wyoming	0.0

RANK ORDER

RANK	STATE	PERCENT
1	Colorado	50.9
2	Hawaii	40.7
3	Alabama	34.5
4	Nebraska	33.2
5	Minnesota	32.9
6	Tennessee	31.8
7	Texas	28.7
8	Illinois	24.4
9	Washington	24.1
10	California	23.4
11	Mississippi	22.8
12	Missouri	22.5
13	Florida	22.2
14	Maryland	21.1
15	Ohio	19.7
16	Nevada	18.5
17	Arizona	16.5
18	Indiana	15.9
19	Oregon	15.6
20	Louisiana	15.5
21	Kansas	15.1
22	Pennsylvania	13.8
23	Georgia	13.3
24	New Jersey	13.1
25	Oklahoma	12.9
26	Kentucky	11.6
26	South Carolina	11.6
28	North Carolina	11.2
28	Wisconsin	11.2
30	Rhode Island	9.6
31	Iowa	8.9
32	Utah	8.6
33	Virginia	7.9
34	Michigan	7.7
35	Massachusetts	7.6
36	Connecticut	4.6
37	West Virginia	4.2
38	New York	3.8
39	New Hampshire	3.3
40	Alaska	3.1
41	Arkansas	2.5
42	New Mexico	2.4
43	South Dakota	1.6
44	Delaware	1.2
45	Maine	0.8
46	Vermont	0.3
47	Idaho	0.2
47	Montana	0.2
49	North Dakota	0.0
49	Wyoming	0.0
	District of Columbia	9.9

Source: American Managed Care and Review Association, Washington, D.C. (reprinted with permission)
    "AMCRA Foundation Managed Health Care Database"
*As of December 31, 1993. National rate includes enrollees for whom state of resident is not known but excludes enrollees in Puerto Rico.

Percent of Insured Population in a Preferred Provider Organization (PPO) in 1993

National Percent = 27.5% of Insured Population*

ALPHA ORDER			RANK ORDER		
RANK	STATE	PERCENT	RANK	STATE	PERCENT
3	Alabama	41.7	1	Colorado	58.2
39	Alaska	3.4	2	Hawaii	45.8
16	Arizona	20.7	3	Alabama	41.7
40	Arkansas	3.2	4	Nebraska	37.6
8	California	29.1	5	Minnesota	36.7
1	Colorado	58.2	5	Tennessee	36.7
36	Connecticut	5.1	5	Texas	36.7
44	Delaware	1.4	8	California	29.1
10	Florida	27.6	9	Illinois	27.9
22	Georgia	16.3	10	Florida	27.6
2	Hawaii	45.8	11	Washington	27.5
47	Idaho	0.3	12	Missouri	25.6
9	Illinois	27.9	13	Maryland	24.3
19	Indiana	18.1	14	Nevada	22.6
30	Iowa	9.8	15	Ohio	22.2
20	Kansas	17.2	16	Arizona	20.7
26	Kentucky	13.3	17	Louisiana	20.4
17	Louisiana	20.4	18	Oregon	18.3
45	Maine	0.9	19	Indiana	18.1
13	Maryland	24.3	20	Kansas	17.2
34	Massachusetts	8.6	21	Oklahoma	16.8
33	Michigan	8.8	22	Georgia	16.3
5	Minnesota	36.7	23	Pennsylvania	15.5
42	Mississippi	2.8	24	New Jersey	15.2
12	Missouri	25.6	25	South Carolina	13.9
47	Montana	0.3	26	Kentucky	13.3
4	Nebraska	37.6	27	North Carolina	13.1
14	Nevada	22.6	28	Wisconsin	12.3
38	New Hampshire	3.7	29	Rhode Island	10.7
24	New Jersey	15.2	30	Iowa	9.8
41	New Mexico	3.1	30	Utah	9.8
37	New York	4.5	32	Virginia	9.1
27	North Carolina	13.1	33	Michigan	8.8
49	North Dakota	0.0	34	Massachusetts	8.6
15	Ohio	22.2	35	West Virginia	5.2
21	Oklahoma	16.8	36	Connecticut	5.1
18	Oregon	18.3	37	New York	4.5
23	Pennsylvania	15.5	38	New Hampshire	3.7
29	Rhode Island	10.7	39	Alaska	3.4
25	South Carolina	13.9	40	Arkansas	3.2
43	South Dakota	1.8	41	New Mexico	3.1
5	Tennessee	36.7	42	Mississippi	2.8
5	Texas	36.7	43	South Dakota	1.8
30	Utah	9.8	44	Delaware	1.4
46	Vermont	0.4	45	Maine	0.9
32	Virginia	9.1	46	Vermont	0.4
11	Washington	27.5	47	Idaho	0.3
35	West Virginia	5.2	47	Montana	0.3
28	Wisconsin	12.3	49	North Dakota	0.0
49	Wyoming	0.0	49	Wyoming	0.0
				District of Columbia	12.6

Source: Morgan Quitno Press using data from American Managed Care and Review Association, Washington, D.C.
"AMCRA Foundation Managed Health Care Database" (reprinted with permission)
*As of December 31, 1993. National rate includes enrollees for whom state of resident is not known but excludes enrollees in Puerto Rico.

Civilian Health and Medical Program of the Uniformed Services (CHAMPUS): 1995

National Total = 5,037,115 Eligible to Enroll*

ALPHA ORDER

RANK	STATE	ELIGIBLE	% of USA
11	Alabama	114,573	2.27%
28	Alaska	49,058	0.97%
12	Arizona	110,286	2.19%
30	Arkansas	45,443	0.90%
1	California	631,058	12.53%
10	Colorado	133,773	2.66%
35	Connecticut	31,323	0.62%
44	Delaware	17,505	0.35%
4	Florida	392,000	7.78%
6	Georgia	229,337	4.55%
14	Hawaii	90,230	1.79%
38	Idaho	23,834	0.47%
19	Illinois	83,968	1.67%
33	Indiana	39,603	0.79%
46	Iowa	15,221	0.30%
23	Kansas	69,531	1.38%
20	Kentucky	80,723	1.60%
17	Louisiana	86,526	1.72%
37	Maine	26,194	0.52%
9	Maryland	139,348	2.77%
32	Massachusetts	39,937	0.79%
29	Michigan	46,896	0.93%
41	Minnesota	21,669	0.43%
25	Mississippi	60,799	1.21%
22	Missouri	70,816	1.41%
42	Montana	18,546	0.37%
31	Nebraska	40,478	0.80%
26	Nevada	51,945	1.03%
47	New Hampshire	14,525	0.29%
27	New Jersey	51,002	1.01%
24	New Mexico	61,250	1.22%
18	New York	83,982	1.67%
5	North Carolina	249,067	4.94%
40	North Dakota	22,411	0.44%
16	Ohio	87,223	1.73%
13	Oklahoma	101,353	2.01%
34	Oregon	31,806	0.63%
21	Pennsylvania	72,561	1.44%
45	Rhode Island	16,321	0.32%
8	South Carolina	147,790	2.93%
43	South Dakota	17,918	0.36%
15	Tennessee	87,987	1.75%
3	Texas	459,300	9.12%
36	Utah	30,085	0.60%
50	Vermont	4,066	0.08%
2	Virginia	470,947	9.35%
7	Washington	206,878	4.11%
48	West Virginia	14,433	0.29%
39	Wisconsin	23,542	0.47%
49	Wyoming	12,686	0.25%

RANK ORDER

RANK	STATE	ELIGIBLE	% of USA
1	California	631,058	12.53%
2	Virginia	470,947	9.35%
3	Texas	459,300	9.12%
4	Florida	392,000	7.78%
5	North Carolina	249,067	4.94%
6	Georgia	229,337	4.55%
7	Washington	206,878	4.11%
8	South Carolina	147,790	2.93%
9	Maryland	139,348	2.77%
10	Colorado	133,773	2.66%
11	Alabama	114,573	2.27%
12	Arizona	110,286	2.19%
13	Oklahoma	101,353	2.01%
14	Hawaii	90,230	1.79%
15	Tennessee	87,987	1.75%
16	Ohio	87,223	1.73%
17	Louisiana	86,526	1.72%
18	New York	83,982	1.67%
19	Illinois	83,968	1.67%
20	Kentucky	80,723	1.60%
21	Pennsylvania	72,561	1.44%
22	Missouri	70,816	1.41%
23	Kansas	69,531	1.38%
24	New Mexico	61,250	1.22%
25	Mississippi	60,799	1.21%
26	Nevada	51,945	1.03%
27	New Jersey	51,002	1.01%
28	Alaska	49,058	0.97%
29	Michigan	46,896	0.93%
30	Arkansas	45,443	0.90%
31	Nebraska	40,478	0.80%
32	Massachusetts	39,937	0.79%
33	Indiana	39,603	0.79%
34	Oregon	31,806	0.63%
35	Connecticut	31,323	0.62%
36	Utah	30,085	0.60%
37	Maine	26,194	0.52%
38	Idaho	23,834	0.47%
39	Wisconsin	23,542	0.47%
40	North Dakota	22,411	0.44%
41	Minnesota	21,669	0.43%
42	Montana	18,546	0.37%
43	South Dakota	17,918	0.36%
44	Delaware	17,505	0.35%
45	Rhode Island	16,321	0.32%
46	Iowa	15,221	0.30%
47	New Hampshire	14,525	0.29%
48	West Virginia	14,433	0.29%
49	Wyoming	12,686	0.25%
50	Vermont	4,066	0.08%

	District of Columbia	9,362	0.19%

Source: U.S. Department of Defense, Office of CHAMPUS
"Defense Enrollment Eligibility Reporting System (DEERS) Report" (February 23, 1995)
*As of February 21, 1995. National total does not include 27,285 eligible in U.S. territories and possessions. CHAMPUS provides health care coverage for current or former U.S. military personnel and their dependents.

Percent of Population Eligible for CHAMPUS in 1995

National Percent = 1.93% of Population Eligible*

ALPHA ORDER				RANK ORDER		
RANK	STATE	PERCENT		RANK	STATE	PERCENT
15	Alabama	2.72		1	Alaska	8.10
1	Alaska	8.10		2	Hawaii	7.65
17	Arizona	2.71		3	Virginia	7.19
30	Arkansas	1.85		4	South Carolina	4.03
28	California	2.01		5	Washington	3.87
7	Colorado	3.66		6	New Mexico	3.70
37	Connecticut	0.96		7	Colorado	3.66
22	Delaware	2.48		8	Nevada	3.57
13	Florida	2.81		9	North Carolina	3.52
11	Georgia	3.25		10	North Dakota	3.51
2	Hawaii	7.65		11	Georgia	3.25
27	Idaho	2.10		12	Oklahoma	3.11
40	Illinois	0.71		13	Florida	2.81
42	Indiana	0.69		14	Maryland	2.78
46	Iowa	0.54		15	Alabama	2.72
15	Kansas	2.72		15	Kansas	2.72
25	Kentucky	2.11		17	Arizona	2.71
28	Louisiana	2.01		18	Wyoming	2.67
25	Maine	2.11		19	Texas	2.50
14	Maryland	2.78		20	Nebraska	2.49
43	Massachusetts	0.66		20	South Dakota	2.49
47	Michigan	0.49		22	Delaware	2.48
48	Minnesota	0.47		23	Mississippi	2.28
23	Mississippi	2.28		24	Montana	2.17
34	Missouri	1.34		25	Kentucky	2.11
24	Montana	2.17		25	Maine	2.11
20	Nebraska	2.49		27	Idaho	2.10
8	Nevada	3.57		28	California	2.01
35	New Hampshire	1.28		28	Louisiana	2.01
44	New Jersey	0.65		30	Arkansas	1.85
6	New Mexico	3.70		31	Tennessee	1.70
49	New York	0.46		32	Rhode Island	1.64
9	North Carolina	3.52		33	Utah	1.58
10	North Dakota	3.51		34	Missouri	1.34
38	Ohio	0.79		35	New Hampshire	1.28
12	Oklahoma	3.11		36	Oregon	1.03
36	Oregon	1.03		37	Connecticut	0.96
45	Pennsylvania	0.60		38	Ohio	0.79
32	Rhode Island	1.64		38	West Virginia	0.79
4	South Carolina	4.03		40	Illinois	0.71
20	South Dakota	2.49		41	Vermont	0.70
31	Tennessee	1.70		42	Indiana	0.69
19	Texas	2.50		43	Massachusetts	0.66
33	Utah	1.58		44	New Jersey	0.65
41	Vermont	0.70		45	Pennsylvania	0.60
3	Virginia	7.19		46	Iowa	0.54
5	Washington	3.87		47	Michigan	0.49
38	West Virginia	0.79		48	Minnesota	0.47
49	Wisconsin	0.46		49	New York	0.46
18	Wyoming	2.67		49	Wisconsin	0.46
					District of Columbia	1.64

Source: Morgan Quitno Press using data from U.S. Department of Defense, Office of CHAMPUS
"Defense Enrollment Eligibility Reporting System (DEERS) Report" (February 23, 1995)
*As of February 21, 1995. CHAMPUS is the Civilian Health and Medical Program of the Uniformed Services. Percentages calculated using Census estimates as of 12/31/94. National percent does not include eligibles in U.S. territories and possessions.

Health Care Expenditures in 1993

National Total = $846,400,000,000*

<u>ALPHA ORDER</u>

RANK	STATE	EXPENDITURES	% of USA
22	Alabama	$12,898,000,000	1.52%
48	Alaska	1,775,000,000	0.21%
25	Arizona	11,425,000,000	1.35%
31	Arkansas	7,691,000,000	0.91%
1	California	105,317,000,000	12.44%
26	Colorado	10,911,000,000	1.29%
24	Connecticut	11,889,000,000	1.40%
45	Delaware	2,455,000,000	0.29%
4	Florida	46,827,000,000	5.53%
11	Georgia	21,458,000,000	2.54%
39	Hawaii	3,609,000,000	0.43%
44	Idaho	2,531,000,000	0.30%
6	Illinois	38,096,000,000	4.50%
15	Indiana	17,771,000,000	2.10%
29	Iowa	8,756,000,000	1.03%
32	Kansas	7,690,000,000	0.91%
23	Kentucky	12,256,000,000	1.45%
20	Louisiana	15,003,000,000	1.77%
40	Maine	3,568,000,000	0.42%
17	Maryland	16,385,000,000	1.94%
10	Massachusetts	25,030,000,000	2.96%
8	Michigan	30,153,000,000	3.56%
21	Minnesota	14,358,000,000	1.70%
33	Mississippi	7,266,000,000	0.86%
13	Missouri	18,231,000,000	2.15%
43	Montana	2,577,000,000	0.30%
35	Nebraska	4,811,000,000	0.57%
38	Nevada	3,643,000,000	0.43%
42	New Hampshire	3,075,000,000	0.36%
9	New Jersey	27,000,000,000	3.19%
37	New Mexico	4,707,000,000	0.56%
2	New York	72,889,000,000	8.61%
12	North Carolina	19,871,000,000	2.35%
46	North Dakota	2,250,000,000	0.27%
7	Ohio	36,777,000,000	4.35%
28	Oklahoma	9,595,000,000	1.13%
30	Oregon	8,579,000,000	1.01%
5	Pennsylvania	41,847,000,000	4.94%
41	Rhode Island	3,388,000,000	0.40%
27	South Carolina	9,981,000,000	1.18%
47	South Dakota	2,180,000,000	0.26%
16	Tennessee	17,717,000,000	2.09%
3	Texas	53,558,000,000	6.33%
36	Utah	4,801,000,000	0.57%
49	Vermont	1,626,000,000	0.19%
14	Virginia	18,057,000,000	2.13%
18	Washington	15,425,000,000	1.82%
34	West Virginia	5,778,000,000	0.68%
19	Wisconsin	15,070,000,000	1.78%
50	Wyoming	1,277,000,000	0.15%

<u>RANK ORDER</u>

RANK	STATE	EXPENDITURES	% of USA
1	California	$105,317,000,000	12.44%
2	New York	72,889,000,000	8.61%
3	Texas	53,558,000,000	6.33%
4	Florida	46,827,000,000	5.53%
5	Pennsylvania	41,847,000,000	4.94%
6	Illinois	38,096,000,000	4.50%
7	Ohio	36,777,000,000	4.35%
8	Michigan	30,153,000,000	3.56%
9	New Jersey	27,000,000,000	3.19%
10	Massachusetts	25,030,000,000	2.96%
11	Georgia	21,458,000,000	2.54%
12	North Carolina	19,871,000,000	2.35%
13	Missouri	18,231,000,000	2.15%
14	Virginia	18,057,000,000	2.13%
15	Indiana	17,771,000,000	2.10%
16	Tennessee	17,717,000,000	2.09%
17	Maryland	16,385,000,000	1.94%
18	Washington	15,425,000,000	1.82%
19	Wisconsin	15,070,000,000	1.78%
20	Louisiana	15,003,000,000	1.77%
21	Minnesota	14,358,000,000	1.70%
22	Alabama	12,898,000,000	1.52%
23	Kentucky	12,256,000,000	1.45%
24	Connecticut	11,889,000,000	1.40%
25	Arizona	11,425,000,000	1.35%
26	Colorado	10,911,000,000	1.29%
27	South Carolina	9,981,000,000	1.18%
28	Oklahoma	9,595,000,000	1.13%
29	Iowa	8,756,000,000	1.03%
30	Oregon	8,579,000,000	1.01%
31	Arkansas	7,691,000,000	0.91%
32	Kansas	7,690,000,000	0.91%
33	Mississippi	7,266,000,000	0.86%
34	West Virginia	5,778,000,000	0.68%
35	Nebraska	4,811,000,000	0.57%
36	Utah	4,801,000,000	0.57%
37	New Mexico	4,707,000,000	0.56%
38	Nevada	3,643,000,000	0.43%
39	Hawaii	3,609,000,000	0.43%
40	Maine	3,568,000,000	0.42%
41	Rhode Island	3,388,000,000	0.40%
42	New Hampshire	3,075,000,000	0.36%
43	Montana	2,577,000,000	0.30%
44	Idaho	2,531,000,000	0.30%
45	Delaware	2,455,000,000	0.29%
46	North Dakota	2,250,000,000	0.27%
47	South Dakota	2,180,000,000	0.26%
48	Alaska	1,775,000,000	0.21%
49	Vermont	1,626,000,000	0.19%
50	Wyoming	1,277,000,000	0.15%

District of Columbia**	NA	NA

Source: Lewin-VHI, Inc. as reported by Families USA Foundation

"Skyrocketing Health Inflation" (November 1993) *This "expenditure" number represents the amount actually spent on health care in each state. Other tables in this section refer to health care "payments." Payments represent the health care payments made by residents of a given state whether the funds were spent in that state or not. For example, medicare payroll taxes paid by residents of one state may end being spent on another state's resident. See beginning of this chapter for other definitions. **Not available.

247

Health Care Expenditures as a Percent of Gross State Product in 1993

National Percent = 14.3% of Gross Domestic Product*

ALPHA ORDER			RANK ORDER		
RANK	**STATE**	**PERCENT**	**RANK**	**STATE**	**PERCENT**
6	Alabama	15.8	1	West Virginia	17.5
50	Alaska	6.0	2	Arkansas	17.1
12	Arizona	14.8	3	Montana	16.7
2	Arkansas	17.1	4	Florida	16.6
35	California	12.3	5	Tennessee	16.1
25	Colorado	13.4	6	Alabama	15.8
47	Connecticut	10.7	6	North Dakota	15.8
46	Delaware	10.8	8	Mississippi	15.7
4	Florida	16.6	9	Kentucky	15.6
19	Georgia	13.7	10	New Mexico	15.4
45	Hawaii	10.9	11	Missouri	15.1
41	Idaho	11.9	12	Arizona	14.8
40	Illinois	12.0	13	Oklahoma	14.7
19	Indiana	13.7	14	Pennsylvania	14.6
27	Iowa	13.3	15	South Dakota	14.3
31	Kansas	12.9	16	Louisiana	14.2
9	Kentucky	15.6	16	Ohio	14.2
16	Louisiana	14.2	18	Massachusetts	13.8
29	Maine	13.1	19	Georgia	13.7
30	Maryland	13.0	19	Indiana	13.7
18	Massachusetts	13.8	19	Michigan	13.7
19	Michigan	13.7	19	Rhode Island	13.7
35	Minnesota	12.3	19	Utah	13.7
8	Mississippi	15.7	24	South Carolina	13.5
11	Missouri	15.1	25	Colorado	13.4
3	Montana	16.7	25	Oregon	13.4
35	Nebraska	12.3	27	Iowa	13.3
48	Nevada	10.6	27	New York	13.3
43	New Hampshire	11.1	29	Maine	13.1
42	New Jersey	11.2	30	Maryland	13.0
10	New Mexico	15.4	31	Kansas	12.9
27	New York	13.3	32	Wisconsin	12.8
39	North Carolina	12.1	33	Texas	12.5
6	North Dakota	15.8	34	Vermont	12.4
16	Ohio	14.2	35	California	12.3
13	Oklahoma	14.7	35	Minnesota	12.3
25	Oregon	13.4	35	Nebraska	12.3
14	Pennsylvania	14.6	35	Washington	12.3
19	Rhode Island	13.7	39	North Carolina	12.1
24	South Carolina	13.5	40	Illinois	12.0
15	South Dakota	14.3	41	Idaho	11.9
5	Tennessee	16.1	42	New Jersey	11.2
33	Texas	12.5	43	New Hampshire	11.1
19	Utah	13.7	43	Virginia	11.1
34	Vermont	12.4	45	Hawaii	10.9
43	Virginia	11.1	46	Delaware	10.8
35	Washington	12.3	47	Connecticut	10.7
1	West Virginia	17.5	48	Nevada	10.6
32	Wisconsin	12.8	49	Wyoming	8.7
49	Wyoming	8.7	50	Alaska	6.0

District of Columbia**   NA

Source: Lewin-VHI, Inc. (Fairfax, Virginia)
  "Health Care Problems: Variation Across States" (December 1994)
Data on gross state product from "Survey of Current Business" (December 1991)
**Not available.*

248

Total Health Care Payments in 1993

National Total = $846,773,000,000*

ALPHA ORDER					RANK ORDER			

RANK	STATE	PAYMENTS	% of USA		RANK	STATE	PAYMENTS	% of USA
23	Alabama	$12,165,000,000	1.44%		1	California	$108,520,000,000	12.82%
48	Alaska	1,974,000,000	0.23%		2	New York	74,631,000,000	8.81%
25	Arizona	11,354,000,000	1.34%		3	Texas	54,077,000,000	6.39%
32	Arkansas	7,358,000,000	0.87%		4	Florida	43,206,000,000	5.10%
1	California	108,520,000,000	12.82%		5	Pennsylvania	39,216,000,000	4.63%
26	Colorado	11,352,000,000	1.34%		6	Illinois	39,087,000,000	4.62%
22	Connecticut	12,726,000,000	1.50%		7	Ohio	36,419,000,000	4.30%
43	Delaware	2,765,000,000	0.33%		8	Michigan	30,498,000,000	3.60%
4	Florida	43,206,000,000	5.10%		9	New Jersey	27,908,000,000	3.30%
11	Georgia	21,429,000,000	2.53%		10	Massachusetts	25,017,000,000	2.95%
38	Hawaii	3,818,000,000	0.45%		11	Georgia	21,429,000,000	2.53%
44	Idaho	2,576,000,000	0.30%		12	North Carolina	19,983,000,000	2.36%
6	Illinois	39,087,000,000	4.62%		13	Virginia	18,485,000,000	2.18%
14	Indiana	17,671,000,000	2.09%		14	Indiana	17,671,000,000	2.09%
30	Iowa	8,642,000,000	1.02%		15	Missouri	17,506,000,000	2.07%
31	Kansas	7,692,000,000	0.91%		16	Tennessee	16,896,000,000	2.00%
24	Kentucky	11,610,000,000	1.37%		17	Maryland	16,573,000,000	1.96%
21	Louisiana	14,378,000,000	1.70%		18	Washington	15,828,000,000	1.87%
40	Maine	3,485,000,000	0.41%		19	Wisconsin	15,449,000,000	1.82%
17	Maryland	16,573,000,000	1.96%		20	Minnesota	15,376,000,000	1.82%
10	Massachusetts	25,017,000,000	2.95%		21	Louisiana	14,378,000,000	1.70%
8	Michigan	30,498,000,000	3.60%		22	Connecticut	12,726,000,000	1.50%
20	Minnesota	15,376,000,000	1.82%		23	Alabama	12,165,000,000	1.44%
33	Mississippi	6,779,000,000	0.80%		24	Kentucky	11,610,000,000	1.37%
15	Missouri	17,506,000,000	2.07%		25	Arizona	11,354,000,000	1.34%
45	Montana	2,502,000,000	0.30%		26	Colorado	11,352,000,000	1.34%
36	Nebraska	4,844,000,000	0.57%		27	South Carolina	10,028,000,000	1.18%
39	Nevada	3,676,000,000	0.43%		28	Oklahoma	9,353,000,000	1.10%
42	New Hampshire	3,264,000,000	0.39%		29	Oregon	8,775,000,000	1.04%
9	New Jersey	27,908,000,000	3.30%		30	Iowa	8,642,000,000	1.02%
37	New Mexico	4,727,000,000	0.56%		31	Kansas	7,692,000,000	0.91%
2	New York	74,631,000,000	8.81%		32	Arkansas	7,358,000,000	0.87%
12	North Carolina	19,983,000,000	2.36%		33	Mississippi	6,779,000,000	0.80%
46	North Dakota	2,136,000,000	0.25%		34	West Virginia	5,375,000,000	0.63%
7	Ohio	36,419,000,000	4.30%		35	Utah	4,865,000,000	0.57%
28	Oklahoma	9,353,000,000	1.10%		36	Nebraska	4,844,000,000	0.57%
29	Oregon	8,775,000,000	1.04%		37	New Mexico	4,727,000,000	0.56%
5	Pennsylvania	39,216,000,000	4.63%		38	Hawaii	3,818,000,000	0.45%
41	Rhode Island	3,318,000,000	0.39%		39	Nevada	3,676,000,000	0.43%
27	South Carolina	10,028,000,000	1.18%		40	Maine	3,485,000,000	0.41%
47	South Dakota	2,107,000,000	0.25%		41	Rhode Island	3,318,000,000	0.39%
16	Tennessee	16,896,000,000	2.00%		42	New Hampshire	3,264,000,000	0.39%
3	Texas	54,077,000,000	6.39%		43	Delaware	2,765,000,000	0.33%
35	Utah	4,865,000,000	0.57%		44	Idaho	2,576,000,000	0.30%
49	Vermont	1,670,000,000	0.20%		45	Montana	2,502,000,000	0.30%
13	Virginia	18,485,000,000	2.18%		46	North Dakota	2,136,000,000	0.25%
18	Washington	15,828,000,000	1.87%		47	South Dakota	2,107,000,000	0.25%
34	West Virginia	5,375,000,000	0.63%		48	Alaska	1,974,000,000	0.23%
19	Wisconsin	15,449,000,000	1.82%		49	Vermont	1,670,000,000	0.20%
50	Wyoming	1,328,000,000	0.16%		50	Wyoming	1,328,000,000	0.16%
						District of Columbia**	NA	NA

Source: Lewin-VHI, Inc. (Fairfax, Virginia)
    unpublished data
Payments by both families and business for health care. See beginning of this chapter for definitions.
**Not available.*

Per Capita Health Care Payments in 1993

National Per Capita = $3,285*

ALPHA ORDER

RANK	STATE	PER CAPITA
36	Alabama	$2,910
15	Alaska	3,301
41	Arizona	2,878
28	Arkansas	3,033
6	California	3,476
20	Colorado	3,185
4	Connecticut	3,882
3	Delaware	3,961
21	Florida	3,148
22	Georgia	3,105
17	Hawaii	3,274
50	Idaho	2,342
10	Illinois	3,345
23	Indiana	3,097
24	Iowa	3,063
27	Kansas	3,034
26	Kentucky	3,060
9	Louisiana	3,352
45	Maine	2,810
12	Maryland	3,343
1	Massachusetts	4,157
19	Michigan	3,224
7	Minnesota	3,399
49	Mississippi	2,568
11	Missouri	3,344
32	Montana	2,975
30	Nebraska	3,003
47	Nevada	2,660
37	New Hampshire	2,904
5	New Jersey	3,551
35	New Mexico	2,925
2	New York	4,111
42	North Carolina	2,874
8	North Dakota	3,353
16	Ohio	3,293
39	Oklahoma	2,893
40	Oregon	2,891
18	Pennsylvania	3,260
13	Rhode Island	3,318
46	South Carolina	2,763
34	South Dakota	2,943
14	Tennessee	3,317
31	Texas	3,001
48	Utah	2,616
38	Vermont	2,899
43	Virginia	2,856
29	Washington	3,010
33	West Virginia	2,957
24	Wisconsin	3,063
44	Wyoming	2,826

RANK ORDER

RANK	STATE	PER CAPITA
1	Massachusetts	$4,157
2	New York	4,111
3	Delaware	3,961
4	Connecticut	3,882
5	New Jersey	3,551
6	California	3,476
7	Minnesota	3,399
8	North Dakota	3,353
9	Louisiana	3,352
10	Illinois	3,345
11	Missouri	3,344
12	Maryland	3,343
13	Rhode Island	3,318
14	Tennessee	3,317
15	Alaska	3,301
16	Ohio	3,293
17	Hawaii	3,274
18	Pennsylvania	3,260
19	Michigan	3,224
20	Colorado	3,185
21	Florida	3,148
22	Georgia	3,105
23	Indiana	3,097
24	Iowa	3,063
24	Wisconsin	3,063
26	Kentucky	3,060
27	Kansas	3,034
28	Arkansas	3,033
29	Washington	3,010
30	Nebraska	3,003
31	Texas	3,001
32	Montana	2,975
33	West Virginia	2,957
34	South Dakota	2,943
35	New Mexico	2,925
36	Alabama	2,910
37	New Hampshire	2,904
38	Vermont	2,899
39	Oklahoma	2,893
40	Oregon	2,891
41	Arizona	2,878
42	North Carolina	2,874
43	Virginia	2,856
44	Wyoming	2,826
45	Maine	2,810
46	South Carolina	2,763
47	Nevada	2,660
48	Utah	2,616
49	Mississippi	2,568
50	Idaho	2,342

District of Columbia**   NA

Source: Morgan Quitno Press using data from Lewin-VHI, Inc. (Fairfax, Virginia)
unpublished data

*Payments by both families and business for health care divided by updated 1993 Census population estimates.

**Not available.

Total Health Care Payments per Family in 1993

National Average = $7,739 per Family*

ALPHA ORDER

RANK	STATE	PER FAMILY
24	Alabama	$7,453
8	Alaska	8,092
33	Arizona	7,069
26	Arkansas	7,343
9	California	7,996
32	Colorado	7,084
5	Connecticut	8,257
12	Delaware	7,851
17	Florida	7,663
15	Georgia	7,743
16	Hawaii	7,717
50	Idaho	5,941
22	Illinois	7,536
30	Indiana	7,211
40	Iowa	6,843
35	Kansas	6,980
19	Kentucky	7,622
3	Louisiana	8,554
45	Maine	6,510
20	Maryland	7,561
1	Massachusetts	9,352
23	Michigan	7,514
28	Minnesota	7,245
43	Mississippi	6,673
11	Missouri	7,958
29	Montana	7,218
39	Nebraska	6,852
46	Nevada	6,477
49	New Hampshire	6,186
7	New Jersey	8,165
27	New Mexico	7,274
2	New York	9,185
42	North Carolina	6,832
6	North Dakota	8,205
14	Ohio	7,806
41	Oklahoma	6,840
47	Oregon	6,445
10	Pennsylvania	7,972
18	Rhode Island	7,655
36	South Carolina	6,916
31	South Dakota	7,143
4	Tennessee	8,307
21	Texas	7,547
13	Utah	7,824
48	Vermont	6,299
38	Virginia	6,871
37	Washington	6,873
25	West Virginia	7,369
34	Wisconsin	7,012
44	Wyoming	6,535

RANK ORDER

RANK	STATE	PER FAMILY
1	Massachusetts	$9,352
2	New York	9,185
3	Louisiana	8,554
4	Tennessee	8,307
5	Connecticut	8,257
6	North Dakota	8,205
7	New Jersey	8,165
8	Alaska	8,092
9	California	7,996
10	Pennsylvania	7,972
11	Missouri	7,958
12	Delaware	7,851
13	Utah	7,824
14	Ohio	7,806
15	Georgia	7,743
16	Hawaii	7,717
17	Florida	7,663
18	Rhode Island	7,655
19	Kentucky	7,622
20	Maryland	7,561
21	Texas	7,547
22	Illinois	7,536
23	Michigan	7,514
24	Alabama	7,453
25	West Virginia	7,369
26	Arkansas	7,343
27	New Mexico	7,274
28	Minnesota	7,245
29	Montana	7,218
30	Indiana	7,211
31	South Dakota	7,143
32	Colorado	7,084
33	Arizona	7,069
34	Wisconsin	7,012
35	Kansas	6,980
36	South Carolina	6,916
37	Washington	6,873
38	Virginia	6,871
39	Nebraska	6,852
40	Iowa	6,843
41	Oklahoma	6,840
42	North Carolina	6,832
43	Mississippi	6,673
44	Wyoming	6,535
45	Maine	6,510
46	Nevada	6,477
47	Oregon	6,445
48	Vermont	6,299
49	New Hampshire	6,186
50	Idaho	5,941
	District of Columbia**	NA

Source: Lewin-VHI, Inc. (Fairfax, Virginia)
 unpublished data

*Payments by both families and business for health care. See beginning of this chapter for definitions.

**Not available.

Average Annual Health Care Payments Paid by Families in 1993

National Average = $5,190 per Family*

ALPHA ORDER				RANK ORDER		
RANK	STATE	AVERAGE PAYMENTS		RANK	STATE	AVERAGE PAYMENTS
30	Alabama	$4,860		1	Alaska	$6,760
1	Alaska	6,760		2	New York	6,501
29	Arizona	4,862		3	Massachusetts	6,106
24	Arkansas	4,978		4	Delaware	6,029
10	California	5,392		5	Hawaii	5,893
21	Colorado	5,033		6	North Dakota	5,558
14	Connecticut	5,219		7	Louisiana	5,550
4	Delaware	6,029		8	Maryland	5,507
38	Florida	4,743		9	New Jersey	5,500
11	Georgia	5,369		10	California	5,392
5	Hawaii	5,893		11	Georgia	5,369
49	Idaho	4,054		12	Utah	5,311
19	Illinois	5,100		13	New Mexico	5,257
25	Indiana	4,963		14	Connecticut	5,219
34	Iowa	4,800		15	Missouri	5,215
35	Kansas	4,798		16	Texas	5,169
22	Kentucky	5,026		17	Minnesota	5,160
7	Louisiana	5,550		18	Rhode Island	5,139
47	Maine	4,357		19	Illinois	5,100
8	Maryland	5,507		20	Ohio	5,065
3	Massachusetts	6,106		21	Colorado	5,033
36	Michigan	4,792		22	Kentucky	5,026
17	Minnesota	5,160		23	Virginia	4,979
45	Mississippi	4,405		24	Arkansas	4,978
15	Missouri	5,215		25	Indiana	4,963
32	Montana	4,811		26	South Carolina	4,958
39	Nebraska	4,730		27	South Dakota	4,929
48	Nevada	4,186		28	Oklahoma	4,864
50	New Hampshire	3,742		29	Arizona	4,862
9	New Jersey	5,500		30	Alabama	4,860
13	New Mexico	5,257		31	Washington	4,840
2	New York	6,501		32	Montana	4,811
40	North Carolina	4,722		33	Wyoming	4,806
6	North Dakota	5,558		34	Iowa	4,800
20	Ohio	5,065		35	Kansas	4,798
28	Oklahoma	4,864		36	Michigan	4,792
46	Oregon	4,364		37	Tennessee	4,763
43	Pennsylvania	4,602		38	Florida	4,743
18	Rhode Island	5,139		39	Nebraska	4,730
26	South Carolina	4,958		40	North Carolina	4,722
27	South Dakota	4,929		41	Wisconsin	4,690
37	Tennessee	4,763		42	West Virginia	4,640
16	Texas	5,169		43	Pennsylvania	4,602
12	Utah	5,311		44	Vermont	4,477
44	Vermont	4,477		45	Mississippi	4,405
23	Virginia	4,979		46	Oregon	4,364
31	Washington	4,840		47	Maine	4,357
42	West Virginia	4,640		48	Nevada	4,186
41	Wisconsin	4,690		49	Idaho	4,054
33	Wyoming	4,806		50	New Hampshire	3,742
				District of Columbia**		NA

Source: Lewin-VHI, Inc. as reported by Families USA Foundation
   "Skyrocketing Health Inflation" (November 1993)

*Total annual direct and indirect health care payments by families divided by number of families. See beginning of this chapter for definitions.

**Not available.

Average Annual Direct Health Care Payments Paid by Families in 1993

National Average = $2,321 per Family*

ALPHA ORDER				RANK ORDER		
RANK	STATE	DIRECT PAYMENTS		RANK	STATE	DIRECT PAYMENTS
20	Alabama	$2,319		1	North Dakota	$2,746
35	Alaska	2,150		2	Louisiana	2,691
8	Arizona	2,538		3	Utah	2,635
26	Arkansas	2,249		4	Missouri	2,593
10	California	2,516		5	Massachusetts	2,576
24	Colorado	2,268		6	Tennessee	2,556
28	Connecticut	2,235		7	Texas	2,547
11	Delaware	2,474		8	Arizona	2,538
15	Florida	2,413		9	Georgia	2,531
9	Georgia	2,531		10	California	2,516
32	Hawaii	2,188		11	Delaware	2,474
48	Idaho	1,816		12	Kansas	2,459
16	Illinois	2,405		13	New Jersey	2,441
18	Indiana	2,379		14	Maryland	2,437
17	Iowa	2,392		15	Florida	2,413
12	Kansas	2,459		16	Illinois	2,405
31	Kentucky	2,195		17	Iowa	2,392
2	Louisiana	2,691		18	Indiana	2,379
50	Maine	1,543		19	Wisconsin	2,337
14	Maryland	2,437		20	Alabama	2,319
5	Massachusetts	2,576		21	Virginia	2,295
33	Michigan	2,180		22	Oklahoma	2,284
34	Minnesota	2,154		23	New Mexico	2,270
47	Mississippi	1,865		24	Colorado	2,268
4	Missouri	2,593		25	Montana	2,259
25	Montana	2,259		26	Arkansas	2,249
40	Nebraska	2,056		26	South Dakota	2,249
38	Nevada	2,089		28	Connecticut	2,235
44	New Hampshire	1,975		29	Wyoming	2,224
13	New Jersey	2,441		30	Ohio	2,199
23	New Mexico	2,270		31	Kentucky	2,195
43	New York	2,005		32	Hawaii	2,188
36	North Carolina	2,127		33	Michigan	2,180
1	North Dakota	2,746		34	Minnesota	2,154
30	Ohio	2,199		35	Alaska	2,150
22	Oklahoma	2,284		36	North Carolina	2,127
39	Oregon	2,071		37	Washington	2,104
45	Pennsylvania	1,972		38	Nevada	2,089
46	Rhode Island	1,894		39	Oregon	2,071
41	South Carolina	2,040		40	Nebraska	2,056
26	South Dakota	2,249		41	South Carolina	2,040
6	Tennessee	2,556		42	West Virginia	2,035
7	Texas	2,547		43	New York	2,005
3	Utah	2,635		44	New Hampshire	1,975
49	Vermont	1,763		45	Pennsylvania	1,972
21	Virginia	2,295		46	Rhode Island	1,894
37	Washington	2,104		47	Mississippi	1,865
42	West Virginia	2,035		48	Idaho	1,816
19	Wisconsin	2,337		49	Vermont	1,763
29	Wyoming	2,224		50	Maine	1,543

District of Columbia**　　　　　　　　　　NA

Source: Morgan Quitno Press using data from Lewin-VHI, Inc. as reported by Families USA Foundation
　　"Skyrocketing Health Inflation" (November 1993)
*Consists of out-of-pocket payments and insurance premiums. See beginning of this chapter for definitions.
**Not available.

Average Annual Indirect Health Care Payments Paid by Families in 1993

National Average = $2,868 per Family*

<table>
<tr><td colspan="3">ALPHA ORDER</td><td colspan="3">RANK ORDER</td></tr>
<tr><td>RANK</td><td>STATE</td><td>INDIRECT PAYMENTS</td><td>RANK</td><td>STATE</td><td>INDIRECT PAYMENTS</td></tr>
<tr><td>39</td><td>Alabama</td><td>$2,542</td><td>1</td><td>Alaska</td><td>$4,611</td></tr>
<tr><td>1</td><td>Alaska</td><td>4,611</td><td>2</td><td>New York</td><td>4,496</td></tr>
<tr><td>45</td><td>Arizona</td><td>2,324</td><td>3</td><td>Hawaii</td><td>3,706</td></tr>
<tr><td>22</td><td>Arkansas</td><td>2,728</td><td>4</td><td>Delaware</td><td>3,555</td></tr>
<tr><td>13</td><td>California</td><td>2,876</td><td>5</td><td>Massachusetts</td><td>3,530</td></tr>
<tr><td>20</td><td>Colorado</td><td>2,765</td><td>6</td><td>Rhode Island</td><td>3,246</td></tr>
<tr><td>11</td><td>Connecticut</td><td>2,984</td><td>7</td><td>Maryland</td><td>3,070</td></tr>
<tr><td>4</td><td>Delaware</td><td>3,555</td><td>8</td><td>New Jersey</td><td>3,059</td></tr>
<tr><td>44</td><td>Florida</td><td>2,330</td><td>9</td><td>Minnesota</td><td>3,006</td></tr>
<tr><td>16</td><td>Georgia</td><td>2,838</td><td>10</td><td>New Mexico</td><td>2,987</td></tr>
<tr><td>3</td><td>Hawaii</td><td>3,706</td><td>11</td><td>Connecticut</td><td>2,984</td></tr>
<tr><td>47</td><td>Idaho</td><td>2,239</td><td>12</td><td>South Carolina</td><td>2,918</td></tr>
<tr><td>24</td><td>Illinois</td><td>2,696</td><td>13</td><td>California</td><td>2,876</td></tr>
<tr><td>35</td><td>Indiana</td><td>2,585</td><td>14</td><td>Ohio</td><td>2,867</td></tr>
<tr><td>41</td><td>Iowa</td><td>2,409</td><td>15</td><td>Louisiana</td><td>2,860</td></tr>
<tr><td>43</td><td>Kansas</td><td>2,340</td><td>16</td><td>Georgia</td><td>2,838</td></tr>
<tr><td>17</td><td>Kentucky</td><td>2,830</td><td>17</td><td>Kentucky</td><td>2,830</td></tr>
<tr><td>15</td><td>Louisiana</td><td>2,860</td><td>18</td><td>Maine</td><td>2,814</td></tr>
<tr><td>18</td><td>Maine</td><td>2,814</td><td>19</td><td>North Dakota</td><td>2,812</td></tr>
<tr><td>7</td><td>Maryland</td><td>3,070</td><td>20</td><td>Colorado</td><td>2,765</td></tr>
<tr><td>5</td><td>Massachusetts</td><td>3,530</td><td>21</td><td>Washington</td><td>2,738</td></tr>
<tr><td>32</td><td>Michigan</td><td>2,612</td><td>22</td><td>Arkansas</td><td>2,728</td></tr>
<tr><td>9</td><td>Minnesota</td><td>3,006</td><td>23</td><td>Vermont</td><td>2,714</td></tr>
<tr><td>40</td><td>Mississippi</td><td>2,540</td><td>24</td><td>Illinois</td><td>2,696</td></tr>
<tr><td>31</td><td>Missouri</td><td>2,622</td><td>25</td><td>Virginia</td><td>2,685</td></tr>
<tr><td>38</td><td>Montana</td><td>2,552</td><td>26</td><td>South Dakota</td><td>2,679</td></tr>
<tr><td>28</td><td>Nebraska</td><td>2,674</td><td>27</td><td>Utah</td><td>2,677</td></tr>
<tr><td>49</td><td>Nevada</td><td>2,097</td><td>28</td><td>Nebraska</td><td>2,674</td></tr>
<tr><td>50</td><td>New Hampshire</td><td>1,768</td><td>29</td><td>Pennsylvania</td><td>2,629</td></tr>
<tr><td>8</td><td>New Jersey</td><td>3,059</td><td>30</td><td>Texas</td><td>2,623</td></tr>
<tr><td>10</td><td>New Mexico</td><td>2,987</td><td>31</td><td>Missouri</td><td>2,622</td></tr>
<tr><td>2</td><td>New York</td><td>4,496</td><td>32</td><td>Michigan</td><td>2,612</td></tr>
<tr><td>34</td><td>North Carolina</td><td>2,595</td><td>33</td><td>West Virginia</td><td>2,605</td></tr>
<tr><td>19</td><td>North Dakota</td><td>2,812</td><td>34</td><td>North Carolina</td><td>2,595</td></tr>
<tr><td>14</td><td>Ohio</td><td>2,867</td><td>35</td><td>Indiana</td><td>2,585</td></tr>
<tr><td>37</td><td>Oklahoma</td><td>2,580</td><td>36</td><td>Wyoming</td><td>2,583</td></tr>
<tr><td>46</td><td>Oregon</td><td>2,293</td><td>37</td><td>Oklahoma</td><td>2,580</td></tr>
<tr><td>29</td><td>Pennsylvania</td><td>2,629</td><td>38</td><td>Montana</td><td>2,552</td></tr>
<tr><td>6</td><td>Rhode Island</td><td>3,246</td><td>39</td><td>Alabama</td><td>2,542</td></tr>
<tr><td>12</td><td>South Carolina</td><td>2,918</td><td>40</td><td>Mississippi</td><td>2,540</td></tr>
<tr><td>26</td><td>South Dakota</td><td>2,679</td><td>41</td><td>Iowa</td><td>2,409</td></tr>
<tr><td>48</td><td>Tennessee</td><td>2,208</td><td>42</td><td>Wisconsin</td><td>2,353</td></tr>
<tr><td>30</td><td>Texas</td><td>2,623</td><td>43</td><td>Kansas</td><td>2,340</td></tr>
<tr><td>27</td><td>Utah</td><td>2,677</td><td>44</td><td>Florida</td><td>2,330</td></tr>
<tr><td>23</td><td>Vermont</td><td>2,714</td><td>45</td><td>Arizona</td><td>2,324</td></tr>
<tr><td>25</td><td>Virginia</td><td>2,685</td><td>46</td><td>Oregon</td><td>2,293</td></tr>
<tr><td>21</td><td>Washington</td><td>2,738</td><td>47</td><td>Idaho</td><td>2,239</td></tr>
<tr><td>33</td><td>West Virginia</td><td>2,605</td><td>48</td><td>Tennessee</td><td>2,208</td></tr>
<tr><td>42</td><td>Wisconsin</td><td>2,353</td><td>49</td><td>Nevada</td><td>2,097</td></tr>
<tr><td>36</td><td>Wyoming</td><td>2,583</td><td>50</td><td>New Hampshire</td><td>1,768</td></tr>
<tr><td></td><td></td><td></td><td></td><td>District of Columbia**</td><td>NA</td></tr>
</table>

Source: Morgan Quitno Press using data from Lewin-VHI, Inc. as reported by Families USA Foundation
   "Skyrocketing Health Inflation" (November 1993)
*Consists of medicare payroll taxes, medicare premiums and general taxes. See beginning of this chapter for definitions.
**Not available.

Percent of Average Family Income Spent on Health Care in 1993

National Percent = 13.1% of Family Income*

ALPHA ORDER				RANK ORDER		
RANK	STATE	PERCENT OF INCOME		RANK	STATE	PERCENT OF INCOME
6	Alabama	15.5		1	North Dakota	17.4
13	Alaska	14.7		2	Louisiana	17.0
28	Arizona	13.0		3	Arkansas	16.3
3	Arkansas	16.3		4	Kentucky	15.8
33	California	12.5		5	Delaware	15.6
23	Colorado	13.3		6	Alabama	15.5
50	Connecticut	9.7		6	South Dakota	15.5
5	Delaware	15.6		8	West Virginia	15.3
23	Florida	13.3		9	Montana	15.2
19	Georgia	13.9		9	New Mexico	15.2
41	Hawaii	11.9		11	New York	15.0
37	Idaho	12.2		12	Mississippi	14.8
37	Illinois	12.2		13	Alaska	14.7
14	Indiana	14.4		14	Indiana	14.4
18	Iowa	14.0		15	Tennessee	14.3
31	Kansas	12.6		16	Missouri	14.2
4	Kentucky	15.8		16	Texas	14.2
2	Louisiana	17.0		18	Iowa	14.0
45	Maine	11.3		19	Georgia	13.9
36	Maryland	12.3		19	South Carolina	13.9
28	Massachusetts	13.0		21	Oklahoma	13.8
40	Michigan	12.0		22	Utah	13.6
26	Minnesota	13.2		23	Colorado	13.3
12	Mississippi	14.8		23	Florida	13.3
16	Missouri	14.2		23	Nebraska	13.3
9	Montana	15.2		26	Minnesota	13.2
23	Nebraska	13.3		26	North Carolina	13.2
43	Nevada	11.6		28	Arizona	13.0
49	New Hampshire	9.8		28	Massachusetts	13.0
48	New Jersey	10.8		28	Ohio	13.0
9	New Mexico	15.2		31	Kansas	12.6
11	New York	15.0		31	Rhode Island	12.6
26	North Carolina	13.2		33	California	12.5
1	North Dakota	17.4		33	Wisconsin	12.5
28	Ohio	13.0		35	Wyoming	12.4
21	Oklahoma	13.8		36	Maryland	12.3
42	Oregon	11.8		37	Idaho	12.2
44	Pennsylvania	11.5		37	Illinois	12.2
31	Rhode Island	12.6		39	Washington	12.1
19	South Carolina	13.9		40	Michigan	12.0
6	South Dakota	15.5		41	Hawaii	11.9
15	Tennessee	14.3		42	Oregon	11.8
16	Texas	14.2		43	Nevada	11.6
22	Utah	13.6		44	Pennsylvania	11.5
46	Vermont	11.1		45	Maine	11.3
47	Virginia	10.9		46	Vermont	11.1
39	Washington	12.1		47	Virginia	10.9
8	West Virginia	15.3		48	New Jersey	10.8
33	Wisconsin	12.5		49	New Hampshire	9.8
35	Wyoming	12.4		50	Connecticut	9.7
				District of Columbia**		NA

Source: Lewin-VHI, Inc. as reported by Families USA Foundation
"Skyrocketing Health Inflation" (November 1993)
*See beginning of this chapter for definitions.
**Not available.

Health Care Payments Paid by Business in 1993

National Total = $279,154,000,000*

ALPHA ORDER				RANK ORDER			
RANK	STATE	PAYMENTS	% of USA	RANK	STATE	PAYMENTS	% of USA
23	Alabama	$3,755,000,000	1.35%	1	California	$37,494,000,000	13.43%
49	Alaska	491,000,000	0.18%	2	New York	23,036,000,000	8.25%
26	Arizona	3,496,000,000	1.25%	3	Texas	17,393,000,000	6.23%
32	Arkansas	2,143,000,000	0.77%	4	Pennsylvania	15,062,000,000	5.40%
1	California	37,494,000,000	13.43%	5	Florida	14,226,000,000	5.10%
24	Colorado	3,601,000,000	1.29%	6	Illinois	13,306,000,000	4.77%
18	Connecticut	5,211,000,000	1.87%	7	Ohio	12,556,000,000	4.50%
43	Delaware	880,000,000	0.32%	8	Michigan	11,269,000,000	4.04%
5	Florida	14,226,000,000	5.10%	9	New Jersey	9,721,000,000	3.48%
12	Georgia	6,549,000,000	2.35%	10	Massachusetts	8,675,000,000	3.11%
41	Hawaii	1,062,000,000	0.38%	11	Tennessee	6,737,000,000	2.41%
44	Idaho	849,000,000	0.30%	12	Georgia	6,549,000,000	2.35%
6	Illinois	13,306,000,000	4.77%	13	North Carolina	6,248,000,000	2.24%
15	Indiana	5,441,000,000	1.95%	14	Missouri	5,557,000,000	1.99%
30	Iowa	2,500,000,000	0.90%	15	Indiana	5,441,000,000	1.95%
31	Kansas	2,406,000,000	0.86%	16	Virginia	5,399,000,000	1.93%
25	Kentucky	3,529,000,000	1.26%	17	Wisconsin	5,370,000,000	1.92%
21	Louisiana	4,644,000,000	1.66%	18	Connecticut	5,211,000,000	1.87%
40	Maine	1,097,000,000	0.39%	19	Minnesota	5,151,000,000	1.85%
22	Maryland	4,639,000,000	1.66%	20	Washington	4,965,000,000	1.78%
10	Massachusetts	8,675,000,000	3.11%	21	Louisiana	4,644,000,000	1.66%
8	Michigan	11,269,000,000	4.04%	22	Maryland	4,639,000,000	1.66%
19	Minnesota	5,151,000,000	1.85%	23	Alabama	3,755,000,000	1.35%
33	Mississippi	1,983,000,000	0.71%	24	Colorado	3,601,000,000	1.29%
14	Missouri	5,557,000,000	1.99%	25	Kentucky	3,529,000,000	1.26%
45	Montana	784,000,000	0.28%	26	Arizona	3,496,000,000	1.25%
36	Nebraska	1,523,000,000	0.55%	27	Oregon	2,965,000,000	1.06%
39	Nevada	1,321,000,000	0.47%	28	South Carolina	2,873,000,000	1.03%
37	New Hampshire	1,404,000,000	0.50%	29	Oklahoma	2,530,000,000	0.91%
9	New Jersey	9,721,000,000	3.48%	30	Iowa	2,500,000,000	0.90%
38	New Mexico	1,326,000,000	0.48%	31	Kansas	2,406,000,000	0.86%
2	New York	23,036,000,000	8.25%	32	Arkansas	2,143,000,000	0.77%
13	North Carolina	6,248,000,000	2.24%	33	Mississippi	1,983,000,000	0.71%
46	North Dakota	612,000,000	0.22%	34	West Virginia	1,736,000,000	0.62%
7	Ohio	12,556,000,000	4.50%	35	Utah	1,606,000,000	0.58%
29	Oklahoma	2,530,000,000	0.91%	36	Nebraska	1,523,000,000	0.55%
27	Oregon	2,965,000,000	1.06%	37	New Hampshire	1,404,000,000	0.50%
4	Pennsylvania	15,062,000,000	5.40%	38	New Mexico	1,326,000,000	0.48%
42	Rhode Island	1,043,000,000	0.37%	39	Nevada	1,321,000,000	0.47%
28	South Carolina	2,873,000,000	1.03%	40	Maine	1,097,000,000	0.39%
47	South Dakota	602,000,000	0.22%	41	Hawaii	1,062,000,000	0.38%
11	Tennessee	6,737,000,000	2.41%	42	Rhode Island	1,043,000,000	0.37%
3	Texas	17,393,000,000	6.23%	43	Delaware	880,000,000	0.32%
35	Utah	1,606,000,000	0.58%	44	Idaho	849,000,000	0.30%
48	Vermont	515,000,000	0.18%	45	Montana	784,000,000	0.28%
16	Virginia	5,399,000,000	1.93%	46	North Dakota	612,000,000	0.22%
20	Washington	4,965,000,000	1.78%	47	South Dakota	602,000,000	0.22%
34	West Virginia	1,736,000,000	0.62%	48	Vermont	515,000,000	0.18%
17	Wisconsin	5,370,000,000	1.92%	49	Alaska	491,000,000	0.18%
50	Wyoming	389,000,000	0.14%	50	Wyoming	389,000,000	0.14%
					District of Columbia**	NA	NA

Source: Lewin-VHI, Inc. as reported by Families USA Foundation
"Skyrocketing Health Inflation" (November 1993)
*Total of insurance premiums and indirect health care payments by business. See beginning of this chapter for definitions.
**Not available.

Average Annual Health Care Payment by Business per Family in 1993

National Average = $2,549 per Family*

<u>ALPHA ORDER</u>

RANK	STATE	AVERAGE PAYMENT
16	Alabama	$2,593
50	Alaska	1,331
30	Arizona	2,207
24	Arkansas	2,364
14	California	2,603
38	Colorado	2,052
4	Connecticut	3,038
47	Delaware	1,822
6	Florida	2,921
23	Georgia	2,374
46	Hawaii	1,823
45	Idaho	1,887
20	Illinois	2,436
28	Indiana	2,249
39	Iowa	2,043
31	Kansas	2,182
15	Kentucky	2,596
5	Louisiana	3,004
32	Maine	2,153
37	Maryland	2,054
3	Massachusetts	3,246
10	Michigan	2,722
35	Minnesota	2,086
27	Mississippi	2,268
7	Missouri	2,742
21	Montana	2,407
33	Nebraska	2,122
26	Nevada	2,291
19	New Hampshire	2,443
12	New Jersey	2,665
41	New Mexico	2,017
11	New York	2,683
34	North Carolina	2,110
13	North Dakota	2,647
8	Ohio	2,741
42	Oklahoma	1,976
36	Oregon	2,080
2	Pennsylvania	3,370
17	Rhode Island	2,516
43	South Carolina	1,959
29	South Dakota	2,213
1	Tennessee	3,544
22	Texas	2,378
18	Utah	2,513
47	Vermont	1,822
44	Virginia	1,892
40	Washington	2,032
9	West Virginia	2,728
25	Wisconsin	2,323
49	Wyoming	1,729

<u>RANK ORDER</u>

RANK	STATE	AVERAGE PAYMENT
1	Tennessee	$3,544
2	Pennsylvania	3,370
3	Massachusetts	3,246
4	Connecticut	3,038
5	Louisiana	3,004
6	Florida	2,921
7	Missouri	2,742
8	Ohio	2,741
9	West Virginia	2,728
10	Michigan	2,722
11	New York	2,683
12	New Jersey	2,665
13	North Dakota	2,647
14	California	2,603
15	Kentucky	2,596
16	Alabama	2,593
17	Rhode Island	2,516
18	Utah	2,513
19	New Hampshire	2,443
20	Illinois	2,436
21	Montana	2,407
22	Texas	2,378
23	Georgia	2,374
24	Arkansas	2,364
25	Wisconsin	2,323
26	Nevada	2,291
27	Mississippi	2,268
28	Indiana	2,249
29	South Dakota	2,213
30	Arizona	2,207
31	Kansas	2,182
32	Maine	2,153
33	Nebraska	2,122
34	North Carolina	2,110
35	Minnesota	2,086
36	Oregon	2,080
37	Maryland	2,054
38	Colorado	2,052
39	Iowa	2,043
40	Washington	2,032
41	New Mexico	2,017
42	Oklahoma	1,976
43	South Carolina	1,959
44	Virginia	1,892
45	Idaho	1,887
46	Hawaii	1,823
47	Delaware	1,822
47	Vermont	1,822
49	Wyoming	1,729
50	Alaska	1,331

	District of Columbia**	NA

Source: Lewin-VHI, Inc. as reported by Families USA Foundation
    "Skyrocketing Health Inflation" (November 1993)
*Total annual health care payments by business divided by number of families. See beginning of this chapter for definitions.
**Not available.

Payments by Business for Health Care Insurance Premiums in 1993

National Total = $159,133,000,000*

ALPHA ORDER

RANK	STATE	PAYMENTS	% of USA
22	Alabama	$2,326,000,000	1.46%
50	Alaska	153,000,000	0.10%
24	Arizona	2,171,000,000	1.36%
32	Arkansas	1,122,000,000	0.71%
1	California	21,004,000,000	13.20%
25	Colorado	2,138,000,000	1.34%
20	Connecticut	2,594,000,000	1.63%
44	Delaware	429,000,000	0.27%
5	Florida	8,779,000,000	5.52%
11	Georgia	3,961,000,000	2.49%
40	Hawaii	538,000,000	0.34%
43	Idaho	485,000,000	0.30%
6	Illinois	7,875,000,000	4.95%
14	Indiana	3,410,000,000	2.14%
29	Iowa	1,402,000,000	0.88%
30	Kansas	1,401,000,000	0.88%
26	Kentucky	2,022,000,000	1.27%
23	Louisiana	2,274,000,000	1.43%
42	Maine	509,000,000	0.32%
19	Maryland	2,686,000,000	1.69%
10	Massachusetts	5,329,000,000	3.35%
8	Michigan	6,266,000,000	3.94%
18	Minnesota	2,999,000,000	1.88%
34	Mississippi	1,015,000,000	0.64%
13	Missouri	3,550,000,000	2.23%
45	Montana	372,000,000	0.23%
36	Nebraska	882,000,000	0.55%
37	Nevada	811,000,000	0.51%
39	New Hampshire	665,000,000	0.42%
9	New Jersey	5,466,000,000	3.43%
38	New Mexico	678,000,000	0.43%
2	New York	12,314,000,000	7.74%
12	North Carolina	3,855,000,000	2.42%
48	North Dakota	280,000,000	0.18%
7	Ohio	7,399,000,000	4.65%
31	Oklahoma	1,378,000,000	0.87%
27	Oregon	1,765,000,000	1.11%
4	Pennsylvania	8,831,000,000	5.55%
41	Rhode Island	526,000,000	0.33%
28	South Carolina	1,687,000,000	1.06%
47	South Dakota	295,000,000	0.19%
16	Tennessee	3,311,000,000	2.08%
3	Texas	9,926,000,000	6.24%
33	Utah	1,069,000,000	0.67%
46	Vermont	298,000,000	0.19%
17	Virginia	3,284,000,000	2.06%
21	Washington	2,585,000,000	1.62%
35	West Virginia	990,000,000	0.62%
15	Wisconsin	3,373,000,000	2.12%
49	Wyoming	208,000,000	0.13%

RANK ORDER

RANK	STATE	PAYMENTS	% of USA
1	California	$21,004,000,000	13.20%
2	New York	12,314,000,000	7.74%
3	Texas	9,926,000,000	6.24%
4	Pennsylvania	8,831,000,000	5.55%
5	Florida	8,779,000,000	5.52%
6	Illinois	7,875,000,000	4.95%
7	Ohio	7,399,000,000	4.65%
8	Michigan	6,266,000,000	3.94%
9	New Jersey	5,466,000,000	3.43%
10	Massachusetts	5,329,000,000	3.35%
11	Georgia	3,961,000,000	2.49%
12	North Carolina	3,855,000,000	2.42%
13	Missouri	3,550,000,000	2.23%
14	Indiana	3,410,000,000	2.14%
15	Wisconsin	3,373,000,000	2.12%
16	Tennessee	3,311,000,000	2.08%
17	Virginia	3,284,000,000	2.06%
18	Minnesota	2,999,000,000	1.88%
19	Maryland	2,686,000,000	1.69%
20	Connecticut	2,594,000,000	1.63%
21	Washington	2,585,000,000	1.62%
22	Alabama	2,326,000,000	1.46%
23	Louisiana	2,274,000,000	1.43%
24	Arizona	2,171,000,000	1.36%
25	Colorado	2,138,000,000	1.34%
26	Kentucky	2,022,000,000	1.27%
27	Oregon	1,765,000,000	1.11%
28	South Carolina	1,687,000,000	1.06%
29	Iowa	1,402,000,000	0.88%
30	Kansas	1,401,000,000	0.88%
31	Oklahoma	1,378,000,000	0.87%
32	Arkansas	1,122,000,000	0.71%
33	Utah	1,069,000,000	0.67%
34	Mississippi	1,015,000,000	0.64%
35	West Virginia	990,000,000	0.62%
36	Nebraska	882,000,000	0.55%
37	Nevada	811,000,000	0.51%
38	New Mexico	678,000,000	0.43%
39	New Hampshire	665,000,000	0.42%
40	Hawaii	538,000,000	0.34%
41	Rhode Island	526,000,000	0.33%
42	Maine	509,000,000	0.32%
43	Idaho	485,000,000	0.30%
44	Delaware	429,000,000	0.27%
45	Montana	372,000,000	0.23%
46	Vermont	298,000,000	0.19%
47	South Dakota	295,000,000	0.19%
48	North Dakota	280,000,000	0.18%
49	Wyoming	208,000,000	0.13%
50	Alaska	153,000,000	0.10%
	District of Columbia**	NA	NA

Source: Lewin-VHI, Inc. as reported by Families USA Foundation
"Skyrocketing Health Inflation" (November 1993)
*See beginning of this chapter for definitions.
**Not available.

Payments by Business for Indirect Health Care Costs in 1993

National Total = $120,021,000,000*

ALPHA ORDER

RANK	STATE	PAYMENTS	% of USA
25	Alabama	$1,428,000,000	1.19%
46	Alaska	339,000,000	0.28%
26	Arizona	1,325,000,000	1.10%
31	Arkansas	1,022,000,000	0.85%
1	California	16,490,000,000	13.74%
24	Colorado	1,462,000,000	1.22%
12	Connecticut	2,617,000,000	2.18%
43	Delaware	451,000,000	0.38%
5	Florida	5,446,000,000	4.54%
13	Georgia	2,587,000,000	2.16%
40	Hawaii	525,000,000	0.44%
45	Idaho	364,000,000	0.30%
6	Illinois	5,430,000,000	4.52%
19	Indiana	2,031,000,000	1.69%
30	Iowa	1,098,000,000	0.91%
32	Kansas	1,005,000,000	0.84%
23	Kentucky	1,507,000,000	1.26%
16	Louisiana	2,370,000,000	1.97%
38	Maine	588,000,000	0.49%
22	Maryland	1,954,000,000	1.63%
11	Massachusetts	3,347,000,000	2.79%
8	Michigan	5,003,000,000	4.17%
17	Minnesota	2,152,000,000	1.79%
33	Mississippi	968,000,000	0.81%
20	Missouri	2,007,000,000	1.67%
44	Montana	412,000,000	0.34%
37	Nebraska	640,000,000	0.53%
42	Nevada	511,000,000	0.43%
35	New Hampshire	739,000,000	0.62%
9	New Jersey	4,255,000,000	3.55%
36	New Mexico	647,000,000	0.54%
2	New York	10,722,000,000	8.93%
14	North Carolina	2,393,000,000	1.99%
47	North Dakota	334,000,000	0.28%
7	Ohio	5,158,000,000	4.30%
29	Oklahoma	1,152,000,000	0.96%
27	Oregon	1,201,000,000	1.00%
4	Pennsylvania	6,230,000,000	5.19%
41	Rhode Island	518,000,000	0.43%
28	South Carolina	1,185,000,000	0.99%
48	South Dakota	308,000,000	0.26%
10	Tennessee	3,426,000,000	2.85%
3	Texas	7,467,000,000	6.22%
39	Utah	537,000,000	0.45%
49	Vermont	216,000,000	0.18%
18	Virginia	2,115,000,000	1.76%
15	Washington	2,379,000,000	1.98%
34	West Virginia	746,000,000	0.62%
21	Wisconsin	1,996,000,000	1.66%
50	Wyoming	180,000,000	0.15%

RANK ORDER

RANK	STATE	PAYMENTS	% of USA
1	California	$16,490,000,000	13.74%
2	New York	10,722,000,000	8.93%
3	Texas	7,467,000,000	6.22%
4	Pennsylvania	6,230,000,000	5.19%
5	Florida	5,446,000,000	4.54%
6	Illinois	5,430,000,000	4.52%
7	Ohio	5,158,000,000	4.30%
8	Michigan	5,003,000,000	4.17%
9	New Jersey	4,255,000,000	3.55%
10	Tennessee	3,426,000,000	2.85%
11	Massachusetts	3,347,000,000	2.79%
12	Connecticut	2,617,000,000	2.18%
13	Georgia	2,587,000,000	2.16%
14	North Carolina	2,393,000,000	1.99%
15	Washington	2,379,000,000	1.98%
16	Louisiana	2,370,000,000	1.97%
17	Minnesota	2,152,000,000	1.79%
18	Virginia	2,115,000,000	1.76%
19	Indiana	2,031,000,000	1.69%
20	Missouri	2,007,000,000	1.67%
21	Wisconsin	1,996,000,000	1.66%
22	Maryland	1,954,000,000	1.63%
23	Kentucky	1,507,000,000	1.26%
24	Colorado	1,462,000,000	1.22%
25	Alabama	1,428,000,000	1.19%
26	Arizona	1,325,000,000	1.10%
27	Oregon	1,201,000,000	1.00%
28	South Carolina	1,185,000,000	0.99%
29	Oklahoma	1,152,000,000	0.96%
30	Iowa	1,098,000,000	0.91%
31	Arkansas	1,022,000,000	0.85%
32	Kansas	1,005,000,000	0.84%
33	Mississippi	968,000,000	0.81%
34	West Virginia	746,000,000	0.62%
35	New Hampshire	739,000,000	0.62%
36	New Mexico	647,000,000	0.54%
37	Nebraska	640,000,000	0.53%
38	Maine	588,000,000	0.49%
39	Utah	537,000,000	0.45%
40	Hawaii	525,000,000	0.44%
41	Rhode Island	518,000,000	0.43%
42	Nevada	511,000,000	0.43%
43	Delaware	451,000,000	0.38%
44	Montana	412,000,000	0.34%
45	Idaho	364,000,000	0.30%
46	Alaska	339,000,000	0.28%
47	North Dakota	334,000,000	0.28%
48	South Dakota	308,000,000	0.26%
49	Vermont	216,000,000	0.18%
50	Wyoming	180,000,000	0.15%

District of Columbia**   NA   NA

Source: Morgan Quitno Press using data from Lewin-VHI, Inc. as reported by Families USA Foundation
"Skyrocketing Health Inflation" (November 1993)
*Consists of medicare payroll tax, general taxes and other costs. See beginning of this chapter for definitions.
**Not available.

Expenditures for Physician Services in 1991

National Total = $150,891,000,000*

<table>
<tr><th colspan="4">ALPHA ORDER</th><th colspan="4">RANK ORDER</th></tr>
<tr><th>RANK</th><th>STATE</th><th>EXPENDITURES</th><th>% of USA</th><th>RANK</th><th>STATE</th><th>EXPENDITURES</th><th>% of USA</th></tr>
<tr><td>23</td><td>Alabama</td><td>$2,296,000,000</td><td>1.52%</td><td>1</td><td>California</td><td>$23,108,000,000</td><td>15.31%</td></tr>
<tr><td>48</td><td>Alaska</td><td>312,000,000</td><td>0.21%</td><td>2</td><td>New York</td><td>10,611,000,000</td><td>7.03%</td></tr>
<tr><td>22</td><td>Arizona</td><td>2,321,000,000</td><td>1.54%</td><td>3</td><td>Florida</td><td>9,881,000,000</td><td>6.55%</td></tr>
<tr><td>32</td><td>Arkansas</td><td>1,241,000,000</td><td>0.82%</td><td>4</td><td>Texas</td><td>9,754,000,000</td><td>6.46%</td></tr>
<tr><td>1</td><td>California</td><td>23,108,000,000</td><td>15.31%</td><td>5</td><td>Pennsylvania</td><td>6,680,000,000</td><td>4.43%</td></tr>
<tr><td>25</td><td>Colorado</td><td>2,122,000,000</td><td>1.41%</td><td>6</td><td>Ohio</td><td>6,094,000,000</td><td>4.04%</td></tr>
<tr><td>24</td><td>Connecticut</td><td>2,236,000,000</td><td>1.48%</td><td>7</td><td>Illinois</td><td>5,731,000,000</td><td>3.80%</td></tr>
<tr><td>43</td><td>Delaware</td><td>488,000,000</td><td>0.32%</td><td>8</td><td>Michigan</td><td>5,141,000,000</td><td>3.41%</td></tr>
<tr><td>3</td><td>Florida</td><td>9,881,000,000</td><td>6.55%</td><td>9</td><td>New Jersey</td><td>4,569,000,000</td><td>3.03%</td></tr>
<tr><td>11</td><td>Georgia</td><td>3,902,000,000</td><td>2.59%</td><td>10</td><td>Massachusetts</td><td>4,244,000,000</td><td>2.81%</td></tr>
<tr><td>38</td><td>Hawaii</td><td>719,000,000</td><td>0.48%</td><td>11</td><td>Georgia</td><td>3,902,000,000</td><td>2.59%</td></tr>
<tr><td>45</td><td>Idaho</td><td>397,000,000</td><td>0.26%</td><td>12</td><td>Minnesota</td><td>3,571,000,000</td><td>2.37%</td></tr>
<tr><td>7</td><td>Illinois</td><td>5,731,000,000</td><td>3.80%</td><td>13</td><td>Virginia</td><td>3,464,000,000</td><td>2.30%</td></tr>
<tr><td>18</td><td>Indiana</td><td>2,890,000,000</td><td>1.92%</td><td>14</td><td>Washington</td><td>3,336,000,000</td><td>2.21%</td></tr>
<tr><td>31</td><td>Iowa</td><td>1,294,000,000</td><td>0.86%</td><td>15</td><td>Maryland</td><td>3,284,000,000</td><td>2.18%</td></tr>
<tr><td>30</td><td>Kansas</td><td>1,404,000,000</td><td>0.93%</td><td>16</td><td>North Carolina</td><td>3,200,000,000</td><td>2.12%</td></tr>
<tr><td>26</td><td>Kentucky</td><td>1,814,000,000</td><td>1.20%</td><td>17</td><td>Wisconsin</td><td>3,077,000,000</td><td>2.04%</td></tr>
<tr><td>21</td><td>Louisiana</td><td>2,400,000,000</td><td>1.59%</td><td>18</td><td>Indiana</td><td>2,890,000,000</td><td>1.92%</td></tr>
<tr><td>41</td><td>Maine</td><td>547,000,000</td><td>0.36%</td><td>19</td><td>Tennessee</td><td>2,865,000,000</td><td>1.90%</td></tr>
<tr><td>15</td><td>Maryland</td><td>3,284,000,000</td><td>2.18%</td><td>20</td><td>Missouri</td><td>2,815,000,000</td><td>1.87%</td></tr>
<tr><td>10</td><td>Massachusetts</td><td>4,244,000,000</td><td>2.81%</td><td>21</td><td>Louisiana</td><td>2,400,000,000</td><td>1.59%</td></tr>
<tr><td>8</td><td>Michigan</td><td>5,141,000,000</td><td>3.41%</td><td>22</td><td>Arizona</td><td>2,321,000,000</td><td>1.54%</td></tr>
<tr><td>12</td><td>Minnesota</td><td>3,571,000,000</td><td>2.37%</td><td>23</td><td>Alabama</td><td>2,296,000,000</td><td>1.52%</td></tr>
<tr><td>34</td><td>Mississippi</td><td>923,000,000</td><td>0.61%</td><td>24</td><td>Connecticut</td><td>2,236,000,000</td><td>1.48%</td></tr>
<tr><td>20</td><td>Missouri</td><td>2,815,000,000</td><td>1.87%</td><td>25</td><td>Colorado</td><td>2,122,000,000</td><td>1.41%</td></tr>
<tr><td>47</td><td>Montana</td><td>314,000,000</td><td>0.21%</td><td>26</td><td>Kentucky</td><td>1,814,000,000</td><td>1.20%</td></tr>
<tr><td>37</td><td>Nebraska</td><td>779,000,000</td><td>0.52%</td><td>27</td><td>Oregon</td><td>1,738,000,000</td><td>1.15%</td></tr>
<tr><td>33</td><td>Nevada</td><td>945,000,000</td><td>0.63%</td><td>28</td><td>Oklahoma</td><td>1,471,000,000</td><td>0.97%</td></tr>
<tr><td>40</td><td>New Hampshire</td><td>641,000,000</td><td>0.42%</td><td>29</td><td>South Carolina</td><td>1,455,000,000</td><td>0.96%</td></tr>
<tr><td>9</td><td>New Jersey</td><td>4,569,000,000</td><td>3.03%</td><td>30</td><td>Kansas</td><td>1,404,000,000</td><td>0.93%</td></tr>
<tr><td>39</td><td>New Mexico</td><td>699,000,000</td><td>0.46%</td><td>31</td><td>Iowa</td><td>1,294,000,000</td><td>0.86%</td></tr>
<tr><td>2</td><td>New York</td><td>10,611,000,000</td><td>7.03%</td><td>32</td><td>Arkansas</td><td>1,241,000,000</td><td>0.82%</td></tr>
<tr><td>16</td><td>North Carolina</td><td>3,200,000,000</td><td>2.12%</td><td>33</td><td>Nevada</td><td>945,000,000</td><td>0.63%</td></tr>
<tr><td>44</td><td>North Dakota</td><td>442,000,000</td><td>0.29%</td><td>34</td><td>Mississippi</td><td>923,000,000</td><td>0.61%</td></tr>
<tr><td>6</td><td>Ohio</td><td>6,094,000,000</td><td>4.04%</td><td>35</td><td>West Virginia</td><td>900,000,000</td><td>0.60%</td></tr>
<tr><td>28</td><td>Oklahoma</td><td>1,471,000,000</td><td>0.97%</td><td>36</td><td>Utah</td><td>822,000,000</td><td>0.54%</td></tr>
<tr><td>27</td><td>Oregon</td><td>1,738,000,000</td><td>1.15%</td><td>37</td><td>Nebraska</td><td>779,000,000</td><td>0.52%</td></tr>
<tr><td>5</td><td>Pennsylvania</td><td>6,680,000,000</td><td>4.43%</td><td>38</td><td>Hawaii</td><td>719,000,000</td><td>0.48%</td></tr>
<tr><td>42</td><td>Rhode Island</td><td>543,000,000</td><td>0.36%</td><td>39</td><td>New Mexico</td><td>699,000,000</td><td>0.46%</td></tr>
<tr><td>29</td><td>South Carolina</td><td>1,455,000,000</td><td>0.96%</td><td>40</td><td>New Hampshire</td><td>641,000,000</td><td>0.42%</td></tr>
<tr><td>46</td><td>South Dakota</td><td>342,000,000</td><td>0.23%</td><td>41</td><td>Maine</td><td>547,000,000</td><td>0.36%</td></tr>
<tr><td>19</td><td>Tennessee</td><td>2,865,000,000</td><td>1.90%</td><td>42</td><td>Rhode Island</td><td>543,000,000</td><td>0.36%</td></tr>
<tr><td>4</td><td>Texas</td><td>9,754,000,000</td><td>6.46%</td><td>43</td><td>Delaware</td><td>488,000,000</td><td>0.32%</td></tr>
<tr><td>36</td><td>Utah</td><td>822,000,000</td><td>0.54%</td><td>44</td><td>North Dakota</td><td>442,000,000</td><td>0.29%</td></tr>
<tr><td>49</td><td>Vermont</td><td>243,000,000</td><td>0.16%</td><td>45</td><td>Idaho</td><td>397,000,000</td><td>0.26%</td></tr>
<tr><td>13</td><td>Virginia</td><td>3,464,000,000</td><td>2.30%</td><td>46</td><td>South Dakota</td><td>342,000,000</td><td>0.23%</td></tr>
<tr><td>14</td><td>Washington</td><td>3,336,000,000</td><td>2.21%</td><td>47</td><td>Montana</td><td>314,000,000</td><td>0.21%</td></tr>
<tr><td>35</td><td>West Virginia</td><td>900,000,000</td><td>0.60%</td><td>48</td><td>Alaska</td><td>312,000,000</td><td>0.21%</td></tr>
<tr><td>17</td><td>Wisconsin</td><td>3,077,000,000</td><td>2.04%</td><td>49</td><td>Vermont</td><td>243,000,000</td><td>0.16%</td></tr>
<tr><td>50</td><td>Wyoming</td><td>155,000,000</td><td>0.10%</td><td>50</td><td>Wyoming</td><td>155,000,000</td><td>0.10%</td></tr>
<tr><td></td><td></td><td></td><td></td><td></td><td>District of Columbia</td><td>666,000,000</td><td>0.44%</td></tr>
</table>

Source: U.S. Department of Health and Human Services, Health Care Financing Administration
"Health Spending by State: New Estimates for Policy Making" (Health Affairs, Fall 1993)
*By state of provider.

Percent Change in Expenditures for Physician Services: 1990 to 1991

National Percent Change = 7.2% Increase*

ALPHA ORDER

RANK	STATE	PERCENT CHANGE
9	Alabama	9.6
21	Alaska	8.2
30	Arizona	7.3
36	Arkansas	6.4
37	California	6.3
7	Colorado	10.2
24	Connecticut	7.9
8	Delaware	10.1
40	Florida	6.0
44	Georgia	5.1
41	Hawaii	5.8
34	Idaho	7.0
43	Illinois	5.2
30	Indiana	7.3
14	Iowa	8.8
3	Kansas	13.0
20	Kentucky	8.4
24	Louisiana	7.9
17	Maine	8.6
28	Maryland	7.4
14	Massachusetts	8.8
32	Michigan	7.2
1	Minnesota	13.8
41	Mississippi	5.8
14	Missouri	8.8
45	Montana	5.0
17	Nebraska	8.6
19	Nevada	8.5
22	New Hampshire	8.0
46	New Jersey	4.6
2	New Mexico	13.1
27	New York	7.7
37	North Carolina	6.3
49	North Dakota	1.8
48	Ohio	2.0
50	Oklahoma	1.7
28	Oregon	7.4
22	Pennsylvania	8.0
24	Rhode Island	7.9
11	South Carolina	9.2
35	South Dakota	6.5
10	Tennessee	9.5
39	Texas	6.1
12	Utah	9.0
13	Vermont	8.9
6	Virginia	10.3
4	Washington	12.6
32	West Virginia	7.2
5	Wisconsin	11.0
47	Wyoming	3.6

RANK ORDER

RANK	STATE	PERCENT CHANGE
1	Minnesota	13.8
2	New Mexico	13.1
3	Kansas	13.0
4	Washington	12.6
5	Wisconsin	11.0
6	Virginia	10.3
7	Colorado	10.2
8	Delaware	10.1
9	Alabama	9.6
10	Tennessee	9.5
11	South Carolina	9.2
12	Utah	9.0
13	Vermont	8.9
14	Iowa	8.8
14	Massachusetts	8.8
14	Missouri	8.8
17	Maine	8.6
17	Nebraska	8.6
19	Nevada	8.5
20	Kentucky	8.4
21	Alaska	8.2
22	New Hampshire	8.0
22	Pennsylvania	8.0
24	Connecticut	7.9
24	Louisiana	7.9
24	Rhode Island	7.9
27	New York	7.7
28	Maryland	7.4
28	Oregon	7.4
30	Arizona	7.3
30	Indiana	7.3
32	Michigan	7.2
32	West Virginia	7.2
34	Idaho	7.0
35	South Dakota	6.5
36	Arkansas	6.4
37	California	6.3
37	North Carolina	6.3
39	Texas	6.1
40	Florida	6.0
41	Hawaii	5.8
41	Mississippi	5.8
43	Illinois	5.2
44	Georgia	5.1
45	Montana	5.0
46	New Jersey	4.6
47	Wyoming	3.6
48	Ohio	2.0
49	North Dakota	1.8
50	Oklahoma	1.7
	District of Columbia	9.9

Source: U.S. Department of Health and Human Services, Health Care Financing Administration
"Health Spending by State: New Estimates for Policy Making" (Health Affairs, Fall 1993)
*By state of provider.

Average Annual Change in Expenditures for Physician Services: 1980 to 1991

National Percent = 11.6% Average Annual Increase*

ALPHA ORDER			RANK ORDER		
RANK	STATE	PERCENT	RANK	STATE	PERCENT
16	Alabama	12.4	1	New Hampshire	15.7
29	Alaska	11.3	2	Nevada	14.7
18	Arizona	12.3	3	Massachusetts	14.3
26	Arkansas	11.5	4	Delaware	14.2
23	California	11.6	5	Vermont	13.4
19	Colorado	12.1	6	Florida	13.3
11	Connecticut	12.9	6	Georgia	13.3
4	Delaware	14.2	6	Maryland	13.3
6	Florida	13.3	9	Maine	13.1
6	Georgia	13.3	9	Virginia	13.1
39	Hawaii	10.0	11	Connecticut	12.9
40	Idaho	9.9	11	New Mexico	12.9
46	Illinois	9.4	13	Minnesota	12.6
34	Indiana	11.1	13	North Carolina	12.6
47	Iowa	9.3	13	Washington	12.6
37	Kansas	10.6	16	Alabama	12.4
29	Kentucky	11.3	16	South Carolina	12.4
29	Louisiana	11.3	18	Arizona	12.3
9	Maine	13.1	19	Colorado	12.1
6	Maryland	13.3	20	New York	12.0
3	Massachusetts	14.3	21	Pennsylvania	11.8
48	Michigan	8.7	22	Tennessee	11.7
13	Minnesota	12.6	23	California	11.6
40	Mississippi	9.9	23	New Jersey	11.6
34	Missouri	11.1	23	Utah	11.6
50	Montana	7.8	26	Arkansas	11.5
40	Nebraska	9.9	26	South Dakota	11.5
2	Nevada	14.7	28	Rhode Island	11.4
1	New Hampshire	15.7	29	Alaska	11.3
23	New Jersey	11.6	29	Kentucky	11.3
11	New Mexico	12.9	29	Louisiana	11.3
20	New York	12.0	29	Texas	11.3
13	North Carolina	12.6	29	Wisconsin	11.3
36	North Dakota	11.0	34	Indiana	11.1
40	Ohio	9.9	34	Missouri	11.1
45	Oklahoma	9.5	36	North Dakota	11.0
38	Oregon	10.2	37	Kansas	10.6
21	Pennsylvania	11.8	38	Oregon	10.2
28	Rhode Island	11.4	39	Hawaii	10.0
16	South Carolina	12.4	40	Idaho	9.9
26	South Dakota	11.5	40	Mississippi	9.9
22	Tennessee	11.7	40	Nebraska	9.9
29	Texas	11.3	40	Ohio	9.9
23	Utah	11.6	44	West Virginia	9.6
5	Vermont	13.4	45	Oklahoma	9.5
9	Virginia	13.1	46	Illinois	9.4
13	Washington	12.6	47	Iowa	9.3
44	West Virginia	9.6	48	Michigan	8.7
29	Wisconsin	11.3	49	Wyoming	8.2
49	Wyoming	8.2	50	Montana	7.8
				District of Columbia	9.8

Source: U.S. Department of Health and Human Services, Health Care Financing Administration
"Health Spending by State: New Estimates for Policy Making" (Health Affairs, Fall 1993)
*By state of provider.

Per Capita Expenditures for Physician Services in 1991

National Per Capita = $598*

ALPHA ORDER				RANK ORDER		
RANK	STATE	PER CAPITA		RANK	STATE	PER CAPITA
24	Alabama	$561		1	Minnesota	$806
29	Alaska	548		2	California	761
14	Arizona	619		3	Florida	744
32	Arkansas	523		4	Nevada	736
2	California	761		5	Delaware	718
12	Colorado	628		6	Massachusetts	708
8	Connecticut	679		7	North Dakota	697
5	Delaware	718		8	Connecticut	679
3	Florida	744		9	Maryland	676
16	Georgia	589		10	Washington	665
11	Hawaii	634		11	Hawaii	634
48	Idaho	382		12	Colorado	628
35	Illinois	496		13	Wisconsin	621
33	Indiana	515		14	Arizona	619
41	Iowa	463		15	Oregon	595
22	Kansas	563		16	Georgia	589
36	Kentucky	489		16	New Jersey	589
21	Louisiana	564		18	New York	588
44	Maine	443		19	New Hampshire	581
9	Maryland	676		20	Tennessee	579
6	Massachusetts	708		21	Louisiana	564
28	Michigan	549		22	Kansas	563
1	Minnesota	806		23	Texas	562
49	Mississippi	356		24	Alabama	561
30	Missouri	546		25	Pennsylvania	559
47	Montana	388		26	Ohio	557
36	Nebraska	489		27	Virginia	551
4	Nevada	736		28	Michigan	549
19	New Hampshire	581		29	Alaska	548
16	New Jersey	589		30	Missouri	546
43	New Mexico	452		31	Rhode Island	541
18	New York	588		32	Arkansas	523
39	North Carolina	475		33	Indiana	515
7	North Dakota	697		34	West Virginia	500
26	Ohio	557		35	Illinois	496
41	Oklahoma	463		36	Kentucky	489
15	Oregon	595		36	Nebraska	489
25	Pennsylvania	559		38	South Dakota	487
31	Rhode Island	541		39	North Carolina	475
46	South Carolina	409		40	Utah	464
38	South Dakota	487		41	Iowa	463
20	Tennessee	579		41	Oklahoma	463
23	Texas	562		43	New Mexico	452
40	Utah	464		44	Maine	443
45	Vermont	429		45	Vermont	429
27	Virginia	551		46	South Carolina	409
10	Washington	665		47	Montana	388
34	West Virginia	500		48	Idaho	382
13	Wisconsin	621		49	Mississippi	356
50	Wyoming	337		50	Wyoming	337
				District of Columbia**		1,112

Source: U.S. Department of Health and Human Services, Health Care Financing Administration

"Health Spending by State: New Estimates for Policy Making" (Health Affairs, Fall 1993) and unpublished data
*By state of provider.
**The District of Columbia's per capita is greatly affected by residents of Maryland and Virginia receiving services.

Percent Change in Per Capita Expenditures for Physician Services: 1990 to 1991

National Percent Change = 6.1% Increase*

ALPHA ORDER				RANK ORDER		
RANK	STATE	PERCENT CHANGE		RANK	STATE	PERCENT CHANGE
8	Alabama	8.5		1	Minnesota	12.7
34	Alaska	5.1		2	Kansas	12.4
32	Arizona	5.4		3	New Mexico	11.2
30	Arkansas	5.6		4	Washington	9.9
37	California	4.5		5	Wisconsin	9.8
14	Colorado	8.1		6	Massachusetts	9.1
17	Connecticut	7.8		7	Virginia	8.9
11	Delaware	8.3		8	Alabama	8.5
43	Florida	3.8		9	New Hampshire	8.4
45	Georgia	3.3		9	Vermont	8.4
43	Hawaii	3.8		11	Delaware	8.3
38	Idaho	4.4		12	Iowa	8.2
38	Illinois	4.4		12	Maine	8.2
28	Indiana	6.3		14	Colorado	8.1
12	Iowa	8.2		14	Missouri	8.1
2	Kansas	12.4		14	Tennessee	8.1
17	Kentucky	7.8		17	Connecticut	7.8
24	Louisiana	7.2		17	Kentucky	7.8
12	Maine	8.2		17	Nebraska	7.8
29	Maryland	6.0		17	Rhode Island	7.8
6	Massachusetts	9.1		21	South Carolina	7.5
27	Michigan	6.6		22	New York	7.4
1	Minnesota	12.7		22	Pennsylvania	7.4
33	Mississippi	5.2		24	Louisiana	7.2
14	Missouri	8.1		25	West Virginia	6.8
42	Montana	4.0		26	Utah	6.7
17	Nebraska	7.8		27	Michigan	6.6
46	Nevada	2.9		28	Indiana	6.3
9	New Hampshire	8.4		29	Maryland	6.0
41	New Jersey	4.2		30	Arkansas	5.6
3	New Mexico	11.2		30	South Dakota	5.6
22	New York	7.4		32	Arizona	5.4
36	North Carolina	4.9		33	Mississippi	5.2
48	North Dakota	2.3		34	Alaska	5.1
49	Ohio	1.3		34	Oregon	5.1
50	Oklahoma	1.0		36	North Carolina	4.9
34	Oregon	5.1		37	California	4.5
22	Pennsylvania	7.4		38	Idaho	4.4
17	Rhode Island	7.8		38	Illinois	4.4
21	South Carolina	7.5		40	Texas	4.3
30	South Dakota	5.6		41	New Jersey	4.2
14	Tennessee	8.1		42	Montana	4.0
40	Texas	4.3		43	Florida	3.8
26	Utah	6.7		43	Hawaii	3.8
9	Vermont	8.4		45	Georgia	3.3
7	Virginia	8.9		46	Nevada	2.9
4	Washington	9.9		47	Wyoming	2.5
25	West Virginia	6.8		48	North Dakota	2.3
5	Wisconsin	9.8		49	Ohio	1.3
47	Wyoming	2.5		50	Oklahoma	1.0
					District of Columbia	11.1

Source: U.S. Department of Health and Human Services, Health Care Financing Administration
"Health Spending by State: New Estimates for Policy Making" (Health Affairs, Fall 1993) and unpublished data
*By state of provider.

Average Annual Percent Change in Per Capita Expenditures
For Physician Services: 1980 to 1991
National Percent = 10.5% Average Annual Increase*

ALPHA ORDER

RANK	STATE	PERCENT
7	Alabama	11.9
49	Alaska	7.9
42	Arizona	9.1
19	Arkansas	11.1
42	California	9.1
27	Colorado	10.6
4	Connecticut	12.3
3	Delaware	12.9
31	Florida	10.3
13	Georgia	11.4
48	Hawaii	8.4
45	Idaho	9.0
40	Illinois	9.3
24	Indiana	10.9
36	Iowa	9.7
32	Kansas	10.1
19	Kentucky	11.1
16	Louisiana	11.2
6	Maine	12.2
7	Maryland	11.9
1	Massachusetts	13.9
46	Michigan	8.6
9	Minnesota	11.8
36	Mississippi	9.7
27	Missouri	10.6
50	Montana	7.6
36	Nebraska	9.7
33	Nevada	10.0
2	New Hampshire	13.8
19	New Jersey	11.1
16	New Mexico	11.2
10	New York	11.7
16	North Carolina	11.2
13	North Dakota	11.4
34	Ohio	9.8
42	Oklahoma	9.1
41	Oregon	9.2
10	Pennsylvania	11.7
24	Rhode Island	10.9
19	South Carolina	11.1
13	South Dakota	11.4
23	Tennessee	11.0
39	Texas	9.4
34	Utah	9.8
4	Vermont	12.3
12	Virginia	11.5
27	Washington	10.6
30	West Virginia	10.4
26	Wisconsin	10.7
47	Wyoming	8.5

RANK ORDER

RANK	STATE	PERCENT
1	Massachusetts	13.9
2	New Hampshire	13.8
3	Delaware	12.9
4	Connecticut	12.3
4	Vermont	12.3
6	Maine	12.2
7	Alabama	11.9
7	Maryland	11.9
9	Minnesota	11.8
10	New York	11.7
10	Pennsylvania	11.7
12	Virginia	11.5
13	Georgia	11.4
13	North Dakota	11.4
13	South Dakota	11.4
16	Louisiana	11.2
16	New Mexico	11.2
16	North Carolina	11.2
19	Arkansas	11.1
19	Kentucky	11.1
19	New Jersey	11.1
19	South Carolina	11.1
23	Tennessee	11.0
24	Indiana	10.9
24	Rhode Island	10.9
26	Wisconsin	10.7
27	Colorado	10.6
27	Missouri	10.6
27	Washington	10.6
30	West Virginia	10.4
31	Florida	10.3
32	Kansas	10.1
33	Nevada	10.0
34	Ohio	9.8
34	Utah	9.8
36	Iowa	9.7
36	Mississippi	9.7
36	Nebraska	9.7
39	Texas	9.4
40	Illinois	9.3
41	Oregon	9.2
42	Arizona	9.1
42	California	9.1
42	Oklahoma	9.1
45	Idaho	9.0
46	Michigan	8.6
47	Wyoming	8.5
48	Hawaii	8.4
49	Alaska	7.9
50	Montana	7.6

District of Columbia	10.5

Source: U.S. Department of Health and Human Services, Health Care Financing Administration
"Health Spending by State: New Estimates for Policy Making" (Health Affairs, Fall 1993) and unpublished data
*By state of provider.

Expenditures for Physician Services per Physician in 1991

National Rate = $380,100 Spent per Physician*

ALPHA ORDER				RANK ORDER		
RANK	STATE	PER PHYSICIAN		RANK	STATE	PER PHYSICIAN
4	Alabama	$461,400		1	Nevada	$572,900
5	Alaska	456,100		2	Minnesota	524,200
19	Arizona	385,000		3	North Dakota	476,100
11	Arkansas	425,900		4	Alabama	461,400
9	California	441,600		5	Alaska	456,100
20	Colorado	378,100		6	Delaware	456,000
30	Connecticut	355,200		7	Florida	447,800
6	Delaware	456,000		8	Georgia	446,500
7	Florida	447,800		9	California	441,600
8	Georgia	446,500		10	Wisconsin	429,100
32	Hawaii	353,600		11	Arkansas	425,900
40	Idaho	329,100		12	Texas	419,800
41	Illinois	325,900		13	Indiana	409,200
13	Indiana	409,200		14	Louisiana	407,700
29	Iowa	356,200		15	Washington	402,000
18	Kansas	397,600		16	South Dakota	400,100
24	Kentucky	372,400		17	Tennessee	399,000
14	Louisiana	407,700		18	Kansas	397,600
48	Maine	278,400		19	Arizona	385,000
35	Maryland	346,300		20	Colorado	378,100
23	Massachusetts	373,000		21	Nebraska	375,300
36	Michigan	344,400		22	Virginia	373,200
2	Minnesota	524,200		23	Massachusetts	373,000
38	Mississippi	333,800		24	Kentucky	372,400
34	Missouri	351,800		25	New Hampshire	366,300
49	Montana	262,400		26	West Virginia	362,000
21	Nebraska	375,300		27	North Carolina	361,500
1	Nevada	572,900		28	Ohio	360,300
25	New Hampshire	366,300		29	Iowa	356,200
44	New Jersey	317,600		30	Connecticut	355,200
45	New Mexico	315,800		31	Oregon	354,400
43	New York	318,700		32	Hawaii	353,600
27	North Carolina	361,500		33	Utah	352,400
3	North Dakota	476,100		34	Missouri	351,800
28	Ohio	360,300		35	Maryland	346,300
39	Oklahoma	333,100		36	Michigan	344,400
31	Oregon	354,400		37	South Carolina	343,900
46	Pennsylvania	301,500		38	Mississippi	333,800
42	Rhode Island	321,000		39	Oklahoma	333,100
37	South Carolina	343,900		40	Idaho	329,100
16	South Dakota	400,100		41	Illinois	325,900
17	Tennessee	399,000		42	Rhode Island	321,000
12	Texas	419,800		43	New York	318,700
33	Utah	352,400		44	New Jersey	317,600
50	Vermont	247,400		45	New Mexico	315,800
22	Virginia	373,200		46	Pennsylvania	301,500
15	Washington	402,000		47	Wyoming	278,700
26	West Virginia	362,000		48	Maine	278,400
10	Wisconsin	429,100		49	Montana	262,400
47	Wyoming	278,700		50	Vermont	247,400
					District of Columbia	325,300

Source: U.S. Department of Health and Human Services, Health Care Financing Administration
"Health Spending by State: New Estimates for Policy Making" (Health Affairs, Fall 1993) and unpublished data
By state of provider. Calculated using counts of active nonfederal office-based Doctors of Medicine and Doctors of Osteopathy.

Expenditures for Prescription Drugs in 1991

National Total = $36,377,000,000*

<table>
<tr><td colspan="4">ALPHA ORDER</td><td colspan="4">RANK ORDER</td></tr>
<tr><td>RANK</td><td>STATE</td><td>EXPENDITURES</td><td>% of USA</td><td>RANK</td><td>STATE</td><td>EXPENDITURES</td><td>% of USA</td></tr>
<tr><td>18</td><td>Alabama</td><td>$677,000,000</td><td>1.86%</td><td>1</td><td>California</td><td>$3,904,000,000</td><td>10.73%</td></tr>
<tr><td>49</td><td>Alaska</td><td>56,000,000</td><td>0.15%</td><td>2</td><td>New York</td><td>2,577,000,000</td><td>7.08%</td></tr>
<tr><td>25</td><td>Arizona</td><td>483,000,000</td><td>1.33%</td><td>3</td><td>Texas</td><td>2,382,000,000</td><td>6.55%</td></tr>
<tr><td>30</td><td>Arkansas</td><td>368,000,000</td><td>1.01%</td><td>4</td><td>Florida</td><td>1,956,000,000</td><td>5.38%</td></tr>
<tr><td>1</td><td>California</td><td>3,904,000,000</td><td>10.73%</td><td>5</td><td>Pennsylvania</td><td>1,876,000,000</td><td>5.16%</td></tr>
<tr><td>31</td><td>Colorado</td><td>364,000,000</td><td>1.00%</td><td>6</td><td>Illinois</td><td>1,711,000,000</td><td>4.70%</td></tr>
<tr><td>24</td><td>Connecticut</td><td>520,000,000</td><td>1.43%</td><td>7</td><td>Ohio</td><td>1,613,000,000</td><td>4.43%</td></tr>
<tr><td>44</td><td>Delaware</td><td>91,000,000</td><td>0.25%</td><td>8</td><td>Michigan</td><td>1,578,000,000</td><td>4.34%</td></tr>
<tr><td>4</td><td>Florida</td><td>1,956,000,000</td><td>5.38%</td><td>9</td><td>New Jersey</td><td>1,249,000,000</td><td>3.43%</td></tr>
<tr><td>12</td><td>Georgia</td><td>971,000,000</td><td>2.67%</td><td>10</td><td>Massachusetts</td><td>1,061,000,000</td><td>2.92%</td></tr>
<tr><td>41</td><td>Hawaii</td><td>137,000,000</td><td>0.38%</td><td>11</td><td>North Carolina</td><td>992,000,000</td><td>2.73%</td></tr>
<tr><td>43</td><td>Idaho</td><td>123,000,000</td><td>0.34%</td><td>12</td><td>Georgia</td><td>971,000,000</td><td>2.67%</td></tr>
<tr><td>6</td><td>Illinois</td><td>1,711,000,000</td><td>4.70%</td><td>13</td><td>Virginia</td><td>955,000,000</td><td>2.63%</td></tr>
<tr><td>15</td><td>Indiana</td><td>835,000,000</td><td>2.30%</td><td>14</td><td>Tennessee</td><td>844,000,000</td><td>2.32%</td></tr>
<tr><td>28</td><td>Iowa</td><td>404,000,000</td><td>1.11%</td><td>15</td><td>Indiana</td><td>835,000,000</td><td>2.30%</td></tr>
<tr><td>32</td><td>Kansas</td><td>358,000,000</td><td>0.98%</td><td>16</td><td>Maryland</td><td>829,000,000</td><td>2.28%</td></tr>
<tr><td>21</td><td>Kentucky</td><td>639,000,000</td><td>1.76%</td><td>17</td><td>Missouri</td><td>751,000,000</td><td>2.06%</td></tr>
<tr><td>20</td><td>Louisiana</td><td>658,000,000</td><td>1.81%</td><td>18</td><td>Alabama</td><td>677,000,000</td><td>1.86%</td></tr>
<tr><td>39</td><td>Maine</td><td>162,000,000</td><td>0.45%</td><td>19</td><td>Wisconsin</td><td>675,000,000</td><td>1.86%</td></tr>
<tr><td>16</td><td>Maryland</td><td>829,000,000</td><td>2.28%</td><td>20</td><td>Louisiana</td><td>658,000,000</td><td>1.81%</td></tr>
<tr><td>10</td><td>Massachusetts</td><td>1,061,000,000</td><td>2.92%</td><td>21</td><td>Kentucky</td><td>639,000,000</td><td>1.76%</td></tr>
<tr><td>8</td><td>Michigan</td><td>1,578,000,000</td><td>4.34%</td><td>22</td><td>Washington</td><td>568,000,000</td><td>1.56%</td></tr>
<tr><td>23</td><td>Minnesota</td><td>548,000,000</td><td>1.51%</td><td>23</td><td>Minnesota</td><td>548,000,000</td><td>1.51%</td></tr>
<tr><td>29</td><td>Mississippi</td><td>384,000,000</td><td>1.06%</td><td>24</td><td>Connecticut</td><td>520,000,000</td><td>1.43%</td></tr>
<tr><td>17</td><td>Missouri</td><td>751,000,000</td><td>2.06%</td><td>25</td><td>Arizona</td><td>483,000,000</td><td>1.33%</td></tr>
<tr><td>45</td><td>Montana</td><td>87,000,000</td><td>0.24%</td><td>26</td><td>South Carolina</td><td>479,000,000</td><td>1.32%</td></tr>
<tr><td>35</td><td>Nebraska</td><td>227,000,000</td><td>0.62%</td><td>27</td><td>Oklahoma</td><td>442,000,000</td><td>1.22%</td></tr>
<tr><td>42</td><td>Nevada</td><td>135,000,000</td><td>0.37%</td><td>28</td><td>Iowa</td><td>404,000,000</td><td>1.11%</td></tr>
<tr><td>40</td><td>New Hampshire</td><td>146,000,000</td><td>0.40%</td><td>29</td><td>Mississippi</td><td>384,000,000</td><td>1.06%</td></tr>
<tr><td>9</td><td>New Jersey</td><td>1,249,000,000</td><td>3.43%</td><td>30</td><td>Arkansas</td><td>368,000,000</td><td>1.01%</td></tr>
<tr><td>37</td><td>New Mexico</td><td>179,000,000</td><td>0.49%</td><td>31</td><td>Colorado</td><td>364,000,000</td><td>1.00%</td></tr>
<tr><td>2</td><td>New York</td><td>2,577,000,000</td><td>7.08%</td><td>32</td><td>Kansas</td><td>358,000,000</td><td>0.98%</td></tr>
<tr><td>11</td><td>North Carolina</td><td>992,000,000</td><td>2.73%</td><td>33</td><td>West Virginia</td><td>329,000,000</td><td>0.90%</td></tr>
<tr><td>46</td><td>North Dakota</td><td>84,000,000</td><td>0.23%</td><td>34</td><td>Oregon</td><td>297,000,000</td><td>0.82%</td></tr>
<tr><td>7</td><td>Ohio</td><td>1,613,000,000</td><td>4.43%</td><td>35</td><td>Nebraska</td><td>227,000,000</td><td>0.62%</td></tr>
<tr><td>27</td><td>Oklahoma</td><td>442,000,000</td><td>1.22%</td><td>36</td><td>Utah</td><td>207,000,000</td><td>0.57%</td></tr>
<tr><td>34</td><td>Oregon</td><td>297,000,000</td><td>0.82%</td><td>37</td><td>New Mexico</td><td>179,000,000</td><td>0.49%</td></tr>
<tr><td>5</td><td>Pennsylvania</td><td>1,876,000,000</td><td>5.16%</td><td>38</td><td>Rhode Island</td><td>166,000,000</td><td>0.46%</td></tr>
<tr><td>38</td><td>Rhode Island</td><td>166,000,000</td><td>0.46%</td><td>39</td><td>Maine</td><td>162,000,000</td><td>0.45%</td></tr>
<tr><td>26</td><td>South Carolina</td><td>479,000,000</td><td>1.32%</td><td>40</td><td>New Hampshire</td><td>146,000,000</td><td>0.40%</td></tr>
<tr><td>47</td><td>South Dakota</td><td>80,000,000</td><td>0.22%</td><td>41</td><td>Hawaii</td><td>137,000,000</td><td>0.38%</td></tr>
<tr><td>14</td><td>Tennessee</td><td>844,000,000</td><td>2.32%</td><td>42</td><td>Nevada</td><td>135,000,000</td><td>0.37%</td></tr>
<tr><td>3</td><td>Texas</td><td>2,382,000,000</td><td>6.55%</td><td>43</td><td>Idaho</td><td>123,000,000</td><td>0.34%</td></tr>
<tr><td>36</td><td>Utah</td><td>207,000,000</td><td>0.57%</td><td>44</td><td>Delaware</td><td>91,000,000</td><td>0.25%</td></tr>
<tr><td>48</td><td>Vermont</td><td>79,000,000</td><td>0.22%</td><td>45</td><td>Montana</td><td>87,000,000</td><td>0.24%</td></tr>
<tr><td>13</td><td>Virginia</td><td>955,000,000</td><td>2.63%</td><td>46</td><td>North Dakota</td><td>84,000,000</td><td>0.23%</td></tr>
<tr><td>22</td><td>Washington</td><td>568,000,000</td><td>1.56%</td><td>47</td><td>South Dakota</td><td>80,000,000</td><td>0.22%</td></tr>
<tr><td>33</td><td>West Virginia</td><td>329,000,000</td><td>0.90%</td><td>48</td><td>Vermont</td><td>79,000,000</td><td>0.22%</td></tr>
<tr><td>19</td><td>Wisconsin</td><td>675,000,000</td><td>1.86%</td><td>49</td><td>Alaska</td><td>56,000,000</td><td>0.15%</td></tr>
<tr><td>50</td><td>Wyoming</td><td>49,000,000</td><td>0.13%</td><td>50</td><td>Wyoming</td><td>49,000,000</td><td>0.13%</td></tr>
<tr><td></td><td></td><td></td><td></td><td></td><td>District of Columbia</td><td>93,000,000</td><td>0.26%</td></tr>
</table>

Source: U.S. Department of Health and Human Services, Health Care Financing Administration
"Health Spending by State: New Estimates for Policy Making" (Health Affairs, Fall 1993)
*Purchases in retail outlets. By state of outlet.

Percent Change in Expenditures for Prescription Drugs: 1990 to 1991

National Percent Change = 11.1% Increase*

ALPHA ORDER				RANK ORDER		
RANK	STATE	PERCENT CHANGE		RANK	STATE	PERCENT CHANGE
24	Alabama	11.0		1	Nevada	15.9
2	Alaska	13.2		2	Alaska	13.2
10	Arizona	12.0		3	Idaho	12.8
28	Arkansas	10.8		4	Washington	12.7
13	California	11.8		5	Oregon	12.4
8	Colorado	12.2		5	Utah	12.4
46	Connecticut	10.1		7	Florida	12.3
13	Delaware	11.8		8	Colorado	12.2
7	Florida	12.3		9	Hawaii	12.1
11	Georgia	11.9		10	Arizona	12.0
9	Hawaii	12.1		11	Georgia	11.9
3	Idaho	12.8		11	New Mexico	11.9
28	Illinois	10.8		13	California	11.8
24	Indiana	11.0		13	Delaware	11.8
34	Iowa	10.6		13	South Carolina	11.8
34	Kansas	10.6		13	Texas	11.8
34	Kentucky	10.6		17	Maryland	11.4
34	Louisiana	10.6		17	North Carolina	11.4
42	Maine	10.4		17	Virginia	11.4
17	Maryland	11.4		20	Tennessee	11.3
48	Massachusetts	9.7		21	Minnesota	11.1
34	Michigan	10.6		21	Wisconsin	11.1
21	Minnesota	11.1		21	Wyoming	11.1
34	Mississippi	10.6		24	Alabama	11.0
32	Missouri	10.7		24	Indiana	11.0
24	Montana	11.0		24	Montana	11.0
28	Nebraska	10.8		27	South Dakota	10.9
1	Nevada	15.9		28	Arkansas	10.8
49	New Hampshire	9.6		28	Illinois	10.8
43	New Jersey	10.3		28	Nebraska	10.8
11	New Mexico	11.9		28	Oklahoma	10.8
43	New York	10.3		32	Missouri	10.7
17	North Carolina	11.4		32	Ohio	10.7
50	North Dakota	9.4		34	Iowa	10.6
32	Ohio	10.7		34	Kansas	10.6
28	Oklahoma	10.8		34	Kentucky	10.6
5	Oregon	12.4		34	Louisiana	10.6
34	Pennsylvania	10.6		34	Michigan	10.6
47	Rhode Island	10.0		34	Mississippi	10.6
13	South Carolina	11.8		34	Pennsylvania	10.6
27	South Dakota	10.9		34	Vermont	10.6
20	Tennessee	11.3		42	Maine	10.4
13	Texas	11.8		43	New Jersey	10.3
5	Utah	12.4		43	New York	10.3
34	Vermont	10.6		43	West Virginia	10.3
17	Virginia	11.4		46	Connecticut	10.1
4	Washington	12.7		47	Rhode Island	10.0
43	West Virginia	10.3		48	Massachusetts	9.7
21	Wisconsin	11.1		49	New Hampshire	9.6
21	Wyoming	11.1		50	North Dakota	9.4
					District of Columbia	8.7

Source: U.S. Department of Health and Human Services, Health Care Financing Administration
"Health Spending by State: New Estimates for Policy Making" (Health Affairs, Fall 1993)
*Purchases in retail outlets. By state of outlet.

Average Annual Change in Expenditures for Prescription Drugs: 1980 to 1991

National Percent = 10.6% Average Annual Increase*

ALPHA ORDER

RANK	STATE	PERCENT
29	Alabama	10.1
10	Alaska	12.0
1	Arizona	13.3
48	Arkansas	8.3
23	California	10.5
30	Colorado	10.0
23	Connecticut	10.5
8	Delaware	12.4
6	Florida	12.5
14	Georgia	11.5
18	Hawaii	10.9
35	Idaho	9.8
21	Illinois	10.7
39	Indiana	9.6
45	Iowa	9.0
35	Kansas	9.8
30	Kentucky	10.0
45	Louisiana	9.0
16	Maine	11.0
4	Maryland	12.6
6	Massachusetts	12.5
23	Michigan	10.5
30	Minnesota	10.0
41	Mississippi	9.5
39	Missouri	9.6
35	Montana	9.8
34	Nebraska	9.9
4	Nevada	12.6
3	New Hampshire	12.8
15	New Jersey	11.4
10	New Mexico	12.0
16	New York	11.0
28	North Carolina	10.2
23	North Dakota	10.5
43	Ohio	9.3
47	Oklahoma	8.8
49	Oregon	8.2
21	Pennsylvania	10.7
13	Rhode Island	11.8
18	South Carolina	10.9
43	South Dakota	9.3
27	Tennessee	10.3
35	Texas	9.8
2	Utah	13.0
8	Vermont	12.4
10	Virginia	12.0
42	Washington	9.4
30	West Virginia	10.0
20	Wisconsin	10.8
50	Wyoming	7.2

RANK ORDER

RANK	STATE	PERCENT
1	Arizona	13.3
2	Utah	13.0
3	New Hampshire	12.8
4	Maryland	12.6
4	Nevada	12.6
6	Florida	12.5
6	Massachusetts	12.5
8	Delaware	12.4
8	Vermont	12.4
10	Alaska	12.0
10	New Mexico	12.0
10	Virginia	12.0
13	Rhode Island	11.8
14	Georgia	11.5
15	New Jersey	11.4
16	Maine	11.0
16	New York	11.0
18	Hawaii	10.9
18	South Carolina	10.9
20	Wisconsin	10.8
21	Illinois	10.7
21	Pennsylvania	10.7
23	California	10.5
23	Connecticut	10.5
23	Michigan	10.5
23	North Dakota	10.5
27	Tennessee	10.3
28	North Carolina	10.2
29	Alabama	10.1
30	Colorado	10.0
30	Kentucky	10.0
30	Minnesota	10.0
30	West Virginia	10.0
34	Nebraska	9.9
35	Idaho	9.8
35	Kansas	9.8
35	Montana	9.8
35	Texas	9.8
39	Indiana	9.6
39	Missouri	9.6
41	Mississippi	9.5
42	Washington	9.4
43	Ohio	9.3
43	South Dakota	9.3
45	Iowa	9.0
45	Louisiana	9.0
47	Oklahoma	8.8
48	Arkansas	8.3
49	Oregon	8.2
50	Wyoming	7.2

	District of Columbia	10.3

Source: U.S. Department of Health and Human Services, Health Care Financing Administration
"Health Spending by State: New Estimates for Policy Making" (Health Affairs, Fall 1993)
*Purchases in retail outlets. By state of outlet.

Per Capita Expenditures for Prescription Drugs in 1991

National Per Capita = $144*

Source: U.S. Department of Health and Human Services, Health Care Financing Administration
"Health Spending by State: New Estimates for Policy Making" (Health Affairs, Fall 1993)
*Purchases in retail outlets. By state of outlet.

Percent Change in Per Capita Expenditures for Prescription Drugs: 1990 to 1991

National Percent Change = 9.9% Increase*

ALPHA ORDER				RANK ORDER		
RANK	STATE	PERCENT CHANGE		RANK	STATE	PERCENT CHANGE
26	Alabama	9.9		1	Oregon	10.9
50	Alaska	9.0		2	South Carolina	10.7
9	Arizona	10.3		3	Missouri	10.6
26	Arkansas	9.9		4	Georgia	10.5
9	California	10.3		4	Nevada	10.5
14	Colorado	10.2		4	New Mexico	10.5
35	Connecticut	9.7		7	Indiana	10.4
32	Delaware	9.8		7	Utah	10.4
35	Florida	9.7		9	Arizona	10.3
4	Georgia	10.5		9	California	10.3
21	Hawaii	10.0		9	Maryland	10.3
14	Idaho	10.2		9	New Jersey	10.3
44	Illinois	9.6		9	Wyoming	10.3
7	Indiana	10.4		14	Colorado	10.2
26	Iowa	9.9		14	Idaho	10.2
26	Kansas	9.9		14	Montana	10.2
44	Kentucky	9.6		14	Vermont	10.2
26	Louisiana	9.9		18	Maine	10.1
18	Maine	10.1		18	Nebraska	10.1
9	Maryland	10.3		18	Virginia	10.1
26	Massachusetts	9.9		21	Hawaii	10.0
32	Michigan	9.8		21	New Hampshire	10.0
35	Minnesota	9.7		21	New York	10.0
44	Mississippi	9.6		21	North Dakota	10.0
3	Missouri	10.6		21	Rhode Island	10.0
14	Montana	10.2		26	Alabama	9.9
18	Nebraska	10.1		26	Arkansas	9.9
4	Nevada	10.5		26	Iowa	9.9
21	New Hampshire	10.0		26	Kansas	9.9
9	New Jersey	10.3		26	Louisiana	9.9
4	New Mexico	10.5		26	Massachusetts	9.9
21	New York	10.0		32	Delaware	9.8
35	North Carolina	9.7		32	Michigan	9.8
21	North Dakota	10.0		32	Pennsylvania	9.8
35	Ohio	9.7		35	Connecticut	9.7
49	Oklahoma	9.4		35	Florida	9.7
1	Oregon	10.9		35	Minnesota	9.7
32	Pennsylvania	9.8		35	North Carolina	9.7
21	Rhode Island	10.0		35	Ohio	9.7
2	South Carolina	10.7		35	South Dakota	9.7
35	South Dakota	9.7		35	Tennessee	9.7
35	Tennessee	9.7		35	Washington	9.7
44	Texas	9.6		35	Wisconsin	9.7
7	Utah	10.4		44	Illinois	9.6
14	Vermont	10.2		44	Kentucky	9.6
18	Virginia	10.1		44	Mississippi	9.6
35	Washington	9.7		44	Texas	9.6
44	West Virginia	9.6		44	West Virginia	9.6
35	Wisconsin	9.7		49	Oklahoma	9.4
9	Wyoming	10.3		50	Alaska	9.0
					District of Columbia	9.9

Source: U.S. Department of Health and Human Services, Health Care Financing Administration
"Health Spending by State: New Estimates for Policy Making" (Health Affairs, Fall 1993) and unpublished data
*Purchases in retail outlets. By state of outlet.

Average Annual Percent Change in Per Capita Expenditures
For Prescription Drugs: 1980 to 1991
National Percent = 9.5% Average Annual Increase*

ALPHA ORDER

RANK ORDER

RANK	STATE	PERCENT		RANK	STATE	PERCENT
23	Alabama	9.7		1	Massachusetts	12.0
41	Alaska	8.7		2	Vermont	11.4
18	Arizona	10.1		3	Maryland	11.3
47	Arkansas	7.9		3	Rhode Island	11.3
43	California	8.3		5	Utah	11.1
42	Colorado	8.5		6	New Hampshire	11.0
20	Connecticut	9.9		7	Delaware	10.9
7	Delaware	10.9		8	New Jersey	10.8
27	Florida	9.5		8	North Dakota	10.8
26	Georgia	9.6		8	West Virginia	10.8
29	Hawaii	9.4		11	New York	10.7
37	Idaho	9.0		12	Illinois	10.6
12	Illinois	10.6		12	Pennsylvania	10.6
30	Indiana	9.3		14	Virginia	10.5
30	Iowa	9.3		15	Michigan	10.4
30	Kansas	9.3		15	New Mexico	10.4
20	Kentucky	9.9		15	Wisconsin	10.4
37	Louisiana	9.0		18	Arizona	10.1
19	Maine	10.0		19	Maine	10.0
3	Maryland	11.3		20	Connecticut	9.9
1	Massachusetts	12.0		20	Kentucky	9.9
15	Michigan	10.4		22	Nebraska	9.8
33	Minnesota	9.2		23	Alabama	9.7
33	Mississippi	9.2		23	Montana	9.7
36	Missouri	9.1		23	South Carolina	9.7
23	Montana	9.7		26	Georgia	9.6
22	Nebraska	9.8		27	Florida	9.5
45	Nevada	8.0		27	Tennessee	9.5
6	New Hampshire	11.0		29	Hawaii	9.4
8	New Jersey	10.8		30	Indiana	9.3
15	New Mexico	10.4		30	Iowa	9.3
11	New York	10.7		30	Kansas	9.3
40	North Carolina	8.8		33	Minnesota	9.2
8	North Dakota	10.8		33	Mississippi	9.2
33	Ohio	9.2		33	Ohio	9.2
43	Oklahoma	8.3		36	Missouri	9.1
50	Oregon	7.3		37	Idaho	9.0
12	Pennsylvania	10.6		37	Louisiana	9.0
3	Rhode Island	11.3		37	South Dakota	9.0
23	South Carolina	9.7		40	North Carolina	8.8
37	South Dakota	9.0		41	Alaska	8.7
27	Tennessee	9.5		42	Colorado	8.5
45	Texas	8.0		43	California	8.3
5	Utah	11.1		43	Oklahoma	8.3
2	Vermont	11.4		45	Nevada	8.0
14	Virginia	10.5		45	Texas	8.0
48	Washington	7.6		47	Arkansas	7.9
8	West Virginia	10.8		48	Washington	7.6
15	Wisconsin	10.4		48	Wyoming	7.6
48	Wyoming	7.6		50	Oregon	7.3

District of Columbia 10.9

Source: Morgan Quitno Press using data from US Dept of Health & Human Services, Health Care Financing Administration "Health Spending by State: New Estimates for Policy Making" (Health Affairs, Fall 1993) and unpublished data
Purchases in retail outlets. By state of outlet.

Expenditures for Hospital Care in 1991

National Total = $286,053,000,000*

ALPHA ORDER

RANK	STATE	EXPENDITURES	% of USA
22	Alabama	$4,521,000,000	1.58%
48	Alaska	659,000,000	0.23%
25	Arizona	3,615,000,000	1.26%
33	Arkansas	2,359,000,000	0.82%
1	California	31,128,000,000	10.88%
26	Colorado	3,614,000,000	1.26%
23	Connecticut	4,089,000,000	1.43%
43	Delaware	800,000,000	0.28%
5	Florida	15,210,000,000	5.32%
11	Georgia	7,603,000,000	2.66%
38	Hawaii	1,287,000,000	0.45%
47	Idaho	762,000,000	0.27%
6	Illinois	13,792,000,000	4.82%
16	Indiana	6,024,000,000	2.11%
29	Iowa	2,933,000,000	1.03%
31	Kansas	2,545,000,000	0.89%
24	Kentucky	3,908,000,000	1.37%
17	Louisiana	5,277,000,000	1.84%
39	Maine	1,257,000,000	0.44%
18	Maryland	5,210,000,000	1.82%
9	Massachusetts	9,097,000,000	3.18%
8	Michigan	10,663,000,000	3.73%
20	Minnesota	4,607,000,000	1.61%
32	Mississippi	2,425,000,000	0.85%
13	Missouri	6,660,000,000	2.33%
46	Montana	763,000,000	0.27%
35	Nebraska	1,789,000,000	0.63%
41	Nevada	1,195,000,000	0.42%
42	New Hampshire	1,129,000,000	0.39%
10	New Jersey	8,829,000,000	3.09%
36	New Mexico	1,570,000,000	0.55%
2	New York	25,345,000,000	8.86%
12	North Carolina	6,795,000,000	2.38%
45	North Dakota	796,000,000	0.28%
7	Ohio	12,628,000,000	4.41%
28	Oklahoma	3,016,000,000	1.05%
30	Oregon	2,562,000,000	0.90%
4	Pennsylvania	16,622,000,000	5.81%
40	Rhode Island	1,215,000,000	0.42%
26	South Carolina	3,614,000,000	1.26%
44	South Dakota	799,000,000	0.28%
15	Tennessee	6,239,000,000	2.18%
3	Texas	18,086,000,000	6.32%
37	Utah	1,510,000,000	0.53%
49	Vermont	502,000,000	0.18%
14	Virginia	6,407,000,000	2.24%
21	Washington	4,581,000,000	1.60%
34	West Virginia	2,000,000,000	0.70%
19	Wisconsin	4,981,000,000	1.74%
50	Wyoming	394,000,000	0.14%

RANK ORDER

RANK	STATE	EXPENDITURES	% of USA
1	California	$31,128,000,000	10.88%
2	New York	25,345,000,000	8.86%
3	Texas	18,086,000,000	6.32%
4	Pennsylvania	16,622,000,000	5.81%
5	Florida	15,210,000,000	5.32%
6	Illinois	13,792,000,000	4.82%
7	Ohio	12,628,000,000	4.41%
8	Michigan	10,663,000,000	3.73%
9	Massachusetts	9,097,000,000	3.18%
10	New Jersey	8,829,000,000	3.09%
11	Georgia	7,603,000,000	2.66%
12	North Carolina	6,795,000,000	2.38%
13	Missouri	6,660,000,000	2.33%
14	Virginia	6,407,000,000	2.24%
15	Tennessee	6,239,000,000	2.18%
16	Indiana	6,024,000,000	2.11%
17	Louisiana	5,277,000,000	1.84%
18	Maryland	5,210,000,000	1.82%
19	Wisconsin	4,981,000,000	1.74%
20	Minnesota	4,607,000,000	1.61%
21	Washington	4,581,000,000	1.60%
22	Alabama	4,521,000,000	1.58%
23	Connecticut	4,089,000,000	1.43%
24	Kentucky	3,908,000,000	1.37%
25	Arizona	3,615,000,000	1.26%
26	Colorado	3,614,000,000	1.26%
26	South Carolina	3,614,000,000	1.26%
28	Oklahoma	3,016,000,000	1.05%
29	Iowa	2,933,000,000	1.03%
30	Oregon	2,562,000,000	0.90%
31	Kansas	2,545,000,000	0.89%
32	Mississippi	2,425,000,000	0.85%
33	Arkansas	2,359,000,000	0.82%
34	West Virginia	2,000,000,000	0.70%
35	Nebraska	1,789,000,000	0.63%
36	New Mexico	1,570,000,000	0.55%
37	Utah	1,510,000,000	0.53%
38	Hawaii	1,287,000,000	0.45%
39	Maine	1,257,000,000	0.44%
40	Rhode Island	1,215,000,000	0.42%
41	Nevada	1,195,000,000	0.42%
42	New Hampshire	1,129,000,000	0.39%
43	Delaware	800,000,000	0.28%
44	South Dakota	799,000,000	0.28%
45	North Dakota	796,000,000	0.28%
46	Montana	763,000,000	0.27%
47	Idaho	762,000,000	0.27%
48	Alaska	659,000,000	0.23%
49	Vermont	502,000,000	0.18%
50	Wyoming	394,000,000	0.14%
	District of Columbia	2,641,000,000	0.92%

Source: U.S. Department of Health and Human Services, Health Care Financing Administration
"Health Spending by State: New Estimates for Policy Making" (Health Affairs, Fall 1993)
*By state of provider.

Percent Change in Expenditures for Hospital Care: 1990 to 1991

National Percent Change = 11.9% Increase*

ALPHA ORDER			RANK ORDER		
RANK	STATE	PERCENT CHANGE	RANK	STATE	PERCENT CHANGE
29	Alabama	11.8	1	South Carolina	15.7
5	Alaska	14.1	2	Indiana	15.3
30	Arizona	11.6	3	Washington	14.8
33	Arkansas	11.3	4	Idaho	14.6
43	California	10.7	5	Alaska	14.1
14	Colorado	13.1	6	North Carolina	14.0
38	Connecticut	11.0	7	South Dakota	13.8
20	Delaware	12.3	8	Nevada	13.7
20	Florida	12.3	9	Louisiana	13.6
15	Georgia	12.9	9	New Mexico	13.6
40	Hawaii	10.9	11	Kentucky	13.4
4	Idaho	14.6	11	Utah	13.4
45	Illinois	10.6	13	Wisconsin	13.3
2	Indiana	15.3	14	Colorado	13.1
42	Iowa	10.8	15	Georgia	12.9
32	Kansas	11.5	15	West Virginia	12.9
11	Kentucky	13.4	17	Texas	12.8
9	Louisiana	13.6	18	Tennessee	12.4
28	Maine	11.9	18	Virginia	12.4
36	Maryland	11.1	20	Delaware	12.3
34	Massachusetts	11.2	20	Florida	12.3
30	Michigan	11.6	22	Nebraska	12.2
26	Minnesota	12.0	22	New Jersey	12.2
46	Mississippi	10.4	22	Vermont	12.2
40	Missouri	10.9	25	Oklahoma	12.1
26	Montana	12.0	26	Minnesota	12.0
22	Nebraska	12.2	26	Montana	12.0
8	Nevada	13.7	28	Maine	11.9
50	New Hampshire	6.5	29	Alabama	11.8
22	New Jersey	12.2	30	Arizona	11.6
9	New Mexico	13.6	30	Michigan	11.6
34	New York	11.2	32	Kansas	11.5
6	North Carolina	14.0	33	Arkansas	11.3
48	North Dakota	10.2	34	Massachusetts	11.2
49	Ohio	9.9	34	New York	11.2
25	Oklahoma	12.1	36	Maryland	11.1
38	Oregon	11.0	36	Pennsylvania	11.1
36	Pennsylvania	11.1	38	Connecticut	11.0
43	Rhode Island	10.7	38	Oregon	11.0
1	South Carolina	15.7	40	Hawaii	10.9
7	South Dakota	13.8	40	Missouri	10.9
18	Tennessee	12.4	42	Iowa	10.8
17	Texas	12.8	43	California	10.7
11	Utah	13.4	43	Rhode Island	10.7
22	Vermont	12.2	45	Illinois	10.6
18	Virginia	12.4	46	Mississippi	10.4
3	Washington	14.8	47	Wyoming	10.3
15	West Virginia	12.9	48	North Dakota	10.2
13	Wisconsin	13.3	49	Ohio	9.9
47	Wyoming	10.3	50	New Hampshire	6.5
				District of Columbia	13.7

Source: U.S. Department of Health and Human Services, Health Care Financing Administration
"Health Spending by State: New Estimates for Policy Making" (Health Affairs, Fall 1993) and unpublished data
*By state of provider.

Average Annual Growth in Expenditures for Hospital Care: 1980 to 1991

National Percent = 9.9% Average Annual Growth*

ALPHA ORDER			RANK ORDER		
RANK	STATE	PERCENT	RANK	STATE	PERCENT
27	Alabama	10.0	1	South Carolina	12.7
10	Alaska	11.4	2	New Hampshire	12.4
9	Arizona	11.5	3	Hawaii	12.3
14	Arkansas	11.1	4	Georgia	12.2
33	California	9.4	5	New Mexico	12.1
22	Colorado	10.4	6	Florida	12.0
23	Connecticut	10.3	6	North Carolina	12.0
17	Delaware	10.8	8	Utah	11.6
6	Florida	12.0	9	Arizona	11.5
4	Georgia	12.2	10	Alaska	11.4
3	Hawaii	12.3	10	Texas	11.4
16	Idaho	11.0	10	Washington	11.4
50	Illinois	7.5	13	New Jersey	11.2
28	Indiana	9.9	14	Arkansas	11.1
45	Iowa	8.7	14	Kentucky	11.1
49	Kansas	8.1	16	Idaho	11.0
14	Kentucky	11.1	17	Delaware	10.8
21	Louisiana	10.6	17	Nevada	10.8
32	Maine	9.6	17	Tennessee	10.8
41	Maryland	8.9	17	Virginia	10.8
45	Massachusetts	8.7	21	Louisiana	10.6
48	Michigan	8.2	22	Colorado	10.4
35	Minnesota	9.3	23	Connecticut	10.3
28	Mississippi	9.9	23	South Dakota	10.3
37	Missouri	9.2	25	Vermont	10.2
26	Montana	10.1	26	Montana	10.1
37	Nebraska	9.2	27	Alabama	10.0
17	Nevada	10.8	28	Indiana	9.9
2	New Hampshire	12.4	28	Mississippi	9.9
13	New Jersey	11.2	30	Oregon	9.7
5	New Mexico	12.1	30	Pennsylvania	9.7
35	New York	9.3	32	Maine	9.6
6	North Carolina	12.0	33	California	9.4
43	North Dakota	8.8	33	Wyoming	9.4
37	Ohio	9.2	35	Minnesota	9.3
40	Oklahoma	9.0	35	New York	9.3
30	Oregon	9.7	37	Missouri	9.2
30	Pennsylvania	9.7	37	Nebraska	9.2
43	Rhode Island	8.8	37	Ohio	9.2
1	South Carolina	12.7	40	Oklahoma	9.0
23	South Dakota	10.3	41	Maryland	8.9
17	Tennessee	10.8	41	Wisconsin	8.9
10	Texas	11.4	43	North Dakota	8.8
8	Utah	11.6	43	Rhode Island	8.8
25	Vermont	10.2	45	Iowa	8.7
17	Virginia	10.8	45	Massachusetts	8.7
10	Washington	11.4	47	West Virginia	8.4
47	West Virginia	8.4	48	Michigan	8.2
41	Wisconsin	8.9	49	Kansas	8.1
33	Wyoming	9.4	50	Illinois	7.5
				District of Columbia	9.4

Source: U.S. Department of Health and Human Services, Health Care Financing Administration
"Health Spending by State: New Estimates for Policy Making" (Health Affairs, Fall 1993)
*By state of provider.

Per Capita Expenditures for Hospital Care in 1991

National Per Capita = $1,134*

ALPHA ORDER

RANK	STATE	PER CAPITA
22	Alabama	$1,105
12	Alaska	1,155
40	Arizona	964
39	Arkansas	994
30	California	1,025
25	Colorado	1,070
7	Connecticut	1,242
11	Delaware	1,177
15	Florida	1,146
14	Georgia	1,148
19	Hawaii	1,135
50	Idaho	733
10	Illinois	1,195
23	Indiana	1,074
27	Iowa	1,049
32	Kansas	1,020
26	Kentucky	1,052
8	Louisiana	1,241
34	Maine	1,018
24	Maryland	1,072
1	Massachusetts	1,517
16	Michigan	1,138
29	Minnesota	1,039
43	Mississippi	936
4	Missouri	1,291
42	Montana	944
20	Nebraska	1,123
44	Nevada	930
31	New Hampshire	1,022
16	New Jersey	1,138
36	New Mexico	1,014
2	New York	1,404
37	North Carolina	1,009
6	North Dakota	1,255
13	Ohio	1,154
41	Oklahoma	950
47	Oregon	877
3	Pennsylvania	1,390
9	Rhode Island	1,210
35	South Carolina	1,015
18	South Dakota	1,136
5	Tennessee	1,260
28	Texas	1,042
49	Utah	853
46	Vermont	886
33	Virginia	1,019
45	Washington	913
21	West Virginia	1,111
38	Wisconsin	1,005
48	Wyoming	857

RANK ORDER

RANK	STATE	PER CAPITA
1	Massachusetts	$1,517
2	New York	1,404
3	Pennsylvania	1,390
4	Missouri	1,291
5	Tennessee	1,260
6	North Dakota	1,255
7	Connecticut	1,242
8	Louisiana	1,241
9	Rhode Island	1,210
10	Illinois	1,195
11	Delaware	1,177
12	Alaska	1,155
13	Ohio	1,154
14	Georgia	1,148
15	Florida	1,146
16	Michigan	1,138
16	New Jersey	1,138
18	South Dakota	1,136
19	Hawaii	1,135
20	Nebraska	1,123
21	West Virginia	1,111
22	Alabama	1,105
23	Indiana	1,074
24	Maryland	1,072
25	Colorado	1,070
26	Kentucky	1,052
27	Iowa	1,049
28	Texas	1,042
29	Minnesota	1,039
30	California	1,025
31	New Hampshire	1,022
32	Kansas	1,020
33	Virginia	1,019
34	Maine	1,018
35	South Carolina	1,015
36	New Mexico	1,014
37	North Carolina	1,009
38	Wisconsin	1,005
39	Arkansas	994
40	Arizona	964
41	Oklahoma	950
42	Montana	944
43	Mississippi	936
44	Nevada	930
45	Washington	913
46	Vermont	886
47	Oregon	877
48	Wyoming	857
49	Utah	853
50	Idaho	733
	District of Columbia**	4,415

Source: U.S. Department of Health and Human Services, Health Care Financing Administration
"Health Spending by State: New Estimates for Policy Making" (Health Affairs, Fall 1993) and unpublished data
*By state of provider.
**The District of Columbia's per capita is greatly affected by residents of Maryland and Virginia receiving services.

Percent Change in Per Capita Expenditures for Hospital Care: 1990 to 1991

National Percent Change = 10.6% Increase*

ALPHA ORDER		
RANK	STATE	PERCENT CHANGE
31	Alabama	10.7
24	Alaska	10.9
43	Arizona	9.6
33	Arkansas	10.6
46	California	8.9
24	Colorado	10.9
24	Connecticut	10.9
35	Delaware	10.5
39	Florida	10.0
19	Georgia	11.0
47	Hawaii	8.8
10	Idaho	11.8
40	Illinois	9.7
1	Indiana	14.2
37	Iowa	10.2
24	Kansas	10.9
5	Kentucky	12.7
3	Louisiana	12.9
15	Maine	11.4
40	Maryland	9.7
13	Massachusetts	11.6
24	Michigan	10.9
24	Minnesota	10.9
40	Mississippi	9.7
37	Missouri	10.2
19	Montana	11.0
16	Nebraska	11.3
49	Nevada	7.9
50	New Hampshire	6.9
10	New Jersey	11.8
12	New Mexico	11.7
24	New York	10.9
6	North Carolina	12.5
31	North Dakota	10.7
44	Ohio	9.2
17	Oklahoma	11.2
48	Oregon	8.6
35	Pennsylvania	10.5
33	Rhode Island	10.6
2	South Carolina	13.8
4	South Dakota	12.8
18	Tennessee	11.1
19	Texas	11.0
19	Utah	11.0
13	Vermont	11.6
19	Virginia	11.0
9	Washington	12.0
6	West Virginia	12.5
8	Wisconsin	12.2
44	Wyoming	9.2

RANK ORDER		
RANK	STATE	PERCENT CHANGE
1	Indiana	14.2
2	South Carolina	13.8
3	Louisiana	12.9
4	South Dakota	12.8
5	Kentucky	12.7
6	North Carolina	12.5
6	West Virginia	12.5
8	Wisconsin	12.2
9	Washington	12.0
10	Idaho	11.8
10	New Jersey	11.8
12	New Mexico	11.7
13	Massachusetts	11.6
13	Vermont	11.6
15	Maine	11.4
16	Nebraska	11.3
17	Oklahoma	11.2
18	Tennessee	11.1
19	Georgia	11.0
19	Montana	11.0
19	Texas	11.0
19	Utah	11.0
19	Virginia	11.0
24	Alaska	10.9
24	Colorado	10.9
24	Connecticut	10.9
24	Kansas	10.9
24	Michigan	10.9
24	Minnesota	10.9
24	New York	10.9
31	Alabama	10.7
31	North Dakota	10.7
33	Arkansas	10.6
33	Rhode Island	10.6
35	Delaware	10.5
35	Pennsylvania	10.5
37	Iowa	10.2
37	Missouri	10.2
39	Florida	10.0
40	Illinois	9.7
40	Maryland	9.7
40	Mississippi	9.7
43	Arizona	9.6
44	Ohio	9.2
44	Wyoming	9.2
46	California	8.9
47	Hawaii	8.8
48	Oregon	8.6
49	Nevada	7.9
50	New Hampshire	6.9
	District of Columbia	15.0

Source: U.S. Department of Health and Human Services, Health Care Financing Administration
"Health Spending by State: New Estimates for Policy Making" (Health Affairs, Fall 1993) and unpublished data
*By state of provider.

Average Annual Percent Change in Per Capita Expenditures
For Hospital Care: 1980 to 1991
National Percent = 8.9% Average Annual Increase*

ALPHA ORDER

RANK ORDER

RANK	STATE	PERCENT	RANK	STATE	PERCENT
20	Alabama	9.6	1	South Carolina	11.4
44	Alaska	8.1	2	Kentucky	11.1
39	Arizona	8.5	3	Arkansas	10.8
3	Arkansas	10.8	3	Hawaii	10.8
49	California	7.1	5	Louisiana	10.7
33	Colorado	9.0	5	New Jersey	10.7
15	Connecticut	9.8	5	North Carolina	10.7
24	Delaware	9.5	8	New Hampshire	10.6
31	Florida	9.1	9	New Mexico	10.5
10	Georgia	10.3	10	Georgia	10.3
3	Hawaii	10.8	11	South Dakota	10.2
12	Idaho	10.1	12	Idaho	10.1
48	Illinois	7.5	12	Tennessee	10.1
15	Indiana	9.8	14	Montana	10.0
28	Iowa	9.2	15	Connecticut	9.8
46	Kansas	7.7	15	Indiana	9.8
2	Kentucky	11.1	15	Utah	9.8
5	Louisiana	10.7	15	Wyoming	9.8
37	Maine	8.7	19	Pennsylvania	9.7
47	Maryland	7.6	20	Alabama	9.6
42	Massachusetts	8.3	20	Mississippi	9.6
44	Michigan	8.1	20	Texas	9.6
39	Minnesota	8.5	20	Washington	9.6
20	Mississippi	9.6	24	Delaware	9.5
35	Missouri	8.8	25	Vermont	9.3
14	Montana	10.0	25	Virginia	9.3
28	Nebraska	9.2	25	West Virginia	9.3
50	Nevada	6.4	28	Iowa	9.2
8	New Hampshire	10.6	28	Nebraska	9.2
5	New Jersey	10.7	28	North Dakota	9.2
9	New Mexico	10.5	31	Florida	9.1
33	New York	9.0	31	Ohio	9.1
5	North Carolina	10.7	33	Colorado	9.0
28	North Dakota	9.2	33	New York	9.0
31	Ohio	9.1	35	Missouri	8.8
37	Oklahoma	8.7	35	Oregon	8.8
35	Oregon	8.8	37	Maine	8.7
19	Pennsylvania	9.7	37	Oklahoma	8.7
42	Rhode Island	8.3	39	Arizona	8.5
1	South Carolina	11.4	39	Minnesota	8.5
11	South Dakota	10.2	39	Wisconsin	8.5
12	Tennessee	10.1	42	Massachusetts	8.3
20	Texas	9.6	42	Rhode Island	8.3
15	Utah	9.8	44	Alaska	8.1
25	Vermont	9.3	44	Michigan	8.1
25	Virginia	9.3	46	Kansas	7.7
20	Washington	9.6	47	Maryland	7.6
25	West Virginia	9.3	48	Illinois	7.5
39	Wisconsin	8.5	49	California	7.1
15	Wyoming	9.8	50	Nevada	6.4

District of Columbia 10.1

Source: Morgan Quitno Press using data from US Dept of Health & Human Services, Health Care Financing Administration
"Health Spending by State: New Estimates for Policy Making" (Health Affairs, Fall 1993) and unpublished data
*By state of provider.

Uncompensated Care in Community Hospitals
As a Percent of Total Expenditures in 1991
National Percent = 5.9% of Expenditures Are for Uncompensated Care

ALPHA ORDER

RANK	STATE	PERCENT
6	Alabama	8.8
29	Alaska	5.1
19	Arizona	6.1
8	Arkansas	7.9
27	California	5.5
25	Colorado	5.6
31	Connecticut	5.0
3	Delaware	9.3
9	Florida	7.7
2	Georgia	9.8
42	Hawaii	3.7
37	Idaho	4.1
21	Illinois	6.0
25	Indiana	5.6
37	Iowa	4.1
39	Kansas	4.0
29	Kentucky	5.1
34	Louisiana	4.3
31	Maine	5.0
15	Maryland	6.9
22	Massachusetts	5.8
44	Michigan	3.1
47	Minnesota	2.8
4	Mississippi	9.2
22	Missouri	5.8
41	Montana	3.8
49	Nebraska	2.6
12	Nevada	7.2
22	New Hampshire	5.8
5	New Jersey	8.9
7	New Mexico	8.2
28	New York	5.4
15	North Carolina	6.9
50	North Dakota	2.2
33	Ohio	4.6
11	Oklahoma	7.3
18	Oregon	6.2
45	Pennsylvania	3.0
43	Rhode Island	3.4
10	South Carolina	7.6
46	South Dakota	2.9
19	Tennessee	6.1
1	Texas	10.8
34	Utah	4.3
34	Vermont	4.3
12	Virginia	7.2
40	Washington	3.9
12	West Virginia	7.2
47	Wisconsin	2.8
17	Wyoming	6.4

RANK ORDER

RANK	STATE	PERCENT
1	Texas	10.8
2	Georgia	9.8
3	Delaware	9.3
4	Mississippi	9.2
5	New Jersey	8.9
6	Alabama	8.8
7	New Mexico	8.2
8	Arkansas	7.9
9	Florida	7.7
10	South Carolina	7.6
11	Oklahoma	7.3
12	Nevada	7.2
12	Virginia	7.2
12	West Virginia	7.2
15	Maryland	6.9
15	North Carolina	6.9
17	Wyoming	6.4
18	Oregon	6.2
19	Arizona	6.1
19	Tennessee	6.1
21	Illinois	6.0
22	Massachusetts	5.8
22	Missouri	5.8
22	New Hampshire	5.8
25	Colorado	5.6
25	Indiana	5.6
27	California	5.5
28	New York	5.4
29	Alaska	5.1
29	Kentucky	5.1
31	Connecticut	5.0
31	Maine	5.0
33	Ohio	4.6
34	Louisiana	4.3
34	Utah	4.3
34	Vermont	4.3
37	Idaho	4.1
37	Iowa	4.1
39	Kansas	4.0
40	Washington	3.9
41	Montana	3.8
42	Hawaii	3.7
43	Rhode Island	3.4
44	Michigan	3.1
45	Pennsylvania	3.0
46	South Dakota	2.9
47	Minnesota	2.8
47	Wisconsin	2.8
49	Nebraska	2.6
50	North Dakota	2.2

| District of Columbia | | 12.2 |

Source: Health Insurance Association of America
"Source Book of Health Insurance Data 1993" (based on data from the American Hospital Association)

Medicaid Expenditures in 1993

National Total = $101,708,889,399*

ALPHA ORDER				RANK ORDER			
RANK	STATE	EXPENDITURES	% of USA	RANK	STATE	EXPENDITURES	% of USA
25	Alabama	$1,191,818,404	1.17%	1	New York	$17,557,088,944	17.26%
48	Alaska	217,399,377	0.21%	2	California	9,649,517,851	9.49%
49	Arizona	211,910,126	0.21%	3	Texas	5,574,649,490	5.48%
28	Arkansas	997,814,499	0.98%	4	Ohio	4,666,662,717	4.59%
2	California	9,649,517,851	9.49%	5	Illinois	4,625,248,849	4.55%
29	Colorado	911,335,406	0.90%	6	Florida	4,131,305,669	4.06%
17	Connecticut	1,825,047,783	1.79%	7	Pennsylvania	3,886,201,196	3.82%
46	Delaware	251,564,500	0.25%	8	New Jersey	3,485,064,908	3.43%
6	Florida	4,131,305,669	4.06%	9	Michigan	3,077,140,677	3.03%
13	Georgia	2,440,618,176	2.40%	10	Louisiana	2,873,044,183	2.82%
42	Hawaii	292,508,880	0.29%	11	Massachusetts	2,725,602,358	2.68%
41	Idaho	300,629,716	0.30%	12	North Carolina	2,451,957,053	2.41%
5	Illinois	4,625,248,849	4.55%	13	Georgia	2,440,618,176	2.40%
14	Indiana	2,353,934,283	2.31%	14	Indiana	2,353,934,283	2.31%
30	Iowa	895,794,880	0.88%	15	Tennessee	1,977,468,671	1.94%
35	Kansas	701,670,756	0.69%	16	Minnesota	1,929,619,868	1.90%
20	Kentucky	1,706,895,310	1.68%	17	Connecticut	1,825,047,783	1.79%
10	Louisiana	2,873,044,183	2.82%	18	Wisconsin	1,786,328,158	1.76%
33	Maine	712,571,930	0.70%	19	Maryland	1,720,670,090	1.69%
19	Maryland	1,720,670,090	1.69%	20	Kentucky	1,706,895,310	1.68%
11	Massachusetts	2,725,602,358	2.68%	21	Virginia	1,622,885,677	1.60%
9	Michigan	3,077,140,677	3.03%	22	Missouri	1,548,325,871	1.52%
16	Minnesota	1,929,619,868	1.90%	23	Washington	1,537,056,515	1.51%
31	Mississippi	895,591,469	0.88%	24	South Carolina	1,249,311,570	1.23%
22	Missouri	1,548,325,871	1.52%	25	Alabama	1,191,818,404	1.17%
43	Montana	287,428,709	0.28%	26	West Virginia	1,056,113,210	1.04%
36	Nebraska	552,803,728	0.54%	27	Oklahoma	1,043,449,614	1.03%
40	Nevada	300,920,807	0.30%	28	Arkansas	997,814,499	0.98%
39	New Hampshire	380,342,519	0.37%	29	Colorado	911,335,406	0.90%
8	New Jersey	3,485,064,908	3.43%	30	Iowa	895,794,880	0.88%
37	New Mexico	542,592,891	0.53%	31	Mississippi	895,591,469	0.88%
1	New York	17,557,088,944	17.26%	32	Oregon	831,015,325	0.82%
12	North Carolina	2,451,957,053	2.41%	33	Maine	712,571,930	0.70%
44	North Dakota	272,713,407	0.27%	34	Rhode Island	709,789,379	0.70%
4	Ohio	4,666,662,717	4.59%	35	Kansas	701,670,756	0.69%
27	Oklahoma	1,043,449,614	1.03%	36	Nebraska	552,803,728	0.54%
32	Oregon	831,015,325	0.82%	37	New Mexico	542,592,891	0.53%
7	Pennsylvania	3,886,201,196	3.82%	38	Utah	408,458,430	0.40%
34	Rhode Island	709,789,379	0.70%	39	New Hampshire	380,342,519	0.37%
24	South Carolina	1,249,311,570	1.23%	40	Nevada	300,920,807	0.30%
45	South Dakota	263,859,418	0.26%	41	Idaho	300,629,716	0.30%
15	Tennessee	1,977,468,671	1.94%	42	Hawaii	292,508,880	0.29%
3	Texas	5,574,649,490	5.48%	43	Montana	287,428,709	0.28%
38	Utah	408,458,430	0.40%	44	North Dakota	272,713,407	0.27%
47	Vermont	234,897,152	0.23%	45	South Dakota	263,859,418	0.26%
21	Virginia	1,622,885,677	1.60%	46	Delaware	251,564,500	0.25%
23	Washington	1,537,056,515	1.51%	47	Vermont	234,897,152	0.23%
26	West Virginia	1,056,113,210	1.04%	48	Alaska	217,399,377	0.21%
18	Wisconsin	1,786,328,158	1.76%	49	Arizona	211,910,126	0.21%
50	Wyoming	125,448,070	0.12%	50	Wyoming	125,448,070	0.12%
					District of Columbia	554,518,849	0.55%

Source: U.S. Department of Health and Human Services, Health Care Financing Administration
"Statistical Report on Medical Care: Eligibles, Recipients, Payments and Services" (HCFA-2082)
*For fiscal year ending September 30, 1993. National total includes $158,000,000 for Puerto Rico and $4,282,081 for the Virgin Islands.

Percent Change in Medicaid Expenditures: 1990 to 1993

National Percent Change = 56.82% Increase*

ALPHA ORDER			RANK ORDER		
RANK	**STATE**	**PERCENT CHANGE**	**RANK**	**STATE**	**PERCENT CHANGE**
8	Alabama	95.60	1	West Virginia	192.49
31	Alaska	56.27	2	Louisiana	118.52
NA	Arizona**	NA	3	Wyoming	112.88
21	Arkansas	66.52	4	Delaware	104.23
39	California	48.30	5	Nevada	102.52
12	Colorado	76.72	6	Texas	100.45
37	Connecticut	51.43	7	New Mexico	97.13
4	Delaware	104.23	8	Alabama	95.60
14	Florida	75.00	9	Illinois	90.81
48	Georgia	17.56	10	Idaho	85.36
33	Hawaii	52.89	11	Nebraska	78.72
10	Idaho	85.36	12	Colorado	76.72
9	Illinois	90.81	13	Indiana	75.34
13	Indiana	75.34	14	Florida	75.00
41	Iowa	44.42	15	Kentucky	74.73
43	Kansas	43.03	16	Missouri	72.56
15	Kentucky	74.73	17	North Carolina	71.94
2	Louisiana	118.52	18	Tennessee	70.07
23	Maine	64.94	19	Montana	68.53
29	Maryland	57.82	20	South Carolina	68.13
49	Massachusetts	(0.17)	21	Arkansas	66.52
45	Michigan	40.20	22	Utah	65.60
46	Minnesota	36.82	23	Maine	64.94
34	Mississippi	52.80	24	Virginia	64.75
16	Missouri	72.56	25	Washington	61.38
19	Montana	68.53	26	Rhode Island	60.52
11	Nebraska	78.72	27	Oregon	60.18
5	Nevada	102.52	28	South Dakota	58.89
30	New Hampshire	56.49	29	Maryland	57.82
36	New Jersey	51.65	30	New Hampshire	56.49
7	New Mexico	97.13	31	Alaska	56.27
40	New York	47.82	32	Vermont	53.63
17	North Carolina	71.94	33	Hawaii	52.89
44	North Dakota	40.72	34	Mississippi	52.80
38	Ohio	49.00	35	Oklahoma	51.76
35	Oklahoma	51.76	36	New Jersey	51.65
27	Oregon	60.18	37	Connecticut	51.43
47	Pennsylvania	34.79	38	Ohio	49.00
26	Rhode Island	60.52	39	California	48.30
20	South Carolina	68.13	40	New York	47.82
28	South Dakota	58.89	41	Iowa	44.42
18	Tennessee	70.07	42	Wisconsin	43.09
6	Texas	100.45	43	Kansas	43.03
22	Utah	65.60	44	North Dakota	40.72
32	Vermont	53.63	45	Michigan	40.20
24	Virginia	64.75	46	Minnesota	36.82
25	Washington	61.38	47	Pennsylvania	34.79
1	West Virginia	192.49	48	Georgia	17.56
42	Wisconsin	43.09	49	Massachusetts	(0.17)
3	Wyoming	112.88	NA	Arizona**	NA

District of Columbia   125.65

Source: Morgan Quitno Press using data from US Dept of Health & Human Services, Health Care Financing Administration "Statistical Report on Medical Care: Eligibles, Recipients, Payments and Services" (HCFA-2082)

*For fiscal year ending September 30, 1993.

**Not available.

Medicaid Recipients in 1993

National Total = 33,432,025 Recipients*

<u>ALPHA ORDER</u>

RANK	STATE	RECIPIENTS	% of USA
20	Alabama	521,539	1.56%
48	Alaska	65,079	0.19%
26	Arizona	404,030	1.21%
29	Arkansas	339,451	1.02%
1	California	4,833,824	14.46%
33	Colorado	280,664	0.84%
30	Connecticut	333,685	1.00%
47	Delaware	68,934	0.21%
4	Florida	1,744,945	5.22%
9	Georgia	955,262	2.86%
40	Hawaii	109,970	0.33%
41	Idaho	99,515	0.30%
6	Illinois	1,395,566	4.17%
19	Indiana	564,952	1.69%
32	Iowa	289,211	0.87%
34	Kansas	242,896	0.73%
16	Kentucky	617,759	1.85%
14	Louisiana	751,242	2.25%
37	Maine	168,812	0.50%
24	Maryland	444,673	1.33%
13	Massachusetts	764,933	2.29%
8	Michigan	1,171,548	3.50%
25	Minnesota	425,478	1.27%
21	Mississippi	504,498	1.51%
17	Missouri	609,386	1.82%
42	Montana	89,041	0.27%
38	Nebraska	164,663	0.49%
43	Nevada	88,428	0.26%
45	New Hampshire	79,332	0.24%
12	New Jersey	793,634	2.37%
35	New Mexico	240,690	0.72%
2	New York	2,742,494	8.20%
11	North Carolina	898,416	2.69%
49	North Dakota	62,087	0.19%
5	Ohio	1,490,983	4.46%
27	Oklahoma	386,531	1.16%
31	Oregon	325,233	0.97%
7	Pennsylvania	1,223,080	3.66%
36	Rhode Island	191,138	0.57%
23	South Carolina	470,416	1.41%
46	South Dakota	69,606	0.21%
10	Tennessee	908,943	2.72%
3	Texas	2,308,443	6.90%
39	Utah	148,131	0.44%
44	Vermont	80,564	0.24%
18	Virginia	575,929	1.72%
15	Washington	633,364	1.89%
28	West Virginia	347,014	1.04%
22	Wisconsin	471,103	1.41%
50	Wyoming	46,262	0.14%

<u>RANK ORDER</u>

RANK	STATE	RECIPIENTS	% of USA
1	California	4,833,824	14.46%
2	New York	2,742,494	8.20%
3	Texas	2,308,443	6.90%
4	Florida	1,744,945	5.22%
5	Ohio	1,490,983	4.46%
6	Illinois	1,395,566	4.17%
7	Pennsylvania	1,223,080	3.66%
8	Michigan	1,171,548	3.50%
9	Georgia	955,262	2.86%
10	Tennessee	908,943	2.72%
11	North Carolina	898,416	2.69%
12	New Jersey	793,634	2.37%
13	Massachusetts	764,933	2.29%
14	Louisiana	751,242	2.25%
15	Washington	633,364	1.89%
16	Kentucky	617,759	1.85%
17	Missouri	609,386	1.82%
18	Virginia	575,929	1.72%
19	Indiana	564,952	1.69%
20	Alabama	521,539	1.56%
21	Mississippi	504,498	1.51%
22	Wisconsin	471,103	1.41%
23	South Carolina	470,416	1.41%
24	Maryland	444,673	1.33%
25	Minnesota	425,478	1.27%
26	Arizona	404,030	1.21%
27	Oklahoma	386,531	1.16%
28	West Virginia	347,014	1.04%
29	Arkansas	339,451	1.02%
30	Connecticut	333,685	1.00%
31	Oregon	325,233	0.97%
32	Iowa	289,211	0.87%
33	Colorado	280,664	0.84%
34	Kansas	242,896	0.73%
35	New Mexico	240,690	0.72%
36	Rhode Island	191,138	0.57%
37	Maine	168,812	0.50%
38	Nebraska	164,663	0.49%
39	Utah	148,131	0.44%
40	Hawaii	109,970	0.33%
41	Idaho	99,515	0.30%
42	Montana	89,041	0.27%
43	Nevada	88,428	0.26%
44	Vermont	80,564	0.24%
45	New Hampshire	79,332	0.24%
46	South Dakota	69,606	0.21%
47	Delaware	68,934	0.21%
48	Alaska	65,079	0.19%
49	North Dakota	62,087	0.19%
50	Wyoming	46,262	0.14%
	District of Columbia	120,256	0.36%

Source: U.S. Department of Health and Human Services, Health Care Financing Administration
"Statistical Report on Medical Care: Eligibles, Recipients, Payments and Services" (HCFA-2082)
*For fiscal year ending September 30, 1993. National total includes 757,432 recipients in Puerto Rico and 10,960 recipients in the Virgin Islands.

Percent Change in Number of Medicaid Recipients: 1990 to 1993

National Percent Change = 32.38% Increase*

ALPHA ORDER			RANK ORDER		
RANK	STATE	PERCENT CHANGE	RANK	STATE	PERCENT CHANGE
16	Alabama	48.17	1	Nevada	88.11
7	Alaska	66.64	2	New Mexico	85.35
NA	Arizona**	NA	3	Idaho	82.42
37	Arkansas	28.44	4	New Hampshire	77.01
31	California	33.37	5	Delaware	68.09
17	Colorado	47.23	6	Florida	68.03
30	Connecticut	33.69	7	Alaska	66.64
5	Delaware	68.09	8	Rhode Island	63.30
6	Florida	68.03	9	Indiana	62.40
18	Georgia	46.77	10	Texas	60.08
36	Hawaii	29.42	11	Wyoming	59.85
3	Idaho	82.42	12	North Carolina	59.48
34	Illinois	30.74	13	Virginia	51.78
9	Indiana	62.40	14	South Carolina	48.34
43	Iowa	20.71	15	Tennessee	48.20
41	Kansas	24.96	16	Alabama	48.17
33	Kentucky	32.08	17	Colorado	47.23
38	Louisiana	28.40	18	Georgia	46.77
39	Maine	26.91	19	Montana	45.83
29	Maryland	34.59	20	Oregon	43.15
35	Massachusetts	29.49	21	Washington	41.49
48	Michigan	11.79	22	Oklahoma	41.45
47	Minnesota	11.88	23	South Dakota	41.18
46	Mississippi	16.55	24	New Jersey	40.01
28	Missouri	35.95	25	West Virginia	38.66
19	Montana	45.83	26	Nebraska	38.17
26	Nebraska	38.17	27	Utah	36.84
1	Nevada	88.11	28	Missouri	35.95
4	New Hampshire	77.01	29	Maryland	34.59
24	New Jersey	40.01	30	Connecticut	33.69
2	New Mexico	85.35	31	California	33.37
45	New York	17.73	32	Vermont	33.34
12	North Carolina	59.48	33	Kentucky	32.08
40	North Dakota	26.70	34	Illinois	30.74
42	Ohio	22.13	35	Massachusetts	29.49
22	Oklahoma	41.45	36	Hawaii	29.42
20	Oregon	43.15	37	Arkansas	28.44
49	Pennsylvania	3.90	38	Louisiana	28.40
8	Rhode Island	63.30	39	Maine	26.91
14	South Carolina	48.34	40	North Dakota	26.70
23	South Dakota	41.18	41	Kansas	24.96
15	Tennessee	48.20	42	Ohio	22.13
10	Texas	60.08	43	Iowa	20.71
27	Utah	36.84	44	Wisconsin	19.96
32	Vermont	33.34	45	New York	17.73
13	Virginia	51.78	46	Mississippi	16.55
21	Washington	41.49	47	Minnesota	11.88
25	West Virginia	38.66	48	Michigan	11.79
44	Wisconsin	19.96	49	Pennsylvania	3.90
11	Wyoming	59.85	NA	Arizona**	NA

| | | | District of Columbia | 28.64 |

Source: Morgan Quitno Press using data from US Dept of Health & Human Services, Health Care Financing Administration "Statistical Report on Medical Care: Eligibles, Recipients, Payments and Services" (HCFA-2082)
*For fiscal year ending September 30, 1993.
**Not available.

Medicaid Cost per Recipient in 1993

National Per Capita = $3,042 per Recipient*

ALPHA ORDER

RANK	STATE	PER CAPITA
45	Alabama	$2,285
18	Alaska	3,341
50	Arizona	524
27	Arkansas	2,939
48	California	1,996
20	Colorado	3,247
2	Connecticut	5,469
14	Delaware	3,649
44	Florida	2,368
39	Georgia	2,555
36	Hawaii	2,660
26	Idaho	3,021
19	Illinois	3,314
8	Indiana	4,167
24	Iowa	3,097
29	Kansas	2,889
31	Kentucky	2,763
10	Louisiana	3,824
7	Maine	4,221
9	Maryland	3,870
15	Massachusetts	3,563
38	Michigan	2,627
4	Minnesota	4,535
49	Mississippi	1,775
41	Missouri	2,541
21	Montana	3,228
17	Nebraska	3,357
16	Nevada	3,403
3	New Hampshire	4,794
6	New Jersey	4,391
46	New Mexico	2,254
1	New York	6,402
33	North Carolina	2,729
5	North Dakota	4,392
23	Ohio	3,130
35	Oklahoma	2,700
39	Oregon	2,555
22	Pennsylvania	3,177
13	Rhode Island	3,713
37	South Carolina	2,656
12	South Dakota	3,791
47	Tennessee	2,176
43	Texas	2,415
32	Utah	2,757
28	Vermont	2,916
30	Virginia	2,818
42	Washington	2,427
25	West Virginia	3,043
11	Wisconsin	3,792
34	Wyoming	2,712

RANK ORDER

RANK	STATE	PER CAPITA
1	New York	$6,402
2	Connecticut	5,469
3	New Hampshire	4,794
4	Minnesota	4,535
5	North Dakota	4,392
6	New Jersey	4,391
7	Maine	4,221
8	Indiana	4,167
9	Maryland	3,870
10	Louisiana	3,824
11	Wisconsin	3,792
12	South Dakota	3,791
13	Rhode Island	3,713
14	Delaware	3,649
15	Massachusetts	3,563
16	Nevada	3,403
17	Nebraska	3,357
18	Alaska	3,341
19	Illinois	3,314
20	Colorado	3,247
21	Montana	3,228
22	Pennsylvania	3,177
23	Ohio	3,130
24	Iowa	3,097
25	West Virginia	3,043
26	Idaho	3,021
27	Arkansas	2,939
28	Vermont	2,916
29	Kansas	2,889
30	Virginia	2,818
31	Kentucky	2,763
32	Utah	2,757
33	North Carolina	2,729
34	Wyoming	2,712
35	Oklahoma	2,700
36	Hawaii	2,660
37	South Carolina	2,656
38	Michigan	2,627
39	Georgia	2,555
39	Oregon	2,555
41	Missouri	2,541
42	Washington	2,427
43	Texas	2,415
44	Florida	2,368
45	Alabama	2,285
46	New Mexico	2,254
47	Tennessee	2,176
48	California	1,996
49	Mississippi	1,775
50	Arizona	524

District of Columbia	4,611

Source: Morgan Quitno Press using data from US Dept of Health & Human Services, Health Care Financing Administration "Statistical Report on Medical Care: Eligibles, Recipients, Payments and Services" (HCFA-2082)
*For fiscal year ending September 30, 1993.

Percent Change in Cost per Medicaid Recipient: 1990 to 1993

National Percent Change = 18.46% Increase*

ALPHA ORDER				RANK ORDER		
RANK	STATE	PERCENT CHANGE		RANK	STATE	PERCENT CHANGE
6	Alabama	32.00		1	West Virginia	110.88
46	Alaska	(6.20)		2	Louisiana	70.18
NA	Arizona**	NA		3	Illinois	45.93
10	Arkansas	29.64		4	Wyoming	33.20
34	California	11.20		5	Kentucky	32.26
20	Colorado	20.04		6	Alabama	32.00
31	Connecticut	13.25		7	Mississippi	31.09
18	Delaware	21.47		8	Maine	29.96
43	Florida	4.18		9	Pennsylvania	29.73
48	Georgia	(19.91)		10	Arkansas	29.64
23	Hawaii	18.12		11	Nebraska	29.36
44	Idaho	1.61		12	Missouri	26.92
3	Illinois	45.93		13	New York	25.55
38	Indiana	7.98		14	Michigan	25.45
21	Iowa	19.62		15	Texas	25.26
28	Kansas	14.46		16	Minnesota	22.27
5	Kentucky	32.26		17	Ohio	21.98
2	Louisiana	70.18		18	Delaware	21.47
8	Maine	29.96		19	Utah	20.97
24	Maryland	17.27		20	Colorado	20.04
49	Massachusetts	(22.91)		21	Iowa	19.62
14	Michigan	25.45		22	Wisconsin	19.28
16	Minnesota	22.27		23	Hawaii	18.12
7	Mississippi	31.09		24	Maryland	17.27
12	Missouri	26.92		25	Montana	15.57
25	Montana	15.57		26	Vermont	15.26
11	Nebraska	29.36		27	Tennessee	14.77
40	Nevada	7.66		28	Kansas	14.46
47	New Hampshire	(11.60)		29	Washington	14.05
37	New Jersey	8.31		30	South Carolina	13.36
42	New Mexico	6.32		31	Connecticut	13.25
13	New York	25.55		32	South Dakota	12.56
39	North Carolina	7.82		33	Oregon	11.91
35	North Dakota	11.05		34	California	11.20
17	Ohio	21.98		35	North Dakota	11.05
41	Oklahoma	7.31		36	Virginia	8.55
33	Oregon	11.91		37	New Jersey	8.31
9	Pennsylvania	29.73		38	Indiana	7.98
45	Rhode Island	(1.72)		39	North Carolina	7.82
30	South Carolina	13.36		40	Nevada	7.66
32	South Dakota	12.56		41	Oklahoma	7.31
27	Tennessee	14.77		42	New Mexico	6.32
15	Texas	25.26		43	Florida	4.18
19	Utah	20.97		44	Idaho	1.61
26	Vermont	15.26		45	Rhode Island	(1.72)
36	Virginia	8.55		46	Alaska	(6.20)
29	Washington	14.05		47	New Hampshire	(11.60)
1	West Virginia	110.88		48	Georgia	(19.91)
22	Wisconsin	19.28		49	Massachusetts	(22.91)
4	Wyoming	33.20		NA	Arizona**	NA
					District of Columbia	75.39

Source: Morgan Quitno Press using data from US Dept of Health & Human Services, Health Care Financing Administration
"Statistical Report on Medical Care: Eligibles, Recipients, Payments and Services" (HCFA-2082)
*For fiscal year ending September 30, 1993.
**Not available.

Percent of Population Receiving Medicaid in 1993

National Percent = 12.67% of Population*

ALPHA ORDER			RANK ORDER		
RANK	STATE	PERCENT	RANK	STATE	PERCENT
20	Alabama	12.47	1	Mississippi	19.11
26	Alaska	10.88	1	Rhode Island	19.11
30	Arizona	10.24	3	West Virginia	19.09
10	Arkansas	13.99	4	Tennessee	17.84
7	California	15.48	5	Louisiana	17.51
48	Colorado	7.87	6	Kentucky	16.28
32	Connecticut	10.18	7	California	15.48
36	Delaware	9.88	8	New York	15.11
18	Florida	12.71	9	New Mexico	14.89
12	Georgia	13.84	10	Arkansas	13.99
41	Hawaii	9.43	10	Vermont	13.99
44	Idaho	9.05	12	Georgia	13.84
24	Illinois	11.94	13	Maine	13.61
35	Indiana	9.90	14	Ohio	13.48
29	Iowa	10.25	15	South Carolina	12.96
40	Kansas	9.58	16	North Carolina	12.92
6	Kentucky	16.28	17	Texas	12.81
5	Louisiana	17.51	18	Florida	12.71
13	Maine	13.61	18	Massachusetts	12.71
45	Maryland	8.97	20	Alabama	12.47
18	Massachusetts	12.71	21	Michigan	12.38
21	Michigan	12.38	22	Washington	12.04
42	Minnesota	9.40	23	Oklahoma	11.96
1	Mississippi	19.11	24	Illinois	11.94
25	Missouri	11.64	25	Missouri	11.64
28	Montana	10.59	26	Alaska	10.88
31	Nebraska	10.21	27	Oregon	10.72
50	Nevada	6.40	28	Montana	10.59
49	New Hampshire	7.06	29	Iowa	10.25
34	New Jersey	10.10	30	Arizona	10.24
9	New Mexico	14.89	31	Nebraska	10.21
8	New York	15.11	32	Connecticut	10.18
16	North Carolina	12.92	33	Pennsylvania	10.17
38	North Dakota	9.75	34	New Jersey	10.10
14	Ohio	13.48	35	Indiana	9.90
23	Oklahoma	11.96	36	Delaware	9.88
27	Oregon	10.72	37	Wyoming	9.84
33	Pennsylvania	10.17	38	North Dakota	9.75
1	Rhode Island	19.11	39	South Dakota	9.72
15	South Carolina	12.96	40	Kansas	9.58
39	South Dakota	9.72	41	Hawaii	9.43
4	Tennessee	17.84	42	Minnesota	9.40
17	Texas	12.81	43	Wisconsin	9.34
47	Utah	7.96	44	Idaho	9.05
10	Vermont	13.99	45	Maryland	8.97
46	Virginia	8.90	46	Virginia	8.90
22	Washington	12.04	47	Utah	7.96
3	West Virginia	19.09	48	Colorado	7.87
43	Wisconsin	9.34	49	New Hampshire	7.06
37	Wyoming	9.84	50	Nevada	6.40

District of Columbia   20.77

Source: Morgan Quitno Press using data from US Dept of Health & Human Services, Health Care Financing Administration "Statistical Report on Medical Care: Eligibles, Recipients, Payments and Services" (HCFA-2082)
For fiscal year ending September 30, 1993. National rate does not include population or recipients in U.S. territories.

Federal Medicaid Matching Fund Rate for 1995

National Average = 60.47% of State's Medicaid Funds Matched by Federal Government*

ALPHA ORDER				RANK ORDER		
RANK	STATE	RATE		RANK	STATE	RATE
9	Alabama	70.45		1	Mississippi	78.58
38	Alaska	50.00		2	West Virginia	74.60
16	Arizona	66.40		3	Arkansas	73.75
3	Arkansas	73.75		4	Utah	73.48
38	California	50.00		5	New Mexico	73.31
36	Colorado	53.10		6	Louisiana	72.65
38	Connecticut	50.00		7	Montana	70.81
38	Delaware	50.00		8	South Carolina	70.71
32	Florida	56.28		9	Alabama	70.45
24	Georgia	62.23		10	Idaho	70.14
38	Hawaii	50.00		11	Oklahoma	70.05
10	Idaho	70.14		12	Kentucky	69.58
38	Illinois	50.00		13	North Dakota	68.73
20	Indiana	63.03		14	South Dakota	68.06
22	Iowa	62.62		15	Tennessee	66.52
30	Kansas	58.90		16	Arizona	66.40
12	Kentucky	69.58		17	North Carolina	64.71
6	Louisiana	72.65		18	Texas	63.31
19	Maine	63.30		19	Maine	63.30
38	Maryland	50.00		20	Indiana	63.03
38	Massachusetts	50.00		21	Wyoming	62.87
31	Michigan	56.84		22	Iowa	62.62
34	Minnesota	54.27		23	Oregon	62.36
1	Mississippi	78.58		24	Georgia	62.23
29	Missouri	58.95		25	Vermont	60.92
7	Montana	70.81		26	Ohio	60.69
27	Nebraska	60.40		27	Nebraska	60.40
38	Nevada	50.00		28	Wisconsin	59.81
38	New Hampshire	50.00		29	Missouri	58.95
38	New Jersey	50.00		30	Kansas	58.90
5	New Mexico	73.31		31	Michigan	56.84
38	New York	50.00		32	Florida	56.28
17	North Carolina	64.71		33	Rhode Island	55.49
13	North Dakota	68.73		34	Minnesota	54.27
26	Ohio	60.69		34	Pennsylvania	54.27
11	Oklahoma	70.05		36	Colorado	53.10
23	Oregon	62.36		37	Washington	51.97
34	Pennsylvania	54.27		38	Alaska	50.00
33	Rhode Island	55.49		38	California	50.00
8	South Carolina	70.71		38	Connecticut	50.00
14	South Dakota	68.06		38	Delaware	50.00
15	Tennessee	66.52		38	Hawaii	50.00
18	Texas	63.31		38	Illinois	50.00
4	Utah	73.48		38	Maryland	50.00
25	Vermont	60.92		38	Massachusetts	50.00
38	Virginia	50.00		38	Nevada	50.00
37	Washington	51.97		38	New Hampshire	50.00
2	West Virginia	74.60		38	New Jersey	50.00
28	Wisconsin	59.81		38	New York	50.00
21	Wyoming	62.87		38	Virginia	50.00
					District of Columbia	50.00

*Source: U.S. Department of Health and Human Services, Health Care Financing Administration
unpublished data reported by the Medicaid Bureau*

*50 percent is minimum. National average is a simple average of the 51 individual rates and is not weighted for population or funds.

Medicare Benefit Payments in 1993

National Total = $142,933,727,000*

ALPHA ORDER

RANK	STATE	BENEFITS	% of USA
18	Alabama	$2,460,573,000	1.72%
50	Alaska	97,340,000	0.07%
21	Arizona	2,178,377,000	1.52%
32	Arkansas	1,306,041,000	0.91%
1	California	16,487,553,000	11.54%
29	Colorado	1,429,580,000	1.00%
24	Connecticut	2,052,656,000	1.44%
44	Delaware	368,391,000	0.26%
2	Florida	11,721,988,000	8.20%
11	Georgia	3,301,647,000	2.31%
41	Hawaii	472,706,000	0.33%
46	Idaho	341,832,000	0.24%
6	Illinois	6,136,399,000	4.29%
15	Indiana	2,876,565,000	2.01%
33	Iowa	1,305,372,000	0.91%
30	Kansas	1,350,204,000	0.94%
25	Kentucky	1,958,777,000	1.37%
16	Louisiana	2,607,035,000	1.82%
39	Maine	561,490,000	0.39%
17	Maryland	2,469,631,000	1.73%
10	Massachusetts	4,487,227,000	3.14%
8	Michigan	5,171,403,000	3.62%
23	Minnesota	2,106,232,000	1.47%
31	Mississippi	1,327,867,000	0.93%
14	Missouri	3,122,092,000	2.18%
43	Montana	369,612,000	0.26%
35	Nebraska	689,410,000	0.48%
36	Nevada	663,596,000	0.46%
42	New Hampshire	462,196,000	0.32%
9	New Jersey	4,749,355,000	3.32%
40	New Mexico	556,534,000	0.39%
3	New York	11,447,774,000	8.01%
13	North Carolina	3,242,292,000	2.27%
45	North Dakota	347,160,000	0.24%
7	Ohio	6,086,116,000	4.26%
26	Oklahoma	1,546,624,000	1.08%
27	Oregon	1,443,639,000	1.01%
4	Pennsylvania	9,270,961,000	6.49%
37	Rhode Island	628,236,000	0.44%
28	South Carolina	1,440,252,000	1.01%
47	South Dakota	331,488,000	0.23%
12	Tennessee	3,251,676,000	2.27%
5	Texas	8,007,117,000	5.60%
38	Utah	590,761,000	0.41%
48	Vermont	227,995,000	0.16%
19	Virginia	2,420,279,000	1.69%
22	Washington	2,166,637,000	1.52%
34	West Virginia	1,017,016,000	0.71%
20	Wisconsin	2,305,182,000	1.61%
49	Wyoming	138,637,000	0.10%

RANK ORDER

RANK	STATE	BENEFITS	% of USA
1	California	$16,487,553,000	11.54%
2	Florida	11,721,988,000	8.20%
3	New York	11,447,774,000	8.01%
4	Pennsylvania	9,270,961,000	6.49%
5	Texas	8,007,117,000	5.60%
6	Illinois	6,136,399,000	4.29%
7	Ohio	6,086,116,000	4.26%
8	Michigan	5,171,403,000	3.62%
9	New Jersey	4,749,355,000	3.32%
10	Massachusetts	4,487,227,000	3.14%
11	Georgia	3,301,647,000	2.31%
12	Tennessee	3,251,676,000	2.27%
13	North Carolina	3,242,292,000	2.27%
14	Missouri	3,122,092,000	2.18%
15	Indiana	2,876,565,000	2.01%
16	Louisiana	2,607,035,000	1.82%
17	Maryland	2,469,631,000	1.73%
18	Alabama	2,460,573,000	1.72%
19	Virginia	2,420,279,000	1.69%
20	Wisconsin	2,305,182,000	1.61%
21	Arizona	2,178,377,000	1.52%
22	Washington	2,166,637,000	1.52%
23	Minnesota	2,106,232,000	1.47%
24	Connecticut	2,052,656,000	1.44%
25	Kentucky	1,958,777,000	1.37%
26	Oklahoma	1,546,624,000	1.08%
27	Oregon	1,443,639,000	1.01%
28	South Carolina	1,440,252,000	1.01%
29	Colorado	1,429,580,000	1.00%
30	Kansas	1,350,204,000	0.94%
31	Mississippi	1,327,867,000	0.93%
32	Arkansas	1,306,041,000	0.91%
33	Iowa	1,305,372,000	0.91%
34	West Virginia	1,017,016,000	0.71%
35	Nebraska	689,410,000	0.48%
36	Nevada	663,596,000	0.46%
37	Rhode Island	628,236,000	0.44%
38	Utah	590,761,000	0.41%
39	Maine	561,490,000	0.39%
40	New Mexico	556,534,000	0.39%
41	Hawaii	472,706,000	0.33%
42	New Hampshire	462,196,000	0.32%
43	Montana	369,612,000	0.26%
44	Delaware	368,391,000	0.26%
45	North Dakota	347,160,000	0.24%
46	Idaho	341,832,000	0.24%
47	South Dakota	331,488,000	0.23%
48	Vermont	227,995,000	0.16%
49	Wyoming	138,637,000	0.10%
50	Alaska	97,340,000	0.07%
	District of Columbia	1,111,826,000	0.78%

Source: U.S. Department of Health and Human Services, Health Care Financing Administration
HHS News Release (March 11, 1994)
For fiscal year 1993. Includes payments to aged and disabled enrollees. Total includes $722,377,000 in payments to enrollees in territories, foreign countries and whose residences are unknown.

Medicare Enrollees in 1993

National Total = 36,270,936 Enrollees*

<u>ALPHA ORDER</u>

RANK	STATE	ENROLLEES	% of USA
19	Alabama	618,246	1.70%
50	Alaska	30,098	0.08%
24	Arizona	553,500	1.53%
30	Arkansas	409,902	1.13%
1	California	3,503,976	9.66%
31	Colorado	396,453	1.09%
25	Connecticut	491,055	1.35%
47	Delaware	95,539	0.26%
3	Florida	2,493,700	6.88%
14	Georgia	790,781	2.18%
43	Hawaii	141,124	0.39%
42	Idaho	142,309	0.39%
7	Illinois	1,593,485	4.39%
13	Indiana	802,572	2.21%
28	Iowa	469,081	1.29%
33	Kansas	376,481	1.04%
22	Kentucky	564,958	1.56%
23	Louisiana	562,561	1.55%
37	Maine	194,376	0.54%
21	Maryland	578,311	1.59%
11	Massachusetts	911,420	2.51%
8	Michigan	1,308,694	3.61%
20	Minnesota	615,327	1.70%
32	Mississippi	383,922	1.06%
12	Missouri	814,200	2.24%
44	Montana	125,084	0.34%
35	Nebraska	244,825	0.67%
39	Nevada	169,614	0.47%
41	New Hampshire	148,442	0.41%
9	New Jersey	1,143,658	3.15%
36	New Mexico	198,466	0.55%
2	New York	2,594,326	7.15%
10	North Carolina	971,209	2.68%
46	North Dakota	101,920	0.28%
6	Ohio	1,626,085	4.48%
27	Oklahoma	472,900	1.30%
29	Oregon	452,353	1.25%
4	Pennsylvania	2,039,305	5.62%
40	Rhode Island	164,910	0.45%
26	South Carolina	481,173	1.33%
45	South Dakota	114,514	0.32%
17	Tennessee	737,910	2.03%
5	Texas	1,973,343	5.44%
38	Utah	176,799	0.49%
48	Vermont	79,351	0.22%
15	Virginia	779,006	2.15%
18	Washington	657,780	1.81%
34	West Virginia	321,949	0.89%
16	Wisconsin	744,796	2.05%
49	Wyoming	56,921	0.16%

<u>RANK ORDER</u>

RANK	STATE	ENROLLEES	% of USA
1	California	3,503,976	9.66%
2	New York	2,594,326	7.15%
3	Florida	2,493,700	6.88%
4	Pennsylvania	2,039,305	5.62%
5	Texas	1,973,343	5.44%
6	Ohio	1,626,085	4.48%
7	Illinois	1,593,485	4.39%
8	Michigan	1,308,694	3.61%
9	New Jersey	1,143,658	3.15%
10	North Carolina	971,209	2.68%
11	Massachusetts	911,420	2.51%
12	Missouri	814,200	2.24%
13	Indiana	802,572	2.21%
14	Georgia	790,781	2.18%
15	Virginia	779,006	2.15%
16	Wisconsin	744,796	2.05%
17	Tennessee	737,910	2.03%
18	Washington	657,780	1.81%
19	Alabama	618,246	1.70%
20	Minnesota	615,327	1.70%
21	Maryland	578,311	1.59%
22	Kentucky	564,958	1.56%
23	Louisiana	562,561	1.55%
24	Arizona	553,500	1.53%
25	Connecticut	491,055	1.35%
26	South Carolina	481,173	1.33%
27	Oklahoma	472,900	1.30%
28	Iowa	469,081	1.29%
29	Oregon	452,353	1.25%
30	Arkansas	409,902	1.13%
31	Colorado	396,453	1.09%
32	Mississippi	383,922	1.06%
33	Kansas	376,481	1.04%
34	West Virginia	321,949	0.89%
35	Nebraska	244,825	0.67%
36	New Mexico	198,466	0.55%
37	Maine	194,376	0.54%
38	Utah	176,799	0.49%
39	Nevada	169,614	0.47%
40	Rhode Island	164,910	0.45%
41	New Hampshire	148,442	0.41%
42	Idaho	142,309	0.39%
43	Hawaii	141,124	0.39%
44	Montana	125,084	0.34%
45	South Dakota	114,514	0.32%
46	North Dakota	101,920	0.28%
47	Delaware	95,539	0.26%
48	Vermont	79,351	0.22%
49	Wyoming	56,921	0.16%
50	Alaska	30,098	0.08%
	District of Columbia	78,496	0.22%

Source: U.S. Department of Health and Human Services, Health Care Financing Administration
HHS News Release (March 11, 1994)

As of September 1993. Includes aged and disabled enrollees. Total includes 773,730 enrollees in territories, foreign countries and whose residences are unknown.

Medicare Payments per Enrollee in 1993

National Rate = $3,941 per Enrollee*

ALPHA ORDER				RANK ORDER		
RANK	STATE	PER ENROLLEE		RANK	STATE	PER ENROLLEE
13	Alabama	$3,980		1	Massachusetts	$4,923
34	Alaska	3,234		2	California	4,705
15	Arizona	3,936		3	Florida	4,701
36	Arkansas	3,186		4	Louisiana	4,634
2	California	4,705		5	Pennsylvania	4,546
22	Colorado	3,606		6	New York	4,413
9	Connecticut	4,180		7	Tennessee	4,407
17	Delaware	3,856		8	Maryland	4,270
3	Florida	4,701		9	Connecticut	4,180
10	Georgia	4,175		10	Georgia	4,175
29	Hawaii	3,350		11	New Jersey	4,153
50	Idaho	2,402		12	Texas	4,058
18	Illinois	3,851		13	Alabama	3,980
24	Indiana	3,584		14	Michigan	3,952
48	Iowa	2,783		15	Arizona	3,936
23	Kansas	3,586		16	Nevada	3,912
25	Kentucky	3,467		17	Delaware	3,856
4	Louisiana	4,634		18	Illinois	3,851
44	Maine	2,889		19	Missouri	3,835
8	Maryland	4,270		20	Rhode Island	3,810
1	Massachusetts	4,923		21	Ohio	3,743
14	Michigan	3,952		22	Colorado	3,606
27	Minnesota	3,423		23	Kansas	3,586
26	Mississippi	3,459		24	Indiana	3,584
19	Missouri	3,835		25	Kentucky	3,467
42	Montana	2,955		26	Mississippi	3,459
46	Nebraska	2,816		27	Minnesota	3,423
16	Nevada	3,912		28	North Dakota	3,406
38	New Hampshire	3,114		29	Hawaii	3,350
11	New Jersey	4,153		30	Utah	3,341
47	New Mexico	2,804		31	North Carolina	3,338
6	New York	4,413		32	Washington	3,294
31	North Carolina	3,338		33	Oklahoma	3,271
28	North Dakota	3,406		34	Alaska	3,234
21	Ohio	3,743		35	Oregon	3,191
33	Oklahoma	3,271		36	Arkansas	3,186
35	Oregon	3,191		37	West Virginia	3,159
5	Pennsylvania	4,546		38	New Hampshire	3,114
20	Rhode Island	3,810		39	Virginia	3,107
41	South Carolina	2,993		40	Wisconsin	3,095
43	South Dakota	2,895		41	South Carolina	2,993
7	Tennessee	4,407		42	Montana	2,955
12	Texas	4,058		43	South Dakota	2,895
30	Utah	3,341		44	Maine	2,889
45	Vermont	2,873		45	Vermont	2,873
39	Virginia	3,107		46	Nebraska	2,816
32	Washington	3,294		47	New Mexico	2,804
37	West Virginia	3,159		48	Iowa	2,783
40	Wisconsin	3,095		49	Wyoming	2,436
49	Wyoming	2,436		50	Idaho	2,402
					District of Columbia**	NA

Source: Morgan Quitno Press using data from US Dept of Health & Human Services, Health Care Financing Administration HHS News Release (March 11, 1994)

*As of September 1993. Includes aged and disabled enrollees. National rate includes payments to enrollees in territories, foreign countries and whose residences are unknown. National rate without such payments would be $4,006 per enrollee.

**Not available.

Percent of Population Enrolled in Medicare in 1993

National Percent = 13.77% of Population*

ALPHA ORDER

RANK	STATE	PERCENT
18	Alabama	14.79
50	Alaska	5.03
27	Arizona	14.03
4	Arkansas	16.90
46	California	11.22
47	Colorado	11.12
13	Connecticut	14.98
31	Delaware	13.69
1	Florida	18.17
45	Georgia	11.46
42	Hawaii	12.10
37	Idaho	12.94
32	Illinois	13.64
26	Indiana	14.07
5	Iowa	16.63
17	Kansas	14.85
15	Kentucky	14.89
36	Louisiana	13.11
9	Maine	15.68
44	Maryland	11.66
12	Massachusetts	15.14
29	Michigan	13.83
33	Minnesota	13.60
23	Mississippi	14.54
10	Missouri	15.55
16	Montana	14.87
11	Nebraska	15.18
40	Nevada	12.27
35	New Hampshire	13.21
22	New Jersey	14.55
39	New Mexico	12.28
25	New York	14.29
28	North Carolina	13.97
7	North Dakota	16.00
20	Ohio	14.70
21	Oklahoma	14.63
14	Oregon	14.90
3	Pennsylvania	16.95
6	Rhode Island	16.49
34	South Carolina	13.26
8	South Dakota	15.99
24	Tennessee	14.49
48	Texas	10.95
49	Utah	9.51
30	Vermont	13.78
43	Virginia	12.03
38	Washington	12.51
2	West Virginia	17.71
19	Wisconsin	14.77
41	Wyoming	12.11

RANK ORDER

RANK	STATE	PERCENT
1	Florida	18.17
2	West Virginia	17.71
3	Pennsylvania	16.95
4	Arkansas	16.90
5	Iowa	16.63
6	Rhode Island	16.49
7	North Dakota	16.00
8	South Dakota	15.99
9	Maine	15.68
10	Missouri	15.55
11	Nebraska	15.18
12	Massachusetts	15.14
13	Connecticut	14.98
14	Oregon	14.90
15	Kentucky	14.89
16	Montana	14.87
17	Kansas	14.85
18	Alabama	14.79
19	Wisconsin	14.77
20	Ohio	14.70
21	Oklahoma	14.63
22	New Jersey	14.55
23	Mississippi	14.54
24	Tennessee	14.49
25	New York	14.29
26	Indiana	14.07
27	Arizona	14.03
28	North Carolina	13.97
29	Michigan	13.83
30	Vermont	13.78
31	Delaware	13.69
32	Illinois	13.64
33	Minnesota	13.60
34	South Carolina	13.26
35	New Hampshire	13.21
36	Louisiana	13.11
37	Idaho	12.94
38	Washington	12.51
39	New Mexico	12.28
40	Nevada	12.27
41	Wyoming	12.11
42	Hawaii	12.10
43	Virginia	12.03
44	Maryland	11.66
45	Georgia	11.46
46	California	11.22
47	Colorado	11.12
48	Texas	10.95
49	Utah	9.51
50	Alaska	5.03

District of Columbia   13.56

Source: Morgan Quitno Press using data from US Dept of Health & Human Services, Health Care Financing Administration HHS News Release (March 11, 1994)

As of September 1993. Includes aged and disabled enrollees. National rate is only for residents of the 50 states and the District of Columbia.

Percent of Physicians Participating in Medicare in 1993

National State Average = 59.8% of Physicians Participate in Medicare*

ALPHA ORDER				RANK ORDER		
RANK	STATE	PERCENT		RANK	STATE	PERCENT
1	Alabama	85.1		1	Alabama	85.1
25	Alaska	60.4		2	Nevada	84.9
6	Arizona	76.2		3	Rhode Island	80.9
22	Arkansas	62.1		4	Utah	80.3
20	California	65.9		5	Ohio	76.6
33	Colorado	55.7		6	Arizona	76.2
35	Connecticut	55.4		7	Hawaii	75.9
30	Delaware	57.4		7	West Virginia	75.9
34	Florida	55.6		9	Georgia	74.9
9	Georgia	74.9		10	Kentucky	73.6
7	Hawaii	75.9		11	Kansas	73.2
49	Idaho	37.1		12	North Carolina	72.8
29	Illinois	57.6		13	Maryland	72.5
32	Indiana	55.8		14	Nebraska	70.6
23	Iowa	61.8		15	Tennessee	70.5
11	Kansas	73.2		16	Missouri	67.5
10	Kentucky	73.6		17	South Carolina	67.3
45	Louisiana	44.0		18	New Mexico	66.8
42	Maine	52.0		18	Wisconsin	66.8
13	Maryland	72.5		20	California	65.9
43	Massachusetts	50.2		21	Washington	64.7
28	Michigan	58.1		22	Arkansas	62.1
44	Minnesota	44.4		23	Iowa	61.8
39	Mississippi	53.4		24	Texas	61.3
16	Missouri	67.5		25	Alaska	60.4
37	Montana	54.7		26	Pennsylvania	59.7
14	Nebraska	70.6		27	Oregon	59.2
2	Nevada	84.9		28	Michigan	58.1
46	New Hampshire	43.0		29	Illinois	57.6
47	New Jersey	42.6		30	Delaware	57.4
18	New Mexico	66.8		31	Vermont	56.5
48	New York	40.7		32	Indiana	55.8
12	North Carolina	72.8		33	Colorado	55.7
36	North Dakota	55.0		34	Florida	55.6
5	Ohio	76.6		35	Connecticut	55.4
38	Oklahoma	53.9		36	North Dakota	55.0
27	Oregon	59.2		37	Montana	54.7
26	Pennsylvania	59.7		38	Oklahoma	53.9
3	Rhode Island	80.9		39	Mississippi	53.4
17	South Carolina	67.3		40	Wyoming	53.3
50	South Dakota	31.6		41	Virginia	52.2
15	Tennessee	70.5		42	Maine	52.0
24	Texas	61.3		43	Massachusetts	50.2
4	Utah	80.3		44	Minnesota	44.4
31	Vermont	56.5		45	Louisiana	44.0
41	Virginia	52.2		46	New Hampshire	43.0
21	Washington	64.7		47	New Jersey	42.6
7	West Virginia	75.9		48	New York	40.7
18	Wisconsin	66.8		49	Idaho	37.1
40	Wyoming	53.3		50	South Dakota	31.6
				District of Columbia		50.6

Source: U.S. Department of Health and Human Services, Health Care Financing Administration
"1994 Data Compendium" (Pub. No. 03349, March 1994)
*Medicare Part B. Physicians include MDs, DOs and limited license practitioners.

State Government Expenditures for Health Programs in 1993

National Total = $25,766,959,000*

ALPHA ORDER				RANK ORDER			
RANK	STATE	EXPENDITURES	% of USA	RANK	STATE	EXPENDITURES	% of USA
20	Alabama	$412,456,000	1.60%	1	California	$4,391,129,000	17.04%
34	Alaska	173,336,000	0.67%	2	Florida	1,968,067,000	7.64%
17	Arizona	459,287,000	1.78%	3	New York	1,935,065,000	7.51%
32	Arkansas	200,595,000	0.78%	4	Michigan	1,470,953,000	5.71%
1	California	4,391,129,000	17.04%	5	Pennsylvania	1,228,100,000	4.77%
29	Colorado	220,766,000	0.86%	6	Texas	1,024,134,000	3.97%
26	Connecticut	329,967,000	1.28%	7	Illinois	982,710,000	3.81%
40	Delaware	122,143,000	0.47%	8	Massachusetts	974,112,000	3.78%
2	Florida	1,968,067,000	7.64%	9	Ohio	815,642,000	3.17%
14	Georgia	517,091,000	2.01%	10	Maryland	615,986,000	2.39%
28	Hawaii	275,777,000	1.07%	11	North Carolina	615,288,000	2.39%
46	Idaho	62,893,000	0.24%	12	Washington	539,275,000	2.09%
7	Illinois	982,710,000	3.81%	13	New Jersey	521,286,000	2.02%
25	Indiana	334,833,000	1.30%	14	Georgia	517,091,000	2.01%
37	Iowa	150,963,000	0.59%	15	Virginia	473,415,000	1.84%
36	Kansas	154,432,000	0.60%	16	South Carolina	467,952,000	1.82%
30	Kentucky	219,051,000	0.85%	17	Arizona	459,287,000	1.78%
24	Louisiana	345,153,000	1.34%	18	Wisconsin	456,485,000	1.77%
39	Maine	123,166,000	0.48%	19	Minnesota	429,462,000	1.67%
10	Maryland	615,986,000	2.39%	20	Alabama	412,456,000	1.60%
8	Massachusetts	974,112,000	3.78%	21	Missouri	388,672,000	1.51%
4	Michigan	1,470,953,000	5.71%	22	Tennessee	360,592,000	1.40%
19	Minnesota	429,462,000	1.67%	23	Oregon	357,204,000	1.39%
35	Mississippi	155,442,000	0.60%	24	Louisiana	345,153,000	1.34%
21	Missouri	388,672,000	1.51%	25	Indiana	334,833,000	1.30%
44	Montana	96,446,000	0.37%	26	Connecticut	329,967,000	1.28%
38	Nebraska	150,157,000	0.58%	27	Oklahoma	279,002,000	1.08%
47	Nevada	60,614,000	0.24%	28	Hawaii	275,777,000	1.07%
43	New Hampshire	101,686,000	0.39%	29	Colorado	220,766,000	0.86%
13	New Jersey	521,286,000	2.02%	30	Kentucky	219,051,000	0.85%
31	New Mexico	207,734,000	0.81%	31	New Mexico	207,734,000	0.81%
3	New York	1,935,065,000	7.51%	32	Arkansas	200,595,000	0.78%
11	North Carolina	615,288,000	2.39%	33	Rhode Island	176,159,000	0.68%
49	North Dakota	46,037,000	0.18%	34	Alaska	173,336,000	0.67%
9	Ohio	815,642,000	3.17%	35	Mississippi	155,442,000	0.60%
27	Oklahoma	279,002,000	1.08%	36	Kansas	154,432,000	0.60%
23	Oregon	357,204,000	1.39%	37	Iowa	150,963,000	0.59%
5	Pennsylvania	1,228,100,000	4.77%	38	Nebraska	150,157,000	0.58%
33	Rhode Island	176,159,000	0.68%	39	Maine	123,166,000	0.48%
16	South Carolina	467,952,000	1.82%	40	Delaware	122,143,000	0.47%
48	South Dakota	50,627,000	0.20%	41	Utah	122,069,000	0.47%
22	Tennessee	360,592,000	1.40%	42	West Virginia	102,208,000	0.40%
6	Texas	1,024,134,000	3.97%	43	New Hampshire	101,686,000	0.39%
41	Utah	122,069,000	0.47%	44	Montana	96,446,000	0.37%
50	Vermont	36,007,000	0.14%	45	Wyoming	65,333,000	0.25%
15	Virginia	473,415,000	1.84%	46	Idaho	62,893,000	0.24%
12	Washington	539,275,000	2.09%	47	Nevada	60,614,000	0.24%
42	West Virginia	102,208,000	0.40%	48	South Dakota	50,627,000	0.20%
18	Wisconsin	456,485,000	1.77%	49	North Dakota	46,037,000	0.18%
45	Wyoming	65,333,000	0.25%	50	Vermont	36,007,000	0.14%
					District of Columbia**	NA	NA

Source: U.S. Bureau of the Census
   "State Government Finances: 1993"
*Includes outpatient health services other than hospital care, research and education, categorical health programs, treatment and immunization clinics, nursing and environmental health activities. Includes capital expenditures.
**Not applicable.

Per Capita State Government Expenditures for Health Programs in 1993

National Per Capita = $99.96*

<table>
<tr><td colspan="3">ALPHA ORDER</td><td colspan="3">RANK ORDER</td></tr>
<tr><td>RANK</td><td>STATE</td><td>PER CAPITA</td><td>RANK</td><td>STATE</td><td>PER CAPITA</td></tr>
<tr><td>21</td><td>Alabama</td><td>$98.65</td><td>1</td><td>Alaska</td><td>$289.86</td></tr>
<tr><td>1</td><td>Alaska</td><td>289.86</td><td>2</td><td>Hawaii</td><td>236.52</td></tr>
<tr><td>14</td><td>Arizona</td><td>116.42</td><td>3</td><td>Rhode Island</td><td>176.16</td></tr>
<tr><td>29</td><td>Arkansas</td><td>82.69</td><td>4</td><td>Delaware</td><td>174.99</td></tr>
<tr><td>8</td><td>California</td><td>140.66</td><td>5</td><td>Massachusetts</td><td>161.87</td></tr>
<tr><td>41</td><td>Colorado</td><td>61.94</td><td>6</td><td>Michigan</td><td>155.49</td></tr>
<tr><td>19</td><td>Connecticut</td><td>100.66</td><td>7</td><td>Florida</td><td>143.38</td></tr>
<tr><td>4</td><td>Delaware</td><td>174.99</td><td>8</td><td>California</td><td>140.66</td></tr>
<tr><td>7</td><td>Florida</td><td>143.38</td><td>9</td><td>Wyoming</td><td>139.01</td></tr>
<tr><td>31</td><td>Georgia</td><td>74.92</td><td>10</td><td>South Carolina</td><td>128.91</td></tr>
<tr><td>2</td><td>Hawaii</td><td>236.52</td><td>11</td><td>New Mexico</td><td>128.55</td></tr>
<tr><td>46</td><td>Idaho</td><td>57.18</td><td>12</td><td>Maryland</td><td>124.24</td></tr>
<tr><td>28</td><td>Illinois</td><td>84.09</td><td>13</td><td>Oregon</td><td>117.69</td></tr>
<tr><td>44</td><td>Indiana</td><td>58.68</td><td>14</td><td>Arizona</td><td>116.42</td></tr>
<tr><td>49</td><td>Iowa</td><td>53.51</td><td>15</td><td>Montana</td><td>114.68</td></tr>
<tr><td>42</td><td>Kansas</td><td>60.92</td><td>16</td><td>New York</td><td>106.60</td></tr>
<tr><td>45</td><td>Kentucky</td><td>57.74</td><td>17</td><td>Washington</td><td>102.54</td></tr>
<tr><td>30</td><td>Louisiana</td><td>80.46</td><td>18</td><td>Pennsylvania</td><td>102.09</td></tr>
<tr><td>20</td><td>Maine</td><td>99.33</td><td>19</td><td>Connecticut</td><td>100.66</td></tr>
<tr><td>12</td><td>Maryland</td><td>124.24</td><td>20</td><td>Maine</td><td>99.33</td></tr>
<tr><td>5</td><td>Massachusetts</td><td>161.87</td><td>21</td><td>Alabama</td><td>98.65</td></tr>
<tr><td>6</td><td>Michigan</td><td>155.49</td><td>22</td><td>Minnesota</td><td>94.93</td></tr>
<tr><td>22</td><td>Minnesota</td><td>94.93</td><td>23</td><td>Nebraska</td><td>93.09</td></tr>
<tr><td>43</td><td>Mississippi</td><td>58.88</td><td>24</td><td>Wisconsin</td><td>90.50</td></tr>
<tr><td>32</td><td>Missouri</td><td>74.24</td><td>25</td><td>New Hampshire</td><td>90.47</td></tr>
<tr><td>15</td><td>Montana</td><td>114.68</td><td>26</td><td>North Carolina</td><td>88.51</td></tr>
<tr><td>23</td><td>Nebraska</td><td>93.09</td><td>27</td><td>Oklahoma</td><td>86.30</td></tr>
<tr><td>50</td><td>Nevada</td><td>43.86</td><td>28</td><td>Illinois</td><td>84.09</td></tr>
<tr><td>25</td><td>New Hampshire</td><td>90.47</td><td>29</td><td>Arkansas</td><td>82.69</td></tr>
<tr><td>38</td><td>New Jersey</td><td>66.33</td><td>30</td><td>Louisiana</td><td>80.46</td></tr>
<tr><td>11</td><td>New Mexico</td><td>128.55</td><td>31</td><td>Georgia</td><td>74.92</td></tr>
<tr><td>16</td><td>New York</td><td>106.60</td><td>32</td><td>Missouri</td><td>74.24</td></tr>
<tr><td>26</td><td>North Carolina</td><td>88.51</td><td>33</td><td>Ohio</td><td>73.74</td></tr>
<tr><td>35</td><td>North Dakota</td><td>72.27</td><td>34</td><td>Virginia</td><td>73.14</td></tr>
<tr><td>33</td><td>Ohio</td><td>73.74</td><td>35</td><td>North Dakota</td><td>72.27</td></tr>
<tr><td>27</td><td>Oklahoma</td><td>86.30</td><td>36</td><td>Tennessee</td><td>70.79</td></tr>
<tr><td>13</td><td>Oregon</td><td>117.69</td><td>37</td><td>South Dakota</td><td>70.71</td></tr>
<tr><td>18</td><td>Pennsylvania</td><td>102.09</td><td>38</td><td>New Jersey</td><td>66.33</td></tr>
<tr><td>3</td><td>Rhode Island</td><td>176.16</td><td>39</td><td>Utah</td><td>65.63</td></tr>
<tr><td>10</td><td>South Carolina</td><td>128.91</td><td>40</td><td>Vermont</td><td>62.51</td></tr>
<tr><td>37</td><td>South Dakota</td><td>70.71</td><td>41</td><td>Colorado</td><td>61.94</td></tr>
<tr><td>36</td><td>Tennessee</td><td>70.79</td><td>42</td><td>Kansas</td><td>60.92</td></tr>
<tr><td>47</td><td>Texas</td><td>56.83</td><td>43</td><td>Mississippi</td><td>58.88</td></tr>
<tr><td>39</td><td>Utah</td><td>65.63</td><td>44</td><td>Indiana</td><td>58.68</td></tr>
<tr><td>40</td><td>Vermont</td><td>62.51</td><td>45</td><td>Kentucky</td><td>57.74</td></tr>
<tr><td>34</td><td>Virginia</td><td>73.14</td><td>46</td><td>Idaho</td><td>57.18</td></tr>
<tr><td>17</td><td>Washington</td><td>102.54</td><td>47</td><td>Texas</td><td>56.83</td></tr>
<tr><td>48</td><td>West Virginia</td><td>56.22</td><td>48</td><td>West Virginia</td><td>56.22</td></tr>
<tr><td>24</td><td>Wisconsin</td><td>90.50</td><td>49</td><td>Iowa</td><td>53.51</td></tr>
<tr><td>9</td><td>Wyoming</td><td>139.01</td><td>50</td><td>Nevada</td><td>43.86</td></tr>
<tr><td></td><td></td><td></td><td></td><td>District of Columbia**</td><td>NA</td></tr>
</table>

Source: Morgan Quitno Press using data from U.S. Bureau of the Census
   "State Government Finances: 1993"
*Includes outpatient health services other than hospital care, research and education, categorical health programs, treatment and immunization clinics, nursing and environmental health activities. Includes capital expenditures.
**Not applicable.

State Government Expenditures for Hospitals in 1993

National Total = $27,434,629,000*

ALPHA ORDER

RANK	STATE	EXPENDITURES	% of USA
10	Alabama	$887,835,000	3.24%
46	Alaska	35,341,000	0.13%
39	Arizona	71,652,000	0.26%
34	Arkansas	204,906,000	0.75%
2	California	2,818,232,000	10.27%
36	Colorado	179,713,000	0.66%
11	Connecticut	799,554,000	2.91%
44	Delaware	43,635,000	0.16%
22	Florida	457,908,000	1.67%
16	Georgia	569,756,000	2.08%
35	Hawaii	203,306,000	0.74%
49	Idaho	33,217,000	0.12%
13	Illinois	706,963,000	2.58%
20	Indiana	506,971,000	1.85%
19	Iowa	509,271,000	1.86%
28	Kansas	306,831,000	1.12%
29	Kentucky	295,982,000	1.08%
7	Louisiana	1,024,526,000	3.73%
40	Maine	61,439,000	0.22%
27	Maryland	322,539,000	1.18%
12	Massachusetts	760,360,000	2.77%
6	Michigan	1,097,617,000	4.00%
17	Minnesota	551,989,000	2.01%
31	Mississippi	265,741,000	0.97%
25	Missouri	400,882,000	1.46%
47	Montana	35,289,000	0.13%
33	Nebraska	250,434,000	0.91%
42	Nevada	48,913,000	0.18%
45	New Hampshire	38,164,000	0.14%
9	New Jersey	935,136,000	3.41%
32	New Mexico	257,522,000	0.94%
1	New York	3,484,401,000	12.70%
14	North Carolina	691,506,000	2.52%
41	North Dakota	60,297,000	0.22%
5	Ohio	1,183,524,000	4.31%
26	Oklahoma	328,749,000	1.20%
23	Oregon	447,585,000	1.63%
4	Pennsylvania	1,363,708,000	4.97%
38	Rhode Island	75,568,000	0.28%
15	South Carolina	607,963,000	2.22%
43	South Dakota	43,872,000	0.16%
21	Tennessee	462,828,000	1.69%
3	Texas	1,650,577,000	6.02%
30	Utah	267,195,000	0.97%
50	Vermont	20,596,000	0.08%
8	Virginia	998,622,000	3.64%
18	Washington	527,970,000	1.92%
37	West Virginia	93,704,000	0.34%
24	Wisconsin	410,249,000	1.50%
48	Wyoming	34,091,000	0.12%

RANK ORDER

RANK	STATE	EXPENDITURES	% of USA
1	New York	$3,484,401,000	12.70%
2	California	2,818,232,000	10.27%
3	Texas	1,650,577,000	6.02%
4	Pennsylvania	1,363,708,000	4.97%
5	Ohio	1,183,524,000	4.31%
6	Michigan	1,097,617,000	4.00%
7	Louisiana	1,024,526,000	3.73%
8	Virginia	998,622,000	3.64%
9	New Jersey	935,136,000	3.41%
10	Alabama	887,835,000	3.24%
11	Connecticut	799,554,000	2.91%
12	Massachusetts	760,360,000	2.77%
13	Illinois	706,963,000	2.58%
14	North Carolina	691,506,000	2.52%
15	South Carolina	607,963,000	2.22%
16	Georgia	569,756,000	2.08%
17	Minnesota	551,989,000	2.01%
18	Washington	527,970,000	1.92%
19	Iowa	509,271,000	1.86%
20	Indiana	506,971,000	1.85%
21	Tennessee	462,828,000	1.69%
22	Florida	457,908,000	1.67%
23	Oregon	447,585,000	1.63%
24	Wisconsin	410,249,000	1.50%
25	Missouri	400,882,000	1.46%
26	Oklahoma	328,749,000	1.20%
27	Maryland	322,539,000	1.18%
28	Kansas	306,831,000	1.12%
29	Kentucky	295,982,000	1.08%
30	Utah	267,195,000	0.97%
31	Mississippi	265,741,000	0.97%
32	New Mexico	257,522,000	0.94%
33	Nebraska	250,434,000	0.91%
34	Arkansas	204,906,000	0.75%
35	Hawaii	203,306,000	0.74%
36	Colorado	179,713,000	0.66%
37	West Virginia	93,704,000	0.34%
38	Rhode Island	75,568,000	0.28%
39	Arizona	71,652,000	0.26%
40	Maine	61,439,000	0.22%
41	North Dakota	60,297,000	0.22%
42	Nevada	48,913,000	0.18%
43	South Dakota	43,872,000	0.16%
44	Delaware	43,635,000	0.16%
45	New Hampshire	38,164,000	0.14%
46	Alaska	35,341,000	0.13%
47	Montana	35,289,000	0.13%
48	Wyoming	34,091,000	0.12%
49	Idaho	33,217,000	0.12%
50	Vermont	20,596,000	0.08%
	District of Columbia**	NA	NA

Source: U.S. Bureau of the Census
"State Government Finances: 1993"
*Financing, construction, acquisition, maintenance or operation of hospital facilities, provision of hospital care and support of public or private hospitals.
**Not applicable.

Per Capita State Government Expenditures for Hospitals in 1993

National Per Capita = $106.43*

ALPHA ORDER			RANK ORDER		
RANK	STATE	PER CAPITA	RANK	STATE	PER CAPITA
3	Alabama	$212.35	1	Connecticut	$243.92
40	Alaska	59.10	2	Louisiana	238.82
50	Arizona	18.16	3	Alabama	212.35
29	Arkansas	84.46	4	New York	191.95
27	California	90.28	5	Iowa	180.53
42	Colorado	50.42	6	Hawaii	174.36
1	Connecticut	243.92	7	South Carolina	167.48
37	Delaware	62.51	8	New Mexico	159.36
48	Florida	33.36	9	Nebraska	155.26
30	Georgia	82.55	10	Virginia	154.27
6	Hawaii	174.36	11	Oregon	147.47
49	Idaho	30.20	12	Utah	143.65
39	Illinois	60.50	13	Massachusetts	126.35
28	Indiana	88.85	14	Minnesota	122.01
5	Iowa	180.53	15	Kansas	121.04
15	Kansas	121.04	16	New Jersey	118.99
32	Kentucky	78.01	17	Michigan	116.03
2	Louisiana	238.82	18	Pennsylvania	113.36
43	Maine	49.55	19	Ohio	107.00
36	Maryland	65.05	20	Oklahoma	101.69
13	Massachusetts	126.35	21	Mississippi	100.66
17	Michigan	116.03	22	Washington	100.39
14	Minnesota	122.01	23	North Carolina	99.47
21	Mississippi	100.66	24	North Dakota	94.66
33	Missouri	76.58	25	Texas	91.59
44	Montana	41.96	26	Tennessee	90.86
9	Nebraska	155.26	27	California	90.28
46	Nevada	35.39	28	Indiana	88.85
47	New Hampshire	33.95	29	Arkansas	84.46
16	New Jersey	118.99	30	Georgia	82.55
8	New Mexico	159.36	31	Wisconsin	81.33
4	New York	191.95	32	Kentucky	78.01
23	North Carolina	99.47	33	Missouri	76.58
24	North Dakota	94.66	34	Rhode Island	75.57
19	Ohio	107.00	35	Wyoming	72.53
20	Oklahoma	101.69	36	Maryland	65.05
11	Oregon	147.47	37	Delaware	62.51
18	Pennsylvania	113.36	38	South Dakota	61.27
34	Rhode Island	75.57	39	Illinois	60.50
7	South Carolina	167.48	40	Alaska	59.10
38	South Dakota	61.27	41	West Virginia	51.54
26	Tennessee	90.86	42	Colorado	50.42
25	Texas	91.59	43	Maine	49.55
12	Utah	143.65	44	Montana	41.96
45	Vermont	35.76	45	Vermont	35.76
10	Virginia	154.27	46	Nevada	35.39
22	Washington	100.39	47	New Hampshire	33.95
41	West Virginia	51.54	48	Florida	33.36
31	Wisconsin	81.33	49	Idaho	30.20
35	Wyoming	72.53	50	Arizona	18.16
				District of Columbia**	NA

Source: Morgan Quitno Press using data from U.S. Bureau of the Census
   "State Government Finances: 1993"

Financing, construction, acquisition, maintenance or operation of hospital facilities, provision of hospital care and support of public or private hospitals.

**Not applicable.*

Receipts of Health Services Establishments in 1992

National Total = $623,480,434,000*

<table>
<tr><td colspan="4">ALPHA ORDER</td><td colspan="4">RANK ORDER</td></tr>
<tr><th>RANK</th><th>STATE</th><th>RECEIPTS</th><th>% of USA</th><th>RANK</th><th>STATE</th><th>RECEIPTS</th><th>% of USA</th></tr>
<tr><td>23</td><td>Alabama</td><td>$9,400,816,000</td><td>1.51%</td><td>1</td><td>California</td><td>$79,130,980,000</td><td>12.69%</td></tr>
<tr><td>48</td><td>Alaska</td><td>1,225,327,000</td><td>0.20%</td><td>2</td><td>New York</td><td>53,091,018,000</td><td>8.52%</td></tr>
<tr><td>24</td><td>Arizona</td><td>8,624,782,000</td><td>1.38%</td><td>3</td><td>Texas</td><td>38,769,630,000</td><td>6.22%</td></tr>
<tr><td>32</td><td>Arkansas</td><td>4,791,668,000</td><td>0.77%</td><td>4</td><td>Florida</td><td>36,667,132,000</td><td>5.88%</td></tr>
<tr><td>1</td><td>California</td><td>79,130,980,000</td><td>12.69%</td><td>5</td><td>Pennsylvania</td><td>33,155,698,000</td><td>5.32%</td></tr>
<tr><td>25</td><td>Colorado</td><td>8,000,876,000</td><td>1.28%</td><td>6</td><td>Illinois</td><td>27,961,997,000</td><td>4.48%</td></tr>
<tr><td>22</td><td>Connecticut</td><td>9,932,092,000</td><td>1.59%</td><td>7</td><td>Ohio</td><td>27,492,361,000</td><td>4.41%</td></tr>
<tr><td>43</td><td>Delaware</td><td>1,780,075,000</td><td>0.29%</td><td>8</td><td>Michigan</td><td>21,891,285,000</td><td>3.51%</td></tr>
<tr><td>4</td><td>Florida</td><td>36,667,132,000</td><td>5.88%</td><td>9</td><td>New Jersey</td><td>21,102,821,000</td><td>3.38%</td></tr>
<tr><td>11</td><td>Georgia</td><td>15,774,705,000</td><td>2.53%</td><td>10</td><td>Massachusetts</td><td>19,296,743,000</td><td>3.10%</td></tr>
<tr><td>39</td><td>Hawaii</td><td>2,757,575,000</td><td>0.44%</td><td>11</td><td>Georgia</td><td>15,774,705,000</td><td>2.53%</td></tr>
<tr><td>44</td><td>Idaho</td><td>1,775,447,000</td><td>0.28%</td><td>12</td><td>North Carolina</td><td>14,227,452,000</td><td>2.28%</td></tr>
<tr><td>6</td><td>Illinois</td><td>27,961,997,000</td><td>4.48%</td><td>13</td><td>Virginia</td><td>13,140,339,000</td><td>2.11%</td></tr>
<tr><td>14</td><td>Indiana</td><td>13,010,617,000</td><td>2.09%</td><td>14</td><td>Indiana</td><td>13,010,617,000</td><td>2.09%</td></tr>
<tr><td>30</td><td>Iowa</td><td>5,852,492,000</td><td>0.94%</td><td>15</td><td>Missouri</td><td>12,918,009,000</td><td>2.07%</td></tr>
<tr><td>31</td><td>Kansas</td><td>5,763,990,000</td><td>0.92%</td><td>16</td><td>Tennessee</td><td>12,807,220,000</td><td>2.05%</td></tr>
<tr><td>26</td><td>Kentucky</td><td>7,923,070,000</td><td>1.27%</td><td>17</td><td>Washington</td><td>12,022,436,000</td><td>1.93%</td></tr>
<tr><td>21</td><td>Louisiana</td><td>10,204,980,000</td><td>1.64%</td><td>18</td><td>Maryland</td><td>11,824,018,000</td><td>1.90%</td></tr>
<tr><td>40</td><td>Maine</td><td>2,666,876,000</td><td>0.43%</td><td>19</td><td>Wisconsin</td><td>11,288,091,000</td><td>1.81%</td></tr>
<tr><td>18</td><td>Maryland</td><td>11,824,018,000</td><td>1.90%</td><td>20</td><td>Minnesota</td><td>11,199,561,000</td><td>1.80%</td></tr>
<tr><td>10</td><td>Massachusetts</td><td>19,296,743,000</td><td>3.10%</td><td>21</td><td>Louisiana</td><td>10,204,980,000</td><td>1.64%</td></tr>
<tr><td>8</td><td>Michigan</td><td>21,891,285,000</td><td>3.51%</td><td>22</td><td>Connecticut</td><td>9,932,092,000</td><td>1.59%</td></tr>
<tr><td>20</td><td>Minnesota</td><td>11,199,561,000</td><td>1.80%</td><td>23</td><td>Alabama</td><td>9,400,816,000</td><td>1.51%</td></tr>
<tr><td>33</td><td>Mississippi</td><td>4,605,036,000</td><td>0.74%</td><td>24</td><td>Arizona</td><td>8,624,782,000</td><td>1.38%</td></tr>
<tr><td>15</td><td>Missouri</td><td>12,918,009,000</td><td>2.07%</td><td>25</td><td>Colorado</td><td>8,000,876,000</td><td>1.28%</td></tr>
<tr><td>46</td><td>Montana</td><td>1,589,295,000</td><td>0.25%</td><td>26</td><td>Kentucky</td><td>7,923,070,000</td><td>1.27%</td></tr>
<tr><td>35</td><td>Nebraska</td><td>3,483,096,000</td><td>0.56%</td><td>27</td><td>South Carolina</td><td>6,612,570,000</td><td>1.06%</td></tr>
<tr><td>37</td><td>Nevada</td><td>3,016,118,000</td><td>0.48%</td><td>28</td><td>Oklahoma</td><td>6,268,749,000</td><td>1.01%</td></tr>
<tr><td>41</td><td>New Hampshire</td><td>2,642,095,000</td><td>0.42%</td><td>29</td><td>Oregon</td><td>6,137,525,000</td><td>0.98%</td></tr>
<tr><td>9</td><td>New Jersey</td><td>21,102,821,000</td><td>3.38%</td><td>30</td><td>Iowa</td><td>5,852,492,000</td><td>0.94%</td></tr>
<tr><td>38</td><td>New Mexico</td><td>2,881,524,000</td><td>0.46%</td><td>31</td><td>Kansas</td><td>5,763,990,000</td><td>0.92%</td></tr>
<tr><td>2</td><td>New York</td><td>53,091,018,000</td><td>8.52%</td><td>32</td><td>Arkansas</td><td>4,791,668,000</td><td>0.77%</td></tr>
<tr><td>12</td><td>North Carolina</td><td>14,227,452,000</td><td>2.28%</td><td>33</td><td>Mississippi</td><td>4,605,036,000</td><td>0.74%</td></tr>
<tr><td>45</td><td>North Dakota</td><td>1,651,634,000</td><td>0.26%</td><td>34</td><td>West Virginia</td><td>4,040,621,000</td><td>0.65%</td></tr>
<tr><td>7</td><td>Ohio</td><td>27,492,361,000</td><td>4.41%</td><td>35</td><td>Nebraska</td><td>3,483,096,000</td><td>0.56%</td></tr>
<tr><td>28</td><td>Oklahoma</td><td>6,268,749,000</td><td>1.01%</td><td>36</td><td>Utah</td><td>3,216,121,000</td><td>0.52%</td></tr>
<tr><td>29</td><td>Oregon</td><td>6,137,525,000</td><td>0.98%</td><td>37</td><td>Nevada</td><td>3,016,118,000</td><td>0.48%</td></tr>
<tr><td>5</td><td>Pennsylvania</td><td>33,155,698,000</td><td>5.32%</td><td>38</td><td>New Mexico</td><td>2,881,524,000</td><td>0.46%</td></tr>
<tr><td>42</td><td>Rhode Island</td><td>2,617,386,000</td><td>0.42%</td><td>39</td><td>Hawaii</td><td>2,757,575,000</td><td>0.44%</td></tr>
<tr><td>27</td><td>South Carolina</td><td>6,612,570,000</td><td>1.06%</td><td>40</td><td>Maine</td><td>2,666,876,000</td><td>0.43%</td></tr>
<tr><td>47</td><td>South Dakota</td><td>1,543,627,000</td><td>0.25%</td><td>41</td><td>New Hampshire</td><td>2,642,095,000</td><td>0.42%</td></tr>
<tr><td>16</td><td>Tennessee</td><td>12,807,220,000</td><td>2.05%</td><td>42</td><td>Rhode Island</td><td>2,617,386,000</td><td>0.42%</td></tr>
<tr><td>3</td><td>Texas</td><td>38,769,630,000</td><td>6.22%</td><td>43</td><td>Delaware</td><td>1,780,075,000</td><td>0.29%</td></tr>
<tr><td>36</td><td>Utah</td><td>3,216,121,000</td><td>0.52%</td><td>44</td><td>Idaho</td><td>1,775,447,000</td><td>0.28%</td></tr>
<tr><td>49</td><td>Vermont</td><td>1,121,735,000</td><td>0.18%</td><td>45</td><td>North Dakota</td><td>1,651,634,000</td><td>0.26%</td></tr>
<tr><td>13</td><td>Virginia</td><td>13,140,339,000</td><td>2.11%</td><td>46</td><td>Montana</td><td>1,589,295,000</td><td>0.25%</td></tr>
<tr><td>17</td><td>Washington</td><td>12,022,436,000</td><td>1.93%</td><td>47</td><td>South Dakota</td><td>1,543,627,000</td><td>0.25%</td></tr>
<tr><td>34</td><td>West Virginia</td><td>4,040,621,000</td><td>0.65%</td><td>48</td><td>Alaska</td><td>1,225,327,000</td><td>0.20%</td></tr>
<tr><td>19</td><td>Wisconsin</td><td>11,288,091,000</td><td>1.81%</td><td>49</td><td>Vermont</td><td>1,121,735,000</td><td>0.18%</td></tr>
<tr><td>50</td><td>Wyoming</td><td>708,286,000</td><td>0.11%</td><td>50</td><td>Wyoming</td><td>708,286,000</td><td>0.11%</td></tr>
<tr><td></td><td></td><td></td><td></td><td></td><td>District of Columbia</td><td>3,872,837,000</td><td>0.62%</td></tr>
</table>

Source: Morgan Quitno Press using data from U.S. Bureau of the Census
"1992 Census of Service Industries, Geographic Area Series, United States" (SC92-A-52)
*Includes establishments exempt from as well as subject to the federal income tax. Includes those establishments within the Standard Industry Classification (SIC) 80. These include those primarily engaged in furnishing medical, surgical and other health services to persons. See Facilities Chapter for establishments.

Receipts per Health Service Establishment in 1992

National Rate = $1,339,792 per Establishment*

ALPHA ORDER				RANK ORDER		
RANK	STATE	PER ESTABLISHMENT		RANK	STATE	PER ESTABLISHMENT
4	Alabama	$1,606,428		1	North Dakota	$1,736,734
27	Alaska	1,304,928		2	Massachusetts	1,700,753
40	Arizona	1,155,517		3	Minnesota	1,676,581
31	Arkansas	1,261,297		4	Alabama	1,606,428
33	California	1,251,696		5	New York	1,549,922
44	Colorado	1,081,199		6	North Carolina	1,520,839
10	Connecticut	1,430,931		7	Tennessee	1,478,040
13	Delaware	1,419,518		8	Missouri	1,452,768
38	Florida	1,201,768		9	Wisconsin	1,438,340
19	Georgia	1,375,541		10	Connecticut	1,430,931
39	Hawaii	1,183,509		11	Louisiana	1,430,872
48	Idaho	966,493		12	Pennsylvania	1,420,492
14	Illinois	1,415,296		13	Delaware	1,419,518
15	Indiana	1,392,701		14	Illinois	1,415,296
32	Iowa	1,252,942		15	Indiana	1,392,701
20	Kansas	1,360,073		16	Mississippi	1,391,670
24	Kentucky	1,322,495		17	Ohio	1,388,854
11	Louisiana	1,430,872		18	West Virginia	1,378,111
42	Maine	1,114,449		19	Georgia	1,375,541
35	Maryland	1,244,110		20	Kansas	1,360,073
2	Massachusetts	1,700,753		21	South Carolina	1,357,817
26	Michigan	1,307,333		22	Nebraska	1,348,469
3	Minnesota	1,676,581		23	South Dakota	1,348,146
16	Mississippi	1,391,670		24	Kentucky	1,322,495
8	Missouri	1,452,768		25	New Hampshire	1,312,516
49	Montana	944,323		26	Michigan	1,307,333
22	Nebraska	1,348,469		27	Alaska	1,304,928
29	Nevada	1,274,237		28	Virginia	1,298,581
25	New Hampshire	1,312,516		29	Nevada	1,274,237
36	New Jersey	1,239,884		30	Rhode Island	1,265,661
43	New Mexico	1,109,132		31	Arkansas	1,261,297
5	New York	1,549,922		32	Iowa	1,252,942
6	North Carolina	1,520,839		33	California	1,251,696
1	North Dakota	1,736,734		34	Texas	1,249,666
17	Ohio	1,388,854		35	Maryland	1,244,110
41	Oklahoma	1,116,032		36	New Jersey	1,239,884
45	Oregon	1,041,317		37	Washington	1,237,003
12	Pennsylvania	1,420,492		38	Florida	1,201,768
30	Rhode Island	1,265,661		39	Hawaii	1,183,509
21	South Carolina	1,357,817		40	Arizona	1,155,517
23	South Dakota	1,348,146		41	Oklahoma	1,116,032
7	Tennessee	1,478,040		42	Maine	1,114,449
34	Texas	1,249,666		43	New Mexico	1,109,132
47	Utah	1,021,964		44	Colorado	1,081,199
46	Vermont	1,040,571		45	Oregon	1,041,317
28	Virginia	1,298,581		46	Vermont	1,040,571
37	Washington	1,237,003		47	Utah	1,021,964
18	West Virginia	1,378,111		48	Idaho	966,493
9	Wisconsin	1,438,340		49	Montana	944,323
50	Wyoming	897,701		50	Wyoming	897,701
					District of Columbia	2,639,971

Source: Morgan Quitno Press using data from U.S. Bureau of the Census
"1992 Census of Service Industries, Geographic Area Series, United States" (SC92-A-52)
*Includes establishments exempt from as well as subject to the federal income tax. Includes those establishments within the Standard Industry Classification (SIC) 80. These include those primarily engaged in furnishing medical, surgical and other health services to persons. See Facilities Chapter for establishments.

Receipts of Offices and Clinics of Doctors of Medicine in 1992

National Total = $141,429,109,000*

ALPHA ORDER					RANK ORDER			
RANK	STATE	RECEIPTS	% of USA		RANK	STATE	RECEIPTS	% of USA
23	Alabama	$2,194,200,000	1.55%		1	California	$21,969,551,000	15.53%
48	Alaska	257,847,000	0.18%		2	Florida	10,360,884,000	7.33%
21	Arizona	2,358,063,000	1.67%		3	New York	9,895,040,000	7.00%
31	Arkansas	1,184,434,000	0.84%		4	Texas	9,488,688,000	6.71%
1	California	21,969,551,000	15.53%		5	Illinois	6,252,042,000	4.42%
26	Colorado	1,823,874,000	1.29%		6	Pennsylvania	6,183,845,000	4.37%
22	Connecticut	2,264,576,000	1.60%		7	Ohio	5,703,695,000	4.03%
45	Delaware	402,076,000	0.28%		8	New Jersey	5,079,647,000	3.59%
2	Florida	10,360,884,000	7.33%		9	Georgia	4,096,050,000	2.90%
9	Georgia	4,096,050,000	2.90%		10	Michigan	3,899,622,000	2.76%
38	Hawaii	621,177,000	0.44%		11	Virginia	3,207,044,000	2.27%
43	Idaho	435,493,000	0.31%		12	North Carolina	3,170,587,000	2.24%
5	Illinois	6,252,042,000	4.42%		13	Massachusetts	3,103,826,000	2.19%
16	Indiana	2,829,577,000	2.00%		14	Maryland	3,054,253,000	2.16%
32	Iowa	1,169,464,000	0.83%		15	Tennessee	2,927,905,000	2.07%
30	Kansas	1,269,708,000	0.90%		16	Indiana	2,829,577,000	2.00%
25	Kentucky	1,867,177,000	1.32%		17	Missouri	2,562,807,000	1.81%
20	Louisiana	2,411,609,000	1.71%		18	Wisconsin	2,415,679,000	1.71%
41	Maine	493,897,000	0.35%		19	Washington	2,415,635,000	1.71%
14	Maryland	3,054,253,000	2.16%		20	Louisiana	2,411,609,000	1.71%
13	Massachusetts	3,103,826,000	2.19%		21	Arizona	2,358,063,000	1.67%
10	Michigan	3,899,622,000	2.76%		22	Connecticut	2,264,576,000	1.60%
24	Minnesota	1,964,322,000	1.39%		23	Alabama	2,194,200,000	1.55%
33	Mississippi	968,510,000	0.68%		24	Minnesota	1,964,322,000	1.39%
17	Missouri	2,562,807,000	1.81%		25	Kentucky	1,867,177,000	1.32%
46	Montana	336,865,000	0.24%		26	Colorado	1,823,874,000	1.29%
37	Nebraska	750,417,000	0.53%		27	Oregon	1,491,857,000	1.05%
34	Nevada	947,372,000	0.67%		28	South Carolina	1,491,246,000	1.05%
40	New Hampshire	495,024,000	0.35%		29	Oklahoma	1,366,055,000	0.97%
8	New Jersey	5,079,647,000	3.59%		30	Kansas	1,269,708,000	0.90%
39	New Mexico	620,805,000	0.44%		31	Arkansas	1,184,434,000	0.84%
3	New York	9,895,040,000	7.00%		32	Iowa	1,169,464,000	0.83%
12	North Carolina	3,170,587,000	2.24%		33	Mississippi	968,510,000	0.68%
44	North Dakota	422,058,000	0.30%		34	Nevada	947,372,000	0.67%
7	Ohio	5,703,695,000	4.03%		35	West Virginia	848,606,000	0.60%
29	Oklahoma	1,366,055,000	0.97%		36	Utah	816,997,000	0.58%
27	Oregon	1,491,857,000	1.05%		37	Nebraska	750,417,000	0.53%
6	Pennsylvania	6,183,845,000	4.37%		38	Hawaii	621,177,000	0.44%
42	Rhode Island	458,399,000	0.32%		39	New Mexico	620,805,000	0.44%
28	South Carolina	1,491,246,000	1.05%		40	New Hampshire	495,024,000	0.35%
47	South Dakota	305,158,000	0.22%		41	Maine	493,897,000	0.35%
15	Tennessee	2,927,905,000	2.07%		42	Rhode Island	458,399,000	0.32%
4	Texas	9,488,688,000	6.71%		43	Idaho	435,493,000	0.31%
36	Utah	816,997,000	0.58%		44	North Dakota	422,058,000	0.30%
49	Vermont	187,557,000	0.13%		45	Delaware	402,076,000	0.28%
11	Virginia	3,207,044,000	2.27%		46	Montana	336,865,000	0.24%
19	Washington	2,415,635,000	1.71%		47	South Dakota	305,158,000	0.22%
35	West Virginia	848,606,000	0.60%		48	Alaska	257,847,000	0.18%
18	Wisconsin	2,415,679,000	1.71%		49	Vermont	187,557,000	0.13%
50	Wyoming	148,221,000	0.10%		50	Wyoming	148,221,000	0.10%
					District of Columbia		439,668,000	0.31%

Source: U.S. Bureau of the Census

"1992 Census of Service Industries, Geographic Area Series, United States" (SC92-A-52)

Includes only establishments subject to the federal income tax. See Facilities Chapter for establishments.

Receipts per Office or Clinic of Doctors of Medicine in 1992

National Rate = $715,369 per Establishment*

ALPHA ORDER				RANK ORDER		
RANK	STATE	PER ESTABLISHMENT		RANK	STATE	PER ESTABLISHMENT
9	Alabama	$840,368		1	North Dakota	$1,736,864
19	Alaska	738,817		2	Minnesota	1,327,245
16	Arizona	748,591		3	Wisconsin	948,813
24	Arkansas	711,799		4	Kansas	918,747
13	California	771,024		5	South Dakota	874,378
29	Colorado	676,010		6	Iowa	866,912
17	Connecticut	745,171		7	Nevada	864,391
27	Delaware	684,968		8	Nebraska	846,972
22	Florida	715,185		9	Alabama	840,368
11	Georgia	785,587		10	North Carolina	828,695
45	Hawaii	582,718		11	Georgia	785,587
44	Idaho	598,205		12	Missouri	781,344
18	Illinois	742,170		13	California	771,024
15	Indiana	755,763		14	Tennessee	762,475
6	Iowa	866,912		15	Indiana	755,763
4	Kansas	918,747		16	Arizona	748,591
21	Kentucky	727,944		17	Connecticut	745,171
20	Louisiana	732,344		18	Illinois	742,170
47	Maine	540,369		19	Alaska	738,817
40	Maryland	641,650		20	Louisiana	732,344
26	Massachusetts	686,080		21	Kentucky	727,944
37	Michigan	657,055		22	Florida	715,185
2	Minnesota	1,327,245		23	Ohio	712,606
32	Mississippi	664,273		24	Arkansas	711,799
12	Missouri	781,344		25	Washington	697,354
46	Montana	562,379		26	Massachusetts	686,080
8	Nebraska	846,972		27	Delaware	684,968
7	Nevada	864,391		28	Virginia	678,883
38	New Hampshire	656,531		29	Colorado	676,010
36	New Jersey	658,156		30	South Carolina	672,035
43	New Mexico	600,973		31	Oklahoma	665,719
42	New York	609,826		32	Mississippi	664,273
10	North Carolina	828,695		33	Pennsylvania	661,586
1	North Dakota	1,736,864		34	Texas	660,450
23	Ohio	712,606		35	Oregon	659,239
31	Oklahoma	665,719		36	New Jersey	658,156
35	Oregon	659,239		37	Michigan	657,055
33	Pennsylvania	661,586		38	New Hampshire	656,531
48	Rhode Island	515,634		39	Utah	647,896
30	South Carolina	672,035		40	Maryland	641,650
5	South Dakota	874,378		41	West Virginia	633,288
14	Tennessee	762,475		42	New York	609,826
34	Texas	660,450		43	New Mexico	600,973
39	Utah	647,896		44	Idaho	598,205
50	Vermont	477,244		45	Hawaii	582,718
28	Virginia	678,883		46	Montana	562,379
25	Washington	697,354		47	Maine	540,369
41	West Virginia	633,288		48	Rhode Island	515,634
3	Wisconsin	948,813		49	Wyoming	504,153
49	Wyoming	504,153		50	Vermont	477,244
					District of Columbia	568,781

Source: Morgan Quitno Press using data from U.S. Bureau of the Census
    "1992 Census of Service Industries, Geographic Area Series, United States" (SC92-A-52)
*Includes only establishments subject to the federal income tax. See Facilities Chapter for establishments.

Receipts of Offices and Clinics of Dentists in 1992

National Total = $35,522,953,000*

ALPHA ORDER					RANK ORDER			

RANK	STATE	RECEIPTS	% of USA
25	Alabama	$423,367,000	1.30%
44	Alaska	114,760,000	0.35%
24	Arizona	506,268,000	1.56%
33	Arkansas	226,609,000	0.70%
1	California	5,523,663,000	16.98%
22	Colorado	555,652,000	1.71%
18	Connecticut	669,243,000	2.06%
45	Delaware	102,416,000	0.31%
4	Florida	1,893,179,000	5.82%
19	Georgia	644,777,000	1.98%
34	Hawaii	219,683,000	0.68%
42	Idaho	150,221,000	0.46%
6	Illinois	1,510,700,000	4.65%
12	Indiana	840,283,000	2.58%
30	Iowa	320,371,000	0.99%
31	Kansas	306,171,000	0.94%
28	Kentucky	338,975,000	1.04%
26	Louisiana	409,110,000	1.26%
41	Maine	150,904,000	0.46%
16	Maryland	713,076,000	2.19%
11	Massachusetts	992,382,000	3.05%
7	Michigan	1,475,023,000	4.54%
17	Minnesota	686,914,000	2.11%
36	Mississippi	198,070,000	0.61%
21	Missouri	569,399,000	1.75%
46	Montana	96,335,000	0.30%
37	Nebraska	185,366,000	0.57%
35	Nevada	204,068,000	0.63%
39	New Hampshire	167,595,000	0.52%
8	New Jersey	1,415,884,000	4.35%
40	New Mexico	160,064,000	0.49%
2	New York	2,770,069,000	8.52%
14	North Carolina	760,910,000	2.34%
49	North Dakota	70,632,000	0.22%
9	Ohio	1,337,215,000	4.11%
29	Oklahoma	338,025,000	1.04%
23	Oregon	526,242,000	1.62%
5	Pennsylvania	1,571,424,000	4.83%
43	Rhode Island	148,838,000	0.46%
27	South Carolina	364,380,000	1.12%
47	South Dakota	79,410,000	0.24%
20	Tennessee	572,138,000	1.76%
3	Texas	1,919,816,000	5.90%
32	Utah	257,633,000	0.79%
48	Vermont	78,673,000	0.24%
13	Virginia	811,992,000	2.50%
10	Washington	1,088,396,000	3.35%
38	West Virginia	174,028,000	0.54%
15	Wisconsin	718,189,000	2.21%
50	Wyoming	52,712,000	0.16%

RANK	STATE	RECEIPTS	% of USA
1	California	$5,523,663,000	16.98%
2	New York	2,770,069,000	8.52%
3	Texas	1,919,816,000	5.90%
4	Florida	1,893,179,000	5.82%
5	Pennsylvania	1,571,424,000	4.83%
6	Illinois	1,510,700,000	4.65%
7	Michigan	1,475,023,000	4.54%
8	New Jersey	1,415,884,000	4.35%
9	Ohio	1,337,215,000	4.11%
10	Washington	1,088,396,000	3.35%
11	Massachusetts	992,382,000	3.05%
12	Indiana	840,283,000	2.58%
13	Virginia	811,992,000	2.50%
14	North Carolina	760,910,000	2.34%
15	Wisconsin	718,189,000	2.21%
16	Maryland	713,076,000	2.19%
17	Minnesota	686,914,000	2.11%
18	Connecticut	669,243,000	2.06%
19	Georgia	644,777,000	1.98%
20	Tennessee	572,138,000	1.76%
21	Missouri	569,399,000	1.75%
22	Colorado	555,652,000	1.71%
23	Oregon	526,242,000	1.62%
24	Arizona	506,268,000	1.56%
25	Alabama	423,367,000	1.30%
26	Louisiana	409,110,000	1.26%
27	South Carolina	364,380,000	1.12%
28	Kentucky	338,975,000	1.04%
29	Oklahoma	338,025,000	1.04%
30	Iowa	320,371,000	0.99%
31	Kansas	306,171,000	0.94%
32	Utah	257,633,000	0.79%
33	Arkansas	226,609,000	0.70%
34	Hawaii	219,683,000	0.68%
35	Nevada	204,068,000	0.63%
36	Mississippi	198,070,000	0.61%
37	Nebraska	185,366,000	0.57%
38	West Virginia	174,028,000	0.54%
39	New Hampshire	167,595,000	0.52%
40	New Mexico	160,064,000	0.49%
41	Maine	150,904,000	0.46%
42	Idaho	150,221,000	0.46%
43	Rhode Island	148,838,000	0.46%
44	Alaska	114,760,000	0.35%
45	Delaware	102,416,000	0.31%
46	Montana	96,335,000	0.30%
47	South Dakota	79,410,000	0.24%
48	Vermont	78,673,000	0.24%
49	North Dakota	70,632,000	0.22%
50	Wyoming	52,712,000	0.16%
	District of Columbia	111,703,000	0.34%

Source: U.S. Bureau of the Census
   "1992 Census of Service Industries, Geographic Area Series, United States" (SC92-A-52)
*Includes only establishments subject to the federal income tax. See Facilities Chapter for establishments.

Receipts per Office or Clinic of Dentists in 1992

National Rate = $326,486 per Establishment*

ALPHA ORDER			RANK ORDER		
RANK	STATE	PER ESTABLISHMENT	RANK	STATE	PER ESTABLISHMENT
26	Alabama	$318,082	1	Delaware	$476,353
2	Alaska	438,015	2	Alaska	438,015
16	Arizona	332,633	3	Nevada	426,921
41	Arkansas	275,680	4	Washington	407,029
7	California	373,069	5	Indiana	385,982
36	Colorado	290,765	6	Connecticut	384,622
6	Connecticut	384,622	7	California	373,069
1	Delaware	476,353	8	Rhode Island	366,596
9	Florida	352,285	9	Florida	352,285
43	Georgia	274,841	10	North Carolina	351,947
12	Hawaii	343,255	11	New Jersey	351,075
18	Idaho	330,156	12	Hawaii	343,255
35	Illinois	292,998	13	Minnesota	341,748
5	Indiana	385,982	14	Michigan	339,242
39	Iowa	278,826	15	Massachusetts	337,430
31	Kansas	305,255	16	Arizona	332,633
50	Kentucky	231,857	17	Oregon	331,595
45	Louisiana	264,283	18	Idaho	330,156
19	Maine	329,485	19	Maine	329,485
21	Maryland	324,864	20	New Hampshire	326,060
15	Massachusetts	337,430	21	Maryland	324,864
14	Michigan	339,242	22	New York	323,606
13	Minnesota	341,748	23	Virginia	321,708
47	Mississippi	252,640	24	Wisconsin	321,337
40	Missouri	278,163	25	Vermont	321,114
49	Montana	242,657	26	Alabama	318,082
48	Nebraska	248,147	27	South Carolina	316,028
3	Nevada	426,921	28	West Virginia	309,108
20	New Hampshire	326,060	29	Texas	308,008
11	New Jersey	351,075	30	South Dakota	305,423
32	New Mexico	300,872	31	Kansas	305,255
22	New York	323,606	32	New Mexico	300,872
10	North Carolina	351,947	33	Ohio	297,357
38	North Dakota	282,528	34	Pennsylvania	295,603
33	Ohio	297,357	35	Illinois	292,998
42	Oklahoma	275,041	36	Colorado	290,765
17	Oregon	331,595	37	Tennessee	288,376
34	Pennsylvania	295,603	38	North Dakota	282,528
8	Rhode Island	366,596	39	Iowa	278,826
27	South Carolina	316,028	40	Missouri	278,163
30	South Dakota	305,423	41	Arkansas	275,680
37	Tennessee	288,376	42	Oklahoma	275,041
29	Texas	308,008	43	Georgia	274,841
44	Utah	264,510	44	Utah	264,510
25	Vermont	321,114	45	Louisiana	264,283
23	Virginia	321,708	46	Wyoming	260,950
4	Washington	407,029	47	Mississippi	252,640
28	West Virginia	309,108	48	Nebraska	248,147
24	Wisconsin	321,337	49	Montana	242,657
46	Wyoming	260,950	50	Kentucky	231,857
				District of Columbia	321,911

Source: Morgan Quitno Press using data from U.S. Bureau of the Census
  "1992 Census of Service Industries, Geographic Area Series, United States" (SC92-A-52)
Includes only establishments subject to the federal income tax. See Facilities Chapter for establishments.

Receipts of Offices and Clinics of Doctors of Osteopathy in 1992

National Total = $3,638,144,000*

ALPHA ORDER

ALPHA ORDER

RANK	STATE	RECEIPTS	% of USA
31	Alabama	$10,073,000	0.28%
36	Alaska	5,757,000	0.16%
8	Arizona	141,382,000	3.89%
33	Arkansas	7,486,000	0.21%
9	California	128,791,000	3.54%
13	Colorado	68,206,000	1.87%
NA	Connecticut**	NA	NA
23	Delaware	23,457,000	0.64%
4	Florida	325,522,000	8.95%
17	Georgia	42,184,000	1.16%
NA	Hawaii**	NA	NA
37	Idaho	4,797,000	0.13%
14	Illinois	62,781,000	1.73%
15	Indiana	54,594,000	1.50%
11	Iowa	77,485,000	2.13%
18	Kansas	39,828,000	1.09%
30	Kentucky	10,275,000	0.28%
44	Louisiana	1,804,000	0.05%
20	Maine	36,670,000	1.01%
38	Maryland	4,765,000	0.13%
29	Massachusetts	10,746,000	0.30%
1	Michigan	593,339,000	16.31%
NA	Minnesota**	NA	NA
32	Mississippi	8,865,000	0.24%
7	Missouri	160,312,000	4.41%
41	Montana	3,003,000	0.08%
NA	Nebraska**	NA	NA
27	Nevada	16,329,000	0.45%
42	New Hampshire	2,867,000	0.08%
6	New Jersey	213,199,000	5.86%
25	New Mexico	18,596,000	0.51%
12	New York	74,955,000	2.06%
35	North Carolina	6,445,000	0.18%
NA	North Dakota**	NA	NA
3	Ohio	386,003,000	10.61%
10	Oklahoma	127,260,000	3.50%
22	Oregon	32,862,000	0.90%
2	Pennsylvania	447,326,000	12.30%
26	Rhode Island	16,940,000	0.47%
34	South Carolina	6,489,000	0.18%
39	South Dakota	3,914,000	0.11%
24	Tennessee	22,588,000	0.62%
5	Texas	286,680,000	7.88%
40	Utah	3,446,000	0.09%
45	Vermont	1,074,000	0.03%
28	Virginia	13,366,000	0.37%
16	Washington	46,322,000	1.27%
19	West Virginia	37,666,000	1.04%
21	Wisconsin	36,056,000	0.99%
43	Wyoming	2,617,000	0.07%

RANK ORDER

RANK	STATE	RECEIPTS	% of USA
1	Michigan	$593,339,000	16.31%
2	Pennsylvania	447,326,000	12.30%
3	Ohio	386,003,000	10.61%
4	Florida	325,522,000	8.95%
5	Texas	286,680,000	7.88%
6	New Jersey	213,199,000	5.86%
7	Missouri	160,312,000	4.41%
8	Arizona	141,382,000	3.89%
9	California	128,791,000	3.54%
10	Oklahoma	127,260,000	3.50%
11	Iowa	77,485,000	2.13%
12	New York	74,955,000	2.06%
13	Colorado	68,206,000	1.87%
14	Illinois	62,781,000	1.73%
15	Indiana	54,594,000	1.50%
16	Washington	46,322,000	1.27%
17	Georgia	42,184,000	1.16%
18	Kansas	39,828,000	1.09%
19	West Virginia	37,666,000	1.04%
20	Maine	36,670,000	1.01%
21	Wisconsin	36,056,000	0.99%
22	Oregon	32,862,000	0.90%
23	Delaware	23,457,000	0.64%
24	Tennessee	22,588,000	0.62%
25	New Mexico	18,596,000	0.51%
26	Rhode Island	16,940,000	0.47%
27	Nevada	16,329,000	0.45%
28	Virginia	13,366,000	0.37%
29	Massachusetts	10,746,000	0.30%
30	Kentucky	10,275,000	0.28%
31	Alabama	10,073,000	0.28%
32	Mississippi	8,865,000	0.24%
33	Arkansas	7,486,000	0.21%
34	South Carolina	6,489,000	0.18%
35	North Carolina	6,445,000	0.18%
36	Alaska	5,757,000	0.16%
37	Idaho	4,797,000	0.13%
38	Maryland	4,765,000	0.13%
39	South Dakota	3,914,000	0.11%
40	Utah	3,446,000	0.09%
41	Montana	3,003,000	0.08%
42	New Hampshire	2,867,000	0.08%
43	Wyoming	2,617,000	0.07%
44	Louisiana	1,804,000	0.05%
45	Vermont	1,074,000	0.03%
NA	Connecticut**	NA	NA
NA	Hawaii**	NA	NA
NA	Minnesota**	NA	NA
NA	Nebraska**	NA	NA
NA	North Dakota**	NA	NA
	District of Columbia**	NA	NA

Source: U.S. Bureau of the Census
 "1992 Census of Service Industries, Geographic Area Series, United States" (SC92-A-52)
*Includes only establishments subject to the federal income tax. See Facilities Chapter for establishments.
**Not available.

Receipts per Office or Clinic of Doctors of Osteopathy in 1992

National Rate = $417,793 per Establishment*

RANK	STATE	PER ESTABLISHMENT		RANK	STATE	PER ESTABLISHMENT
ALPHA ORDER				**RANK ORDER**		
32	Alabama	$314,781		1	New Jersey	$534,333
2	Alaska	523,364		2	Alaska	523,364
6	Arizona	446,000		3	Michigan	494,037
40	Arkansas	287,923		4	Ohio	470,162
16	California	399,972		5	Delaware	469,140
29	Colorado	329,498		6	Arizona	446,000
NA	Connecticut**	NA		7	Mississippi	443,250
5	Delaware	469,140		8	South Dakota	434,889
10	Florida	427,194		9	Tennessee	434,385
27	Georgia	340,194		10	Florida	427,194
NA	Hawaii**	NA		11	Pennsylvania	421,211
22	Idaho	369,000		12	West Virginia	418,511
23	Illinois	362,896		13	Kansas	410,598
19	Indiana	384,465		14	Texas	405,488
15	Iowa	401,477		15	Iowa	401,477
13	Kansas	410,598		16	California	399,972
41	Kentucky	270,395		17	Nevada	398,268
37	Louisiana	300,667		18	Oklahoma	387,988
36	Maine	305,583		19	Indiana	384,465
38	Maryland	297,813		20	Wisconsin	375,583
42	Massachusetts	268,650		21	New York	372,910
3	Michigan	494,037		22	Idaho	369,000
NA	Minnesota**	NA		23	Illinois	362,896
7	Mississippi	443,250		24	Missouri	359,444
24	Missouri	359,444		25	Utah	344,600
44	Montana	250,250		26	Virginia	342,718
NA	Nebraska**	NA		27	Georgia	340,194
17	Nevada	398,268		28	North Carolina	339,211
31	New Hampshire	318,556		29	Colorado	329,498
1	New Jersey	534,333		30	New Mexico	326,246
30	New Mexico	326,246		31	New Hampshire	318,556
21	New York	372,910		32	Alabama	314,781
28	North Carolina	339,211		33	Washington	310,886
NA	North Dakota**	NA		34	South Carolina	309,000
4	Ohio	470,162		35	Rhode Island	308,000
18	Oklahoma	387,988		36	Maine	305,583
39	Oregon	293,411		37	Louisiana	300,667
11	Pennsylvania	421,211		38	Maryland	297,813
35	Rhode Island	308,000		39	Oregon	293,411
34	South Carolina	309,000		40	Arkansas	287,923
8	South Dakota	434,889		41	Kentucky	270,395
9	Tennessee	434,385		42	Massachusetts	268,650
14	Texas	405,488		43	Wyoming	261,700
25	Utah	344,600		44	Montana	250,250
45	Vermont	179,000		45	Vermont	179,000
26	Virginia	342,718		NA	Connecticut**	NA
33	Washington	310,886		NA	Hawaii**	NA
12	West Virginia	418,511		NA	Minnesota**	NA
20	Wisconsin	375,583		NA	Nebraska**	NA
43	Wyoming	261,700		NA	North Dakota**	NA
					District of Columbia**	NA

Source: Morgan Quitno Press using data from U.S. Bureau of the Census
"1992 Census of Service Industries, Geographic Area Series, United States" (SC92-A-52)
*Includes only establishments subject to the federal income tax. See Facilities Chapter for establishments.
**Not available.

Receipts of Offices and Clinics of Chiropractors in 1992

National Total = $5,917,909,000*

ALPHA ORDER					RANK ORDER			

RANK	STATE	RECEIPTS	% of USA	RANK	STATE	RECEIPTS	% of USA
31	Alabama	$50,995,000	0.86%	1	California	$972,152,000	16.43%
41	Alaska	21,901,000	0.37%	2	Florida	444,248,000	7.51%
15	Arizona	123,169,000	2.08%	3	New York	388,348,000	6.56%
33	Arkansas	39,365,000	0.67%	4	Texas	331,418,000	5.60%
1	California	972,152,000	16.43%	5	New Jersey	326,710,000	5.52%
17	Colorado	100,648,000	1.70%	6	Pennsylvania	293,051,000	4.95%
16	Connecticut	101,975,000	1.72%	7	Ohio	237,979,000	4.02%
48	Delaware	13,666,000	0.23%	8	Illinois	216,560,000	3.66%
2	Florida	444,248,000	7.51%	9	Massachusetts	163,870,000	2.77%
12	Georgia	154,081,000	2.60%	10	Minnesota	160,994,000	2.72%
34	Hawaii	38,828,000	0.66%	11	Michigan	155,693,000	2.63%
40	Idaho	22,470,000	0.38%	12	Georgia	154,081,000	2.60%
8	Illinois	216,560,000	3.66%	13	Washington	147,177,000	2.49%
19	Indiana	98,161,000	1.66%	14	Wisconsin	142,761,000	2.41%
24	Iowa	68,192,000	1.15%	15	Arizona	123,169,000	2.08%
28	Kansas	58,992,000	1.00%	16	Connecticut	101,975,000	1.72%
30	Kentucky	51,115,000	0.86%	17	Colorado	100,648,000	1.70%
29	Louisiana	58,506,000	0.99%	18	North Carolina	99,116,000	1.67%
38	Maine	26,779,000	0.45%	19	Indiana	98,161,000	1.66%
22	Maryland	76,300,000	1.29%	20	Missouri	89,333,000	1.51%
9	Massachusetts	163,870,000	2.77%	21	Virginia	85,384,000	1.44%
11	Michigan	155,693,000	2.63%	22	Maryland	76,300,000	1.29%
10	Minnesota	160,994,000	2.72%	23	Tennessee	74,113,000	1.25%
44	Mississippi	19,203,000	0.32%	24	Iowa	68,192,000	1.15%
20	Missouri	89,333,000	1.51%	25	Oklahoma	66,456,000	1.12%
46	Montana	16,310,000	0.28%	26	South Carolina	60,285,000	1.02%
36	Nebraska	30,074,000	0.51%	27	Oregon	60,225,000	1.02%
32	Nevada	47,657,000	0.81%	28	Kansas	58,992,000	1.00%
42	New Hampshire	21,688,000	0.37%	29	Louisiana	58,506,000	0.99%
5	New Jersey	326,710,000	5.52%	30	Kentucky	51,115,000	0.86%
35	New Mexico	34,298,000	0.58%	31	Alabama	50,995,000	0.86%
3	New York	388,348,000	6.56%	32	Nevada	47,657,000	0.81%
18	North Carolina	99,116,000	1.67%	33	Arkansas	39,365,000	0.67%
47	North Dakota	14,992,000	0.25%	34	Hawaii	38,828,000	0.66%
7	Ohio	237,979,000	4.02%	35	New Mexico	34,298,000	0.58%
25	Oklahoma	66,456,000	1.12%	36	Nebraska	30,074,000	0.51%
27	Oregon	60,225,000	1.02%	37	Utah	27,714,000	0.47%
6	Pennsylvania	293,051,000	4.95%	38	Maine	26,779,000	0.45%
45	Rhode Island	17,967,000	0.30%	39	West Virginia	24,442,000	0.41%
26	South Carolina	60,285,000	1.02%	40	Idaho	22,470,000	0.38%
43	South Dakota	20,907,000	0.35%	41	Alaska	21,901,000	0.37%
23	Tennessee	74,113,000	1.25%	42	New Hampshire	21,688,000	0.37%
4	Texas	331,418,000	5.60%	43	South Dakota	20,907,000	0.35%
37	Utah	27,714,000	0.47%	44	Mississippi	19,203,000	0.32%
49	Vermont	10,566,000	0.18%	45	Rhode Island	17,967,000	0.30%
21	Virginia	85,384,000	1.44%	46	Montana	16,310,000	0.28%
13	Washington	147,177,000	2.49%	47	North Dakota	14,992,000	0.25%
39	West Virginia	24,442,000	0.41%	48	Delaware	13,666,000	0.23%
14	Wisconsin	142,761,000	2.41%	49	Vermont	10,566,000	0.18%
50	Wyoming	6,966,000	0.12%	50	Wyoming	6,966,000	0.12%
					District of Columbia	4,109,000	0.07%

Source: U.S. Bureau of the Census
  "1992 Census of Service Industries, Geographic Area Series, United States" (SC92-A-52)
*Includes only establishments subject to the federal income tax. See Facilities Chapter for establishments.

Receipts per Office or Clinic of Chiropractors in 1992

National Rate = $216,543 per Establishment*

ALPHA ORDER

RANK	STATE	PER ESTABLISHMENT
37	Alabama	$180,833
3	Alaska	308,465
28	Arizona	198,021
44	Arkansas	166,097
19	California	222,766
39	Colorado	170,879
4	Connecticut	293,876
7	Delaware	273,320
10	Florida	240,524
26	Georgia	202,738
2	Hawaii	326,286
42	Idaho	167,687
25	Illinois	202,772
16	Indiana	225,140
47	Iowa	152,897
34	Kansas	183,776
30	Kentucky	190,019
24	Louisiana	206,007
21	Maine	212,532
1	Maryland	330,303
6	Massachusetts	284,991
45	Michigan	165,984
29	Minnesota	195,381
40	Mississippi	169,938
48	Missouri	149,386
50	Montana	139,402
33	Nebraska	184,503
5	Nevada	287,090
27	New Hampshire	200,815
9	New Jersey	262,418
32	New Mexico	185,395
18	New York	223,060
15	North Carolina	225,777
43	North Dakota	166,578
8	Ohio	273,225
22	Oklahoma	210,304
49	Oregon	140,713
17	Pennsylvania	223,703
14	Rhode Island	227,430
31	South Carolina	188,981
38	South Dakota	177,178
23	Tennessee	208,183
13	Texas	232,411
36	Utah	181,137
46	Vermont	162,554
11	Virginia	240,518
35	Washington	183,056
12	West Virginia	232,781
20	Wisconsin	214,678
41	Wyoming	169,902

RANK ORDER

RANK	STATE	PER ESTABLISHMENT
1	Maryland	$330,303
2	Hawaii	326,286
3	Alaska	308,465
4	Connecticut	293,876
5	Nevada	287,090
6	Massachusetts	284,991
7	Delaware	273,320
8	Ohio	273,225
9	New Jersey	262,418
10	Florida	240,524
11	Virginia	240,518
12	West Virginia	232,781
13	Texas	232,411
14	Rhode Island	227,430
15	North Carolina	225,777
16	Indiana	225,140
17	Pennsylvania	223,703
18	New York	223,060
19	California	222,766
20	Wisconsin	214,678
21	Maine	212,532
22	Oklahoma	210,304
23	Tennessee	208,183
24	Louisiana	206,007
25	Illinois	202,772
26	Georgia	202,738
27	New Hampshire	200,815
28	Arizona	198,021
29	Minnesota	195,381
30	Kentucky	190,019
31	South Carolina	188,981
32	New Mexico	185,395
33	Nebraska	184,503
34	Kansas	183,776
35	Washington	183,056
36	Utah	181,137
37	Alabama	180,833
38	South Dakota	177,178
39	Colorado	170,879
40	Mississippi	169,938
41	Wyoming	169,902
42	Idaho	167,687
43	North Dakota	166,578
44	Arkansas	166,097
45	Michigan	165,984
46	Vermont	162,554
47	Iowa	152,897
48	Missouri	149,386
49	Oregon	140,713
50	Montana	139,402
	District of Columbia	316,077

Source: Morgan Quitno Press using data from U.S. Bureau of the Census
   "1992 Census of Service Industries, Geographic Area Series, United States" (SC92-A-52)
Includes only establishments subject to the federal income tax. See Facilities Chapter for establishments.

Receipts of Offices and Clinics of Optometrists in 1992

National Total = $4,939,521,000*

ALPHA ORDER

RANK	STATE	RECEIPTS	% of USA
27	Alabama	$65,608,000	1.33%
47	Alaska	17,112,000	0.35%
31	Arizona	49,165,000	1.00%
29	Arkansas	56,672,000	1.15%
1	California	754,317,000	15.27%
24	Colorado	73,235,000	1.48%
23	Connecticut	73,960,000	1.50%
49	Delaware	12,873,000	0.26%
5	Florida	221,280,000	4.48%
13	Georgia	102,345,000	2.07%
39	Hawaii	27,647,000	0.56%
40	Idaho	24,607,000	0.50%
7	Illinois	213,734,000	4.33%
11	Indiana	133,059,000	2.69%
19	Iowa	79,034,000	1.60%
20	Kansas	78,371,000	1.59%
25	Kentucky	72,650,000	1.47%
32	Louisiana	48,393,000	0.98%
37	Maine	35,347,000	0.72%
21	Maryland	78,104,000	1.58%
15	Massachusetts	97,781,000	1.98%
8	Michigan	203,832,000	4.13%
26	Minnesota	71,690,000	1.45%
35	Mississippi	37,655,000	0.76%
18	Missouri	88,489,000	1.79%
41	Montana	24,435,000	0.49%
34	Nebraska	38,725,000	0.78%
36	Nevada	36,924,000	0.75%
45	New Hampshire	20,073,000	0.41%
9	New Jersey	147,976,000	3.00%
38	New Mexico	30,091,000	0.61%
4	New York	226,940,000	4.59%
10	North Carolina	146,551,000	2.97%
43	North Dakota	21,635,000	0.44%
6	Ohio	218,608,000	4.43%
22	Oklahoma	76,308,000	1.54%
30	Oregon	51,605,000	1.04%
3	Pennsylvania	246,226,000	4.98%
44	Rhode Island	21,103,000	0.43%
28	South Carolina	58,093,000	1.18%
46	South Dakota	19,165,000	0.39%
14	Tennessee	101,398,000	2.05%
2	Texas	329,294,000	6.67%
42	Utah	21,944,000	0.44%
50	Vermont	11,768,000	0.24%
12	Virginia	115,755,000	2.34%
16	Washington	95,398,000	1.93%
33	West Virginia	43,184,000	0.87%
17	Wisconsin	94,432,000	1.91%
48	Wyoming	15,714,000	0.32%

RANK ORDER

RANK	STATE	RECEIPTS	% of USA
1	California	$754,317,000	15.27%
2	Texas	329,294,000	6.67%
3	Pennsylvania	246,226,000	4.98%
4	New York	226,940,000	4.59%
5	Florida	221,280,000	4.48%
6	Ohio	218,608,000	4.43%
7	Illinois	213,734,000	4.33%
8	Michigan	203,832,000	4.13%
9	New Jersey	147,976,000	3.00%
10	North Carolina	146,551,000	2.97%
11	Indiana	133,059,000	2.69%
12	Virginia	115,755,000	2.34%
13	Georgia	102,345,000	2.07%
14	Tennessee	101,398,000	2.05%
15	Massachusetts	97,781,000	1.98%
16	Washington	95,398,000	1.93%
17	Wisconsin	94,432,000	1.91%
18	Missouri	88,489,000	1.79%
19	Iowa	79,034,000	1.60%
20	Kansas	78,371,000	1.59%
21	Maryland	78,104,000	1.58%
22	Oklahoma	76,308,000	1.54%
23	Connecticut	73,960,000	1.50%
24	Colorado	73,235,000	1.48%
25	Kentucky	72,650,000	1.47%
26	Minnesota	71,690,000	1.45%
27	Alabama	65,608,000	1.33%
28	South Carolina	58,093,000	1.18%
29	Arkansas	56,672,000	1.15%
30	Oregon	51,605,000	1.04%
31	Arizona	49,165,000	1.00%
32	Louisiana	48,393,000	0.98%
33	West Virginia	43,184,000	0.87%
34	Nebraska	38,725,000	0.78%
35	Mississippi	37,655,000	0.76%
36	Nevada	36,924,000	0.75%
37	Maine	35,347,000	0.72%
38	New Mexico	30,091,000	0.61%
39	Hawaii	27,647,000	0.56%
40	Idaho	24,607,000	0.50%
41	Montana	24,435,000	0.49%
42	Utah	21,944,000	0.44%
43	North Dakota	21,635,000	0.44%
44	Rhode Island	21,103,000	0.43%
45	New Hampshire	20,073,000	0.41%
46	South Dakota	19,165,000	0.39%
47	Alaska	17,112,000	0.35%
48	Wyoming	15,714,000	0.32%
49	Delaware	12,873,000	0.26%
50	Vermont	11,768,000	0.24%
	District of Columbia	9,216,000	0.19%

Source: U.S. Bureau of the Census
"1992 Census of Service Industries, Geographic Area Series, United States" (SC92-A-52)
*Includes only establishments subject to the federal income tax. See Facilities Chapter for establishments.

Receipts per Office or Clinic of Optometrists in 1992

National Rate = $288,271 per Establishment*

ALPHA ORDER			RANK ORDER		
RANK	STATE	PER ESTABLISHMENT	RANK	STATE	PER ESTABLISHMENT
24	Alabama	$286,498	1	Alaska	$388,909
1	Alaska	388,909	2	North Dakota	338,047
41	Arizona	260,132	3	Michigan	335,802
28	Arkansas	280,554	4	Nevada	335,673
10	California	316,674	5	Maryland	332,357
26	Colorado	284,961	6	Connecticut	324,386
6	Connecticut	324,386	7	Delaware	321,825
7	Delaware	321,825	8	Nebraska	320,041
42	Florida	259,110	9	Kansas	317,291
32	Georgia	274,383	10	California	316,674
30	Hawaii	279,263	11	Illinois	306,209
39	Idaho	261,777	12	Texas	299,358
11	Illinois	306,209	13	North Carolina	294,279
21	Indiana	287,384	14	Missouri	293,983
18	Iowa	292,719	15	South Carolina	293,399
9	Kansas	317,291	16	Rhode Island	293,097
17	Kentucky	292,944	17	Kentucky	292,944
45	Louisiana	246,903	18	Iowa	292,719
22	Maine	287,374	19	Wyoming	291,000
5	Maryland	332,357	20	New Mexico	289,337
38	Massachusetts	264,273	21	Indiana	287,384
3	Michigan	335,802	22	Maine	287,374
43	Minnesota	255,125	23	New York	286,903
44	Mississippi	254,426	24	Alabama	286,498
14	Missouri	293,983	25	West Virginia	285,987
48	Montana	237,233	26	Colorado	284,961
8	Nebraska	320,041	27	Pennsylvania	283,344
4	Nevada	335,673	28	Arkansas	280,554
34	New Hampshire	271,257	29	Washington	279,760
36	New Jersey	269,047	30	Hawaii	279,263
20	New Mexico	289,337	31	Tennessee	278,566
23	New York	286,903	32	Georgia	274,383
13	North Carolina	294,279	33	Wisconsin	272,138
2	North Dakota	338,047	34	New Hampshire	271,257
40	Ohio	261,493	35	Utah	270,914
46	Oklahoma	240,719	36	New Jersey	269,047
50	Oregon	232,455	37	Virginia	265,493
27	Pennsylvania	283,344	38	Massachusetts	264,273
16	Rhode Island	293,097	39	Idaho	261,777
15	South Carolina	293,399	40	Ohio	261,493
47	South Dakota	239,563	41	Arizona	260,132
31	Tennessee	278,566	42	Florida	259,110
12	Texas	299,358	43	Minnesota	255,125
35	Utah	270,914	44	Mississippi	254,426
49	Vermont	235,360	45	Louisiana	246,903
37	Virginia	265,493	46	Oklahoma	240,719
29	Washington	279,760	47	South Dakota	239,563
25	West Virginia	285,987	48	Montana	237,233
33	Wisconsin	272,138	49	Vermont	235,360
19	Wyoming	291,000	50	Oregon	232,455
				District of Columbia	384,000

Source: Morgan Quitno Press using data from U.S. Bureau of the Census
"1992 Census of Service Industries, Geographic Area Series, United States" (SC92-A-52)
*Includes only establishments subject to the federal income tax. See Facilities Chapter for establishments.

Receipts of Offices and Clinics of Podiatrists in 1992

National Total = $1,920,076,000*

RANK	STATE	RECEIPTS	% of USA
23	Alabama	$15,910,000	0.83%
46	Alaska	2,222,000	0.12%
18	Arizona	27,962,000	1.46%
42	Arkansas	5,017,000	0.26%
1	California	217,602,000	11.33%
22	Colorado	18,980,000	0.99%
11	Connecticut	48,830,000	2.54%
37	Delaware	6,801,000	0.35%
3	Florida	147,168,000	7.66%
12	Georgia	47,600,000	2.48%
43	Hawaii	3,871,000	0.20%
40	Idaho	5,283,000	0.28%
7	Illinois	105,745,000	5.51%
14	Indiana	41,792,000	2.18%
24	Iowa	14,998,000	0.78%
29	Kansas	12,107,000	0.63%
31	Kentucky	10,299,000	0.54%
26	Louisiana	13,876,000	0.72%
38	Maine	6,464,000	0.34%
10	Maryland	56,379,000	2.94%
13	Massachusetts	43,366,000	2.26%
5	Michigan	112,871,000	5.88%
28	Minnesota	12,440,000	0.65%
44	Mississippi	3,801,000	0.20%
20	Missouri	24,462,000	1.27%
45	Montana	3,441,000	0.18%
36	Nebraska	7,020,000	0.37%
35	Nevada	7,995,000	0.42%
41	New Hampshire	5,180,000	0.27%
9	New Jersey	103,924,000	5.41%
34	New Mexico	8,215,000	0.43%
2	New York	209,057,000	10.89%
16	North Carolina	35,032,000	1.82%
48	North Dakota	1,382,000	0.07%
6	Ohio	109,704,000	5.71%
25	Oklahoma	14,850,000	0.77%
27	Oregon	13,796,000	0.72%
4	Pennsylvania	118,882,000	6.19%
30	Rhode Island	11,842,000	0.62%
32	South Carolina	9,906,000	0.52%
47	South Dakota	1,774,000	0.09%
21	Tennessee	23,034,000	1.20%
8	Texas	104,569,000	5.45%
33	Utah	9,326,000	0.49%
49	Vermont	1,157,000	0.06%
15	Virginia	40,402,000	2.10%
17	Washington	31,204,000	1.63%
39	West Virginia	5,602,000	0.29%
19	Wisconsin	27,720,000	1.44%
50	Wyoming	1,035,000	0.05%

RANK	STATE	RECEIPTS	% of USA
1	California	$217,602,000	11.33%
2	New York	209,057,000	10.89%
3	Florida	147,168,000	7.66%
4	Pennsylvania	118,882,000	6.19%
5	Michigan	112,871,000	5.88%
6	Ohio	109,704,000	5.71%
7	Illinois	105,745,000	5.51%
8	Texas	104,569,000	5.45%
9	New Jersey	103,924,000	5.41%
10	Maryland	56,379,000	2.94%
11	Connecticut	48,830,000	2.54%
12	Georgia	47,600,000	2.48%
13	Massachusetts	43,366,000	2.26%
14	Indiana	41,792,000	2.18%
15	Virginia	40,402,000	2.10%
16	North Carolina	35,032,000	1.82%
17	Washington	31,204,000	1.63%
18	Arizona	27,962,000	1.46%
19	Wisconsin	27,720,000	1.44%
20	Missouri	24,462,000	1.27%
21	Tennessee	23,034,000	1.20%
22	Colorado	18,980,000	0.99%
23	Alabama	15,910,000	0.83%
24	Iowa	14,998,000	0.78%
25	Oklahoma	14,850,000	0.77%
26	Louisiana	13,876,000	0.72%
27	Oregon	13,796,000	0.72%
28	Minnesota	12,440,000	0.65%
29	Kansas	12,107,000	0.63%
30	Rhode Island	11,842,000	0.62%
31	Kentucky	10,299,000	0.54%
32	South Carolina	9,906,000	0.52%
33	Utah	9,326,000	0.49%
34	New Mexico	8,215,000	0.43%
35	Nevada	7,995,000	0.42%
36	Nebraska	7,020,000	0.37%
37	Delaware	6,801,000	0.35%
38	Maine	6,464,000	0.34%
39	West Virginia	5,602,000	0.29%
40	Idaho	5,283,000	0.28%
41	New Hampshire	5,180,000	0.27%
42	Arkansas	5,017,000	0.26%
43	Hawaii	3,871,000	0.20%
44	Mississippi	3,801,000	0.20%
45	Montana	3,441,000	0.18%
46	Alaska	2,222,000	0.12%
47	South Dakota	1,774,000	0.09%
48	North Dakota	1,382,000	0.07%
49	Vermont	1,157,000	0.06%
50	Wyoming	1,035,000	0.05%
	District of Columbia	8,181,000	0.43%

Source: U.S. Bureau of the Census
"1992 Census of Service Industries, Geographic Area Series, United States" (SC92-A-52)
*Includes only establishments subject to the federal income tax. See Facilities Chapter for establishments.

Receipts per Office or Clinic of Podiatrists in 1992

National Rate = $241,580 per Establishment*

ALPHA ORDER			RANK ORDER		
RANK	STATE	PER ESTABLISHMENT	RANK	STATE	PER ESTABLISHMENT
3	Alabama	$324,694	1	Alaska	$444,400
1	Alaska	444,400	2	Georgia	342,446
28	Arizona	231,091	3	Alabama	324,694
17	Arkansas	250,850	4	Connecticut	321,250
25	California	233,981	5	Idaho	310,765
35	Colorado	215,682	6	Louisiana	289,083
4	Connecticut	321,250	7	Oklahoma	285,577
11	Delaware	272,040	8	Nevada	285,536
13	Florida	260,936	9	Michigan	282,178
2	Georgia	342,446	10	Texas	273,741
23	Hawaii	241,938	11	Delaware	272,040
5	Idaho	310,765	12	Maryland	267,199
15	Illinois	252,375	13	Florida	260,936
16	Indiana	251,759	14	Tennessee	255,933
46	Iowa	199,973	15	Illinois	252,375
33	Kansas	220,127	16	Indiana	251,759
30	Kentucky	223,891	17	Arkansas	250,850
6	Louisiana	289,083	18	North Carolina	250,229
48	Maine	179,556	19	Missouri	249,612
12	Maryland	267,199	20	New Mexico	248,939
41	Massachusetts	208,490	21	South Carolina	247,650
9	Michigan	282,178	22	Virginia	246,354
42	Minnesota	207,333	23	Hawaii	241,938
40	Mississippi	211,167	24	Rhode Island	236,840
19	Missouri	249,612	25	California	233,981
37	Montana	215,063	26	Wisconsin	232,941
44	Nebraska	206,471	27	New Jersey	231,457
8	Nevada	285,536	28	Arizona	231,091
34	New Hampshire	215,833	29	Oregon	226,164
27	New Jersey	231,457	30	Kentucky	223,891
20	New Mexico	248,939	31	Ohio	223,886
32	New York	222,875	32	New York	222,875
18	North Carolina	250,229	33	Kansas	220,127
47	North Dakota	197,429	34	New Hampshire	215,833
31	Ohio	223,886	35	Colorado	215,682
7	Oklahoma	285,577	36	West Virginia	215,462
29	Oregon	226,164	37	Montana	215,063
45	Pennsylvania	201,837	38	Washington	213,726
24	Rhode Island	236,840	39	Utah	211,955
21	South Carolina	247,650	40	Mississippi	211,167
50	South Dakota	126,714	41	Massachusetts	208,490
14	Tennessee	255,933	42	Minnesota	207,333
10	Texas	273,741	43	Wyoming	207,000
39	Utah	211,955	44	Nebraska	206,471
49	Vermont	128,556	45	Pennsylvania	201,837
22	Virginia	246,354	46	Iowa	199,973
38	Washington	213,726	47	North Dakota	197,429
36	West Virginia	215,462	48	Maine	179,556
26	Wisconsin	232,941	49	Vermont	128,556
43	Wyoming	207,000	50	South Dakota	126,714
				District of Columbia	255,656

Source: Morgan Quitno Press using data from U.S. Bureau of the Census
"1992 Census of Service Industries, Geographic Area Series, United States" (SC92-A-52)
*Includes only establishments subject to the federal income tax. See Facilities Chapter for establishments.

Receipts of Offices and Clinics of Other Health Practitioners in 1992

National Total = $6,148,059,000*

ALPHA ORDER

RANK	STATE	RECEIPTS	% of USA
29	Alabama	$52,156,000	0.85%
46	Alaska	12,434,000	0.20%
21	Arizona	96,707,000	1.57%
31	Arkansas	40,313,000	0.66%
1	California	1,034,853,000	16.83%
17	Colorado	108,367,000	1.76%
16	Connecticut	109,057,000	1.77%
40	Delaware	24,546,000	0.40%
3	Florida	426,622,000	6.94%
12	Georgia	161,961,000	2.63%
36	Hawaii	30,940,000	0.50%
45	Idaho	14,480,000	0.24%
7	Illinois	224,938,000	3.66%
23	Indiana	84,829,000	1.38%
32	Iowa	38,347,000	0.62%
33	Kansas	38,115,000	0.62%
26	Kentucky	59,948,000	0.98%
24	Louisiana	80,487,000	1.31%
41	Maine	23,413,000	0.38%
10	Maryland	179,434,000	2.92%
13	Massachusetts	158,543,000	2.58%
8	Michigan	212,093,000	3.45%
18	Minnesota	100,371,000	1.63%
39	Mississippi	26,287,000	0.43%
19	Missouri	99,140,000	1.61%
44	Montana	14,602,000	0.24%
38	Nebraska	27,517,000	0.45%
27	Nevada	55,463,000	0.90%
34	New Hampshire	36,653,000	0.60%
9	New Jersey	211,576,000	3.44%
37	New Mexico	30,081,000	0.49%
5	New York	365,739,000	5.95%
14	North Carolina	138,366,000	2.25%
50	North Dakota	6,543,000	0.11%
6	Ohio	241,548,000	3.93%
28	Oklahoma	53,332,000	0.87%
25	Oregon	71,873,000	1.17%
4	Pennsylvania	374,184,000	6.09%
43	Rhode Island	16,002,000	0.26%
30	South Carolina	43,318,000	0.70%
48	South Dakota	9,805,000	0.16%
20	Tennessee	97,742,000	1.59%
2	Texas	430,380,000	7.00%
35	Utah	36,264,000	0.59%
47	Vermont	10,822,000	0.18%
15	Virginia	135,154,000	2.20%
11	Washington	162,891,000	2.65%
42	West Virginia	18,885,000	0.31%
22	Wisconsin	93,109,000	1.51%
49	Wyoming	7,307,000	0.12%

RANK ORDER

RANK	STATE	RECEIPTS	% of USA
1	California	$1,034,853,000	16.83%
2	Texas	430,380,000	7.00%
3	Florida	426,622,000	6.94%
4	Pennsylvania	374,184,000	6.09%
5	New York	365,739,000	5.95%
6	Ohio	241,548,000	3.93%
7	Illinois	224,938,000	3.66%
8	Michigan	212,093,000	3.45%
9	New Jersey	211,576,000	3.44%
10	Maryland	179,434,000	2.92%
11	Washington	162,891,000	2.65%
12	Georgia	161,961,000	2.63%
13	Massachusetts	158,543,000	2.58%
14	North Carolina	138,366,000	2.25%
15	Virginia	135,154,000	2.20%
16	Connecticut	109,057,000	1.77%
17	Colorado	108,367,000	1.76%
18	Minnesota	100,371,000	1.63%
19	Missouri	99,140,000	1.61%
20	Tennessee	97,742,000	1.59%
21	Arizona	96,707,000	1.57%
22	Wisconsin	93,109,000	1.51%
23	Indiana	84,829,000	1.38%
24	Louisiana	80,487,000	1.31%
25	Oregon	71,873,000	1.17%
26	Kentucky	59,948,000	0.98%
27	Nevada	55,463,000	0.90%
28	Oklahoma	53,332,000	0.87%
29	Alabama	52,156,000	0.85%
30	South Carolina	43,318,000	0.70%
31	Arkansas	40,313,000	0.66%
32	Iowa	38,347,000	0.62%
33	Kansas	38,115,000	0.62%
34	New Hampshire	36,653,000	0.60%
35	Utah	36,264,000	0.59%
36	Hawaii	30,940,000	0.50%
37	New Mexico	30,081,000	0.49%
38	Nebraska	27,517,000	0.45%
39	Mississippi	26,287,000	0.43%
40	Delaware	24,546,000	0.40%
41	Maine	23,413,000	0.38%
42	West Virginia	18,885,000	0.31%
43	Rhode Island	16,002,000	0.26%
44	Montana	14,602,000	0.24%
45	Idaho	14,480,000	0.24%
46	Alaska	12,434,000	0.20%
47	Vermont	10,822,000	0.18%
48	South Dakota	9,805,000	0.16%
49	Wyoming	7,307,000	0.12%
50	North Dakota	6,543,000	0.11%
	District of Columbia	20,522,000	0.33%

Source: U.S. Bureau of the Census
"1992 Census of Service Industries, Geographic Area Series, United States" (SC92-A-52)
*Includes only establishments subject to the federal income tax. Includes health practitioners not otherwise classified such as acupuncturists, midwives, nutritionists, physical and occupational therapists and psychologists. See Facilities Chapter for establishments.

Receipts per Office or Clinic of Other Health Practitioners in 1992

National Rate = $276,193 per Establishment*

ALPHA ORDER				RANK ORDER		
RANK	STATE	PER ESTABLISHMENT		RANK	STATE	PER ESTABLISHMENT
11	Alabama	$299,747		1	Nevada	$426,638
44	Alaska	207,233		2	Pennsylvania	416,222
40	Arizona	216,347		3	Connecticut	349,542
29	Arkansas	258,417		4	Delaware	322,974
27	California	261,723		5	New Jersey	317,682
42	Colorado	210,421		6	Michigan	317,030
3	Connecticut	349,542		7	Illinois	311,548
4	Delaware	322,974		8	Indiana	308,469
28	Florida	259,502		9	Maryland	303,098
12	Georgia	297,722		10	Massachusetts	301,413
30	Hawaii	257,833		11	Alabama	299,747
47	Idaho	183,291		12	Georgia	297,722
7	Illinois	311,548		13	Tennessee	296,188
8	Indiana	308,469		14	New Hampshire	286,352
35	Iowa	245,814		15	Kentucky	282,774
37	Kansas	241,234		16	Ohio	280,870
15	Kentucky	282,774		17	Virginia	278,668
34	Louisiana	248,417		18	North Carolina	278,402
43	Maine	209,045		19	Minnesota	278,036
9	Maryland	303,098		20	Wisconsin	273,850
10	Massachusetts	301,413		21	West Virginia	273,696
6	Michigan	317,030		22	New York	272,127
19	Minnesota	278,036		23	Missouri	265,080
31	Mississippi	257,716		24	South Dakota	265,000
23	Missouri	265,080		25	Texas	263,068
49	Montana	169,791		26	Washington	262,727
32	Nebraska	257,168		27	California	261,723
1	Nevada	426,638		28	Florida	259,502
14	New Hampshire	286,352		29	Arkansas	258,417
5	New Jersey	317,682		30	Hawaii	257,833
48	New Mexico	180,126		31	Mississippi	257,716
22	New York	272,127		32	Nebraska	257,168
18	North Carolina	278,402		33	South Carolina	256,320
41	North Dakota	211,065		34	Louisiana	248,417
16	Ohio	280,870		35	Iowa	245,814
38	Oklahoma	233,912		36	Rhode Island	242,455
45	Oregon	199,094		37	Kansas	241,234
2	Pennsylvania	416,222		38	Oklahoma	233,912
36	Rhode Island	242,455		39	Utah	218,458
33	South Carolina	256,320		40	Arizona	216,347
24	South Dakota	265,000		41	North Dakota	211,065
13	Tennessee	296,188		42	Colorado	210,421
25	Texas	263,068		43	Maine	209,045
39	Utah	218,458		44	Alaska	207,233
50	Vermont	156,841		45	Oregon	199,094
17	Virginia	278,668		46	Wyoming	197,486
26	Washington	262,727		47	Idaho	183,291
21	West Virginia	273,696		48	New Mexico	180,126
20	Wisconsin	273,850		49	Montana	169,791
46	Wyoming	197,486		50	Vermont	156,841
					District of Columbia	301,794

Source: Morgan Quitno Press using data from U.S. Bureau of the Census
   "1992 Census of Service Industries, Geographic Area Series, United States" (SC92-A-52)
*Includes only establishments subject to the federal income tax. Includes health practitioners not otherwise classified such as acupuncturists, midwives, nutritionists, physical and occupational therapists and psychologists. See Facilities Chapter for establishments.

Receipts of Hospitals in 1992

National Total = $310,818,211,000*

ALPHA ORDER					RANK ORDER			
RANK	STATE	RECEIPTS	% of USA		RANK	STATE	RECEIPTS	% of USA
21	Alabama	$5,114,698,000	1.65%		1	California	$34,552,067,000	11.12%
NA	Alaska**	NA	NA		2	New York	27,722,480,000	8.92%
23	Arizona	4,064,528,000	1.31%		3	Texas	20,081,248,000	6.46%
30	Arkansas	2,601,895,000	0.84%		4	Pennsylvania	18,019,449,000	5.80%
1	California	34,552,067,000	11.12%		5	Florida	16,528,209,000	5.32%
24	Colorado	3,876,008,000	1.25%		6	Illinois	14,715,279,000	4.73%
NA	Connecticut**	NA	NA		7	Ohio	13,998,840,000	4.50%
37	Delaware	903,055,000	0.29%		8	Michigan	11,444,321,000	3.68%
5	Florida	16,528,209,000	5.32%		9	New Jersey	9,842,808,000	3.17%
11	Georgia	8,079,353,000	2.60%		10	Massachusetts	9,714,787,000	3.13%
NA	Hawaii**	NA	NA		11	Georgia	8,079,353,000	2.60%
38	Idaho	880,530,000	0.28%		12	North Carolina	7,408,964,000	2.38%
6	Illinois	14,715,279,000	4.73%		13	Missouri	7,217,462,000	2.32%
16	Indiana	6,590,871,000	2.12%		14	Virginia	6,793,601,000	2.19%
NA	Iowa**	NA	NA		15	Tennessee	6,770,631,000	2.18%
27	Kansas	2,856,257,000	0.92%		16	Indiana	6,590,871,000	2.12%
22	Kentucky	4,185,657,000	1.35%		17	Louisiana	5,658,657,000	1.82%
17	Louisiana	5,658,657,000	1.82%		18	Maryland	5,440,457,000	1.75%
NA	Maine**	NA	NA		19	Wisconsin	5,262,803,000	1.69%
18	Maryland	5,440,457,000	1.75%		20	Washington	5,193,838,000	1.67%
10	Massachusetts	9,714,787,000	3.13%		21	Alabama	5,114,698,000	1.65%
8	Michigan	11,444,321,000	3.68%		22	Kentucky	4,185,657,000	1.35%
NA	Minnesota**	NA	NA		23	Arizona	4,064,528,000	1.31%
29	Mississippi	2,627,692,000	0.85%		24	Colorado	3,876,008,000	1.25%
13	Missouri	7,217,462,000	2.32%		25	South Carolina	3,833,754,000	1.23%
39	Montana	864,812,000	0.28%		26	Oklahoma	3,232,112,000	1.04%
NA	Nebraska**	NA	NA		27	Kansas	2,856,257,000	0.92%
34	Nevada	1,296,942,000	0.42%		28	Oregon	2,835,585,000	0.91%
36	New Hampshire	1,250,889,000	0.40%		29	Mississippi	2,627,692,000	0.85%
9	New Jersey	9,842,808,000	3.17%		30	Arkansas	2,601,895,000	0.84%
33	New Mexico	1,558,035,000	0.50%		31	West Virginia	2,243,147,000	0.72%
2	New York	27,722,480,000	8.92%		32	Utah	1,626,872,000	0.52%
12	North Carolina	7,408,964,000	2.38%		33	New Mexico	1,558,035,000	0.50%
NA	North Dakota**	NA	NA		34	Nevada	1,296,942,000	0.42%
7	Ohio	13,998,840,000	4.50%		35	Rhode Island	1,257,773,000	0.40%
26	Oklahoma	3,232,112,000	1.04%		36	New Hampshire	1,250,889,000	0.40%
28	Oregon	2,835,585,000	0.91%		37	Delaware	903,055,000	0.29%
4	Pennsylvania	18,019,449,000	5.80%		38	Idaho	880,530,000	0.28%
35	Rhode Island	1,257,773,000	0.40%		39	Montana	864,812,000	0.28%
25	South Carolina	3,833,754,000	1.23%		40	Vermont	545,676,000	0.18%
NA	South Dakota**	NA	NA		NA	Alaska**	NA	NA
15	Tennessee	6,770,631,000	2.18%		NA	Connecticut**	NA	NA
3	Texas	20,081,248,000	6.46%		NA	Hawaii**	NA	NA
32	Utah	1,626,872,000	0.52%		NA	Iowa**	NA	NA
40	Vermont	545,676,000	0.18%		NA	Maine**	NA	NA
14	Virginia	6,793,601,000	2.19%		NA	Minnesota**	NA	NA
20	Washington	5,193,838,000	1.67%		NA	Nebraska**	NA	NA
31	West Virginia	2,243,147,000	0.72%		NA	North Dakota**	NA	NA
19	Wisconsin	5,262,803,000	1.69%		NA	South Dakota**	NA	NA
NA	Wyoming**	NA	NA		NA	Wyoming**	NA	NA
					District of Columbia**		NA	NA

Source: Morgan Quitno Press using data from U.S. Bureau of the Census
  "1992 Census of Service Industries, Geographic Area Series, United States" (SC92-A-52)
*Includes establishments exempt from as well as subject to the federal income tax. Includes general medical and surgical hospitals, psychiatric hospitals and other specialty hospitals. Includes government owned hospitals.
**Not available.

Receipts per Hospital in 1992

National Rate = $43,654,243 per Hospital*

ALPHA ORDER

RANK	STATE	PER HOSPITAL
24	Alabama	$36,533,557
NA	Alaska**	NA
18	Arizona	40,645,280
34	Arkansas	25,508,775
9	California	57,205,409
21	Colorado	38,760,080
NA	Connecticut**	NA
10	Delaware	56,440,938
12	Florida	50,237,717
23	Georgia	38,473,110
NA	Hawaii**	NA
39	Idaho	16,306,111
8	Illinois	57,257,895
20	Indiana	40,434,791
NA	Iowa**	NA
38	Kansas	17,631,216
28	Kentucky	32,700,445
31	Louisiana	30,422,887
NA	Maine**	NA
3	Maryland	64,005,376
4	Massachusetts	60,717,419
11	Michigan	52,257,174
NA	Minnesota**	NA
36	Mississippi	22,268,576
16	Missouri	41,242,640
40	Montana	13,304,800
NA	Nebraska**	NA
19	Nevada	40,529,438
30	New Hampshire	30,509,488
2	New Jersey	72,909,689
35	New Mexico	23,254,254
1	New York	85,038,282
15	North Carolina	42,580,253
NA	North Dakota**	NA
6	Ohio	57,608,395
37	Oklahoma	21,547,413
25	Oregon	35,893,481
7	Pennsylvania	57,386,780
5	Rhode Island	59,893,952
17	South Carolina	41,223,161
NA	South Dakota**	NA
22	Tennessee	38,689,320
26	Texas	34,326,920
33	Utah	29,051,286
32	Vermont	30,315,333
13	Virginia	48,525,721
14	Washington	43,645,697
29	West Virginia	31,154,819
27	Wisconsin	33,521,038
NA	Wyoming**	NA

RANK ORDER

RANK	STATE	PER HOSPITAL
1	New York	$85,038,282
2	New Jersey	72,909,689
3	Maryland	64,005,376
4	Massachusetts	60,717,419
5	Rhode Island	59,893,952
6	Ohio	57,608,395
7	Pennsylvania	57,386,780
8	Illinois	57,257,895
9	California	57,205,409
10	Delaware	56,440,938
11	Michigan	52,257,174
12	Florida	50,237,717
13	Virginia	48,525,721
14	Washington	43,645,697
15	North Carolina	42,580,253
16	Missouri	41,242,640
17	South Carolina	41,223,161
18	Arizona	40,645,280
19	Nevada	40,529,438
20	Indiana	40,434,791
21	Colorado	38,760,080
22	Tennessee	38,689,320
23	Georgia	38,473,110
24	Alabama	36,533,557
25	Oregon	35,893,481
26	Texas	34,326,920
27	Wisconsin	33,521,038
28	Kentucky	32,700,445
29	West Virginia	31,154,819
30	New Hampshire	30,509,488
31	Louisiana	30,422,887
32	Vermont	30,315,333
33	Utah	29,051,286
34	Arkansas	25,508,775
35	New Mexico	23,254,254
36	Mississippi	22,268,576
37	Oklahoma	21,547,413
38	Kansas	17,631,216
39	Idaho	16,306,111
40	Montana	13,304,800
NA	Alaska**	NA
NA	Connecticut**	NA
NA	Hawaii**	NA
NA	Iowa**	NA
NA	Maine**	NA
NA	Minnesota**	NA
NA	Nebraska**	NA
NA	North Dakota**	NA
NA	South Dakota**	NA
NA	Wyoming**	NA
	District of Columbia**	NA

Source: Morgan Quitno Press using data from U.S. Bureau of the Census
  "1992 Census of Service Industries, Geographic Area Series, United States" (SC92-A-52)
*Calculated using Census Bureau count of 7,120 hospitals. Includes establishments exempt from as well as subject to the federal income tax. Includes general medical and surgical hospitals, psychiatric hospitals and other specialty hospitals. Includes government owned hospitals.
**Not available.

V. INCIDENCE OF DISEASE

V. INCIDENCE OF DISEASE (Continued)

Estimated New Cancer Cases in 1995

National Estimated Total = 1,252,000 New Cases*

ALPHA ORDER

RANK	STATE	CASES	% of USA
20	Alabama	21,400	1.71%
50	Alaska	1,200	0.10%
24	Arizona	18,500	1.48%
30	Arkansas	14,100	1.13%
1	California	120,000	9.58%
32	Colorado	13,300	1.06%
27	Connecticut	16,200	1.29%
45	Delaware	3,800	0.30%
2	Florida	88,700	7.08%
15	Georgia	28,400	2.27%
43	Hawaii	4,200	0.34%
42	Idaho	4,400	0.35%
6	Illinois	58,500	4.67%
13	Indiana	28,600	2.28%
29	Iowa	14,700	1.17%
33	Kansas	12,800	1.02%
21	Kentucky	21,300	1.70%
22	Louisiana	21,200	1.69%
36	Maine	7,100	0.57%
18	Maryland	24,100	1.92%
11	Massachusetts	32,300	2.58%
8	Michigan	46,100	3.68%
23	Minnesota	20,200	1.61%
31	Mississippi	13,600	1.09%
14	Missouri	28,500	2.28%
44	Montana	4,100	0.33%
35	Nebraska	7,700	0.62%
37	Nevada	6,400	0.51%
40	New Hampshire	5,200	0.42%
9	New Jersey	43,300	3.46%
38	New Mexico	6,000	0.48%
3	New York	88,100	7.04%
10	North Carolina	34,500	2.76%
46	North Dakota	3,400	0.27%
7	Ohio	57,600	4.60%
26	Oklahoma	16,400	1.31%
28	Oregon	15,500	1.24%
5	Pennsylvania	71,500	5.71%
39	Rhode Island	5,700	0.46%
25	South Carolina	17,600	1.41%
46	South Dakota	3,400	0.27%
16	Tennessee	26,300	2.10%
4	Texas	74,600	5.96%
41	Utah	5,000	0.40%
48	Vermont	2,700	0.22%
12	Virginia	29,200	2.33%
19	Washington	23,000	1.84%
34	West Virginia	10,900	0.87%
17	Wisconsin	25,300	2.02%
49	Wyoming	1,900	0.15%

RANK ORDER

RANK	STATE	CASES	% of USA
1	California	120,000	9.58%
2	Florida	88,700	7.08%
3	New York	88,100	7.04%
4	Texas	74,600	5.96%
5	Pennsylvania	71,500	5.71%
6	Illinois	58,500	4.67%
7	Ohio	57,600	4.60%
8	Michigan	46,100	3.68%
9	New Jersey	43,300	3.46%
10	North Carolina	34,500	2.76%
11	Massachusetts	32,300	2.58%
12	Virginia	29,200	2.33%
13	Indiana	28,600	2.28%
14	Missouri	28,500	2.28%
15	Georgia	28,400	2.27%
16	Tennessee	26,300	2.10%
17	Wisconsin	25,300	2.02%
18	Maryland	24,100	1.92%
19	Washington	23,000	1.84%
20	Alabama	21,400	1.71%
21	Kentucky	21,300	1.70%
22	Louisiana	21,200	1.69%
23	Minnesota	20,200	1.61%
24	Arizona	18,500	1.48%
25	South Carolina	17,600	1.41%
26	Oklahoma	16,400	1.31%
27	Connecticut	16,200	1.29%
28	Oregon	15,500	1.24%
29	Iowa	14,700	1.17%
30	Arkansas	14,100	1.13%
31	Mississippi	13,600	1.09%
32	Colorado	13,300	1.06%
33	Kansas	12,800	1.02%
34	West Virginia	10,900	0.87%
35	Nebraska	7,700	0.62%
36	Maine	7,100	0.57%
37	Nevada	6,400	0.51%
38	New Mexico	6,000	0.48%
39	Rhode Island	5,700	0.46%
40	New Hampshire	5,200	0.42%
41	Utah	5,000	0.40%
42	Idaho	4,400	0.35%
43	Hawaii	4,200	0.34%
44	Montana	4,100	0.33%
45	Delaware	3,800	0.30%
46	North Dakota	3,400	0.27%
46	South Dakota	3,400	0.27%
48	Vermont	2,700	0.22%
49	Wyoming	1,900	0.15%
50	Alaska	1,200	0.10%
	District of Columbia	3,500	0.28%

Source: American Cancer Society

"Cancer Facts & Figures-1995" (Copyright 1995, Reprinted with permission from the American Cancer Society)
*These estimates are offered as a rough guide and should not be regarded as definitive. They are calculated according to the distribution of estimated 1995 cancer deaths by state. Totals do not include carcinoma in situ or basal and squamous cell skin cancers.

Estimated Rate of New Cancer Cases in 1995

National Estimated Rate = 480.91 New Cases per 100,000 Population*

ALPHA ORDER			RANK ORDER		
RANK	**STATE**	**RATE**	**RANK**	**STATE**	**RATE**
17	Alabama	507.23	1	Florida	635.71
50	Alaska	198.02	2	West Virginia	598.24
36	Arizona	453.99	3	Pennsylvania	593.26
4	Arkansas	574.81	4	Arkansas	574.81
45	California	381.79	5	Maine	572.58
46	Colorado	363.79	6	Rhode Island	571.72
24	Connecticut	494.66	7	Kentucky	556.57
10	Delaware	538.24	8	New Jersey	547.82
1	Florida	635.71	9	Missouri	539.98
42	Georgia	402.55	10	Delaware	538.24
48	Hawaii	356.23	11	Massachusetts	534.68
44	Idaho	388.35	12	North Dakota	532.92
22	Illinois	497.79	13	Iowa	519.62
23	Indiana	497.22	14	Ohio	518.83
13	Iowa	519.62	15	Mississippi	509.55
20	Kansas	501.17	16	Tennessee	508.21
7	Kentucky	556.57	17	Alabama	507.23
25	Louisiana	491.31	18	Oklahoma	503.38
5	Maine	572.58	19	Oregon	502.27
29	Maryland	481.42	20	Kansas	501.17
11	Massachusetts	534.68	21	Wisconsin	497.84
27	Michigan	485.47	22	Illinois	497.79
38	Minnesota	442.30	23	Indiana	497.22
15	Mississippi	509.55	24	Connecticut	494.66
9	Missouri	539.98	25	Louisiana	491.31
31	Montana	478.97	26	North Carolina	487.98
32	Nebraska	474.43	27	Michigan	485.47
39	Nevada	439.26	28	New York	484.89
35	New Hampshire	457.34	29	Maryland	481.42
8	New Jersey	547.82	30	South Carolina	480.35
47	New Mexico	362.76	31	Montana	478.97
28	New York	484.89	32	Nebraska	474.43
26	North Carolina	487.98	33	South Dakota	471.57
12	North Dakota	532.92	34	Vermont	465.52
14	Ohio	518.83	35	New Hampshire	457.34
18	Oklahoma	503.38	36	Arizona	453.99
19	Oregon	502.27	37	Virginia	445.67
3	Pennsylvania	593.26	38	Minnesota	442.30
6	Rhode Island	571.72	39	Nevada	439.26
30	South Carolina	480.35	40	Washington	430.47
33	South Dakota	471.57	41	Texas	405.92
16	Tennessee	508.21	42	Georgia	402.55
41	Texas	405.92	43	Wyoming	399.16
49	Utah	262.05	44	Idaho	388.35
34	Vermont	465.52	45	California	381.79
37	Virginia	445.67	46	Colorado	363.79
40	Washington	430.47	47	New Mexico	362.76
2	West Virginia	598.24	48	Hawaii	356.23
21	Wisconsin	497.84	49	Utah	262.05
43	Wyoming	399.16	50	Alaska	198.02
				District of Columbia	614.04

Source: Morgan Quitno Press using data from American Cancer Society
"Cancer Facts & Figures-1995" (Copyright 1995, Reprinted with permission from the American Cancer Society)
*These estimates are offered as a rough guide and should not be regarded as definitive. They are calculated according to the distribution of estimated 1995 cancer deaths by state. Totals do not include carcinoma in situ or basal and squamous cell skin cancers. Rates calculated using 1994 Census resident population estimates.

Estimated New Cases of Bladder Cancer in 1995

National Estimated Total = 50,500 New Cases*

<u>ALPHA ORDER</u>

RANK	STATE	CASES	% of USA
26	Alabama	640	1.27%
49	Alaska	60	0.12%
21	Arizona	830	1.64%
30	Arkansas	550	1.09%
1	California	4,900	9.70%
29	Colorado	570	1.13%
22	Connecticut	800	1.58%
40	Delaware	210	0.42%
2	Florida	4,300	8.51%
19	Georgia	900	1.78%
47	Hawaii	110	0.22%
47	Idaho	110	0.22%
7	Illinois	2,100	4.16%
12	Indiana	1,200	2.38%
25	Iowa	680	1.35%
35	Kansas	330	0.65%
24	Kentucky	700	1.39%
32	Louisiana	430	0.85%
33	Maine	370	0.73%
16	Maryland	980	1.94%
10	Massachusetts	1,700	3.37%
9	Michigan	1,900	3.76%
20	Minnesota	840	1.66%
33	Mississippi	370	0.73%
14	Missouri	1,000	1.98%
45	Montana	130	0.26%
36	Nebraska	290	0.57%
44	Nevada	160	0.32%
38	New Hampshire	230	0.46%
7	New Jersey	2,100	4.16%
38	New Mexico	230	0.46%
3	New York	3,900	7.72%
11	North Carolina	1,300	2.57%
46	North Dakota	120	0.24%
6	Ohio	2,400	4.75%
27	Oklahoma	610	1.21%
28	Oregon	600	1.19%
4	Pennsylvania	3,000	5.94%
37	Rhode Island	280	0.55%
23	South Carolina	710	1.41%
41	South Dakota	200	0.40%
18	Tennessee	920	1.82%
5	Texas	2,700	5.35%
42	Utah	180	0.36%
43	Vermont	170	0.34%
14	Virginia	1,000	1.98%
17	Washington	930	1.84%
31	West Virginia	470	0.93%
13	Wisconsin	1,100	2.18%
49	Wyoming	60	0.12%

<u>RANK ORDER</u>

RANK	STATE	CASES	% of USA
1	California	4,900	9.70%
2	Florida	4,300	8.51%
3	New York	3,900	7.72%
4	Pennsylvania	3,000	5.94%
5	Texas	2,700	5.35%
6	Ohio	2,400	4.75%
7	Illinois	2,100	4.16%
7	New Jersey	2,100	4.16%
9	Michigan	1,900	3.76%
10	Massachusetts	1,700	3.37%
11	North Carolina	1,300	2.57%
12	Indiana	1,200	2.38%
13	Wisconsin	1,100	2.18%
14	Missouri	1,000	1.98%
14	Virginia	1,000	1.98%
16	Maryland	980	1.94%
17	Washington	930	1.84%
18	Tennessee	920	1.82%
19	Georgia	900	1.78%
20	Minnesota	840	1.66%
21	Arizona	830	1.64%
22	Connecticut	800	1.58%
23	South Carolina	710	1.41%
24	Kentucky	700	1.39%
25	Iowa	680	1.35%
26	Alabama	640	1.27%
27	Oklahoma	610	1.21%
28	Oregon	600	1.19%
29	Colorado	570	1.13%
30	Arkansas	550	1.09%
31	West Virginia	470	0.93%
32	Louisiana	430	0.85%
33	Maine	370	0.73%
33	Mississippi	370	0.73%
35	Kansas	330	0.65%
36	Nebraska	290	0.57%
37	Rhode Island	280	0.55%
38	New Hampshire	230	0.46%
38	New Mexico	230	0.46%
40	Delaware	210	0.42%
41	South Dakota	200	0.40%
42	Utah	180	0.36%
43	Vermont	170	0.34%
44	Nevada	160	0.32%
45	Montana	130	0.26%
46	North Dakota	120	0.24%
47	Hawaii	110	0.22%
47	Idaho	110	0.22%
49	Alaska	60	0.12%
49	Wyoming	60	0.12%
	District of Columbia	130	0.26%

Source: American Cancer Society
"Cancer Facts & Figures–1995" (Copyright 1995, Reprinted with permission from the American Cancer Society)
*These estimates are offered as a rough guide and should not be regarded as definitive. They are calculated according to the distribution of estimated 1995 cancer deaths by state.

Estimated Rate of New Cases of Bladder Cancer in 1995

National Estimated Rate = 19.40 New Cases per 100,000 Population*

ALPHA ORDER			RANK ORDER		
RANK	STATE	RATE	RANK	STATE	RATE
38	Alabama	15.17	1	Florida	30.82
47	Alaska	9.90	2	Maine	29.84
18	Arizona	20.37	3	Delaware	29.75
13	Arkansas	22.42	4	Vermont	29.31
34	California	15.59	5	Massachusetts	28.14
34	Colorado	15.59	6	Rhode Island	28.08
11	Connecticut	24.43	7	South Dakota	27.74
3	Delaware	29.75	8	New Jersey	26.57
1	Florida	30.82	9	West Virginia	25.80
43	Georgia	12.76	10	Pennsylvania	24.89
50	Hawaii	9.33	11	Connecticut	24.43
48	Idaho	9.71	12	Iowa	24.04
30	Illinois	17.87	13	Arkansas	22.42
17	Indiana	20.86	14	Wisconsin	21.65
12	Iowa	24.04	15	Ohio	21.62
42	Kansas	12.92	16	New York	21.47
29	Kentucky	18.29	17	Indiana	20.86
46	Louisiana	9.97	18	Arizona	20.37
2	Maine	29.84	19	New Hampshire	20.23
21	Maryland	19.58	20	Michigan	20.01
5	Massachusetts	28.14	21	Maryland	19.58
20	Michigan	20.01	22	Oregon	19.44
27	Minnesota	18.39	23	South Carolina	19.38
41	Mississippi	13.86	24	Missouri	18.95
24	Missouri	18.95	25	North Dakota	18.81
37	Montana	15.19	26	Oklahoma	18.72
30	Nebraska	17.87	27	Minnesota	18.39
45	Nevada	10.98	27	North Carolina	18.39
19	New Hampshire	20.23	29	Kentucky	18.29
8	New Jersey	26.57	30	Illinois	17.87
40	New Mexico	13.91	30	Nebraska	17.87
16	New York	21.47	32	Tennessee	17.78
27	North Carolina	18.39	33	Washington	17.41
25	North Dakota	18.81	34	California	15.59
15	Ohio	21.62	34	Colorado	15.59
26	Oklahoma	18.72	36	Virginia	15.26
22	Oregon	19.44	37	Montana	15.19
10	Pennsylvania	24.89	38	Alabama	15.17
6	Rhode Island	28.08	39	Texas	14.69
23	South Carolina	19.38	40	New Mexico	13.91
7	South Dakota	27.74	41	Mississippi	13.86
32	Tennessee	17.78	42	Kansas	12.92
39	Texas	14.69	43	Georgia	12.76
49	Utah	9.43	44	Wyoming	12.61
4	Vermont	29.31	45	Nevada	10.98
36	Virginia	15.26	46	Louisiana	9.97
33	Washington	17.41	47	Alaska	9.90
9	West Virginia	25.80	48	Idaho	9.71
14	Wisconsin	21.65	49	Utah	9.43
44	Wyoming	12.61	50	Hawaii	9.33
				District of Columbia	22.81

Source: Morgan Quitno Press using data from American Cancer Society
    "Cancer Facts & Figures-1995" (Copyright 1995, Reprinted with permission from the American Cancer Society)
*These estimates are offered as a rough guide and should not be regarded as definitive. They are calculated according to
the distribution of estimated 1995 cancer deaths by state. Rates calculated using 1994 Census resident population
estimates.

Estimated New Female Breast Cancer Cases in 1995

National Estimated Total = 182,000 New Cases*

ALPHA ORDER						RANK ORDER			

RANK	STATE	CASES	% of USA
22	Alabama	3,000	1.65%
50	Alaska	130	0.07%
24	Arizona	2,500	1.37%
31	Arkansas	1,800	0.99%
1	California	17,600	9.67%
28	Colorado	2,100	1.15%
26	Connecticut	2,300	1.26%
43	Delaware	570	0.31%
3	Florida	11,800	6.48%
15	Georgia	3,900	2.14%
46	Hawaii	440	0.24%
42	Idaho	700	0.38%
6	Illinois	9,200	5.05%
14	Indiana	4,100	2.25%
27	Iowa	2,200	1.21%
31	Kansas	1,800	0.99%
25	Kentucky	2,400	1.32%
20	Louisiana	3,200	1.76%
36	Maine	910	0.50%
18	Maryland	3,500	1.92%
10	Massachusetts	5,000	2.75%
9	Michigan	6,800	3.74%
21	Minnesota	3,100	1.70%
33	Mississippi	1,700	0.93%
13	Missouri	4,200	2.31%
44	Montana	560	0.31%
35	Nebraska	1,200	0.66%
41	Nevada	780	0.43%
37	New Hampshire	880	0.48%
8	New Jersey	7,000	3.85%
40	New Mexico	800	0.44%
2	New York	14,500	7.97%
11	North Carolina	4,600	2.53%
45	North Dakota	480	0.26%
7	Ohio	8,400	4.62%
28	Oklahoma	2,100	1.15%
30	Oregon	2,000	1.10%
4	Pennsylvania	11,200	6.15%
37	Rhode Island	880	0.48%
23	South Carolina	2,700	1.48%
47	South Dakota	420	0.23%
17	Tennessee	3,600	1.98%
5	Texas	9,800	5.38%
39	Utah	850	0.47%
48	Vermont	390	0.21%
12	Virginia	4,500	2.47%
19	Washington	3,400	1.87%
34	West Virginia	1,300	0.71%
16	Wisconsin	3,800	2.09%
49	Wyoming	290	0.16%

RANK	STATE	CASES	% of USA
1	California	17,600	9.67%
2	New York	14,500	7.97%
3	Florida	11,800	6.48%
4	Pennsylvania	11,200	6.15%
5	Texas	9,800	5.38%
6	Illinois	9,200	5.05%
7	Ohio	8,400	4.62%
8	New Jersey	7,000	3.85%
9	Michigan	6,800	3.74%
10	Massachusetts	5,000	2.75%
11	North Carolina	4,600	2.53%
12	Virginia	4,500	2.47%
13	Missouri	4,200	2.31%
14	Indiana	4,100	2.25%
15	Georgia	3,900	2.14%
16	Wisconsin	3,800	2.09%
17	Tennessee	3,600	1.98%
18	Maryland	3,500	1.92%
19	Washington	3,400	1.87%
20	Louisiana	3,200	1.76%
21	Minnesota	3,100	1.70%
22	Alabama	3,000	1.65%
23	South Carolina	2,700	1.48%
24	Arizona	2,500	1.37%
25	Kentucky	2,400	1.32%
26	Connecticut	2,300	1.26%
27	Iowa	2,200	1.21%
28	Colorado	2,100	1.15%
28	Oklahoma	2,100	1.15%
30	Oregon	2,000	1.10%
31	Arkansas	1,800	0.99%
31	Kansas	1,800	0.99%
33	Mississippi	1,700	0.93%
34	West Virginia	1,300	0.71%
35	Nebraska	1,200	0.66%
36	Maine	910	0.50%
37	New Hampshire	880	0.48%
37	Rhode Island	880	0.48%
39	Utah	850	0.47%
40	New Mexico	800	0.44%
41	Nevada	780	0.43%
42	Idaho	700	0.38%
43	Delaware	570	0.31%
44	Montana	560	0.31%
45	North Dakota	480	0.26%
46	Hawaii	440	0.24%
47	South Dakota	420	0.23%
48	Vermont	390	0.21%
49	Wyoming	290	0.16%
50	Alaska	130	0.07%
	District of Columbia	620	0.34%

Source: American Cancer Society

"Cancer Facts & Figures–1995" (Copyright 1995, Reprinted with permission from the American Cancer Society)
*These estimates are offered as a rough guide and should not be regarded as definitive. They are calculated according to the distribution of estimated 1995 cancer deaths by state.

Estimated Rate of New Female Breast Cancer Cases in 1995

National Estimated Rate = 136.57 New Cases per 100,000 Female Population*

ALPHA ORDER

RANK	STATE	RATE
24	Alabama	136.65
50	Alaska	45.35
40	Arizona	121.29
19	Arkansas	141.78
43	California	112.03
42	Colorado	113.87
25	Connecticut	136.25
6	Delaware	157.10
4	Florida	164.01
45	Georgia	107.56
49	Hawaii	75.63
36	Idaho	123.22
9	Illinois	152.44
22	Indiana	138.58
11	Iowa	151.26
21	Kansas	138.62
39	Kentucky	121.69
17	Louisiana	142.91
16	Maine	142.98
26	Maryland	135.92
5	Massachusetts	159.56
20	Michigan	139.36
29	Minnesota	133.54
38	Mississippi	122.28
7	Missouri	153.90
31	Montana	130.07
15	Nebraska	144.53
44	Nevada	109.03
10	New Hampshire	151.93
2	New Jersey	171.56
47	New Mexico	95.35
8	New York	153.68
33	North Carolina	126.37
12	North Dakota	149.96
14	Ohio	146.26
35	Oklahoma	125.83
32	Oregon	127.78
1	Pennsylvania	178.76
3	Rhode Island	169.94
18	South Carolina	142.56
41	South Dakota	114.76
28	Tennessee	134.30
46	Texas	105.18
48	Utah	88.62
30	Vermont	132.08
27	Virginia	134.57
34	Washington	126.34
23	West Virginia	137.58
13	Wisconsin	146.74
37	Wyoming	122.49

RANK ORDER

RANK	STATE	RATE
1	Pennsylvania	178.76
2	New Jersey	171.56
3	Rhode Island	169.94
4	Florida	164.01
5	Massachusetts	159.56
6	Delaware	157.10
7	Missouri	153.90
8	New York	153.68
9	Illinois	152.44
10	New Hampshire	151.93
11	Iowa	151.26
12	North Dakota	149.96
13	Wisconsin	146.74
14	Ohio	146.26
15	Nebraska	144.53
16	Maine	142.98
17	Louisiana	142.91
18	South Carolina	142.56
19	Arkansas	141.78
20	Michigan	139.36
21	Kansas	138.62
22	Indiana	138.58
23	West Virginia	137.58
24	Alabama	136.65
25	Connecticut	136.25
26	Maryland	135.92
27	Virginia	134.57
28	Tennessee	134.30
29	Minnesota	133.54
30	Vermont	132.08
31	Montana	130.07
32	Oregon	127.78
33	North Carolina	126.37
34	Washington	126.34
35	Oklahoma	125.83
36	Idaho	123.22
37	Wyoming	122.49
38	Mississippi	122.28
39	Kentucky	121.69
40	Arizona	121.29
41	South Dakota	114.76
42	Colorado	113.87
43	California	112.03
44	Nevada	109.03
45	Georgia	107.56
46	Texas	105.18
47	New Mexico	95.35
48	Utah	88.62
49	Hawaii	75.63
50	Alaska	45.35

District of Columbia 203.86

Source: Morgan Quitno Press using data from American Cancer Society
"Cancer Facts & Figures–1995" (Copyright 1995, Reprinted with permission from the American Cancer Society)
*These estimates are offered as a rough guide and should not be regarded as definitive. They are calculated according to the distribution of estimated 1995 cancer deaths by state. Rates calculated using 1994 Census female resident population estimates.

Percent of Women Age 40 and Older
Who Have Had a Breast Exam and Mammogram as of 1993
National Median = 73.41 % of Women 40 Years and Older

RANK	STATE	PERCENT	RANK	STATE	PERCENT
35	Alabama	71.89	1	Washington	81.75
6	Alaska	78.90	2	Minnesota	80.26
43	Arizona	68.62	3	Oregon	80.08
47	Arkansas	65.74	4	California	79.56
4	California	79.56	5	Colorado	79.15
5	Colorado	79.15	6	Alaska	78.90
11	Connecticut	77.18	7	Massachusetts	78.87
10	Delaware	77.65	8	New Hampshire	78.02
37	Florida	71.12	9	Hawaii	77.66
17	Georgia	74.92	10	Delaware	77.65
9	Hawaii	77.66	11	Connecticut	77.18
30	Idaho	72.73	12	North Dakota	76.92
42	Illinois	69.47	13	New York	76.47
40	Indiana	70.14	14	Maryland	76.34
32	Iowa	72.40	15	Maine	76.16
36	Kansas	71.78	16	Rhode Island	75.30
46	Kentucky	65.90	17	Georgia	74.92
48	Louisiana	64.52	18	Wisconsin	74.51
15	Maine	76.16	19	South Dakota	74.42
14	Maryland	76.34	20	North Carolina	74.21
7	Massachusetts	78.87	21	Missouri	73.99
28	Michigan	73.14	22	Montana	73.79
2	Minnesota	80.26	23	New Mexico	73.57
49	Mississippi	63.79	24	Ohio	73.48
21	Missouri	73.99	24	South Carolina	73.48
22	Montana	73.79	26	Vermont	73.35
41	Nebraska	69.56	27	Utah	73.20
29	Nevada	72.77	28	Michigan	73.14
8	New Hampshire	78.02	29	Nevada	72.77
31	New Jersey	72.62	30	Idaho	72.73
23	New Mexico	73.57	31	New Jersey	72.62
13	New York	76.47	32	Iowa	72.40
20	North Carolina	74.21	33	Texas	72.35
12	North Dakota	76.92	34	Oklahoma	71.98
24	Ohio	73.48	35	Alabama	71.89
34	Oklahoma	71.98	36	Kansas	71.78
3	Oregon	80.08	37	Florida	71.12
44	Pennsylvania	68.50	38	West Virginia	70.43
16	Rhode Island	75.30	39	Virginia	70.32
24	South Carolina	73.48	40	Indiana	70.14
19	South Dakota	74.42	41	Nebraska	69.56
45	Tennessee	66.03	42	Illinois	69.47
33	Texas	72.35	43	Arizona	68.62
27	Utah	73.20	44	Pennsylvania	68.50
26	Vermont	73.35	45	Tennessee	66.03
39	Virginia	70.32	46	Kentucky	65.90
1	Washington	81.75	47	Arkansas	65.74
38	West Virginia	70.43	48	Louisiana	64.52
18	Wisconsin	74.51	49	Mississippi	63.79
NA	Wyoming*	NA	NA	Wyoming*	NA
			District of Columbia		63.59

Source: U.S. Department of Health and Human Services, Centers for Disease Control and Prevention
"1993 Behavioral Risk Factor Surveillance Summary Prevalence Report" (October 1, 1994)
*Not available.

Estimated New Colon and Rectum Cancer Cases in 1995

National Estimated Total = 138,200 New Cases*

ALPHA ORDER

ALPHA ORDER

RANK	STATE	CASES	% of USA
22	Alabama	2,000	1.45%
50	Alaska	140	0.10%
26	Arizona	1,800	1.30%
29	Arkansas	1,600	1.16%
1	California	12,200	8.83%
30	Colorado	1,500	1.09%
22	Connecticut	2,000	1.45%
42	Delaware	480	0.35%
3	Florida	9,300	6.73%
18	Georgia	2,600	1.88%
43	Hawaii	470	0.34%
43	Idaho	470	0.34%
6	Illinois	6,900	4.99%
12	Indiana	3,300	2.39%
26	Iowa	1,800	1.30%
30	Kansas	1,500	1.09%
19	Kentucky	2,400	1.74%
22	Louisiana	2,000	1.45%
36	Maine	790	0.57%
14	Maryland	2,900	2.10%
10	Massachusetts	4,200	3.04%
8	Michigan	5,300	3.84%
19	Minnesota	2,400	1.74%
33	Mississippi	1,400	1.01%
12	Missouri	3,300	2.39%
47	Montana	410	0.30%
35	Nebraska	860	0.62%
38	Nevada	560	0.41%
45	New Hampshire	460	0.33%
8	New Jersey	5,300	3.84%
38	New Mexico	560	0.41%
2	New York	10,700	7.74%
11	North Carolina	3,500	2.53%
41	North Dakota	500	0.36%
7	Ohio	6,600	4.78%
28	Oklahoma	1,700	1.23%
30	Oregon	1,500	1.09%
4	Pennsylvania	8,300	6.01%
37	Rhode Island	690	0.50%
25	South Carolina	1,900	1.37%
46	South Dakota	430	0.31%
17	Tennessee	2,800	2.03%
5	Texas	7,900	5.72%
40	Utah	530	0.38%
48	Vermont	310	0.22%
14	Virginia	2,900	2.10%
21	Washington	2,200	1.59%
34	West Virginia	1,300	0.94%
14	Wisconsin	2,900	2.10%
49	Wyoming	200	0.14%

RANK ORDER

RANK	STATE	CASES	% of USA
1	California	12,200	8.83%
2	New York	10,700	7.74%
3	Florida	9,300	6.73%
4	Pennsylvania	8,300	6.01%
5	Texas	7,900	5.72%
6	Illinois	6,900	4.99%
7	Ohio	6,600	4.78%
8	Michigan	5,300	3.84%
8	New Jersey	5,300	3.84%
10	Massachusetts	4,200	3.04%
11	North Carolina	3,500	2.53%
12	Indiana	3,300	2.39%
12	Missouri	3,300	2.39%
14	Maryland	2,900	2.10%
14	Virginia	2,900	2.10%
14	Wisconsin	2,900	2.10%
17	Tennessee	2,800	2.03%
18	Georgia	2,600	1.88%
19	Kentucky	2,400	1.74%
19	Minnesota	2,400	1.74%
21	Washington	2,200	1.59%
22	Alabama	2,000	1.45%
22	Connecticut	2,000	1.45%
22	Louisiana	2,000	1.45%
25	South Carolina	1,900	1.37%
26	Arizona	1,800	1.30%
26	Iowa	1,800	1.30%
28	Oklahoma	1,700	1.23%
29	Arkansas	1,600	1.16%
30	Colorado	1,500	1.09%
30	Kansas	1,500	1.09%
30	Oregon	1,500	1.09%
33	Mississippi	1,400	1.01%
34	West Virginia	1,300	0.94%
35	Nebraska	860	0.62%
36	Maine	790	0.57%
37	Rhode Island	690	0.50%
38	Nevada	560	0.41%
38	New Mexico	560	0.41%
40	Utah	530	0.38%
41	North Dakota	500	0.36%
42	Delaware	480	0.35%
43	Hawaii	470	0.34%
43	Idaho	470	0.34%
45	New Hampshire	460	0.33%
46	South Dakota	430	0.31%
47	Montana	410	0.30%
48	Vermont	310	0.22%
49	Wyoming	200	0.14%
50	Alaska	140	0.10%
	District of Columbia	440	0.32%

Source: American Cancer Society

"Cancer Facts & Figures-1995" (Copyright 1995, Reprinted with permission from the American Cancer Society)
These estimates are offered as a rough guide and should not be regarded as definitive. They are calculated according to the distribution of estimated 1995 cancer deaths by state.

Estimated Rate of New Colon and Rectum Cancer Cases in 1995

National Estimated Rate = 53.08 New Cases per 100,000 Population*

ALPHA ORDER

RANK ORDER

RANK	STATE	RATE		RANK	STATE	RATE
34	Alabama	47.40		1	North Dakota	78.37
50	Alaska	23.10		2	West Virginia	71.35
37	Arizona	44.17		3	Massachusetts	69.52
9	Arkansas	65.23		4	Rhode Island	69.21
45	California	38.82		5	Pennsylvania	68.87
42	Colorado	41.03		6	Delaware	67.99
14	Connecticut	61.07		7	New Jersey	67.05
6	Delaware	67.99		8	Florida	66.65
8	Florida	66.65		9	Arkansas	65.23
47	Georgia	36.85		10	Maine	63.71
44	Hawaii	39.86		11	Iowa	63.63
40	Idaho	41.48		12	Kentucky	62.71
19	Illinois	58.71		13	Missouri	62.52
21	Indiana	57.37		14	Connecticut	61.07
11	Iowa	63.63		15	South Dakota	59.64
18	Kansas	58.73		16	Ohio	59.45
12	Kentucky	62.71		17	New York	58.89
35	Louisiana	46.35		18	Kansas	58.73
10	Maine	63.71		19	Illinois	58.71
20	Maryland	57.93		20	Maryland	57.93
3	Massachusetts	69.52		21	Indiana	57.37
23	Michigan	55.81		22	Wisconsin	57.06
27	Minnesota	52.55		23	Michigan	55.81
28	Mississippi	52.45		24	Tennessee	54.11
13	Missouri	62.52		25	Vermont	53.45
33	Montana	47.90		26	Nebraska	52.99
26	Nebraska	52.99		27	Minnesota	52.55
46	Nevada	38.44		28	Mississippi	52.45
43	New Hampshire	40.46		29	Oklahoma	52.18
7	New Jersey	67.05		30	South Carolina	51.86
48	New Mexico	33.86		31	North Carolina	49.50
17	New York	58.89		32	Oregon	48.61
31	North Carolina	49.50		33	Montana	47.90
1	North Dakota	78.37		34	Alabama	47.40
16	Ohio	59.45		35	Louisiana	46.35
29	Oklahoma	52.18		36	Virginia	44.26
32	Oregon	48.61		37	Arizona	44.17
5	Pennsylvania	68.87		38	Texas	42.99
4	Rhode Island	69.21		39	Wyoming	42.02
30	South Carolina	51.86		40	Idaho	41.48
15	South Dakota	59.64		41	Washington	41.18
24	Tennessee	54.11		42	Colorado	41.03
38	Texas	42.99		43	New Hampshire	40.46
49	Utah	27.78		44	Hawaii	39.86
25	Vermont	53.45		45	California	38.82
36	Virginia	44.26		46	Nevada	38.44
41	Washington	41.18		47	Georgia	36.85
2	West Virginia	71.35		48	New Mexico	33.86
22	Wisconsin	57.06		49	Utah	27.78
39	Wyoming	42.02		50	Alaska	23.10

District of Columbia   77.19

Source: Morgan Quitno Press using data from American Cancer Society
"Cancer Facts & Figures–1995" (Copyright 1995, Reprinted with permission from the American Cancer Society)
*These estimates are offered as a rough guide and should not be regarded as definitive. They are calculated according to the distribution of estimated 1995 cancer deaths by state. Rates calculated using 1994 Census resident population estimates.

Estimated New Cases of Leukemia in 1995

National Estimated Total = 25,700 New Cases*

ALPHA ORDER				RANK ORDER			
RANK	STATE	CASES	% of USA	RANK	STATE	CASES	% of USA
20	Alabama	460	1.79%	1	California	2,600	10.12%
50	Alaska	10	0.04%	2	Florida	1,700	6.61%
23	Arizona	430	1.67%	2	New York	1,700	6.61%
30	Arkansas	290	1.13%	4	Texas	1,600	6.23%
1	California	2,600	10.12%	5	Pennsylvania	1,400	5.45%
32	Colorado	280	1.09%	6	Illinois	1,300	5.06%
25	Connecticut	360	1.40%	7	Ohio	1,200	4.67%
46	Delaware	70	0.27%	8	Michigan	1,000	3.89%
2	Florida	1,700	6.61%	9	New Jersey	750	2.92%
13	Georgia	590	2.30%	10	North Carolina	680	2.65%
44	Hawaii	80	0.31%	11	Missouri	640	2.49%
40	Idaho	110	0.43%	12	Wisconsin	600	2.33%
6	Illinois	1,300	5.06%	13	Georgia	590	2.30%
16	Indiana	530	2.06%	13	Virginia	590	2.30%
27	Iowa	320	1.25%	15	Massachusetts	550	2.14%
29	Kansas	300	1.17%	16	Indiana	530	2.06%
21	Kentucky	440	1.71%	16	Tennessee	530	2.06%
23	Louisiana	430	1.67%	18	Minnesota	510	1.98%
40	Maine	110	0.43%	18	Washington	510	1.98%
21	Maryland	440	1.71%	20	Alabama	460	1.79%
15	Massachusetts	550	2.14%	21	Kentucky	440	1.71%
8	Michigan	1,000	3.89%	21	Maryland	440	1.71%
18	Minnesota	510	1.98%	23	Arizona	430	1.67%
33	Mississippi	270	1.05%	23	Louisiana	430	1.67%
11	Missouri	640	2.49%	25	Connecticut	360	1.40%
42	Montana	90	0.35%	26	Oregon	340	1.32%
35	Nebraska	150	0.58%	27	Iowa	320	1.25%
39	Nevada	120	0.47%	27	Oklahoma	320	1.25%
42	New Hampshire	90	0.35%	29	Kansas	300	1.17%
9	New Jersey	750	2.92%	30	Arkansas	290	1.13%
35	New Mexico	150	0.58%	30	South Carolina	290	1.13%
2	New York	1,700	6.61%	32	Colorado	280	1.09%
10	North Carolina	680	2.65%	33	Mississippi	270	1.05%
46	North Dakota	70	0.27%	34	West Virginia	200	0.78%
7	Ohio	1,200	4.67%	35	Nebraska	150	0.58%
27	Oklahoma	320	1.25%	35	New Mexico	150	0.58%
26	Oregon	340	1.32%	37	Rhode Island	130	0.51%
5	Pennsylvania	1,400	5.45%	37	Utah	130	0.51%
37	Rhode Island	130	0.51%	39	Nevada	120	0.47%
30	South Carolina	290	1.13%	40	Idaho	110	0.43%
44	South Dakota	80	0.31%	40	Maine	110	0.43%
16	Tennessee	530	2.06%	42	Montana	90	0.35%
4	Texas	1,600	6.23%	42	New Hampshire	90	0.35%
37	Utah	130	0.51%	44	Hawaii	80	0.31%
48	Vermont	60	0.23%	44	South Dakota	80	0.31%
13	Virginia	590	2.30%	46	Delaware	70	0.27%
18	Washington	510	1.98%	46	North Dakota	70	0.27%
34	West Virginia	200	0.78%	48	Vermont	60	0.23%
12	Wisconsin	600	2.33%	49	Wyoming	40	0.16%
49	Wyoming	40	0.16%	50	Alaska	10	0.04%
					District of Columbia	60	0.23%

Source: American Cancer Society

"Cancer Facts & Figures-1995" (Copyright 1995, Reprinted with permission from the American Cancer Society)
These estimates are offered as a rough guide and should not be regarded as definitive. They are calculated according to the distribution of estimated 1995 cancer deaths by state.

Estimated Rate of New Leukemia Cases in 1995

National Estimated Rate = 9.87 New Cases per 100,000 Population*

ALPHA ORDER

RANK ORDER

RANK	STATE	RATE
17	Alabama	10.90
50	Alaska	1.65
19	Arizona	10.55
4	Arkansas	11.82
43	California	8.27
47	Colorado	7.66
14	Connecticut	10.99
26	Delaware	9.92
2	Florida	12.18
42	Georgia	8.36
49	Hawaii	6.79
28	Idaho	9.71
12	Illinois	11.06
34	Indiana	9.21
9	Iowa	11.31
6	Kansas	11.75
8	Kentucky	11.50
25	Louisiana	9.97
38	Maine	8.87
39	Maryland	8.79
35	Massachusetts	9.10
20	Michigan	10.53
10	Minnesota	11.17
24	Mississippi	10.12
3	Missouri	12.13
21	Montana	10.51
33	Nebraska	9.24
44	Nevada	8.24
45	New Hampshire	7.92
31	New Jersey	9.49
36	New Mexico	9.07
32	New York	9.36
29	North Carolina	9.62
16	North Dakota	10.97
18	Ohio	10.81
27	Oklahoma	9.82
13	Oregon	11.02
7	Pennsylvania	11.62
1	Rhode Island	13.04
46	South Carolina	7.91
11	South Dakota	11.10
23	Tennessee	10.24
40	Texas	8.71
48	Utah	6.81
22	Vermont	10.34
37	Virginia	9.00
30	Washington	9.55
15	West Virginia	10.98
5	Wisconsin	11.81
41	Wyoming	8.40

RANK	STATE	RATE
1	Rhode Island	13.04
2	Florida	12.18
3	Missouri	12.13
4	Arkansas	11.82
5	Wisconsin	11.81
6	Kansas	11.75
7	Pennsylvania	11.62
8	Kentucky	11.50
9	Iowa	11.31
10	Minnesota	11.17
11	South Dakota	11.10
12	Illinois	11.06
13	Oregon	11.02
14	Connecticut	10.99
15	West Virginia	10.98
16	North Dakota	10.97
17	Alabama	10.90
18	Ohio	10.81
19	Arizona	10.55
20	Michigan	10.53
21	Montana	10.51
22	Vermont	10.34
23	Tennessee	10.24
24	Mississippi	10.12
25	Louisiana	9.97
26	Delaware	9.92
27	Oklahoma	9.82
28	Idaho	9.71
29	North Carolina	9.62
30	Washington	9.55
31	New Jersey	9.49
32	New York	9.36
33	Nebraska	9.24
34	Indiana	9.21
35	Massachusetts	9.10
36	New Mexico	9.07
37	Virginia	9.00
38	Maine	8.87
39	Maryland	8.79
40	Texas	8.71
41	Wyoming	8.40
42	Georgia	8.36
43	California	8.27
44	Nevada	8.24
45	New Hampshire	7.92
46	South Carolina	7.91
47	Colorado	7.66
48	Utah	6.81
49	Hawaii	6.79
50	Alaska	1.65

District of Columbia   10.53

Source: Morgan Quitno Press using data from American Cancer Society
   "Cancer Facts & Figures–1995" (Copyright 1995, Reprinted with permission from the American Cancer Society)
*These estimates are offered as a rough guide and should not be regarded as definitive. They are calculated according to the distribution of estimated 1995 cancer deaths by state. Rates calculated using 1994 Census resident population estimates.

Estimated New Lung Cancer Cases in 1995

National Estimated Total = 169,900 New Cases*

ALPHA ORDER					RANK ORDER			
RANK	STATE		CASES	% of USA	RANK	STATE	CASES	% of USA
21	Alabama		3,100	1.82%	1	California	15,600	9.18%
50	Alaska		170	0.10%	2	Florida	13,000	7.65%
23	Arizona		2,500	1.47%	3	New York	11,200	6.59%
26	Arkansas		2,300	1.35%	4	Texas	10,800	6.36%
1	California		15,600	9.18%	5	Pennsylvania	9,200	5.41%
34	Colorado		1,500	0.88%	6	Ohio	8,100	4.77%
29	Connecticut		2,100	1.24%	7	Illinois	7,400	4.36%
41	Delaware		560	0.33%	8	Michigan	6,100	3.59%
2	Florida		13,000	7.65%	9	New Jersey	5,300	3.12%
11	Georgia		4,200	2.47%	10	North Carolina	4,900	2.88%
43	Hawaii		520	0.31%	11	Georgia	4,200	2.47%
44	Idaho		500	0.29%	11	Indiana	4,200	2.47%
7	Illinois		7,400	4.36%	11	Missouri	4,200	2.47%
11	Indiana		4,200	2.47%	14	Tennessee	4,000	2.35%
30	Iowa		1,900	1.12%	14	Virginia	4,000	2.35%
32	Kansas		1,700	1.00%	16	Massachusetts	3,900	2.30%
17	Kentucky		3,600	2.12%	17	Kentucky	3,600	2.12%
19	Louisiana		3,200	1.88%	18	Maryland	3,300	1.94%
35	Maine		1,000	0.59%	19	Louisiana	3,200	1.88%
18	Maryland		3,300	1.94%	19	Washington	3,200	1.88%
16	Massachusetts		3,900	2.30%	21	Alabama	3,100	1.82%
8	Michigan		6,100	3.59%	22	Wisconsin	2,900	1.71%
26	Minnesota		2,300	1.35%	23	Arizona	2,500	1.47%
30	Mississippi		1,900	1.12%	23	Oklahoma	2,500	1.47%
11	Missouri		4,200	2.47%	23	South Carolina	2,500	1.47%
42	Montana		540	0.32%	26	Arkansas	2,300	1.35%
37	Nebraska		940	0.55%	26	Minnesota	2,300	1.35%
35	Nevada		1,000	0.59%	28	Oregon	2,200	1.29%
39	New Hampshire		700	0.41%	29	Connecticut	2,100	1.24%
9	New Jersey		5,300	3.12%	30	Iowa	1,900	1.12%
39	New Mexico		700	0.41%	30	Mississippi	1,900	1.12%
3	New York		11,200	6.59%	32	Kansas	1,700	1.00%
10	North Carolina		4,900	2.88%	32	West Virginia	1,700	1.00%
47	North Dakota		360	0.21%	34	Colorado	1,500	0.88%
6	Ohio		8,100	4.77%	35	Maine	1,000	0.59%
23	Oklahoma		2,500	1.47%	35	Nevada	1,000	0.59%
28	Oregon		2,200	1.29%	37	Nebraska	940	0.55%
5	Pennsylvania		9,200	5.41%	38	Rhode Island	710	0.42%
38	Rhode Island		710	0.42%	39	New Hampshire	700	0.41%
23	South Carolina		2,500	1.47%	39	New Mexico	700	0.41%
46	South Dakota		380	0.22%	41	Delaware	560	0.33%
14	Tennessee		4,000	2.35%	42	Montana	540	0.32%
4	Texas		10,800	6.36%	43	Hawaii	520	0.31%
45	Utah		410	0.24%	44	Idaho	500	0.29%
48	Vermont		320	0.19%	45	Utah	410	0.24%
14	Virginia		4,000	2.35%	46	South Dakota	380	0.22%
19	Washington		3,200	1.88%	47	North Dakota	360	0.21%
32	West Virginia		1,700	1.00%	48	Vermont	320	0.19%
22	Wisconsin		2,900	1.71%	49	Wyoming	230	0.14%
49	Wyoming		230	0.14%	50	Alaska	170	0.10%
						District of Columbia	360	0.21%

Source: American Cancer Society
"Cancer Facts & Figures-1995" (Copyright 1995, Reprinted with permission from the American Cancer Society)
These estimates are offered as a rough guide and should not be regarded as definitive. They are calculated according to the distribution of estimated 1995 cancer deaths by state.

Estimated Rate of New Lung Cancer Cases in 1995

National Estimated Rate = 65.26 New Cases per 100,000 Population*

ALPHA ORDER			RANK ORDER		
RANK	STATE	RATE	RANK	STATE	RATE
12	Alabama	73.48	1	Kentucky	94.07
49	Alaska	28.05	2	Arkansas	93.76
32	Arizona	61.35	3	West Virginia	93.30
2	Arkansas	93.76	4	Florida	93.17
43	California	49.63	5	Maine	80.65
48	Colorado	41.03	6	Missouri	79.58
27	Connecticut	64.12	7	Delaware	79.32
7	Delaware	79.32	8	Tennessee	77.29
4	Florida	93.17	9	Oklahoma	76.73
35	Georgia	59.53	10	Pennsylvania	76.34
46	Hawaii	44.11	11	Louisiana	74.16
45	Idaho	44.13	12	Alabama	73.48
29	Illinois	62.97	13	Indiana	73.02
13	Indiana	73.02	14	Ohio	72.96
21	Iowa	67.16	15	Oregon	71.29
23	Kansas	66.56	16	Rhode Island	71.21
1	Kentucky	94.07	17	Mississippi	71.19
11	Louisiana	74.16	18	North Carolina	69.31
5	Maine	80.65	19	Nevada	68.63
24	Maryland	65.92	20	South Carolina	68.23
25	Massachusetts	64.56	21	Iowa	67.16
26	Michigan	64.24	22	New Jersey	67.05
42	Minnesota	50.36	23	Kansas	66.56
17	Mississippi	71.19	24	Maryland	65.92
6	Missouri	79.58	25	Massachusetts	64.56
28	Montana	63.08	26	Michigan	64.24
37	Nebraska	57.92	27	Connecticut	64.12
19	Nevada	68.63	28	Montana	63.08
31	New Hampshire	61.57	29	Illinois	62.97
22	New Jersey	67.05	30	New York	61.64
47	New Mexico	42.32	31	New Hampshire	61.57
30	New York	61.64	32	Arizona	61.35
18	North Carolina	69.31	33	Virginia	61.05
39	North Dakota	56.43	34	Washington	59.89
14	Ohio	72.96	35	Georgia	59.53
9	Oklahoma	76.73	36	Texas	58.77
15	Oregon	71.29	37	Nebraska	57.92
10	Pennsylvania	76.34	38	Wisconsin	57.06
16	Rhode Island	71.21	39	North Dakota	56.43
20	South Carolina	68.23	40	Vermont	55.17
41	South Dakota	52.70	41	South Dakota	52.70
8	Tennessee	77.29	42	Minnesota	50.36
36	Texas	58.77	43	California	49.63
50	Utah	21.49	44	Wyoming	48.32
40	Vermont	55.17	45	Idaho	44.13
33	Virginia	61.05	46	Hawaii	44.11
34	Washington	59.89	47	New Mexico	42.32
3	West Virginia	93.30	48	Colorado	41.03
38	Wisconsin	57.06	49	Alaska	28.05
44	Wyoming	48.32	50	Utah	21.49
				District of Columbia	63.16

Source: Morgan Quitno Press using data from American Cancer Society
"Cancer Facts & Figures–1995" (Copyright 1995, Reprinted with permission from the American Cancer Society)
*These estimates are offered as a rough guide and should not be regarded as definitive. They are calculated according to the distribution of estimated 1995 cancer deaths by state. Rates calculated using 1994 Census resident population estimates.

Estimated New Oral Cancer Cases in 1995

National Estimated Total = 28,150 New Cases*

ALPHA ORDER

RANK	STATE	CASES	% of USA
30	Alabama	320	1.14%
44	Alaska	70	0.25%
25	Arizona	390	1.39%
34	Arkansas	200	0.71%
1	California	3,000	10.66%
28	Colorado	330	1.17%
24	Connecticut	420	1.49%
41	Delaware	110	0.39%
2	Florida	2,300	8.17%
12	Georgia	680	2.42%
38	Hawaii	140	0.50%
42	Idaho	90	0.32%
5	Illinois	1,400	4.97%
15	Indiana	550	1.95%
32	Iowa	240	0.85%
28	Kansas	330	1.17%
22	Kentucky	440	1.56%
15	Louisiana	550	1.95%
36	Maine	160	0.57%
14	Maryland	590	2.10%
11	Massachusetts	710	2.52%
10	Michigan	860	3.06%
23	Minnesota	430	1.53%
26	Mississippi	370	1.31%
20	Missouri	500	1.78%
46	Montana	50	0.18%
35	Nebraska	180	0.64%
40	Nevada	130	0.46%
38	New Hampshire	140	0.50%
8	New Jersey	990	3.52%
36	New Mexico	160	0.57%
3	New York	2,000	7.10%
9	North Carolina	930	3.30%
44	North Dakota	70	0.25%
7	Ohio	1,100	3.91%
31	Oklahoma	280	0.99%
26	Oregon	370	1.31%
6	Pennsylvania	1,300	4.62%
43	Rhode Island	80	0.28%
21	South Carolina	490	1.74%
49	South Dakota	30	0.11%
17	Tennessee	540	1.92%
3	Texas	2,000	7.10%
47	Utah	40	0.14%
47	Vermont	40	0.14%
13	Virginia	630	2.24%
17	Washington	540	1.92%
32	West Virginia	240	0.85%
19	Wisconsin	530	1.88%
50	Wyoming	20	0.07%

RANK ORDER

RANK	STATE	CASES	% of USA
1	California	3,000	10.66%
2	Florida	2,300	8.17%
3	New York	2,000	7.10%
3	Texas	2,000	7.10%
5	Illinois	1,400	4.97%
6	Pennsylvania	1,300	4.62%
7	Ohio	1,100	3.91%
8	New Jersey	990	3.52%
9	North Carolina	930	3.30%
10	Michigan	860	3.06%
11	Massachusetts	710	2.52%
12	Georgia	680	2.42%
13	Virginia	630	2.24%
14	Maryland	590	2.10%
15	Indiana	550	1.95%
15	Louisiana	550	1.95%
17	Tennessee	540	1.92%
17	Washington	540	1.92%
19	Wisconsin	530	1.88%
20	Missouri	500	1.78%
21	South Carolina	490	1.74%
22	Kentucky	440	1.56%
23	Minnesota	430	1.53%
24	Connecticut	420	1.49%
25	Arizona	390	1.39%
26	Mississippi	370	1.31%
26	Oregon	370	1.31%
28	Colorado	330	1.17%
28	Kansas	330	1.17%
30	Alabama	320	1.14%
31	Oklahoma	280	0.99%
32	Iowa	240	0.85%
32	West Virginia	240	0.85%
34	Arkansas	200	0.71%
35	Nebraska	180	0.64%
36	Maine	160	0.57%
36	New Mexico	160	0.57%
38	Hawaii	140	0.50%
38	New Hampshire	140	0.50%
40	Nevada	130	0.46%
41	Delaware	110	0.39%
42	Idaho	90	0.32%
43	Rhode Island	80	0.28%
44	Alaska	70	0.25%
44	North Dakota	70	0.25%
46	Montana	50	0.18%
47	Utah	40	0.14%
47	Vermont	40	0.14%
49	South Dakota	30	0.11%
50	Wyoming	20	0.07%
	District of Columbia	90	0.32%

Source: American Cancer Society

"Cancer Facts & Figures–1995" (Copyright 1995, Reprinted with permission from the American Cancer Society)
These estimates are offered as a rough guide and should not be regarded as definitive. They are calculated according to the distribution of estimated 1995 cancer deaths by state.

328

Estimated Rate of New Oral Cancer Cases in 1995

National Estimated Rate = 10.81 New Cases per 100,000 Population*

ALPHA ORDER			RANK ORDER		
RANK	STATE	RATE	RANK	STATE	RATE
45	Alabama	7.58	1	Florida	16.48
18	Alaska	11.55	2	Delaware	15.58
32	Arizona	9.57	3	Mississippi	13.86
42	Arkansas	8.15	4	South Carolina	13.37
34	California	9.54	5	West Virginia	13.17
38	Colorado	9.03	6	North Carolina	13.15
9	Connecticut	12.82	7	Kansas	12.92
2	Delaware	15.58	8	Maine	12.90
1	Florida	16.48	9	Connecticut	12.82
30	Georgia	9.64	10	Louisiana	12.75
15	Hawaii	11.87	11	New Jersey	12.53
44	Idaho	7.94	12	New Hampshire	12.31
14	Illinois	11.91	13	Oregon	11.99
33	Indiana	9.56	14	Illinois	11.91
41	Iowa	8.48	15	Hawaii	11.87
7	Kansas	12.92	16	Maryland	11.79
19	Kentucky	11.50	17	Massachusetts	11.75
10	Louisiana	12.75	18	Alaska	11.55
8	Maine	12.90	19	Kentucky	11.50
16	Maryland	11.79	20	Nebraska	11.09
17	Massachusetts	11.75	21	New York	11.01
37	Michigan	9.06	22	North Dakota	10.97
36	Minnesota	9.42	23	Texas	10.88
3	Mississippi	13.86	24	Pennsylvania	10.79
35	Missouri	9.47	25	Tennessee	10.43
47	Montana	5.84	25	Wisconsin	10.43
20	Nebraska	11.09	27	Washington	10.11
39	Nevada	8.92	28	Ohio	9.91
12	New Hampshire	12.31	29	New Mexico	9.67
11	New Jersey	12.53	30	Georgia	9.64
29	New Mexico	9.67	31	Virginia	9.62
21	New York	11.01	32	Arizona	9.57
6	North Carolina	13.15	33	Indiana	9.56
22	North Dakota	10.97	34	California	9.54
28	Ohio	9.91	35	Missouri	9.47
40	Oklahoma	8.59	36	Minnesota	9.42
13	Oregon	11.99	37	Michigan	9.06
24	Pennsylvania	10.79	38	Colorado	9.03
43	Rhode Island	8.02	39	Nevada	8.92
4	South Carolina	13.37	40	Oklahoma	8.59
49	South Dakota	4.16	41	Iowa	8.48
25	Tennessee	10.43	42	Arkansas	8.15
23	Texas	10.88	43	Rhode Island	8.02
50	Utah	2.10	44	Idaho	7.94
46	Vermont	6.90	45	Alabama	7.58
31	Virginia	9.62	46	Vermont	6.90
27	Washington	10.11	47	Montana	5.84
5	West Virginia	13.17	48	Wyoming	4.20
25	Wisconsin	10.43	49	South Dakota	4.16
48	Wyoming	4.20	50	Utah	2.10
				District of Columbia	15.79

Source: Morgan Quitno Press using data from American Cancer Society
"Cancer Facts & Figures–1995" (Copyright 1995, Reprinted with permission from the American Cancer Society)
These estimates are offered as a rough guide and should not be regarded as definitive. They are calculated according to the distribution of estimated 1995 cancer deaths by state. Rates calculated using 1994 Census resident population estimates.

Estimated New Prostate Cancer Cases in 1995

National Estimated Total = 244,000 New Cases*

<u>ALPHA ORDER</u>

RANK	STATE	CASES	% of USA
23	Alabama	3,900	1.60%
50	Alaska	180	0.07%
22	Arizona	4,000	1.64%
30	Arkansas	3,000	1.23%
1	California	23,100	9.47%
28	Colorado	3,100	1.27%
30	Connecticut	3,000	1.23%
48	Delaware	520	0.21%
2	Florida	19,000	7.79%
13	Georgia	5,700	2.34%
45	Hawaii	790	0.32%
38	Idaho	1,100	0.45%
6	Illinois	11,500	4.71%
17	Indiana	4,800	1.97%
26	Iowa	3,200	1.31%
33	Kansas	2,600	1.07%
25	Kentucky	3,500	1.43%
21	Louisiana	4,200	1.72%
37	Maine	1,400	0.57%
16	Maryland	4,900	2.01%
11	Massachusetts	5,900	2.42%
8	Michigan	8,700	3.57%
17	Minnesota	4,800	1.97%
30	Mississippi	3,000	1.23%
19	Missouri	4,700	1.93%
46	Montana	780	0.32%
35	Nebraska	1,600	0.66%
38	Nevada	1,100	0.45%
42	New Hampshire	980	0.40%
9	New Jersey	8,100	3.32%
38	New Mexico	1,100	0.45%
3	New York	16,100	6.60%
10	North Carolina	7,500	3.07%
41	North Dakota	1,000	0.41%
7	Ohio	10,500	4.30%
28	Oklahoma	3,100	1.27%
26	Oregon	3,200	1.31%
4	Pennsylvania	13,800	5.66%
43	Rhode Island	950	0.39%
24	South Carolina	3,700	1.52%
44	South Dakota	840	0.34%
15	Tennessee	5,000	2.05%
5	Texas	13,000	5.33%
36	Utah	1,500	0.61%
47	Vermont	570	0.23%
12	Virginia	5,800	2.38%
20	Washington	4,600	1.89%
34	West Virginia	1,700	0.70%
13	Wisconsin	5,700	2.34%
49	Wyoming	410	0.17%

<u>RANK ORDER</u>

RANK	STATE	CASES	% of USA
1	California	23,100	9.47%
2	Florida	19,000	7.79%
3	New York	16,100	6.60%
4	Pennsylvania	13,800	5.66%
5	Texas	13,000	5.33%
6	Illinois	11,500	4.71%
7	Ohio	10,500	4.30%
8	Michigan	8,700	3.57%
9	New Jersey	8,100	3.32%
10	North Carolina	7,500	3.07%
11	Massachusetts	5,900	2.42%
12	Virginia	5,800	2.38%
13	Georgia	5,700	2.34%
13	Wisconsin	5,700	2.34%
15	Tennessee	5,000	2.05%
16	Maryland	4,900	2.01%
17	Indiana	4,800	1.97%
17	Minnesota	4,800	1.97%
19	Missouri	4,700	1.93%
20	Washington	4,600	1.89%
21	Louisiana	4,200	1.72%
22	Arizona	4,000	1.64%
23	Alabama	3,900	1.60%
24	South Carolina	3,700	1.52%
25	Kentucky	3,500	1.43%
26	Iowa	3,200	1.31%
26	Oregon	3,200	1.31%
28	Colorado	3,100	1.27%
28	Oklahoma	3,100	1.27%
30	Arkansas	3,000	1.23%
30	Connecticut	3,000	1.23%
30	Mississippi	3,000	1.23%
33	Kansas	2,600	1.07%
34	West Virginia	1,700	0.70%
35	Nebraska	1,600	0.66%
36	Utah	1,500	0.61%
37	Maine	1,400	0.57%
38	Idaho	1,100	0.45%
38	Nevada	1,100	0.45%
38	New Mexico	1,100	0.45%
41	North Dakota	1,000	0.41%
42	New Hampshire	980	0.40%
43	Rhode Island	950	0.39%
44	South Dakota	840	0.34%
45	Hawaii	790	0.32%
46	Montana	780	0.32%
47	Vermont	570	0.23%
48	Delaware	520	0.21%
49	Wyoming	410	0.17%
50	Alaska	180	0.07%
	District of Columbia	780	0.32%

Source: American Cancer Society

"Cancer Facts & Figures–1995" (Copyright 1995, Reprinted with permission from the American Cancer Society)

*These estimates are offered as a rough guide and should not be regarded as definitive. They are calculated according to the distribution of estimated 1995 cancer deaths by state.

Estimated Rate of New Prostate Cancer Cases in 1995

National Estimated Rate = 192.01 New Cases per 100,000 Male Population*

ALPHA ORDER			RANK ORDER		
RANK	STATE	RATE	RANK	STATE	RATE
29	Alabama	192.74	1	North Dakota	314.57
50	Alaska	56.32	2	Florida	281.14
23	Arizona	198.63	3	Arkansas	253.57
3	Arkansas	253.57	4	Pennsylvania	238.47
46	California	146.94	5	South Dakota	236.49
41	Colorado	171.13	6	Mississippi	234.59
30	Connecticut	189.01	7	Iowa	232.76
44	Delaware	151.37	8	Maine	231.88
2	Florida	281.14	9	Wisconsin	228.72
42	Georgia	166.21	10	North Carolina	218.68
49	Hawaii	132.37	11	Minnesota	213.73
27	Idaho	194.71	12	New Jersey	211.83
20	Illinois	201.17	13	Oregon	210.39
39	Indiana	171.82	14	South Carolina	209.03
7	Iowa	232.76	15	Kansas	207.08
15	Kansas	207.08	16	Massachusetts	202.92
31	Kentucky	188.72	17	Louisiana	202.32
17	Louisiana	202.32	18	Nebraska	201.87
8	Maine	231.88	19	Maryland	201.55
19	Maryland	201.55	20	Illinois	201.17
16	Massachusetts	202.92	21	Tennessee	200.43
32	Michigan	188.44	22	Vermont	200.05
11	Minnesota	213.73	23	Arizona	198.63
6	Mississippi	234.59	24	Rhode Island	198.36
33	Missouri	184.41	25	Ohio	195.93
35	Montana	183.31	26	Oklahoma	195.08
18	Nebraska	201.87	27	Idaho	194.71
45	Nevada	148.33	28	West Virginia	193.82
37	New Hampshire	175.76	29	Alabama	192.74
12	New Jersey	211.83	30	Connecticut	189.01
48	New Mexico	135.05	31	Kentucky	188.72
34	New York	184.33	32	Michigan	188.44
10	North Carolina	218.68	33	Missouri	184.41
1	North Dakota	314.57	34	New York	184.33
25	Ohio	195.93	35	Montana	183.31
26	Oklahoma	195.08	36	Virginia	180.82
13	Oregon	210.39	37	New Hampshire	175.76
4	Pennsylvania	238.47	38	Washington	173.46
24	Rhode Island	198.36	39	Indiana	171.82
14	South Carolina	209.03	40	Wyoming	171.39
5	South Dakota	236.49	41	Colorado	171.13
21	Tennessee	200.43	42	Georgia	166.21
47	Texas	143.48	43	Utah	158.09
43	Utah	158.09	44	Delaware	151.37
22	Vermont	200.05	45	Nevada	148.33
36	Virginia	180.82	46	California	146.94
38	Washington	173.46	47	Texas	143.48
28	West Virginia	193.82	48	New Mexico	135.05
9	Wisconsin	228.72	49	Hawaii	132.37
40	Wyoming	171.39	50	Alaska	56.32
				District of Columbia	293.18

Source: Morgan Quitno Press using data from American Cancer Society
"Cancer Facts & Figures–1995" (Copyright 1995, Reprinted with permission from the American Cancer Society)
*These estimates are offered as a rough guide and should not be regarded as definitive. They are calculated according to the distribution of estimated 1995 cancer deaths by state. Rates calculated using 1994 Census male resident population estimates.

Estimated New Skin Melanoma Cases in 1995

National Estimated Total = 34,100 New Cases*

ALPHA ORDER					RANK ORDER			
RANK	STATE	CASES	% of USA		RANK	STATE	CASES	% of USA
22	Alabama	530	1.55%		1	California	4,500	13.20%
47	Alaska	70	0.21%		2	Florida	2,300	6.74%
19	Arizona	590	1.73%		3	New York	2,100	6.16%
31	Arkansas	360	1.06%		4	Texas	1,800	5.28%
1	California	4,500	13.20%		5	Pennsylvania	1,700	4.99%
25	Colorado	510	1.50%		6	Illinois	1,400	4.11%
30	Connecticut	410	1.20%		6	Ohio	1,400	4.11%
42	Delaware	150	0.44%		8	New Jersey	1,100	3.23%
2	Florida	2,300	6.74%		8	North Carolina	1,100	3.23%
15	Georgia	730	2.14%		10	Michigan	1,000	2.93%
48	Hawaii	50	0.15%		11	Massachusetts	940	2.76%
43	Idaho	140	0.41%		12	Missouri	810	2.38%
6	Illinois	1,400	4.11%		12	Virginia	810	2.38%
17	Indiana	670	1.96%		14	Tennessee	750	2.20%
26	Iowa	490	1.44%		15	Georgia	730	2.14%
28	Kansas	430	1.26%		16	Washington	680	1.99%
24	Kentucky	520	1.52%		17	Indiana	670	1.96%
32	Louisiana	350	1.03%		18	Wisconsin	650	1.91%
38	Maine	200	0.59%		19	Arizona	590	1.73%
20	Maryland	580	1.70%		20	Maryland	580	1.70%
11	Massachusetts	940	2.76%		21	Minnesota	550	1.61%
10	Michigan	1,000	2.93%		22	Alabama	530	1.55%
21	Minnesota	550	1.61%		22	Oklahoma	530	1.55%
33	Mississippi	300	0.88%		24	Kentucky	520	1.52%
12	Missouri	810	2.38%		25	Colorado	510	1.50%
43	Montana	140	0.41%		26	Iowa	490	1.44%
39	Nebraska	180	0.53%		27	Oregon	460	1.35%
36	Nevada	230	0.67%		28	Kansas	430	1.26%
39	New Hampshire	180	0.53%		28	South Carolina	430	1.26%
8	New Jersey	1,100	3.23%		30	Connecticut	410	1.20%
37	New Mexico	210	0.62%		31	Arkansas	360	1.06%
3	New York	2,100	6.16%		32	Louisiana	350	1.03%
8	North Carolina	1,100	3.23%		33	Mississippi	300	0.88%
49	North Dakota	40	0.12%		33	Utah	300	0.88%
6	Ohio	1,400	4.11%		35	West Virginia	280	0.82%
22	Oklahoma	530	1.55%		36	Nevada	230	0.67%
27	Oregon	460	1.35%		37	New Mexico	210	0.62%
5	Pennsylvania	1,700	4.99%		38	Maine	200	0.59%
39	Rhode Island	180	0.53%		39	Nebraska	180	0.53%
28	South Carolina	430	1.26%		39	New Hampshire	180	0.53%
46	South Dakota	100	0.29%		39	Rhode Island	180	0.53%
14	Tennessee	750	2.20%		42	Delaware	150	0.44%
4	Texas	1,800	5.28%		43	Idaho	140	0.41%
33	Utah	300	0.88%		43	Montana	140	0.41%
45	Vermont	110	0.32%		45	Vermont	110	0.32%
12	Virginia	810	2.38%		46	South Dakota	100	0.29%
16	Washington	680	1.99%		47	Alaska	70	0.21%
35	West Virginia	280	0.82%		48	Hawaii	50	0.15%
18	Wisconsin	650	1.91%		49	North Dakota	40	0.12%
49	Wyoming	40	0.12%		49	Wyoming	40	0.12%
						District of Columbia	20	0.06%

Source: American Cancer Society
"Cancer Facts & Figures-1995" (Copyright 1995, Reprinted with permission from the American Cancer Society)
*These estimates are offered as a rough guide and should not be regarded as definitive. They are calculated according to the distribution of estimated 1995 cancer deaths by state.

Estimated Rate of New Skin Melanoma Cases in 1995

National Estimate Rate = 13.10 New Cases per 100,000 Population*

ALPHA ORDER

RANK	STATE	RATE
31	Alabama	12.56
41	Alaska	11.55
20	Arizona	14.48
18	Arkansas	14.68
21	California	14.32
23	Colorado	13.95
32	Connecticut	12.52
1	Delaware	21.25
6	Florida	16.48
45	Georgia	10.35
50	Hawaii	4.24
33	Idaho	12.36
36	Illinois	11.91
38	Indiana	11.65
4	Iowa	17.32
5	Kansas	16.84
26	Kentucky	13.59
48	Louisiana	8.11
9	Maine	16.13
39	Maryland	11.59
13	Massachusetts	15.56
44	Michigan	10.53
35	Minnesota	12.04
42	Mississippi	11.24
16	Missouri	15.35
7	Montana	16.36
43	Nebraska	11.09
11	Nevada	15.79
10	New Hampshire	15.83
24	New Jersey	13.92
29	New Mexico	12.70
40	New York	11.56
13	North Carolina	15.56
49	North Dakota	6.27
30	Ohio	12.61
8	Oklahoma	16.27
17	Oregon	14.91
22	Pennsylvania	14.11
3	Rhode Island	18.05
37	South Carolina	11.74
25	South Dakota	13.87
19	Tennessee	14.49
46	Texas	9.79
12	Utah	15.72
2	Vermont	18.97
33	Virginia	12.36
28	Washington	12.73
15	West Virginia	15.37
27	Wisconsin	12.79
47	Wyoming	8.40

RANK ORDER

RANK	STATE	RATE
1	Delaware	21.25
2	Vermont	18.97
3	Rhode Island	18.05
4	Iowa	17.32
5	Kansas	16.84
6	Florida	16.48
7	Montana	16.36
8	Oklahoma	16.27
9	Maine	16.13
10	New Hampshire	15.83
11	Nevada	15.79
12	Utah	15.72
13	Massachusetts	15.56
13	North Carolina	15.56
15	West Virginia	15.37
16	Missouri	15.35
17	Oregon	14.91
18	Arkansas	14.68
19	Tennessee	14.49
20	Arizona	14.48
21	California	14.32
22	Pennsylvania	14.11
23	Colorado	13.95
24	New Jersey	13.92
25	South Dakota	13.87
26	Kentucky	13.59
27	Wisconsin	12.79
28	Washington	12.73
29	New Mexico	12.70
30	Ohio	12.61
31	Alabama	12.56
32	Connecticut	12.52
33	Idaho	12.36
33	Virginia	12.36
35	Minnesota	12.04
36	Illinois	11.91
37	South Carolina	11.74
38	Indiana	11.65
39	Maryland	11.59
40	New York	11.56
41	Alaska	11.55
42	Mississippi	11.24
43	Nebraska	11.09
44	Michigan	10.53
45	Georgia	10.35
46	Texas	9.79
47	Wyoming	8.40
48	Louisiana	8.11
49	North Dakota	6.27
50	Hawaii	4.24

District of Columbia   3.51

Source: Morgan Quitno Press using data from American Cancer Society
"Cancer Facts & Figures-1995" (Copyright 1995, Reprinted with permission from the American Cancer Society)
These estimates are offered as a rough guide and should not be regarded as definitive. They are calculated according to the distribution of estimated 1995 cancer deaths by state. Rates calculated using 1994 Census resident population estimates.

Estimated New Cancer of the Uterus Cases in 1995

National Estimated Total = 48,600 New Cases*

RANK	STATE	CASES	% of USA	RANK	STATE	CASES	% of USA
21	Alabama	810	1.67%	1	California	4,800	9.88%
50	Alaska	30	0.06%	2	New York	3,900	8.02%
30	Arizona	540	1.11%	3	Florida	3,300	6.79%
27	Arkansas	600	1.23%	4	Texas	3,200	6.58%
1	California	4,800	9.88%	5	Pennsylvania	3,100	6.38%
29	Colorado	560	1.15%	6	Illinois	2,400	4.94%
24	Connecticut	630	1.30%	7	Ohio	2,200	4.53%
39	Delaware	190	0.39%	8	Michigan	1,700	3.50%
3	Florida	3,300	6.79%	8	New Jersey	1,700	3.50%
19	Georgia	850	1.75%	10	North Carolina	1,400	2.88%
44	Hawaii	110	0.23%	11	Missouri	1,200	2.47%
47	Idaho	80	0.16%	11	Wisconsin	1,200	2.47%
6	Illinois	2,400	4.94%	13	Indiana	1,100	2.26%
13	Indiana	1,100	2.26%	13	Virginia	1,100	2.26%
31	Iowa	500	1.03%	15	Maryland	980	2.02%
27	Kansas	600	1.23%	15	Massachusetts	980	2.02%
18	Kentucky	910	1.87%	17	Tennessee	950	1.95%
26	Louisiana	610	1.26%	18	Kentucky	910	1.87%
41	Maine	160	0.33%	19	Georgia	850	1.75%
15	Maryland	980	2.02%	20	Washington	820	1.69%
15	Massachusetts	980	2.02%	21	Alabama	810	1.67%
8	Michigan	1,700	3.50%	22	South Carolina	760	1.56%
23	Minnesota	680	1.40%	23	Minnesota	680	1.40%
33	Mississippi	440	0.91%	24	Connecticut	630	1.30%
11	Missouri	1,200	2.47%	24	Oklahoma	630	1.30%
45	Montana	100	0.21%	26	Louisiana	610	1.26%
35	Nebraska	360	0.74%	27	Arkansas	600	1.23%
37	Nevada	220	0.45%	27	Kansas	600	1.23%
40	New Hampshire	180	0.37%	29	Colorado	560	1.15%
8	New Jersey	1,700	3.50%	30	Arizona	540	1.11%
36	New Mexico	330	0.68%	31	Iowa	500	1.03%
2	New York	3,900	8.02%	32	Oregon	460	0.95%
10	North Carolina	1,400	2.88%	33	Mississippi	440	0.91%
42	North Dakota	140	0.29%	34	West Virginia	420	0.86%
7	Ohio	2,200	4.53%	35	Nebraska	360	0.74%
24	Oklahoma	630	1.30%	36	New Mexico	330	0.68%
32	Oregon	460	0.95%	37	Nevada	220	0.45%
5	Pennsylvania	3,100	6.38%	38	Utah	200	0.41%
45	Rhode Island	100	0.21%	39	Delaware	190	0.39%
22	South Carolina	760	1.56%	40	New Hampshire	180	0.37%
42	South Dakota	140	0.29%	41	Maine	160	0.33%
17	Tennessee	950	1.95%	42	North Dakota	140	0.29%
4	Texas	3,200	6.58%	42	South Dakota	140	0.29%
38	Utah	200	0.41%	44	Hawaii	110	0.23%
48	Vermont	70	0.14%	45	Montana	100	0.21%
13	Virginia	1,100	2.26%	45	Rhode Island	100	0.21%
20	Washington	820	1.69%	47	Idaho	80	0.16%
34	West Virginia	420	0.86%	48	Vermont	70	0.14%
11	Wisconsin	1,200	2.47%	49	Wyoming	60	0.12%
49	Wyoming	60	0.12%	50	Alaska	30	0.06%
					District of Columbia	100	0.21%

ALPHA ORDER — RANK ORDER

Source: American Cancer Society
"Cancer Facts & Figures-1995" (Copyright 1995, Reprinted with permission from the American Cancer Society)
These estimates are offered as a rough guide and should not be regarded as definitive. They are calculated according to the distribution of estimated 1995 cancer deaths by state.

Estimated Rate of New Cancer of the Uterus Cases in 1995

National Estimate Rate = 36.47 New Cases per 100,000 Female Population*

ALPHA ORDER				RANK ORDER		
RANK	STATE	RATE		RANK	STATE	RATE
24	Alabama	36.90		1	Delaware	52.37
50	Alaska	10.46		2	Pennsylvania	49.48
40	Arizona	26.20		3	Arkansas	47.26
3	Arkansas	47.26		4	Wisconsin	46.34
34	California	30.55		5	Kansas	46.21
36	Colorado	30.37		6	Kentucky	46.14
22	Connecticut	37.32		7	Florida	45.87
1	Delaware	52.37		8	West Virginia	44.45
7	Florida	45.87		9	Missouri	43.97
44	Georgia	23.44		10	North Dakota	43.74
48	Hawaii	18.91		11	Nebraska	43.36
49	Idaho	14.08		12	New Jersey	41.67
15	Illinois	39.77		13	New York	41.34
23	Indiana	37.18		14	South Carolina	40.13
27	Iowa	34.38		15	Illinois	39.77
5	Kansas	46.21		16	New Mexico	39.33
6	Kentucky	46.14		17	North Carolina	38.46
39	Louisiana	27.24		18	Ohio	38.31
42	Maine	25.14		19	South Dakota	38.25
20	Maryland	38.06		20	Maryland	38.06
31	Massachusetts	31.27		21	Oklahoma	37.75
26	Michigan	34.84		22	Connecticut	37.32
38	Minnesota	29.29		23	Indiana	37.18
30	Mississippi	31.65		24	Alabama	36.90
9	Missouri	43.97		25	Tennessee	35.44
45	Montana	23.23		26	Michigan	34.84
11	Nebraska	43.36		27	Iowa	34.38
33	Nevada	30.75		28	Texas	34.34
32	New Hampshire	31.08		29	Virginia	32.90
12	New Jersey	41.67		30	Mississippi	31.65
16	New Mexico	39.33		31	Massachusetts	31.27
13	New York	41.34		32	New Hampshire	31.08
17	North Carolina	38.46		33	Nevada	30.75
10	North Dakota	43.74		34	California	30.55
18	Ohio	38.31		35	Washington	30.47
21	Oklahoma	37.75		36	Colorado	30.37
37	Oregon	29.39		37	Oregon	29.39
2	Pennsylvania	49.48		38	Minnesota	29.29
47	Rhode Island	19.31		39	Louisiana	27.24
14	South Carolina	40.13		40	Arizona	26.20
19	South Dakota	38.25		41	Wyoming	25.34
25	Tennessee	35.44		42	Maine	25.14
28	Texas	34.34		43	Vermont	23.71
46	Utah	20.85		44	Georgia	23.44
43	Vermont	23.71		45	Montana	23.23
29	Virginia	32.90		46	Utah	20.85
35	Washington	30.47		47	Rhode Island	19.31
8	West Virginia	44.45		48	Hawaii	18.91
4	Wisconsin	46.34		49	Idaho	14.08
41	Wyoming	25.34		50	Alaska	10.46
					District of Columbia	32.88

Source: Morgan Quitno Press using data from American Cancer Society
   "Cancer Facts & Figures-1995" (Copyright 1995, Reprinted with permission from the American Cancer Society)
*These estimates are offered as a rough guide and should not be regarded as definitive. They are calculated according to the distribution of estimated 1995 cancer deaths by state. Rates calculated using 1994 Census female resident population estimates.

Percent of Women 18 and Older
Who Had A Pap Smear Within the Past Two Years: 1993
National Median = 79.86% of Women 18 Years and Older

ALPHA ORDER

RANK ORDER

RANK	STATE	PERCENT	RANK	STATE	PERCENT
2	Alabama	86.84	1	Alaska	87.22
1	Alaska	87.22	2	Alabama	86.84
5	Arizona	83.85	3	Georgia	85.24
45	Arkansas	73.62	4	Washington	84.96
19	California	80.85	5	Arizona	83.85
18	Colorado	80.92	6	South Carolina	82.94
33	Connecticut	78.97	7	Kansas	82.68
8	Delaware	82.11	8	Delaware	82.11
37	Florida	78.19	9	Maryland	82.10
3	Georgia	85.24	10	Louisiana	81.95
23	Hawaii	80.17	11	Missouri	81.53
40	Idaho	77.22	12	Nebraska	81.44
39	Illinois	77.57	13	Maine	81.43
38	Indiana	77.97	14	New Mexico	81.39
20	Iowa	80.39	15	Ohio	81.27
7	Kansas	82.68	16	Virginia	81.26
47	Kentucky	73.08	17	Oregon	81.05
10	Louisiana	81.95	18	Colorado	80.92
13	Maine	81.43	19	California	80.85
9	Maryland	82.10	20	Iowa	80.39
27	Massachusetts	79.55	20	Texas	80.39
34	Michigan	78.60	22	North Carolina	80.20
24	Minnesota	80.02	23	Hawaii	80.17
46	Mississippi	73.59	24	Minnesota	80.02
11	Missouri	81.53	25	Vermont	79.90
30	Montana	79.07	26	Tennessee	79.83
12	Nebraska	81.44	27	Massachusetts	79.55
28	Nevada	79.47	28	Nevada	79.47
29	New Hampshire	79.17	29	New Hampshire	79.17
43	New Jersey	75.51	30	Montana	79.07
14	New Mexico	81.39	31	New York	79.02
31	New York	79.02	32	North Dakota	78.99
22	North Carolina	80.20	33	Connecticut	78.97
32	North Dakota	78.99	34	Michigan	78.60
15	Ohio	81.27	35	South Dakota	78.38
42	Oklahoma	75.74	36	Rhode Island	78.34
17	Oregon	81.05	37	Florida	78.19
49	Pennsylvania	71.62	38	Indiana	77.97
36	Rhode Island	78.34	39	Illinois	77.57
6	South Carolina	82.94	40	Idaho	77.22
35	South Dakota	78.38	41	Utah	76.03
26	Tennessee	79.83	42	Oklahoma	75.74
20	Texas	80.39	43	New Jersey	75.51
41	Utah	76.03	44	West Virginia	74.35
25	Vermont	79.90	45	Arkansas	73.62
16	Virginia	81.26	46	Mississippi	73.59
4	Washington	84.96	47	Kentucky	73.08
44	West Virginia	74.35	48	Wisconsin	72.00
48	Wisconsin	72.00	49	Pennsylvania	71.62
NA	Wyoming*	NA	NA	Wyoming*	NA
				District of Columbia	75.72

Source: U.S. Department of Health and Human Services, Centers for Disease Control and Prevention
"1993 Behavioral Risk Factor Surveillance Summary Prevalence Report" (October 1, 1994)
*Not available.

AIDS Cases Reported in 1994

National Total = 78,126 New AIDS Cases*

ALPHA ORDER

RANK	STATE	CASES	% of USA
25	Alabama	582	0.74%
45	Alaska	59	0.08%
23	Arizona	612	0.78%
31	Arkansas	284	0.36%
2	California	12,136	15.53%
19	Colorado	816	1.04%
18	Connecticut	912	1.17%
33	Delaware	271	0.35%
3	Florida	8,617	11.03%
9	Georgia	2,245	2.87%
36	Hawaii	216	0.28%
44	Idaho	61	0.08%
6	Illinois	3,104	3.97%
22	Indiana	622	0.80%
39	Iowa	130	0.17%
35	Kansas	245	0.31%
30	Kentucky	320	0.41%
11	Louisiana	1,239	1.59%
40	Maine	117	0.15%
7	Maryland	2,722	3.48%
10	Massachusetts	1,401	1.79%
16	Michigan	1,035	1.32%
27	Minnesota	422	0.54%
26	Mississippi	433	0.55%
21	Missouri	713	0.91%
47	Montana	30	0.04%
43	Nebraska	89	0.11%
28	Nevada	387	0.50%
42	New Hampshire	92	0.12%
5	New Jersey	4,993	6.39%
37	New Mexico	211	0.27%
1	New York	14,944	19.13%
12	North Carolina	1,187	1.52%
48	North Dakota	20	0.03%
13	Ohio	1,184	1.52%
34	Oklahoma	269	0.34%
24	Oregon	606	0.78%
8	Pennsylvania	2,528	3.24%
32	Rhode Island	276	0.35%
15	South Carolina	1,158	1.48%
49	South Dakota	19	0.02%
20	Tennessee	764	0.98%
4	Texas	5,879	7.53%
38	Utah	152	0.19%
46	Vermont	38	0.05%
14	Virginia	1,162	1.49%
17	Washington	932	1.19%
41	West Virginia	96	0.12%
29	Wisconsin	379	0.49%
50	Wyoming	18	0.02%

RANK ORDER

RANK	STATE	CASES	% of USA
1	New York	14,944	19.13%
2	California	12,136	15.53%
3	Florida	8,617	11.03%
4	Texas	5,879	7.53%
5	New Jersey	4,993	6.39%
6	Illinois	3,104	3.97%
7	Maryland	2,722	3.48%
8	Pennsylvania	2,528	3.24%
9	Georgia	2,245	2.87%
10	Massachusetts	1,401	1.79%
11	Louisiana	1,239	1.59%
12	North Carolina	1,187	1.52%
13	Ohio	1,184	1.52%
14	Virginia	1,162	1.49%
15	South Carolina	1,158	1.48%
16	Michigan	1,035	1.32%
17	Washington	932	1.19%
18	Connecticut	912	1.17%
19	Colorado	816	1.04%
20	Tennessee	764	0.98%
21	Missouri	713	0.91%
22	Indiana	622	0.80%
23	Arizona	612	0.78%
24	Oregon	606	0.78%
25	Alabama	582	0.74%
26	Mississippi	433	0.55%
27	Minnesota	422	0.54%
28	Nevada	387	0.50%
29	Wisconsin	379	0.49%
30	Kentucky	320	0.41%
31	Arkansas	284	0.36%
32	Rhode Island	276	0.35%
33	Delaware	271	0.35%
34	Oklahoma	269	0.34%
35	Kansas	245	0.31%
36	Hawaii	216	0.28%
37	New Mexico	211	0.27%
38	Utah	152	0.19%
39	Iowa	130	0.17%
40	Maine	117	0.15%
41	West Virginia	96	0.12%
42	New Hampshire	92	0.12%
43	Nebraska	89	0.11%
44	Idaho	61	0.08%
45	Alaska	59	0.08%
46	Vermont	38	0.05%
47	Montana	30	0.04%
48	North Dakota	20	0.03%
49	South Dakota	19	0.02%
50	Wyoming	18	0.02%
	District of Columbia	1,399	1.79%

Source: U.S. Department of Health and Human Services, National Center for Health Statistics "Morbidity and Mortality Weekly Report" (January 6, 1995, Vol. 43, Nos. 51 & 52)
*Updated through December 31, 1994. AIDS is Acquired Immunodeficiency Syndrome.

AIDS Rate in 1994

National Rate = 30.01 New AIDS Cases Reported per 100,000 Population*

ALPHA ORDER				RANK ORDER		
RANK	STATE	RATE		RANK	STATE	RATE
26	Alabama	13.79		1	New York	82.25
33	Alaska	9.74		2	New Jersey	63.17
24	Arizona	15.02		3	Florida	61.76
29	Arkansas	11.58		4	Maryland	54.37
5	California	38.61		5	California	38.61
16	Colorado	22.32		6	Delaware	38.39
11	Connecticut	27.85		7	Texas	31.99
6	Delaware	38.39		8	Georgia	31.82
3	Florida	61.76		9	South Carolina	31.60
8	Georgia	31.82		10	Louisiana	28.71
19	Hawaii	18.32		11	Connecticut	27.85
44	Idaho	5.38		12	Rhode Island	27.68
14	Illinois	26.41		13	Nevada	26.56
31	Indiana	10.81		14	Illinois	26.41
46	Iowa	4.60		15	Massachusetts	23.19
34	Kansas	9.59		16	Colorado	22.32
37	Kentucky	8.36		17	Pennsylvania	20.98
10	Louisiana	28.71		18	Oregon	19.64
35	Maine	9.44		19	Hawaii	18.32
4	Maryland	54.37		20	Virginia	17.74
15	Massachusetts	23.19		21	Washington	17.44
30	Michigan	10.90		22	North Carolina	16.79
36	Minnesota	9.24		23	Mississippi	16.22
23	Mississippi	16.22		24	Arizona	15.02
27	Missouri	13.51		25	Tennessee	14.76
48	Montana	3.50		26	Alabama	13.79
43	Nebraska	5.48		27	Missouri	13.51
13	Nevada	26.56		28	New Mexico	12.76
39	New Hampshire	8.09		29	Arkansas	11.58
2	New Jersey	63.17		30	Michigan	10.90
28	New Mexico	12.76		31	Indiana	10.81
1	New York	82.25		32	Ohio	10.66
22	North Carolina	16.79		33	Alaska	9.74
49	North Dakota	3.13		34	Kansas	9.59
32	Ohio	10.66		35	Maine	9.44
38	Oklahoma	8.26		36	Minnesota	9.24
18	Oregon	19.64		37	Kentucky	8.36
17	Pennsylvania	20.98		38	Oklahoma	8.26
12	Rhode Island	27.68		39	New Hampshire	8.09
9	South Carolina	31.60		40	Utah	7.97
50	South Dakota	2.64		41	Wisconsin	7.46
25	Tennessee	14.76		42	Vermont	6.55
7	Texas	31.99		43	Nebraska	5.48
40	Utah	7.97		44	Idaho	5.38
42	Vermont	6.55		45	West Virginia	5.27
20	Virginia	17.74		46	Iowa	4.60
21	Washington	17.44		47	Wyoming	3.78
45	West Virginia	5.27		48	Montana	3.50
41	Wisconsin	7.46		49	North Dakota	3.13
47	Wyoming	3.78		50	South Dakota	2.64

District of Columbia 245.44

Source: Morgan Quitno Press using data from U.S. Dept of Health & Human Serv's, National Center for Health Statistics
"Morbidity and Mortality Weekly Report" (January 6, 1995, Vol. 43, Nos. 51 & 52)
*Updated through December 31, 1994. AIDS is Acquired Immunodeficiency Syndrome.

AIDS Cases Through July 1994

National Total = 388,365 AIDS Cases*

ALPHA ORDER				RANK ORDER			
RANK	STATE	CASES	% of USA	RANK	STATE	CASES	% of USA
24	Alabama	2,756	0.71%	1	New York	76,345	19.66%
45	Alaska	225	0.06%	2	California	72,433	18.65%
21	Arizona	3,517	0.91%	3	Florida	38,855	10.00%
31	Arkansas	1,463	0.38%	4	Texas	27,951	7.20%
2	California	72,433	18.65%	5	New Jersey	22,496	5.79%
19	Colorado	4,227	1.09%	6	Illinois	12,735	3.28%
16	Connecticut	5,399	1.39%	7	Pennsylvania	11,375	2.93%
36	Delaware	1,035	0.27%	8	Georgia	11,001	2.83%
3	Florida	38,855	10.00%	9	Maryland	8,897	2.29%
8	Georgia	11,001	2.83%	10	Massachusetts	8,672	2.23%
32	Hawaii	1,420	0.37%	11	Louisiana	5,986	1.54%
44	Idaho	250	0.06%	12	Ohio	5,908	1.52%
6	Illinois	12,735	3.28%	13	Virginia	5,814	1.50%
23	Indiana	3,048	0.78%	14	Michigan	5,739	1.48%
39	Iowa	656	0.17%	15	Washington	5,496	1.42%
34	Kansas	1,239	0.32%	16	Connecticut	5,399	1.39%
33	Kentucky	1,372	0.35%	17	Missouri	5,294	1.36%
11	Louisiana	5,986	1.54%	18	North Carolina	4,885	1.26%
41	Maine	511	0.13%	19	Colorado	4,227	1.09%
9	Maryland	8,897	2.29%	20	South Carolina	3,892	1.00%
10	Massachusetts	8,672	2.23%	21	Arizona	3,517	0.91%
14	Michigan	5,739	1.48%	22	Tennessee	3,384	0.87%
26	Minnesota	2,138	0.55%	23	Indiana	3,048	0.78%
30	Mississippi	1,790	0.46%	24	Alabama	2,756	0.71%
17	Missouri	5,294	1.36%	25	Oregon	2,662	0.69%
47	Montana	154	0.04%	26	Minnesota	2,138	0.55%
40	Nebraska	536	0.14%	27	Oklahoma	2,064	0.53%
29	Nevada	1,978	0.51%	28	Wisconsin	1,981	0.51%
42	New Hampshire	452	0.12%	29	Nevada	1,978	0.51%
5	New Jersey	22,496	5.79%	30	Mississippi	1,790	0.46%
37	New Mexico	951	0.24%	31	Arkansas	1,463	0.38%
1	New York	76,345	19.66%	32	Hawaii	1,420	0.37%
18	North Carolina	4,885	1.26%	33	Kentucky	1,372	0.35%
50	North Dakota	57	0.01%	34	Kansas	1,239	0.32%
12	Ohio	5,908	1.52%	35	Rhode Island	1,049	0.27%
27	Oklahoma	2,064	0.53%	36	Delaware	1,035	0.27%
25	Oregon	2,662	0.69%	37	New Mexico	951	0.24%
7	Pennsylvania	11,375	2.93%	38	Utah	941	0.24%
35	Rhode Island	1,049	0.27%	39	Iowa	656	0.17%
20	South Carolina	3,892	1.00%	40	Nebraska	536	0.14%
49	South Dakota	75	0.02%	41	Maine	511	0.13%
22	Tennessee	3,384	0.87%	42	New Hampshire	452	0.12%
4	Texas	27,951	7.20%	43	West Virginia	430	0.11%
38	Utah	941	0.24%	44	Idaho	250	0.06%
46	Vermont	215	0.06%	45	Alaska	225	0.06%
13	Virginia	5,814	1.50%	46	Vermont	215	0.06%
15	Washington	5,496	1.42%	47	Montana	154	0.04%
43	West Virginia	430	0.11%	48	Wyoming	112	0.03%
28	Wisconsin	1,981	0.51%	49	South Dakota	75	0.02%
48	Wyoming	112	0.03%	50	North Dakota	57	0.01%
					District of Columbia	6,504	1.67%

Source: U.S. Department of Health and Human Services, Centers for Disease Control and Prevention
  "HIV/AIDS Surveillance Report" (Vol. 6, No.1, 1994)

*Cumulative total through July 1994. AIDS is Acquired Immunodeficiency Syndrome. It is a specific group of diseases or conditions which are indicative of severe immunosuppression related to infection with the Human Immunodeficiency Virus (HIV). National total does not include 12,845 cases in Puerto Rico and 194 cases in other U.S. territories.

AIDS Cases in Children 12 Years and Younger Through July 1994

National Total = 5,426 Juvenile AIDS Cases*

ALPHA ORDER

RANK	STATE	CASES	% of USA
17	Alabama	46	0.85%
43	Alaska	3	0.06%
28	Arizona	16	0.29%
23	Arkansas	22	0.41%
4	California	398	7.34%
23	Colorado	22	0.41%
10	Connecticut	127	2.34%
36	Delaware	10	0.18%
2	Florida	876	16.14%
11	Georgia	114	2.10%
34	Hawaii	12	0.22%
47	Idaho	2	0.04%
7	Illinois	153	2.82%
22	Indiana	25	0.46%
38	Iowa	7	0.13%
37	Kansas	8	0.15%
32	Kentucky	13	0.24%
13	Louisiana	83	1.53%
42	Maine	4	0.07%
6	Maryland	193	3.56%
9	Massachusetts	145	2.67%
16	Michigan	69	1.27%
31	Minnesota	15	0.28%
21	Mississippi	26	0.48%
19	Missouri	37	0.68%
47	Montana	2	0.04%
39	Nebraska	6	0.11%
28	Nevada	16	0.29%
39	New Hampshire	6	0.11%
3	New Jersey	522	9.62%
43	New Mexico	3	0.06%
1	New York	1,531	28.22%
14	North Carolina	76	1.40%
49	North Dakota	0	0.00%
15	Ohio	73	1.35%
28	Oklahoma	16	0.29%
35	Oregon	11	0.20%
8	Pennsylvania	151	2.78%
32	Rhode Island	13	0.24%
18	South Carolina	44	0.81%
43	South Dakota	3	0.06%
20	Tennessee	31	0.57%
5	Texas	237	4.37%
26	Utah	20	0.37%
43	Vermont	3	0.06%
12	Virginia	99	1.82%
26	Washington	20	0.37%
41	West Virginia	5	0.09%
23	Wisconsin	22	0.41%
49	Wyoming	0	0.00%

RANK ORDER

RANK	STATE	CASES	% of USA
1	New York	1,531	28.22%
2	Florida	876	16.14%
3	New Jersey	522	9.62%
4	California	398	7.34%
5	Texas	237	4.37%
6	Maryland	193	3.56%
7	Illinois	153	2.82%
8	Pennsylvania	151	2.78%
9	Massachusetts	145	2.67%
10	Connecticut	127	2.34%
11	Georgia	114	2.10%
12	Virginia	99	1.82%
13	Louisiana	83	1.53%
14	North Carolina	76	1.40%
15	Ohio	73	1.35%
16	Michigan	69	1.27%
17	Alabama	46	0.85%
18	South Carolina	44	0.81%
19	Missouri	37	0.68%
20	Tennessee	31	0.57%
21	Mississippi	26	0.48%
22	Indiana	25	0.46%
23	Arkansas	22	0.41%
23	Colorado	22	0.41%
23	Wisconsin	22	0.41%
26	Utah	20	0.37%
26	Washington	20	0.37%
28	Arizona	16	0.29%
28	Nevada	16	0.29%
28	Oklahoma	16	0.29%
31	Minnesota	15	0.28%
32	Kentucky	13	0.24%
32	Rhode Island	13	0.24%
34	Hawaii	12	0.22%
35	Oregon	11	0.20%
36	Delaware	10	0.18%
37	Kansas	8	0.15%
38	Iowa	7	0.13%
39	Nebraska	6	0.11%
39	New Hampshire	6	0.11%
41	West Virginia	5	0.09%
42	Maine	4	0.07%
43	Alaska	3	0.06%
43	New Mexico	3	0.06%
43	South Dakota	3	0.06%
43	Vermont	3	0.06%
47	Idaho	2	0.04%
47	Montana	2	0.04%
49	North Dakota	0	0.00%
49	Wyoming	0	0.00%
	District of Columbia	90	1.66%

Source: U.S. Department of Health and Human Services, Centers for Disease Control and Prevention
    "HIV/AIDS Surveillance Report" (Vol. 6, No.1, 1994)
*Cumulative total through July 1994. AIDS is Acquired Immunodeficiency Syndrome. It is a specific group of diseases or conditions which are indicative of severe immunosuppression related to infection with the Human Immunodeficiency Virus (HIV). National total does not include 299 cases in Puerto Rico and 6 cases in the Virgin Islands.

Aseptic Meningitis Cases Reported in 1994

National Total = 8,050 Cases*

<u>ALPHA ORDER</u>

RANK	STATE	CASES	% of USA
14	Alabama	174	2.16%
39	Alaska	18	0.22%
22	Arizona	77	0.96%
25	Arkansas	51	0.63%
1	California	1,315	16.34%
17	Colorado	138	1.71%
46	Connecticut	0	0.00%
30	Delaware	38	0.47%
4	Florida	553	6.87%
26	Georgia	50	0.62%
18	Hawaii	131	1.63%
43	Idaho	6	0.07%
6	Illinois	402	4.99%
12	Indiana	204	2.53%
19	Iowa	121	1.50%
23	Kansas	76	0.94%
13	Kentucky	180	2.24%
34	Louisiana	34	0.42%
35	Maine	33	0.41%
10	Maryland	244	3.03%
21	Massachusetts	92	1.14%
5	Michigan	537	6.67%
37	Minnesota	27	0.34%
27	Mississippi	49	0.61%
15	Missouri	160	1.99%
41	Montana	8	0.10%
31	Nebraska	37	0.46%
28	Nevada	46	0.57%
33	New Hampshire	35	0.43%
46	New Jersey	0	0.00%
38	New Mexico	20	0.25%
3	New York	599	7.44%
11	North Carolina	240	2.98%
40	North Dakota	13	0.16%
7	Ohio	399	4.96%
46	Oklahoma	0	0.00%
46	Oregon	0	0.00%
8	Pennsylvania	334	4.15%
20	Rhode Island	120	1.49%
36	South Carolina	31	0.39%
45	South Dakota	3	0.04%
16	Tennessee	146	1.81%
2	Texas	790	9.81%
24	Utah	56	0.70%
32	Vermont	36	0.45%
9	Virginia	324	4.02%
46	Washington	0	0.00%
29	West Virginia	39	0.48%
42	Wisconsin	7	0.09%
44	Wyoming	4	0.05%

<u>RANK ORDER</u>

RANK	STATE	CASES	% of USA
1	California	1,315	16.34%
2	Texas	790	9.81%
3	New York	599	7.44%
4	Florida	553	6.87%
5	Michigan	537	6.67%
6	Illinois	402	4.99%
7	Ohio	399	4.96%
8	Pennsylvania	334	4.15%
9	Virginia	324	4.02%
10	Maryland	244	3.03%
11	North Carolina	240	2.98%
12	Indiana	204	2.53%
13	Kentucky	180	2.24%
14	Alabama	174	2.16%
15	Missouri	160	1.99%
16	Tennessee	146	1.81%
17	Colorado	138	1.71%
18	Hawaii	131	1.63%
19	Iowa	121	1.50%
20	Rhode Island	120	1.49%
21	Massachusetts	92	1.14%
22	Arizona	77	0.96%
23	Kansas	76	0.94%
24	Utah	56	0.70%
25	Arkansas	51	0.63%
26	Georgia	50	0.62%
27	Mississippi	49	0.61%
28	Nevada	46	0.57%
29	West Virginia	39	0.48%
30	Delaware	38	0.47%
31	Nebraska	37	0.46%
32	Vermont	36	0.45%
33	New Hampshire	35	0.43%
34	Louisiana	34	0.42%
35	Maine	33	0.41%
36	South Carolina	31	0.39%
37	Minnesota	27	0.34%
38	New Mexico	20	0.25%
39	Alaska	18	0.22%
40	North Dakota	13	0.16%
41	Montana	8	0.10%
42	Wisconsin	7	0.09%
43	Idaho	6	0.07%
44	Wyoming	4	0.05%
45	South Dakota	3	0.04%
46	Connecticut	0	0.00%
46	New Jersey	0	0.00%
46	Oklahoma	0	0.00%
46	Oregon	0	0.00%
46	Washington	0	0.00%
	District of Columbia	53	0.66%

Source: U.S. Department of Health and Human Services, National Center for Health Statistics
"Morbidity and Mortality Weekly Report" (January 6, 1995, Vol. 43, Nos. 51 & 52)
*An inflammation of the membranes that envelope the brain and spinal cord.

Aseptic Meningitis Rate in 1994

National Rate = 3.09 Cases Reported per 100,000 Population*

ALPHA ORDER

RANK	STATE	RATE
12	Alabama	4.12
24	Alaska	2.97
33	Arizona	1.89
31	Arkansas	2.08
11	California	4.18
14	Colorado	3.77
46	Connecticut	0.00
5	Delaware	5.38
13	Florida	3.96
41	Georgia	0.71
2	Hawaii	11.11
43	Idaho	0.53
17	Illinois	3.42
16	Indiana	3.55
10	Iowa	4.28
23	Kansas	2.98
8	Kentucky	4.70
40	Louisiana	0.79
28	Maine	2.66
7	Maryland	4.87
35	Massachusetts	1.52
4	Michigan	5.66
42	Minnesota	0.59
34	Mississippi	1.84
22	Missouri	3.03
37	Montana	0.93
29	Nebraska	2.28
20	Nevada	3.16
21	New Hampshire	3.08
46	New Jersey	0.00
36	New Mexico	1.21
19	New York	3.30
18	North Carolina	3.39
32	North Dakota	2.04
15	Ohio	3.59
46	Oklahoma	0.00
46	Oregon	0.00
27	Pennsylvania	2.77
1	Rhode Island	12.04
38	South Carolina	0.85
44	South Dakota	0.42
26	Tennessee	2.82
9	Texas	4.30
25	Utah	2.94
3	Vermont	6.21
6	Virginia	4.95
46	Washington	0.00
30	West Virginia	2.14
45	Wisconsin	0.14
39	Wyoming	0.84

RANK ORDER

RANK	STATE	RATE
1	Rhode Island	12.04
2	Hawaii	11.11
3	Vermont	6.21
4	Michigan	5.66
5	Delaware	5.38
6	Virginia	4.95
7	Maryland	4.87
8	Kentucky	4.70
9	Texas	4.30
10	Iowa	4.28
11	California	4.18
12	Alabama	4.12
13	Florida	3.96
14	Colorado	3.77
15	Ohio	3.59
16	Indiana	3.55
17	Illinois	3.42
18	North Carolina	3.39
19	New York	3.30
20	Nevada	3.16
21	New Hampshire	3.08
22	Missouri	3.03
23	Kansas	2.98
24	Alaska	2.97
25	Utah	2.94
26	Tennessee	2.82
27	Pennsylvania	2.77
28	Maine	2.66
29	Nebraska	2.28
30	West Virginia	2.14
31	Arkansas	2.08
32	North Dakota	2.04
33	Arizona	1.89
34	Mississippi	1.84
35	Massachusetts	1.52
36	New Mexico	1.21
37	Montana	0.93
38	South Carolina	0.85
39	Wyoming	0.84
40	Louisiana	0.79
41	Georgia	0.71
42	Minnesota	0.59
43	Idaho	0.53
44	South Dakota	0.42
45	Wisconsin	0.14
46	Connecticut	0.00
46	New Jersey	0.00
46	Oklahoma	0.00
46	Oregon	0.00
46	Washington	0.00

District of Columbia 9.30

Source: Morgan Quitno Press using data from U.S. Dept of Health & Human Serv's, National Center for Health Statistics
"Morbidity and Mortality Weekly Report" (January 6, 1995, Vol. 43, Nos. 51 & 52)
*An inflammation of the membranes that envelope the brain and spinal cord.

Chickenpox (Varicella) Cases Reported in 1993

National Total = 134,722 Cases*

ALPHA ORDER					RANK ORDER			
RANK	STATE		CASES	% of USA	RANK	STATE	CASES	% of USA
NA	Alabama*		NA	NA	1	Michigan	32,461	24.09%
NA	Alaska*		NA	NA	2	Illinois	26,447	19.63%
5	Arizona		6,811	5.06%	3	Texas	14,291	10.61%
NA	Arkansas*		NA	NA	4	Missouri	9,609	7.13%
NA	California*		NA	NA	5	Arizona	6,811	5.06%
NA	Colorado*		NA	NA	6	Massachusetts	6,619	4.91%
NA	Connecticut*		NA	NA	7	Ohio	5,472	4.06%
25	Delaware		3	0.00%	8	West Virginia	5,288	3.93%
NA	Florida*		NA	NA	9	Iowa	5,057	3.75%
NA	Georgia*		NA	NA	10	New York*	4,773	3.54%
14	Hawaii		2,303	1.71%	11	Virginia	2,917	2.17%
NA	Idaho*		NA	NA	12	Rhode Island	2,668	1.98%
2	Illinois		26,447	19.63%	13	Tennessee	2,552	1.89%
NA	Indiana*		NA	NA	14	Hawaii	2,303	1.71%
9	Iowa		5,057	3.75%	15	Maine	1,733	1.29%
16	Kansas		1,687	1.25%	16	Kansas	1,687	1.25%
18	Kentucky		1,429	1.06%	17	New Hampshire	1,635	1.21%
NA	Louisiana*		NA	NA	18	Kentucky	1,429	1.06%
15	Maine		1,733	1.29%	19	South Dakota	420	0.31%
NA	Maryland*		NA	NA	20	Utah	297	0.22%
6	Massachusetts		6,619	4.91%	21	South Carolina	120	0.09%
1	Michigan		32,461	24.09%	22	Montana	84	0.06%
NA	Minnesota*		NA	NA	23	North Dakota	37	0.03%
NA	Mississippi*		NA	NA	24	Nebraska	4	0.00%
4	Missouri		9,609	7.13%	25	Delaware	3	0.00%
22	Montana		84	0.06%	NA	Alabama*	NA	NA
24	Nebraska		4	0.00%	NA	Alaska*	NA	NA
NA	Nevada*		NA	NA	NA	Arkansas*	NA	NA
17	New Hampshire		1,635	1.21%	NA	California*	NA	NA
NA	New Jersey*		NA	NA	NA	Colorado*	NA	NA
NA	New Mexico*		NA	NA	NA	Connecticut*	NA	NA
10	New York*		4,773	3.54%	NA	Florida*	NA	NA
NA	North Carolina*		NA	NA	NA	Georgia*	NA	NA
23	North Dakota		37	0.03%	NA	Idaho*	NA	NA
7	Ohio		5,472	4.06%	NA	Indiana*	NA	NA
NA	Oklahoma*		NA	NA	NA	Louisiana*	NA	NA
NA	Oregon*		NA	NA	NA	Maryland*	NA	NA
NA	Pennsylvania*		NA	NA	NA	Minnesota*	NA	NA
12	Rhode Island		2,668	1.98%	NA	Mississippi*	NA	NA
21	South Carolina		120	0.09%	NA	Nevada*	NA	NA
19	South Dakota		420	0.31%	NA	New Jersey*	NA	NA
13	Tennessee		2,552	1.89%	NA	New Mexico*	NA	NA
3	Texas		14,291	10.61%	NA	North Carolina*	NA	NA
20	Utah		297	0.22%	NA	Oklahoma*	NA	NA
NA	Vermont*		NA	NA	NA	Oregon*	NA	NA
11	Virginia		2,917	2.17%	NA	Pennsylvania*	NA	NA
NA	Washington*		NA	NA	NA	Vermont*	NA	NA
8	West Virginia		5,288	3.93%	NA	Washington*	NA	NA
NA	Wisconsin*		NA	NA	NA	Wisconsin*	NA	NA
NA	Wyoming*		NA	NA	NA	Wyoming*	NA	NA
						District of Columbia	4	0.00%

Source: U.S. Department of Health and Human Services, National Center for Health Statistics
"Morbidity and Mortality Weekly Report" (October 21, 1994, Vol. 42, No. 53)
*Chickenpox is not reportable in states marked "NA" except in Wisconsin where data are not available. New York data are for New York City only. National total does not include cases for states not reporting.

Chickenpox (Varicella) Rate in 1993

National Rate = 111.14 Cases per 100,000 Population*

ALPHA ORDER			RANK ORDER		
RANK	STATE	RATE	RANK	STATE	RATE
NA	Alabama*	NA	1	Michigan	343.14
NA	Alaska*	NA	2	West Virginia	290.87
8	Arizona	172.65	3	Rhode Island	266.80
NA	Arkansas*	NA	4	Illinois	226.31
NA	California*	NA	5	Hawaii	197.51
NA	Colorado*	NA	6	Missouri	183.55
NA	Connecticut*	NA	7	Iowa	179.26
24	Delaware	0.43	8	Arizona	172.65
NA	Florida*	NA	9	New Hampshire	145.46
NA	Georgia*	NA	10	Maine	139.76
5	Hawaii	197.51	11	Massachusetts	109.99
NA	Idaho*	NA	12	Texas	79.30
4	Illinois	226.31	13	Kansas	66.55
NA	Indiana*	NA	14	South Dakota	58.66
7	Iowa	179.26	15	Tennessee	50.10
13	Kansas	66.55	16	Ohio	49.47
18	Kentucky	37.66	17	Virginia	45.06
NA	Louisiana*	NA	18	Kentucky	37.66
10	Maine	139.76	19	New York*	26.29
NA	Maryland*	NA	20	Utah	15.97
11	Massachusetts	109.99	21	Montana	9.99
1	Michigan	343.14	22	North Dakota	5.81
NA	Minnesota*	NA	23	South Carolina	3.31
NA	Mississippi*	NA	24	Delaware	0.43
6	Missouri	183.55	25	Nebraska	0.25
21	Montana	9.99	NA	Alabama*	NA
25	Nebraska	0.25	NA	Alaska*	NA
NA	Nevada*	NA	NA	Arkansas*	NA
9	New Hampshire	145.46	NA	California*	NA
NA	New Jersey*	NA	NA	Colorado*	NA
NA	New Mexico*	NA	NA	Connecticut*	NA
19	New York*	26.29	NA	Florida*	NA
NA	North Carolina*	NA	NA	Georgia*	NA
22	North Dakota	5.81	NA	Idaho*	NA
16	Ohio	49.47	NA	Indiana*	NA
NA	Oklahoma*	NA	NA	Louisiana*	NA
NA	Oregon*	NA	NA	Maryland*	NA
NA	Pennsylvania*	NA	NA	Minnesota*	NA
3	Rhode Island	266.80	NA	Mississippi*	NA
23	South Carolina	3.31	NA	Nevada*	NA
14	South Dakota	58.66	NA	New Jersey*	NA
15	Tennessee	50.10	NA	New Mexico*	NA
12	Texas	79.30	NA	North Carolina*	NA
20	Utah	15.97	NA	Oklahoma*	NA
NA	Vermont*	NA	NA	Oregon*	NA
17	Virginia	45.06	NA	Pennsylvania*	NA
NA	Washington*	NA	NA	Vermont*	NA
2	West Virginia	290.87	NA	Washington*	NA
NA	Wisconsin*	NA	NA	Wisconsin*	NA
NA	Wyoming*	NA	NA	Wyoming*	NA
				District of Columbia	0.69

Source: Morgan Quitno Press using data from U.S. Dept of Health & Human Serv's, National Center for Health Statistics "Morbidity and Mortality Weekly Report" (October 21, 1994, Vol. 42, No. 53)
Chickenpox is not reportable in states marked "NA" except in Wisconsin where data are not available. New York data are for New York City only. National total does not include cases for states not reporting. National rate does not include cases or population for states not reporting.

Encephalitis Cases Reported in 1994

National Total = 781 Cases*

<u>ALPHA ORDER</u>

RANK	STATE	CASES	% of USA
17	Alabama	10	1.28%
31	Alaska	3	0.38%
35	Arizona	2	0.26%
41	Arkansas	0	0.00%
1	California	133	17.03%
31	Colorado	3	0.38%
41	Connecticut	0	0.00%
38	Delaware	1	0.13%
12	Florida	21	2.69%
38	Georgia	1	0.13%
38	Hawaii	1	0.13%
41	Idaho	0	0.00%
2	Illinois	62	7.94%
14	Indiana	13	1.66%
35	Iowa	2	0.26%
22	Kansas	7	0.90%
13	Kentucky	18	2.30%
20	Louisiana	8	1.02%
23	Maine	5	0.64%
10	Maryland	32	4.10%
18	Massachusetts	9	1.15%
6	Michigan	50	6.40%
18	Minnesota	9	1.15%
24	Mississippi	4	0.51%
15	Missouri	12	1.54%
41	Montana	0	0.00%
20	Nebraska	8	1.02%
24	Nevada	4	0.51%
35	New Hampshire	2	0.26%
41	New Jersey	0	0.00%
41	New Mexico	0	0.00%
4	New York	51	6.53%
8	North Carolina	45	5.76%
24	North Dakota	4	0.51%
3	Ohio	59	7.55%
41	Oklahoma	0	0.00%
41	Oregon	0	0.00%
11	Pennsylvania	30	3.84%
24	Rhode Island	4	0.51%
41	South Carolina	0	0.00%
24	South Dakota	4	0.51%
15	Tennessee	12	1.54%
7	Texas	47	6.02%
31	Utah	3	0.38%
31	Vermont	3	0.38%
9	Virginia	39	4.99%
41	Washington	0	0.00%
4	West Virginia	51	6.53%
24	Wisconsin	4	0.51%
24	Wyoming	4	0.51%

<u>RANK ORDER</u>

RANK	STATE	CASES	% of USA
1	California	133	17.03%
2	Illinois	62	7.94%
3	Ohio	59	7.55%
4	New York	51	6.53%
4	West Virginia	51	6.53%
6	Michigan	50	6.40%
7	Texas	47	6.02%
8	North Carolina	45	5.76%
9	Virginia	39	4.99%
10	Maryland	32	4.10%
11	Pennsylvania	30	3.84%
12	Florida	21	2.69%
13	Kentucky	18	2.30%
14	Indiana	13	1.66%
15	Missouri	12	1.54%
15	Tennessee	12	1.54%
17	Alabama	10	1.28%
18	Massachusetts	9	1.15%
18	Minnesota	9	1.15%
20	Louisiana	8	1.02%
20	Nebraska	8	1.02%
22	Kansas	7	0.90%
23	Maine	5	0.64%
24	Mississippi	4	0.51%
24	Nevada	4	0.51%
24	North Dakota	4	0.51%
24	Rhode Island	4	0.51%
24	South Dakota	4	0.51%
24	Wisconsin	4	0.51%
24	Wyoming	4	0.51%
31	Alaska	3	0.38%
31	Colorado	3	0.38%
31	Utah	3	0.38%
31	Vermont	3	0.38%
35	Arizona	2	0.26%
35	Iowa	2	0.26%
35	New Hampshire	2	0.26%
38	Delaware	1	0.13%
38	Georgia	1	0.13%
38	Hawaii	1	0.13%
41	Arkansas	0	0.00%
41	Connecticut	0	0.00%
41	Idaho	0	0.00%
41	Montana	0	0.00%
41	New Jersey	0	0.00%
41	New Mexico	0	0.00%
41	Oklahoma	0	0.00%
41	Oregon	0	0.00%
41	South Carolina	0	0.00%
41	Washington	0	0.00%
	District of Columbia	1	0.13%

Source: U.S. Department of Health and Human Services, National Center for Health Statistics
"Morbidity and Mortality Weekly Report" (January 6, 1995, Vol. 43, Nos. 51 & 52)
*Inflammation of the brain. Includes Primary and Post-infectious cases.

Encephalitis Rate in 1994

National Rate = 0.30 Cases Reported per 100,000 Population*

ALPHA ORDER

RANK ORDER

RANK	STATE	RATE
23	Alabama	0.24
12	Alaska	0.50
39	Arizona	0.05
41	Arkansas	0.00
15	California	0.42
35	Colorado	0.08
41	Connecticut	0.00
34	Delaware	0.14
31	Florida	0.15
40	Georgia	0.01
35	Hawaii	0.08
41	Idaho	0.00
8	Illinois	0.53
24	Indiana	0.23
38	Iowa	0.07
19	Kansas	0.27
14	Kentucky	0.47
28	Louisiana	0.19
16	Maine	0.40
3	Maryland	0.64
31	Massachusetts	0.15
8	Michigan	0.53
27	Minnesota	0.20
31	Mississippi	0.15
24	Missouri	0.23
41	Montana	0.00
13	Nebraska	0.49
19	Nevada	0.27
29	New Hampshire	0.18
41	New Jersey	0.00
41	New Mexico	0.00
18	New York	0.28
3	North Carolina	0.64
5	North Dakota	0.63
8	Ohio	0.53
41	Oklahoma	0.00
41	Oregon	0.00
22	Pennsylvania	0.25
16	Rhode Island	0.40
41	South Carolina	0.00
7	South Dakota	0.55
24	Tennessee	0.23
21	Texas	0.26
30	Utah	0.16
11	Vermont	0.52
6	Virginia	0.60
41	Washington	0.00
1	West Virginia	2.80
35	Wisconsin	0.08
2	Wyoming	0.84

RANK	STATE	RATE
1	West Virginia	2.80
2	Wyoming	0.84
3	Maryland	0.64
3	North Carolina	0.64
5	North Dakota	0.63
6	Virginia	0.60
7	South Dakota	0.55
8	Illinois	0.53
8	Michigan	0.53
8	Ohio	0.53
11	Vermont	0.52
12	Alaska	0.50
13	Nebraska	0.49
14	Kentucky	0.47
15	California	0.42
16	Maine	0.40
16	Rhode Island	0.40
18	New York	0.28
19	Kansas	0.27
19	Nevada	0.27
21	Texas	0.26
22	Pennsylvania	0.25
23	Alabama	0.24
24	Indiana	0.23
24	Missouri	0.23
24	Tennessee	0.23
27	Minnesota	0.20
28	Louisiana	0.19
29	New Hampshire	0.18
30	Utah	0.16
31	Florida	0.15
31	Massachusetts	0.15
31	Mississippi	0.15
34	Delaware	0.14
35	Colorado	0.08
35	Hawaii	0.08
35	Wisconsin	0.08
38	Iowa	0.07
39	Arizona	0.05
40	Georgia	0.01
41	Arkansas	0.00
41	Connecticut	0.00
41	Idaho	0.00
41	Montana	0.00
41	New Jersey	0.00
41	New Mexico	0.00
41	Oklahoma	0.00
41	Oregon	0.00
41	South Carolina	0.00
41	Washington	0.00

District of Columbia 0.18

Source: Morgan Quitno Press using data from U.S. Dept of Health & Human Serv's, National Center for Health Statistics
"Morbidity and Mortality Weekly Report" (January 6, 1995, Vol. 43, Nos. 51 & 52)
*Inflammation of the brain. Includes Primary and Post-infectious cases.

German Measles (Rubella) Cases Reported in 1994

National Total = 209 Cases

<u>ALPHA ORDER</u>

RANK	STATE	CASES	% of USA
18	Alabama	0	0.00%
15	Alaska	1	0.48%
18	Arizona	0	0.00%
18	Arkansas	0	0.00%
2	California	28	13.40%
18	Colorado	0	0.00%
9	Connecticut	3	1.44%
18	Delaware	0	0.00%
3	Florida	9	4.31%
13	Georgia	2	0.96%
6	Hawaii	4	1.91%
18	Idaho	0	0.00%
9	Illinois	3	1.44%
18	Indiana	0	0.00%
18	Iowa	0	0.00%
18	Kansas	0	0.00%
18	Kentucky	0	0.00%
18	Louisiana	0	0.00%
18	Maine	0	0.00%
18	Maryland	0	0.00%
1	Massachusetts	125	59.81%
3	Michigan	9	4.31%
18	Minnesota	0	0.00%
18	Mississippi	0	0.00%
13	Missouri	2	0.96%
18	Montana	0	0.00%
18	Nebraska	0	0.00%
15	Nevada	1	0.48%
18	New Hampshire	0	0.00%
15	New Jersey	1	0.48%
18	New Mexico	0	0.00%
5	New York	7	3.35%
18	North Carolina	0	0.00%
18	North Dakota	0	0.00%
18	Ohio	0	0.00%
6	Oklahoma	4	1.91%
9	Oregon	3	1.44%
18	Pennsylvania	0	0.00%
9	Rhode Island	3	1.44%
18	South Carolina	0	0.00%
18	South Dakota	0	0.00%
18	Tennessee	0	0.00%
18	Texas	0	0.00%
6	Utah	4	1.91%
18	Vermont	0	0.00%
18	Virginia	0	0.00%
18	Washington	0	0.00%
18	West Virginia	0	0.00%
18	Wisconsin	0	0.00%
18	Wyoming	0	0.00%

<u>RANK ORDER</u>

RANK	STATE	CASES	% of USA
1	Massachusetts	125	59.81%
2	California	28	13.40%
3	Florida	9	4.31%
3	Michigan	9	4.31%
5	New York	7	3.35%
6	Hawaii	4	1.91%
6	Oklahoma	4	1.91%
6	Utah	4	1.91%
9	Connecticut	3	1.44%
9	Illinois	3	1.44%
9	Oregon	3	1.44%
9	Rhode Island	3	1.44%
13	Georgia	2	0.96%
13	Missouri	2	0.96%
15	Alaska	1	0.48%
15	Nevada	1	0.48%
15	New Jersey	1	0.48%
18	Alabama	0	0.00%
18	Arizona	0	0.00%
18	Arkansas	0	0.00%
18	Colorado	0	0.00%
18	Delaware	0	0.00%
18	Idaho	0	0.00%
18	Indiana	0	0.00%
18	Iowa	0	0.00%
18	Kansas	0	0.00%
18	Kentucky	0	0.00%
18	Louisiana	0	0.00%
18	Maine	0	0.00%
18	Maryland	0	0.00%
18	Minnesota	0	0.00%
18	Mississippi	0	0.00%
18	Montana	0	0.00%
18	Nebraska	0	0.00%
18	New Hampshire	0	0.00%
18	New Mexico	0	0.00%
18	North Carolina	0	0.00%
18	North Dakota	0	0.00%
18	Ohio	0	0.00%
18	Pennsylvania	0	0.00%
18	South Carolina	0	0.00%
18	South Dakota	0	0.00%
18	Tennessee	0	0.00%
18	Texas	0	0.00%
18	Vermont	0	0.00%
18	Virginia	0	0.00%
18	Washington	0	0.00%
18	West Virginia	0	0.00%
18	Wisconsin	0	0.00%
18	Wyoming	0	0.00%
	District of Columbia	0	0.00%

Source: U.S. Department of Health and Human Services, National Center for Health Statistics
"Morbidity and Mortality Weekly Report" (January 6, 1995, Vol. 43, Nos. 51 & 52)

German Measles (Rubella) Rate in 1994

National Rate = 0.08 Cases per 100,000 Population

ALPHA ORDER				RANK ORDER		
RANK	STATE	RATE		RANK	STATE	RATE
18	Alabama	0.00		1	Massachusetts	2.07
5	Alaska	0.17		2	Hawaii	0.34
18	Arizona	0.00		3	Rhode Island	0.30
18	Arkansas	0.00		4	Utah	0.21
8	California	0.09		5	Alaska	0.17
18	Colorado	0.00		6	Oklahoma	0.12
8	Connecticut	0.09		7	Oregon	0.10
18	Delaware	0.00		8	California	0.09
12	Florida	0.06		8	Connecticut	0.09
15	Georgia	0.03		8	Michigan	0.09
2	Hawaii	0.34		11	Nevada	0.07
18	Idaho	0.00		12	Florida	0.06
15	Illinois	0.03		13	Missouri	0.04
18	Indiana	0.00		13	New York	0.04
18	Iowa	0.00		15	Georgia	0.03
18	Kansas	0.00		15	Illinois	0.03
18	Kentucky	0.00		17	New Jersey	0.01
18	Louisiana	0.00		18	Alabama	0.00
18	Maine	0.00		18	Arizona	0.00
18	Maryland	0.00		18	Arkansas	0.00
1	Massachusetts	2.07		18	Colorado	0.00
8	Michigan	0.09		18	Delaware	0.00
18	Minnesota	0.00		18	Idaho	0.00
18	Mississippi	0.00		18	Indiana	0.00
13	Missouri	0.04		18	Iowa	0.00
18	Montana	0.00		18	Kansas	0.00
18	Nebraska	0.00		18	Kentucky	0.00
11	Nevada	0.07		18	Louisiana	0.00
18	New Hampshire	0.00		18	Maine	0.00
17	New Jersey	0.01		18	Maryland	0.00
18	New Mexico	0.00		18	Minnesota	0.00
13	New York	0.04		18	Mississippi	0.00
18	North Carolina	0.00		18	Montana	0.00
18	North Dakota	0.00		18	Nebraska	0.00
18	Ohio	0.00		18	New Hampshire	0.00
6	Oklahoma	0.12		18	New Mexico	0.00
7	Oregon	0.10		18	North Carolina	0.00
18	Pennsylvania	0.00		18	North Dakota	0.00
3	Rhode Island	0.30		18	Ohio	0.00
18	South Carolina	0.00		18	Pennsylvania	0.00
18	South Dakota	0.00		18	South Carolina	0.00
18	Tennessee	0.00		18	South Dakota	0.00
18	Texas	0.00		18	Tennessee	0.00
4	Utah	0.21		18	Texas	0.00
18	Vermont	0.00		18	Vermont	0.00
18	Virginia	0.00		18	Virginia	0.00
18	Washington	0.00		18	Washington	0.00
18	West Virginia	0.00		18	West Virginia	0.00
18	Wisconsin	0.00		18	Wisconsin	0.00
18	Wyoming	0.00		18	Wyoming	0.00
					District of Columbia	0.00

Source: Morgan Quitno Press using data from U.S. Dept of Health & Human Serv's, National Center for Health Statistics "Morbidity and Mortality Weekly Report" (January 6, 1995, Vol. 43, Nos. 51 & 52)

Gonorrhea Cases Reported in 1994

National Total = 400,592 Cases

<u>ALPHA ORDER</u>

RANK	STATE	CASES	% of USA
10	Alabama	15,920	3.97%
37	Alaska	884	0.22%
27	Arizona	3,543	0.88%
20	Arkansas	6,439	1.61%
5	California	23,690	5.91%
26	Colorado	3,616	0.90%
24	Connecticut	4,402	1.10%
32	Delaware	2,000	0.50%
6	Florida	23,412	5.84%
23	Georgia	4,420	1.10%
39	Hawaii	636	0.16%
45	Idaho	99	0.02%
7	Illinois	20,017	5.00%
18	Indiana	9,175	2.29%
33	Iowa	1,662	0.41%
25	Kansas	3,708	0.93%
21	Kentucky	5,127	1.28%
16	Louisiana	11,932	2.98%
46	Maine	90	0.02%
8	Maryland	18,239	4.55%
30	Massachusetts	3,215	0.80%
9	Michigan	18,099	4.52%
27	Minnesota	3,543	0.88%
17	Mississippi	11,256	2.81%
15	Missouri	12,277	3.06%
48	Montana	87	0.02%
36	Nebraska	1,060	0.26%
34	Nevada	1,619	0.40%
44	New Hampshire	105	0.03%
22	New Jersey	5,089	1.27%
35	New Mexico	1,088	0.27%
3	New York	25,810	6.44%
1	North Carolina	29,520	7.37%
50	North Dakota	34	0.01%
4	Ohio	24,742	6.18%
29	Oklahoma	3,259	0.81%
40	Oregon	571	0.14%
13	Pennsylvania	13,418	3.35%
41	Rhode Island	478	0.12%
14	South Carolina	12,898	3.22%
43	South Dakota	216	0.05%
11	Tennessee	15,247	3.81%
2	Texas	25,925	6.47%
42	Utah	239	0.06%
49	Vermont	40	0.01%
12	Virginia	13,668	3.41%
31	Washington	2,896	0.72%
38	West Virginia	847	0.21%
19	Wisconsin	7,172	1.79%
47	Wyoming	88	0.02%

<u>RANK ORDER</u>

RANK	STATE	CASES	% of USA
1	North Carolina	29,520	7.37%
2	Texas	25,925	6.47%
3	New York	25,810	6.44%
4	Ohio	24,742	6.18%
5	California	23,690	5.91%
6	Florida	23,412	5.84%
7	Illinois	20,017	5.00%
8	Maryland	18,239	4.55%
9	Michigan	18,099	4.52%
10	Alabama	15,920	3.97%
11	Tennessee	15,247	3.81%
12	Virginia	13,668	3.41%
13	Pennsylvania	13,418	3.35%
14	South Carolina	12,898	3.22%
15	Missouri	12,277	3.06%
16	Louisiana	11,932	2.98%
17	Mississippi	11,256	2.81%
18	Indiana	9,175	2.29%
19	Wisconsin	7,172	1.79%
20	Arkansas	6,439	1.61%
21	Kentucky	5,127	1.28%
22	New Jersey	5,089	1.27%
23	Georgia	4,420	1.10%
24	Connecticut	4,402	1.10%
25	Kansas	3,708	0.93%
26	Colorado	3,616	0.90%
27	Arizona	3,543	0.88%
27	Minnesota	3,543	0.88%
29	Oklahoma	3,259	0.81%
30	Massachusetts	3,215	0.80%
31	Washington	2,896	0.72%
32	Delaware	2,000	0.50%
33	Iowa	1,662	0.41%
34	Nevada	1,619	0.40%
35	New Mexico	1,088	0.27%
36	Nebraska	1,060	0.26%
37	Alaska	884	0.22%
38	West Virginia	847	0.21%
39	Hawaii	636	0.16%
40	Oregon	571	0.14%
41	Rhode Island	478	0.12%
42	Utah	239	0.06%
43	South Dakota	216	0.05%
44	New Hampshire	105	0.03%
45	Idaho	99	0.02%
46	Maine	90	0.02%
47	Wyoming	88	0.02%
48	Montana	87	0.02%
49	Vermont	40	0.01%
50	North Dakota	34	0.01%
	District of Columbia	7,075	1.77%

Source: U.S. Department of Health and Human Services, National Center for Health Statistics
"Morbidity and Mortality Weekly Report" (January 6, 1995, Vol. 43, Nos. 51 & 52)

Gonorrhea Rate in 1994

National Rate = 153.87 Cases Reported per 100,000 Population

ALPHA ORDER				RANK ORDER		
RANK	**STATE**	**RATE**		**RANK**	**STATE**	**RATE**
3	Alabama	377.34		1	Mississippi	421.73
17	Alaska	145.87		2	North Carolina	417.54
28	Arizona	86.94		3	Alabama	377.34
9	Arkansas	262.49		4	Maryland	364.34
30	California	75.37		5	South Carolina	352.02
27	Colorado	98.91		6	Tennessee	294.63
22	Connecticut	134.41		7	Delaware	283.29
7	Delaware	283.29		8	Louisiana	276.52
15	Florida	167.79		9	Arkansas	262.49
34	Georgia	62.65		10	Missouri	232.61
37	Hawaii	53.94		11	Ohio	222.86
47	Idaho	8.74		12	Virginia	208.61
14	Illinois	170.33		13	Michigan	190.60
16	Indiana	159.51		14	Illinois	170.33
35	Iowa	58.75		15	Florida	167.79
18	Kansas	145.18		16	Indiana	159.51
23	Kentucky	133.97		17	Alaska	145.87
8	Louisiana	276.52		18	Kansas	145.18
48	Maine	7.26		19	New York	142.06
4	Maryland	364.34		20	Wisconsin	141.13
38	Massachusetts	53.22		21	Texas	141.07
13	Michigan	190.60		22	Connecticut	134.41
29	Minnesota	77.58		23	Kentucky	133.97
1	Mississippi	421.73		24	Pennsylvania	111.33
10	Missouri	232.61		25	Nevada	111.12
45	Montana	10.16		26	Oklahoma	100.03
32	Nebraska	65.31		27	Colorado	98.91
25	Nevada	111.12		28	Arizona	86.94
46	New Hampshire	9.23		29	Minnesota	77.58
33	New Jersey	64.39		30	California	75.37
31	New Mexico	65.78		31	New Mexico	65.78
19	New York	142.06		32	Nebraska	65.31
2	North Carolina	417.54		33	New Jersey	64.39
50	North Dakota	5.33		34	Georgia	62.65
11	Ohio	222.86		35	Iowa	58.75
26	Oklahoma	100.03		36	Washington	54.20
42	Oregon	18.50		37	Hawaii	53.94
24	Pennsylvania	111.33		38	Massachusetts	53.22
39	Rhode Island	47.94		39	Rhode Island	47.94
5	South Carolina	352.02		40	West Virginia	46.49
41	South Dakota	29.96		41	South Dakota	29.96
6	Tennessee	294.63		42	Oregon	18.50
21	Texas	141.07		43	Wyoming	18.49
44	Utah	12.53		44	Utah	12.53
49	Vermont	6.90		45	Montana	10.16
12	Virginia	208.61		46	New Hampshire	9.23
36	Washington	54.20		47	Idaho	8.74
40	West Virginia	46.49		48	Maine	7.26
20	Wisconsin	141.13		49	Vermont	6.90
43	Wyoming	18.49		50	North Dakota	5.33

District of Columbia 1,241.23

Source: Morgan Quitno Press using data from U.S. Dept of Health & Human Serv's, National Center for Health Statistics "Morbidity and Mortality Weekly Report" (January 6, 1995, Vol. 43, Nos. 51 & 52)

Hepatitis (Viral) Cases Reported in 1994

National Total = 39,551 Cases Reported*

ALPHA ORDER

RANK	STATE	CASES	% of USA
32	Alabama	251	0.63%
34	Alaska	215	0.54%
6	Arizona	1,653	4.18%
31	Arkansas	257	0.65%
1	California	8,901	22.51%
14	Colorado	795	2.01%
35	Connecticut	186	0.47%
48	Delaware	23	0.06%
5	Florida	1,820	4.60%
15	Georgia	756	1.91%
40	Hawaii	95	0.24%
21	Idaho	530	1.34%
16	Illinois	750	1.90%
20	Indiana	554	1.40%
38	Iowa	116	0.29%
37	Kansas	147	0.37%
29	Kentucky	302	0.76%
22	Louisiana	529	1.34%
47	Maine	35	0.09%
18	Maryland	597	1.51%
25	Massachusetts	405	1.02%
12	Michigan	997	2.52%
28	Minnesota	319	0.81%
42	Mississippi	72	0.18%
9	Missouri	1,113	2.81%
43	Montana	62	0.16%
36	Nebraska	161	0.41%
27	Nevada	344	0.87%
45	New Hampshire	46	0.12%
13	New Jersey	846	2.14%
7	New Mexico	1,410	3.57%
3	New York	2,235	5.65%
24	North Carolina	489	1.24%
50	North Dakota	7	0.02%
8	Ohio	1,394	3.52%
10	Oklahoma	1,059	2.68%
11	Oregon	1,012	2.56%
19	Pennsylvania	575	1.45%
44	Rhode Island	60	0.15%
41	South Carolina	83	0.21%
46	South Dakota	43	0.11%
4	Tennessee	2,220	5.61%
2	Texas	3,762	9.51%
17	Utah	742	1.88%
49	Vermont	14	0.04%
26	Virginia	357	0.90%
23	Washington	500	1.26%
39	West Virginia	114	0.29%
30	Wisconsin	291	0.74%
33	Wyoming	219	0.55%

RANK ORDER

RANK	STATE	CASES	% of USA
1	California	8,901	22.51%
2	Texas	3,762	9.51%
3	New York	2,235	5.65%
4	Tennessee	2,220	5.61%
5	Florida	1,820	4.60%
6	Arizona	1,653	4.18%
7	New Mexico	1,410	3.57%
8	Ohio	1,394	3.52%
9	Missouri	1,113	2.81%
10	Oklahoma	1,059	2.68%
11	Oregon	1,012	2.56%
12	Michigan	997	2.52%
13	New Jersey	846	2.14%
14	Colorado	795	2.01%
15	Georgia	756	1.91%
16	Illinois	750	1.90%
17	Utah	742	1.88%
18	Maryland	597	1.51%
19	Pennsylvania	575	1.45%
20	Indiana	554	1.40%
21	Idaho	530	1.34%
22	Louisiana	529	1.34%
23	Washington	500	1.26%
24	North Carolina	489	1.24%
25	Massachusetts	405	1.02%
26	Virginia	357	0.90%
27	Nevada	344	0.87%
28	Minnesota	319	0.81%
29	Kentucky	302	0.76%
30	Wisconsin	291	0.74%
31	Arkansas	257	0.65%
32	Alabama	251	0.63%
33	Wyoming	219	0.55%
34	Alaska	215	0.54%
35	Connecticut	186	0.47%
36	Nebraska	161	0.41%
37	Kansas	147	0.37%
38	Iowa	116	0.29%
39	West Virginia	114	0.29%
40	Hawaii	95	0.24%
41	South Carolina	83	0.21%
42	Mississippi	72	0.18%
43	Montana	62	0.16%
44	Rhode Island	60	0.15%
45	New Hampshire	46	0.12%
46	South Dakota	43	0.11%
47	Maine	35	0.09%
48	Delaware	23	0.06%
49	Vermont	14	0.04%
50	North Dakota	7	0.02%
	District of Columbia	88	0.22%

Source: U.S. Department of Health and Human Services, National Center for Health Statistics
"Morbidity and Mortality Weekly Report" (January 6, 1995, Vol. 43, Nos. 51 & 52)
*An inflammation of the liver. Includes types A, B, NA, NB and unspecified.

Hepatitis (Viral) Rate in 1994

National Rate = 15.19 Cases Reported per 100,000 Population*

ALPHA ORDER			RANK ORDER		
RANK	STATE	RATE	RANK	STATE	RATE
37	Alabama	5.95	1	New Mexico	85.25
7	Alaska	35.48	2	Idaho	46.78
5	Arizona	40.56	3	Wyoming	46.01
23	Arkansas	10.48	4	Tennessee	42.90
10	California	28.32	5	Arizona	40.56
12	Colorado	21.75	6	Utah	38.89
40	Connecticut	5.68	7	Alaska	35.48
45	Delaware	3.26	8	Oregon	32.79
15	Florida	13.04	9	Oklahoma	32.50
20	Georgia	10.72	10	California	28.32
27	Hawaii	8.06	11	Nevada	23.61
2	Idaho	46.78	12	Colorado	21.75
33	Illinois	6.38	13	Missouri	21.09
25	Indiana	9.63	14	Texas	20.47
43	Iowa	4.10	15	Florida	13.04
38	Kansas	5.76	16	Ohio	12.56
28	Kentucky	7.89	17	New York	12.30
18	Louisiana	12.26	18	Louisiana	12.26
46	Maine	2.82	19	Maryland	11.93
19	Maryland	11.93	20	Georgia	10.72
32	Massachusetts	6.70	21	New Jersey	10.70
22	Michigan	10.50	22	Michigan	10.50
30	Minnesota	6.98	23	Arkansas	10.48
47	Mississippi	2.70	24	Nebraska	9.92
13	Missouri	21.09	25	Indiana	9.63
29	Montana	7.24	26	Washington	9.36
24	Nebraska	9.92	27	Hawaii	8.06
11	Nevada	23.61	28	Kentucky	7.89
44	New Hampshire	4.05	29	Montana	7.24
21	New Jersey	10.70	30	Minnesota	6.98
1	New Mexico	85.25	31	North Carolina	6.92
17	New York	12.30	32	Massachusetts	6.70
31	North Carolina	6.92	33	Illinois	6.38
50	North Dakota	1.10	34	West Virginia	6.26
16	Ohio	12.56	35	Rhode Island	6.02
9	Oklahoma	32.50	36	South Dakota	5.96
8	Oregon	32.79	37	Alabama	5.95
42	Pennsylvania	4.77	38	Kansas	5.76
35	Rhode Island	6.02	39	Wisconsin	5.73
49	South Carolina	2.27	40	Connecticut	5.68
36	South Dakota	5.96	41	Virginia	5.45
4	Tennessee	42.90	42	Pennsylvania	4.77
14	Texas	20.47	43	Iowa	4.10
6	Utah	38.89	44	New Hampshire	4.05
48	Vermont	2.41	45	Delaware	3.26
41	Virginia	5.45	46	Maine	2.82
26	Washington	9.36	47	Mississippi	2.70
34	West Virginia	6.26	48	Vermont	2.41
39	Wisconsin	5.73	49	South Carolina	2.27
3	Wyoming	46.01	50	North Dakota	1.10
				District of Columbia	15.44

Source: Morgan Quitno Press using data from U.S. Dept of Health & Human Serv's, National Center for Health Statistics
"Morbidity and Mortality Weekly Report" (January 6, 1995, Vol. 43, Nos. 51 & 52)
*An inflammation of the liver. Includes types A, B, NA, NB and unspecified.

Legionellosis Cases Reported in 1994

National Total = 1,535 Cases*

ALPHA ORDER

RANK	STATE	CASES	% of USA
25	Alabama	13	0.85%
47	Alaska	0	0.00%
17	Arizona	29	1.89%
31	Arkansas	10	0.65%
7	California	78	5.08%
22	Colorado	21	1.37%
47	Connecticut	0	0.00%
19	Delaware	26	1.69%
10	Florida	55	3.58%
4	Georgia	100	6.51%
38	Hawaii	5	0.33%
43	Idaho	2	0.13%
15	Illinois	31	2.02%
3	Indiana	106	6.91%
14	Iowa	34	2.21%
36	Kansas	6	0.39%
33	Kentucky	9	0.59%
24	Louisiana	14	0.91%
38	Maine	5	0.33%
5	Maryland	85	5.54%
9	Massachusetts	56	3.65%
6	Michigan	82	5.34%
43	Minnesota	2	0.13%
25	Mississippi	13	0.85%
13	Missouri	38	2.48%
23	Montana	16	1.04%
31	Nebraska	10	0.65%
19	Nevada	26	1.69%
47	New Hampshire	0	0.00%
12	New Jersey	43	2.80%
40	New Mexico	4	0.26%
8	New York	71	4.63%
18	North Carolina	28	1.82%
40	North Dakota	4	0.26%
1	Ohio	194	12.64%
30	Oklahoma	11	0.72%
47	Oregon	0	0.00%
2	Pennsylvania	134	8.73%
25	Rhode Island	13	0.85%
21	South Carolina	22	1.43%
45	South Dakota	1	0.07%
11	Tennessee	45	2.93%
29	Texas	12	0.78%
35	Utah	7	0.46%
45	Vermont	1	0.07%
25	Virginia	13	0.85%
34	Washington	8	0.52%
40	West Virginia	4	0.26%
16	Wisconsin	30	1.95%
36	Wyoming	6	0.39%

RANK ORDER

RANK	STATE	CASES	% of USA
1	Ohio	194	12.64%
2	Pennsylvania	134	8.73%
3	Indiana	106	6.91%
4	Georgia	100	6.51%
5	Maryland	85	5.54%
6	Michigan	82	5.34%
7	California	78	5.08%
8	New York	71	4.63%
9	Massachusetts	56	3.65%
10	Florida	55	3.58%
11	Tennessee	45	2.93%
12	New Jersey	43	2.80%
13	Missouri	38	2.48%
14	Iowa	34	2.21%
15	Illinois	31	2.02%
16	Wisconsin	30	1.95%
17	Arizona	29	1.89%
18	North Carolina	28	1.82%
19	Delaware	26	1.69%
19	Nevada	26	1.69%
21	South Carolina	22	1.43%
22	Colorado	21	1.37%
23	Montana	16	1.04%
24	Louisiana	14	0.91%
25	Alabama	13	0.85%
25	Mississippi	13	0.85%
25	Rhode Island	13	0.85%
25	Virginia	13	0.85%
29	Texas	12	0.78%
30	Oklahoma	11	0.72%
31	Arkansas	10	0.65%
31	Nebraska	10	0.65%
33	Kentucky	9	0.59%
34	Washington	8	0.52%
35	Utah	7	0.46%
36	Kansas	6	0.39%
36	Wyoming	6	0.39%
38	Hawaii	5	0.33%
38	Maine	5	0.33%
40	New Mexico	4	0.26%
40	North Dakota	4	0.26%
40	West Virginia	4	0.26%
43	Idaho	2	0.13%
43	Minnesota	2	0.13%
45	South Dakota	1	0.07%
45	Vermont	1	0.07%
47	Alaska	0	0.00%
47	Connecticut	0	0.00%
47	New Hampshire	0	0.00%
47	Oregon	0	0.00%
	District of Columbia	12	0.78%

Source: U.S. Department of Health and Human Services, National Center for Health Statistics
"Morbidity and Mortality Weekly Report" (January 6, 1995, Vol. 43, Nos. 51 & 52)
*A pneumonia-like disease (Legionnaire's Disease).

Legionellosis Rate in 1994

National Rate = 0.59 Cases Reported per 100,000 Population*

<table>
<tr><td colspan="3">ALPHA ORDER</td><td colspan="3">RANK ORDER</td></tr>
<tr><td>RANK</td><td>STATE</td><td>RATE</td><td>RANK</td><td>STATE</td><td>RATE</td></tr>
<tr><td>33</td><td>Alabama</td><td>0.31</td><td>1</td><td>Delaware</td><td>3.68</td></tr>
<tr><td>47</td><td>Alaska</td><td>0.00</td><td>2</td><td>Montana</td><td>1.87</td></tr>
<tr><td>16</td><td>Arizona</td><td>0.71</td><td>3</td><td>Indiana</td><td>1.84</td></tr>
<tr><td>25</td><td>Arkansas</td><td>0.41</td><td>4</td><td>Nevada</td><td>1.78</td></tr>
<tr><td>35</td><td>California</td><td>0.25</td><td>5</td><td>Ohio</td><td>1.75</td></tr>
<tr><td>21</td><td>Colorado</td><td>0.57</td><td>6</td><td>Maryland</td><td>1.70</td></tr>
<tr><td>47</td><td>Connecticut</td><td>0.00</td><td>7</td><td>Georgia</td><td>1.42</td></tr>
<tr><td>1</td><td>Delaware</td><td>3.68</td><td>8</td><td>Rhode Island</td><td>1.30</td></tr>
<tr><td>28</td><td>Florida</td><td>0.39</td><td>9</td><td>Wyoming</td><td>1.26</td></tr>
<tr><td>7</td><td>Georgia</td><td>1.42</td><td>10</td><td>Iowa</td><td>1.20</td></tr>
<tr><td>24</td><td>Hawaii</td><td>0.42</td><td>11</td><td>Pennsylvania</td><td>1.11</td></tr>
<tr><td>41</td><td>Idaho</td><td>0.18</td><td>12</td><td>Massachusetts</td><td>0.93</td></tr>
<tr><td>34</td><td>Illinois</td><td>0.26</td><td>13</td><td>Tennessee</td><td>0.87</td></tr>
<tr><td>3</td><td>Indiana</td><td>1.84</td><td>14</td><td>Michigan</td><td>0.86</td></tr>
<tr><td>10</td><td>Iowa</td><td>1.20</td><td>15</td><td>Missouri</td><td>0.72</td></tr>
<tr><td>38</td><td>Kansas</td><td>0.23</td><td>16</td><td>Arizona</td><td>0.71</td></tr>
<tr><td>36</td><td>Kentucky</td><td>0.24</td><td>17</td><td>North Dakota</td><td>0.63</td></tr>
<tr><td>32</td><td>Louisiana</td><td>0.32</td><td>18</td><td>Nebraska</td><td>0.62</td></tr>
<tr><td>26</td><td>Maine</td><td>0.40</td><td>19</td><td>South Carolina</td><td>0.60</td></tr>
<tr><td>6</td><td>Maryland</td><td>1.70</td><td>20</td><td>Wisconsin</td><td>0.59</td></tr>
<tr><td>12</td><td>Massachusetts</td><td>0.93</td><td>21</td><td>Colorado</td><td>0.57</td></tr>
<tr><td>14</td><td>Michigan</td><td>0.86</td><td>22</td><td>New Jersey</td><td>0.54</td></tr>
<tr><td>46</td><td>Minnesota</td><td>0.04</td><td>23</td><td>Mississippi</td><td>0.49</td></tr>
<tr><td>23</td><td>Mississippi</td><td>0.49</td><td>24</td><td>Hawaii</td><td>0.42</td></tr>
<tr><td>15</td><td>Missouri</td><td>0.72</td><td>25</td><td>Arkansas</td><td>0.41</td></tr>
<tr><td>2</td><td>Montana</td><td>1.87</td><td>26</td><td>Maine</td><td>0.40</td></tr>
<tr><td>18</td><td>Nebraska</td><td>0.62</td><td>26</td><td>North Carolina</td><td>0.40</td></tr>
<tr><td>4</td><td>Nevada</td><td>1.78</td><td>28</td><td>Florida</td><td>0.39</td></tr>
<tr><td>47</td><td>New Hampshire</td><td>0.00</td><td>28</td><td>New York</td><td>0.39</td></tr>
<tr><td>22</td><td>New Jersey</td><td>0.54</td><td>30</td><td>Utah</td><td>0.37</td></tr>
<tr><td>36</td><td>New Mexico</td><td>0.24</td><td>31</td><td>Oklahoma</td><td>0.34</td></tr>
<tr><td>28</td><td>New York</td><td>0.39</td><td>32</td><td>Louisiana</td><td>0.32</td></tr>
<tr><td>26</td><td>North Carolina</td><td>0.40</td><td>33</td><td>Alabama</td><td>0.31</td></tr>
<tr><td>17</td><td>North Dakota</td><td>0.63</td><td>34</td><td>Illinois</td><td>0.26</td></tr>
<tr><td>5</td><td>Ohio</td><td>1.75</td><td>35</td><td>California</td><td>0.25</td></tr>
<tr><td>31</td><td>Oklahoma</td><td>0.34</td><td>36</td><td>Kentucky</td><td>0.24</td></tr>
<tr><td>47</td><td>Oregon</td><td>0.00</td><td>36</td><td>New Mexico</td><td>0.24</td></tr>
<tr><td>11</td><td>Pennsylvania</td><td>1.11</td><td>38</td><td>Kansas</td><td>0.23</td></tr>
<tr><td>8</td><td>Rhode Island</td><td>1.30</td><td>39</td><td>West Virginia</td><td>0.22</td></tr>
<tr><td>19</td><td>South Carolina</td><td>0.60</td><td>40</td><td>Virginia</td><td>0.20</td></tr>
<tr><td>44</td><td>South Dakota</td><td>0.14</td><td>41</td><td>Idaho</td><td>0.18</td></tr>
<tr><td>13</td><td>Tennessee</td><td>0.87</td><td>42</td><td>Vermont</td><td>0.17</td></tr>
<tr><td>45</td><td>Texas</td><td>0.07</td><td>43</td><td>Washington</td><td>0.15</td></tr>
<tr><td>30</td><td>Utah</td><td>0.37</td><td>44</td><td>South Dakota</td><td>0.14</td></tr>
<tr><td>42</td><td>Vermont</td><td>0.17</td><td>45</td><td>Texas</td><td>0.07</td></tr>
<tr><td>40</td><td>Virginia</td><td>0.20</td><td>46</td><td>Minnesota</td><td>0.04</td></tr>
<tr><td>43</td><td>Washington</td><td>0.15</td><td>47</td><td>Alaska</td><td>0.00</td></tr>
<tr><td>39</td><td>West Virginia</td><td>0.22</td><td>47</td><td>Connecticut</td><td>0.00</td></tr>
<tr><td>20</td><td>Wisconsin</td><td>0.59</td><td>47</td><td>New Hampshire</td><td>0.00</td></tr>
<tr><td>9</td><td>Wyoming</td><td>1.26</td><td>47</td><td>Oregon</td><td>0.00</td></tr>
<tr><td></td><td></td><td></td><td></td><td>District of Columbia</td><td>2.11</td></tr>
</table>

Source: Morgan Quitno Press using data from U.S. Dept of Health & Human Serv's, National Center for Health Statistics
"Morbidity and Mortality Weekly Report" (January 6, 1995, Vol. 43, Nos. 51 & 52)
*A pneumonia-like disease (Legionnaire's Disease).

Lyme Disease Cases Reported in 1994

National Total = 11,424 Cases*

ALPHA ORDER

RANK	STATE	CASES	% of USA
33	Alabama	6	0.05%
41	Alaska	0	0.00%
41	Arizona	0	0.00%
30	Arkansas	8	0.07%
12	California	84	0.74%
39	Colorado	1	0.01%
2	Connecticut	1,762	15.42%
13	Delaware	81	0.71%
21	Florida	27	0.24%
10	Georgia	108	0.95%
41	Hawaii	0	0.00%
35	Idaho	3	0.03%
29	Illinois	11	0.10%
26	Indiana	14	0.12%
24	Iowa	17	0.15%
24	Kansas	17	0.15%
23	Kentucky	23	0.20%
37	Louisiana	2	0.02%
20	Maine	28	0.25%
5	Maryland	492	4.31%
7	Massachusetts	267	2.34%
18	Michigan	33	0.29%
8	Minnesota	165	1.44%
41	Mississippi	0	0.00%
11	Missouri	87	0.76%
41	Montana	0	0.00%
37	Nebraska	2	0.02%
39	Nevada	1	0.01%
19	New Hampshire	31	0.27%
4	New Jersey	1,320	11.55%
30	New Mexico	8	0.07%
1	New York	4,532	39.67%
15	North Carolina	77	0.67%
41	North Dakota	0	0.00%
14	Ohio	79	0.69%
16	Oklahoma	76	0.67%
41	Oregon	0	0.00%
3	Pennsylvania	1,337	11.70%
6	Rhode Island	471	4.12%
32	South Carolina	7	0.06%
41	South Dakota	0	0.00%
27	Tennessee	13	0.11%
17	Texas	46	0.40%
35	Utah	3	0.03%
27	Vermont	13	0.11%
9	Virginia	131	1.15%
41	Washington	0	0.00%
21	West Virginia	27	0.24%
41	Wisconsin	0	0.00%
34	Wyoming	5	0.04%

RANK ORDER

RANK	STATE	CASES	% of USA
1	New York	4,532	39.67%
2	Connecticut	1,762	15.42%
3	Pennsylvania	1,337	11.70%
4	New Jersey	1,320	11.55%
5	Maryland	492	4.31%
6	Rhode Island	471	4.12%
7	Massachusetts	267	2.34%
8	Minnesota	165	1.44%
9	Virginia	131	1.15%
10	Georgia	108	0.95%
11	Missouri	87	0.76%
12	California	84	0.74%
13	Delaware	81	0.71%
14	Ohio	79	0.69%
15	North Carolina	77	0.67%
16	Oklahoma	76	0.67%
17	Texas	46	0.40%
18	Michigan	33	0.29%
19	New Hampshire	31	0.27%
20	Maine	28	0.25%
21	Florida	27	0.24%
21	West Virginia	27	0.24%
23	Kentucky	23	0.20%
24	Iowa	17	0.15%
24	Kansas	17	0.15%
26	Indiana	14	0.12%
27	Tennessee	13	0.11%
27	Vermont	13	0.11%
29	Illinois	11	0.10%
30	Arkansas	8	0.07%
30	New Mexico	8	0.07%
32	South Carolina	7	0.06%
33	Alabama	6	0.05%
34	Wyoming	5	0.04%
35	Idaho	3	0.03%
35	Utah	3	0.03%
37	Louisiana	2	0.02%
37	Nebraska	2	0.02%
39	Colorado	1	0.01%
39	Nevada	1	0.01%
41	Alaska	0	0.00%
41	Arizona	0	0.00%
41	Hawaii	0	0.00%
41	Mississippi	0	0.00%
41	Montana	0	0.00%
41	North Dakota	0	0.00%
41	Oregon	0	0.00%
41	South Dakota	0	0.00%
41	Washington	0	0.00%
41	Wisconsin	0	0.00%
	District of Columbia	9	0.08%

Source: U.S. Department of Health and Human Services, National Center for Health Statistics
"Morbidity and Mortality Weekly Report" (January 6, 1995, Vol. 43, Nos. 51 & 52)
*Caused by ticks--lesions, followed by arthritis of large joints, myalgia, malaise and neurologic and cardiac manifestations. Named after Old Lyme, CT, where the disease was first reported.

Lyme Disease Rate in 1994

National Rate = 4.39 Cases Reported per 100,000 Population*

ALPHA ORDER

RANK	STATE	RATE
35	Alabama	0.14
41	Alaska	0.00
41	Arizona	0.00
26	Arkansas	0.33
27	California	0.27
40	Colorado	0.03
1	Connecticut	53.80
5	Delaware	11.47
32	Florida	0.19
16	Georgia	1.53
41	Hawaii	0.00
28	Idaho	0.26
37	Illinois	0.09
31	Indiana	0.24
22	Iowa	0.60
21	Kansas	0.67
22	Kentucky	0.60
39	Louisiana	0.05
12	Maine	2.26
7	Maryland	9.83
8	Massachusetts	4.42
25	Michigan	0.35
9	Minnesota	3.61
41	Mississippi	0.00
15	Missouri	1.65
41	Montana	0.00
36	Nebraska	0.12
38	Nevada	0.07
10	New Hampshire	2.73
4	New Jersey	16.70
24	New Mexico	0.48
3	New York	24.94
18	North Carolina	1.09
41	North Dakota	0.00
20	Ohio	0.71
11	Oklahoma	2.33
41	Oregon	0.00
6	Pennsylvania	11.09
2	Rhode Island	47.24
32	South Carolina	0.19
41	South Dakota	0.00
29	Tennessee	0.25
29	Texas	0.25
34	Utah	0.16
13	Vermont	2.24
14	Virginia	2.00
41	Washington	0.00
17	West Virginia	1.48
41	Wisconsin	0.00
19	Wyoming	1.05

RANK ORDER

RANK	STATE	RATE
1	Connecticut	53.80
2	Rhode Island	47.24
3	New York	24.94
4	New Jersey	16.70
5	Delaware	11.47
6	Pennsylvania	11.09
7	Maryland	9.83
8	Massachusetts	4.42
9	Minnesota	3.61
10	New Hampshire	2.73
11	Oklahoma	2.33
12	Maine	2.26
13	Vermont	2.24
14	Virginia	2.00
15	Missouri	1.65
16	Georgia	1.53
17	West Virginia	1.48
18	North Carolina	1.09
19	Wyoming	1.05
20	Ohio	0.71
21	Kansas	0.67
22	Iowa	0.60
22	Kentucky	0.60
24	New Mexico	0.48
25	Michigan	0.35
26	Arkansas	0.33
27	California	0.27
28	Idaho	0.26
29	Tennessee	0.25
29	Texas	0.25
31	Indiana	0.24
32	Florida	0.19
32	South Carolina	0.19
34	Utah	0.16
35	Alabama	0.14
36	Nebraska	0.12
37	Illinois	0.09
38	Nevada	0.07
39	Louisiana	0.05
40	Colorado	0.03
41	Alaska	0.00
41	Arizona	0.00
41	Hawaii	0.00
41	Mississippi	0.00
41	Montana	0.00
41	North Dakota	0.00
41	Oregon	0.00
41	South Dakota	0.00
41	Washington	0.00
41	Wisconsin	0.00

District of Columbia   1.58

Source: Morgan Quitno Press using data from U.S. Dept of Health & Human Serv's, National Center for Health Statistics "Morbidity and Mortality Weekly Report" (January 6, 1995, Vol. 43, Nos. 51 & 52)
*Caused by ticks--lesions, followed by arthritis of large joints, myalgia, malaise and neurologic and cardiac manifestations. Named after Old Lyme, CT, where the disease was first reported.

Malaria Cases Reported in 1994

National Total = 1,065 Cases*

ALPHA ORDER					RANK ORDER			

RANK	STATE	CASES	% of USA		RANK	STATE	CASES	% of USA
27	Alabama	9	0.85%		1	California	197	18.50%
41	Alaska	2	0.19%		2	New York	144	13.52%
27	Arizona	9	0.85%		3	Maryland	86	8.08%
36	Arkansas	3	0.28%		4	Texas	56	5.26%
1	California	197	18.50%		5	New Jersey	54	5.07%
15	Colorado	19	1.78%		6	Illinois	39	3.66%
13	Connecticut	23	2.16%		7	Virginia	37	3.47%
36	Delaware	3	0.28%		8	Massachusetts	34	3.19%
11	Florida	29	2.72%		9	Michigan	31	2.91%
12	Georgia	26	2.44%		9	Pennsylvania	31	2.91%
17	Hawaii	15	1.41%		11	Florida	29	2.72%
41	Idaho	2	0.19%		12	Georgia	26	2.44%
6	Illinois	39	3.66%		13	Connecticut	23	2.16%
17	Indiana	15	1.41%		14	Ohio	20	1.88%
32	Iowa	5	0.47%		15	Colorado	19	1.78%
29	Kansas	7	0.66%		16	Washington	16	1.50%
22	Kentucky	12	1.13%		17	Hawaii	15	1.41%
24	Louisiana	10	0.94%		17	Indiana	15	1.41%
31	Maine	6	0.56%		19	Minnesota	14	1.31%
3	Maryland	86	8.08%		19	Oregon	14	1.31%
8	Massachusetts	34	3.19%		21	Missouri	13	1.22%
9	Michigan	31	2.91%		22	Kentucky	12	1.13%
19	Minnesota	14	1.31%		22	North Carolina	12	1.13%
45	Mississippi	1	0.09%		24	Louisiana	10	0.94%
21	Missouri	13	1.22%		24	Rhode Island	10	0.94%
48	Montana	0	0.00%		24	Tennessee	10	0.94%
32	Nebraska	5	0.47%		27	Alabama	9	0.85%
41	Nevada	2	0.19%		27	Arizona	9	0.85%
36	New Hampshire	3	0.28%		29	Kansas	7	0.66%
5	New Jersey	54	5.07%		29	Oklahoma	7	0.66%
36	New Mexico	3	0.28%		31	Maine	6	0.56%
2	New York	144	13.52%		32	Iowa	5	0.47%
22	North Carolina	12	1.13%		32	Nebraska	5	0.47%
45	North Dakota	1	0.09%		32	South Carolina	5	0.47%
14	Ohio	20	1.88%		35	Utah	4	0.38%
29	Oklahoma	7	0.66%		36	Arkansas	3	0.28%
19	Oregon	14	1.31%		36	Delaware	3	0.28%
9	Pennsylvania	31	2.91%		36	New Hampshire	3	0.28%
24	Rhode Island	10	0.94%		36	New Mexico	3	0.28%
32	South Carolina	5	0.47%		36	Vermont	3	0.28%
48	South Dakota	0	0.00%		41	Alaska	2	0.19%
24	Tennessee	10	0.94%		41	Idaho	2	0.19%
4	Texas	56	5.26%		41	Nevada	2	0.19%
35	Utah	4	0.38%		41	Wisconsin	2	0.19%
36	Vermont	3	0.28%		45	Mississippi	1	0.09%
7	Virginia	37	3.47%		45	North Dakota	1	0.09%
16	Washington	16	1.50%		45	Wyoming	1	0.09%
48	West Virginia	0	0.00%		48	Montana	0	0.00%
41	Wisconsin	2	0.19%		48	South Dakota	0	0.00%
45	Wyoming	1	0.09%		48	West Virginia	0	0.00%
						District of Columbia	15	1.41%

Source: U.S. Department of Health and Human Services, National Center for Health Statistics
   "Morbidity and Mortality Weekly Report" (January 6, 1995, Vol. 43, Nos. 51 & 52)
*Infectious disease usually transmitted by bites of infected mosquitoes. Symptoms include high fever, shaking chills, sweating and anemia.

Malaria Rate in 1994

National Rate = 0.41 Cases Reported per 100,000 Population*

ALPHA ORDER			RANK ORDER		
RANK	STATE	RATE	RANK	STATE	RATE
31	Alabama	0.21	1	Maryland	1.72
16	Alaska	0.33	2	Hawaii	1.27
30	Arizona	0.22	3	Rhode Island	1.00
45	Arkansas	0.12	4	New York	0.79
7	California	0.63	5	Connecticut	0.70
10	Colorado	0.52	6	New Jersey	0.68
5	Connecticut	0.70	7	California	0.63
14	Delaware	0.42	8	Massachusetts	0.56
31	Florida	0.21	8	Virginia	0.56
15	Georgia	0.37	10	Colorado	0.52
2	Hawaii	1.27	10	Vermont	0.52
37	Idaho	0.18	12	Maine	0.48
16	Illinois	0.33	13	Oregon	0.45
25	Indiana	0.26	14	Delaware	0.42
37	Iowa	0.18	15	Georgia	0.37
24	Kansas	0.27	16	Alaska	0.33
19	Kentucky	0.31	16	Illinois	0.33
29	Louisiana	0.23	16	Michigan	0.33
12	Maine	0.48	19	Kentucky	0.31
1	Maryland	1.72	19	Minnesota	0.31
8	Massachusetts	0.56	19	Nebraska	0.31
16	Michigan	0.33	22	Texas	0.30
19	Minnesota	0.31	22	Washington	0.30
46	Mississippi	0.04	24	Kansas	0.27
28	Missouri	0.25	25	Indiana	0.26
48	Montana	0.00	25	New Hampshire	0.26
19	Nebraska	0.31	25	Pennsylvania	0.26
43	Nevada	0.14	28	Missouri	0.25
25	New Hampshire	0.26	29	Louisiana	0.23
6	New Jersey	0.68	30	Arizona	0.22
37	New Mexico	0.18	31	Alabama	0.21
4	New York	0.79	31	Florida	0.21
41	North Carolina	0.17	31	Oklahoma	0.21
42	North Dakota	0.16	31	Utah	0.21
37	Ohio	0.18	31	Wyoming	0.21
31	Oklahoma	0.21	36	Tennessee	0.19
13	Oregon	0.45	37	Idaho	0.18
25	Pennsylvania	0.26	37	Iowa	0.18
3	Rhode Island	1.00	37	New Mexico	0.18
43	South Carolina	0.14	37	Ohio	0.18
48	South Dakota	0.00	41	North Carolina	0.17
36	Tennessee	0.19	42	North Dakota	0.16
22	Texas	0.30	43	Nevada	0.14
31	Utah	0.21	43	South Carolina	0.14
10	Vermont	0.52	45	Arkansas	0.12
8	Virginia	0.56	46	Mississippi	0.04
22	Washington	0.30	46	Wisconsin	0.04
48	West Virginia	0.00	48	Montana	0.00
46	Wisconsin	0.04	48	South Dakota	0.00
31	Wyoming	0.21	48	West Virginia	0.00

District of Columbia   2.63

Source: Morgan Quitno Press using data from U.S. Dept of Health & Human Serv's, National Center for Health Statistics "Morbidity and Mortality Weekly Report" (January 6, 1995, Vol. 43, Nos. 51 & 52)
*Infectious disease usually transmitted by bites of infected mosquitoes. Symptoms include high fever, shaking chills, sweating and anemia.

Measles (Rubeola) Cases Reported in 1994

National Total = 895 Cases*

ALPHA ORDER

RANK	STATE	CASES	% of USA
39	Alabama	0	0.00%
14	Alaska	16	1.79%
17	Arizona	9	1.01%
33	Arkansas	1	0.11%
4	California	65	7.26%
10	Colorado	20	2.23%
24	Connecticut	4	0.45%
39	Delaware	0	0.00%
11	Florida	18	2.01%
25	Georgia	3	0.34%
15	Hawaii	12	1.34%
33	Idaho	1	0.11%
5	Illinois	56	6.26%
33	Indiana	1	0.11%
20	Iowa	7	0.78%
33	Kansas	1	0.11%
39	Kentucky	0	0.00%
33	Louisiana	1	0.11%
22	Maine	5	0.56%
22	Maryland	5	0.56%
19	Massachusetts	8	0.89%
9	Michigan	26	2.91%
39	Minnesota	0	0.00%
39	Mississippi	0	0.00%
1	Missouri	160	17.88%
39	Montana	0	0.00%
30	Nebraska	2	0.22%
16	Nevada	11	1.23%
33	New Hampshire	1	0.11%
2	New Jersey	156	17.43%
30	New Mexico	2	0.22%
6	New York	42	4.69%
25	North Carolina	3	0.34%
39	North Dakota	0	0.00%
12	Ohio	17	1.90%
39	Oklahoma	0	0.00%
30	Oregon	2	0.22%
17	Pennsylvania	9	1.01%
20	Rhode Island	7	0.78%
39	South Carolina	0	0.00%
39	South Dakota	0	0.00%
8	Tennessee	28	3.13%
12	Texas	17	1.90%
3	Utah	134	14.97%
25	Vermont	3	0.34%
25	Virginia	3	0.34%
39	Washington	0	0.00%
7	West Virginia	36	4.02%
25	Wisconsin	3	0.34%
39	Wyoming	0	0.00%

RANK ORDER

RANK	STATE	CASES	% of USA
1	Missouri	160	17.88%
2	New Jersey	156	17.43%
3	Utah	134	14.97%
4	California	65	7.26%
5	Illinois	56	6.26%
6	New York	42	4.69%
7	West Virginia	36	4.02%
8	Tennessee	28	3.13%
9	Michigan	26	2.91%
10	Colorado	20	2.23%
11	Florida	18	2.01%
12	Ohio	17	1.90%
12	Texas	17	1.90%
14	Alaska	16	1.79%
15	Hawaii	12	1.34%
16	Nevada	11	1.23%
17	Arizona	9	1.01%
17	Pennsylvania	9	1.01%
19	Massachusetts	8	0.89%
20	Iowa	7	0.78%
20	Rhode Island	7	0.78%
22	Maine	5	0.56%
22	Maryland	5	0.56%
24	Connecticut	4	0.45%
25	Georgia	3	0.34%
25	North Carolina	3	0.34%
25	Vermont	3	0.34%
25	Virginia	3	0.34%
25	Wisconsin	3	0.34%
30	Nebraska	2	0.22%
30	New Mexico	2	0.22%
30	Oregon	2	0.22%
33	Arkansas	1	0.11%
33	Idaho	1	0.11%
33	Indiana	1	0.11%
33	Kansas	1	0.11%
33	Louisiana	1	0.11%
33	New Hampshire	1	0.11%
39	Alabama	0	0.00%
39	Delaware	0	0.00%
39	Kentucky	0	0.00%
39	Minnesota	0	0.00%
39	Mississippi	0	0.00%
39	Montana	0	0.00%
39	North Dakota	0	0.00%
39	Oklahoma	0	0.00%
39	South Carolina	0	0.00%
39	South Dakota	0	0.00%
39	Washington	0	0.00%
39	Wyoming	0	0.00%
	District of Columbia	0	0.00%

Source: U.S. Department of Health and Human Services, National Center for Health Statistics
"Morbidity and Mortality Weekly Report" (January 6, 1995, Vol. 43, Nos. 51 & 52)
*Includes indigenous and imported cases.

Measles (Rubeola) Rate in 1994

National Rate = 0.34 Cases Reported per 100,000 Population*

ALPHA ORDER			RANK ORDER		
RANK	**STATE**	**RATE**	**RANK**	**STATE**	**RATE**
39	Alabama	0.00	1	Utah	7.02
3	Alaska	2.64	2	Missouri	3.03
17	Arizona	0.22	3	Alaska	2.64
33	Arkansas	0.04	4	West Virginia	1.98
18	California	0.21	5	New Jersey	1.97
9	Colorado	0.55	6	Hawaii	1.02
22	Connecticut	0.12	7	Nevada	0.75
39	Delaware	0.00	8	Rhode Island	0.70
20	Florida	0.13	9	Colorado	0.55
33	Georgia	0.04	10	Tennessee	0.54
6	Hawaii	1.02	11	Vermont	0.52
26	Idaho	0.09	12	Illinois	0.48
12	Illinois	0.48	13	Maine	0.40
37	Indiana	0.02	14	Michigan	0.27
15	Iowa	0.25	15	Iowa	0.25
33	Kansas	0.04	16	New York	0.23
39	Kentucky	0.00	17	Arizona	0.22
37	Louisiana	0.02	18	California	0.21
13	Maine	0.40	19	Ohio	0.15
25	Maryland	0.10	20	Florida	0.13
20	Massachusetts	0.13	20	Massachusetts	0.13
14	Michigan	0.27	22	Connecticut	0.12
39	Minnesota	0.00	22	Nebraska	0.12
39	Mississippi	0.00	22	New Mexico	0.12
2	Missouri	3.03	25	Maryland	0.10
39	Montana	0.00	26	Idaho	0.09
22	Nebraska	0.12	26	New Hampshire	0.09
7	Nevada	0.75	26	Texas	0.09
26	New Hampshire	0.09	29	Pennsylvania	0.07
5	New Jersey	1.97	30	Oregon	0.06
22	New Mexico	0.12	30	Wisconsin	0.06
16	New York	0.23	32	Virginia	0.05
33	North Carolina	0.04	33	Arkansas	0.04
39	North Dakota	0.00	33	Georgia	0.04
19	Ohio	0.15	33	Kansas	0.04
39	Oklahoma	0.00	33	North Carolina	0.04
30	Oregon	0.06	37	Indiana	0.02
29	Pennsylvania	0.07	37	Louisiana	0.02
8	Rhode Island	0.70	39	Alabama	0.00
39	South Carolina	0.00	39	Delaware	0.00
39	South Dakota	0.00	39	Kentucky	0.00
10	Tennessee	0.54	39	Minnesota	0.00
26	Texas	0.09	39	Mississippi	0.00
1	Utah	7.02	39	Montana	0.00
11	Vermont	0.52	39	North Dakota	0.00
32	Virginia	0.05	39	Oklahoma	0.00
39	Washington	0.00	39	South Carolina	0.00
4	West Virginia	1.98	39	South Dakota	0.00
30	Wisconsin	0.06	39	Washington	0.00
39	Wyoming	0.00	39	Wyoming	0.00
				District of Columbia	0.00

Source: Morgan Quitno Press using data from U.S. Dept of Health & Human Serv's, National Center for Health Statistics
"Morbidity and Mortality Weekly Report" (January 6, 1995, Vol. 43, Nos. 51 & 52)
*Includes indigenous and imported cases.

Mumps Cases Reported in 1994

National Total = 1,322 Cases*

ALPHA ORDER

RANK	STATE	CASES	% of USA
21	Alabama	12	0.91%
35	Alaska	4	0.30%
4	Arizona	95	7.19%
31	Arkansas	5	0.38%
1	California	248	18.76%
38	Colorado	3	0.23%
21	Connecticut	12	0.91%
43	Delaware	0	0.00%
14	Florida	33	2.50%
24	Georgia	9	0.68%
17	Hawaii	19	1.44%
23	Idaho	10	0.76%
3	Illinois	106	8.02%
28	Indiana	7	0.53%
19	Iowa	16	1.21%
43	Kansas	0	0.00%
43	Kentucky	0	0.00%
13	Louisiana	35	2.65%
38	Maine	3	0.23%
6	Maryland	67	5.07%
38	Massachusetts	3	0.23%
7	Michigan	59	4.46%
31	Minnesota	5	0.38%
28	Mississippi	7	0.53%
11	Missouri	41	3.10%
43	Montana	0	0.00%
42	Nebraska	1	0.08%
18	Nevada	18	1.36%
35	New Hampshire	4	0.30%
28	New Jersey	7	0.53%
NA	New Mexico*	NA	NA
9	New York	48	3.63%
12	North Carolina	36	2.72%
31	North Dakota	5	0.38%
5	Ohio	77	5.82%
16	Oklahoma	23	1.74%
NA	Oregon*	NA	NA
8	Pennsylvania	58	4.39%
35	Rhode Island	4	0.30%
26	South Carolina	8	0.61%
43	South Dakota	0	0.00%
26	Tennessee	8	0.61%
2	Texas	121	9.15%
15	Utah	26	1.97%
43	Vermont	0	0.00%
10	Virginia	47	3.56%
24	Washington	9	0.68%
31	West Virginia	5	0.38%
20	Wisconsin	14	1.06%
38	Wyoming	3	0.23%

RANK ORDER

RANK	STATE	CASES	% of USA
1	California	248	18.76%
2	Texas	121	9.15%
3	Illinois	106	8.02%
4	Arizona	95	7.19%
5	Ohio	77	5.82%
6	Maryland	67	5.07%
7	Michigan	59	4.46%
8	Pennsylvania	58	4.39%
9	New York	48	3.63%
10	Virginia	47	3.56%
11	Missouri	41	3.10%
12	North Carolina	36	2.72%
13	Louisiana	35	2.65%
14	Florida	33	2.50%
15	Utah	26	1.97%
16	Oklahoma	23	1.74%
17	Hawaii	19	1.44%
18	Nevada	18	1.36%
19	Iowa	16	1.21%
20	Wisconsin	14	1.06%
21	Alabama	12	0.91%
21	Connecticut	12	0.91%
23	Idaho	10	0.76%
24	Georgia	9	0.68%
24	Washington	9	0.68%
26	South Carolina	8	0.61%
26	Tennessee	8	0.61%
28	Indiana	7	0.53%
28	Mississippi	7	0.53%
28	New Jersey	7	0.53%
31	Arkansas	5	0.38%
31	Minnesota	5	0.38%
31	North Dakota	5	0.38%
31	West Virginia	5	0.38%
35	Alaska	4	0.30%
35	New Hampshire	4	0.30%
35	Rhode Island	4	0.30%
38	Colorado	3	0.23%
38	Maine	3	0.23%
38	Massachusetts	3	0.23%
38	Wyoming	3	0.23%
42	Nebraska	1	0.08%
43	Delaware	0	0.00%
43	Kansas	0	0.00%
43	Kentucky	0	0.00%
43	Montana	0	0.00%
43	South Dakota	0	0.00%
43	Vermont	0	0.00%
NA	New Mexico*	NA	NA
NA	Oregon*	NA	NA
	District of Columbia	0	0.00%

Source: U.S. Department of Health and Human Services, National Center for Health Statistics
"Morbidity and Mortality Weekly Report" (January 6, 1995, Vol. 43, Nos. 51 & 52)
*Mumps is not a notifiable disease in New Mexico and Oregon.

Mumps Rate in 1994

National Rate = 0.51 Cases Reported per 100,000 Population*

ALPHA ORDER			RANK ORDER		
RANK	STATE	RATE	RANK	STATE	RATE
25	Alabama	0.28	1	Arizona	2.33
15	Alaska	0.66	2	Hawaii	1.61
1	Arizona	2.33	3	Utah	1.36
33	Arkansas	0.20	4	Maryland	1.34
9	California	0.79	5	Nevada	1.24
40	Colorado	0.08	6	Illinois	0.90
23	Connecticut	0.37	7	Idaho	0.88
43	Delaware	0.00	8	Louisiana	0.81
30	Florida	0.24	9	California	0.79
36	Georgia	0.13	10	Missouri	0.78
2	Hawaii	1.61	10	North Dakota	0.78
7	Idaho	0.88	12	Virginia	0.72
6	Illinois	0.90	13	Oklahoma	0.71
37	Indiana	0.12	14	Ohio	0.69
19	Iowa	0.57	15	Alaska	0.66
43	Kansas	0.00	15	Texas	0.66
43	Kentucky	0.00	17	Wyoming	0.63
8	Louisiana	0.81	18	Michigan	0.62
30	Maine	0.24	19	Iowa	0.57
4	Maryland	1.34	20	North Carolina	0.51
42	Massachusetts	0.05	21	Pennsylvania	0.48
18	Michigan	0.62	22	Rhode Island	0.40
38	Minnesota	0.11	23	Connecticut	0.37
28	Mississippi	0.26	24	New Hampshire	0.35
10	Missouri	0.78	25	Alabama	0.28
43	Montana	0.00	25	Wisconsin	0.28
41	Nebraska	0.06	27	West Virginia	0.27
5	Nevada	1.24	28	Mississippi	0.26
24	New Hampshire	0.35	28	New York	0.26
39	New Jersey	0.09	30	Florida	0.24
NA	New Mexico*	NA	30	Maine	0.24
28	New York	0.26	32	South Carolina	0.22
20	North Carolina	0.51	33	Arkansas	0.20
10	North Dakota	0.78	34	Washington	0.17
14	Ohio	0.69	35	Tennessee	0.15
13	Oklahoma	0.71	36	Georgia	0.13
NA	Oregon*	NA	37	Indiana	0.12
21	Pennsylvania	0.48	38	Minnesota	0.11
22	Rhode Island	0.40	39	New Jersey	0.09
32	South Carolina	0.22	40	Colorado	0.08
43	South Dakota	0.00	41	Nebraska	0.06
35	Tennessee	0.15	42	Massachusetts	0.05
15	Texas	0.66	43	Delaware	0.00
3	Utah	1.36	43	Kansas	0.00
43	Vermont	0.00	43	Kentucky	0.00
12	Virginia	0.72	43	Montana	0.00
34	Washington	0.17	43	South Dakota	0.00
27	West Virginia	0.27	43	Vermont	0.00
25	Wisconsin	0.28	NA	New Mexico*	NA
17	Wyoming	0.63	NA	Oregon*	NA
				District of Columbia	0.00

Source: Morgan Quitno Press using data from U.S. Dept of Health & Human Serv's, National Center for Health Statistics "Morbidity and Mortality Weekly Report" (January 6, 1995, Vol. 43, Nos. 51 & 52)
*Mumps is not a notifiable disease in New Mexico and Oregon.

Rabies (Animal) Cases Reported in 1994

National Total = 7,347 Cases

ALPHA ORDER

RANK	STATE	CASES	% of USA
17	Alabama	126	1.71%
27	Alaska	30	0.41%
22	Arizona	45	0.61%
30	Arkansas	25	0.34%
10	California	237	3.23%
36	Colorado	15	0.20%
2	Connecticut	744	10.13%
24	Delaware	41	0.56%
12	Florida	188	2.56%
7	Georgia	366	4.98%
46	Hawaii	0	0.00%
45	Idaho	3	0.04%
32	Illinois	19	0.26%
38	Indiana	13	0.18%
18	Iowa	91	1.24%
26	Kansas	35	0.48%
28	Kentucky	26	0.35%
21	Louisiana	69	0.94%
46	Maine	0	0.00%
4	Maryland	520	7.08%
3	Massachusetts	730	9.94%
37	Michigan	14	0.19%
34	Minnesota	17	0.23%
46	Mississippi	0	0.00%
28	Missouri	26	0.35%
31	Montana	22	0.30%
46	Nebraska	0	0.00%
42	Nevada	10	0.14%
11	New Hampshire	212	2.89%
8	New Jersey	275	3.74%
43	New Mexico	8	0.11%
1	New York	1,312	17.86%
13	North Carolina	177	2.41%
40	North Dakota	12	0.16%
44	Ohio	4	0.05%
23	Oklahoma	43	0.59%
40	Oregon	12	0.16%
9	Pennsylvania	252	3.43%
16	Rhode Island	129	1.76%
13	South Carolina	177	2.41%
25	South Dakota	39	0.53%
20	Tennessee	71	0.97%
5	Texas	508	6.91%
38	Utah	13	0.18%
15	Vermont	143	1.95%
6	Virginia	428	5.83%
46	Washington	0	0.00%
19	West Virginia	82	1.12%
35	Wisconsin	16	0.22%
32	Wyoming	19	0.26%

RANK ORDER

RANK	STATE	CASES	% of USA
1	New York	1,312	17.86%
2	Connecticut	744	10.13%
3	Massachusetts	730	9.94%
4	Maryland	520	7.08%
5	Texas	508	6.91%
6	Virginia	428	5.83%
7	Georgia	366	4.98%
8	New Jersey	275	3.74%
9	Pennsylvania	252	3.43%
10	California	237	3.23%
11	New Hampshire	212	2.89%
12	Florida	188	2.56%
13	North Carolina	177	2.41%
13	South Carolina	177	2.41%
15	Vermont	143	1.95%
16	Rhode Island	129	1.76%
17	Alabama	126	1.71%
18	Iowa	91	1.24%
19	West Virginia	82	1.12%
20	Tennessee	71	0.97%
21	Louisiana	69	0.94%
22	Arizona	45	0.61%
23	Oklahoma	43	0.59%
24	Delaware	41	0.56%
25	South Dakota	39	0.53%
26	Kansas	35	0.48%
27	Alaska	30	0.41%
28	Kentucky	26	0.35%
28	Missouri	26	0.35%
30	Arkansas	25	0.34%
31	Montana	22	0.30%
32	Illinois	19	0.26%
32	Wyoming	19	0.26%
34	Minnesota	17	0.23%
35	Wisconsin	16	0.22%
36	Colorado	15	0.20%
37	Michigan	14	0.19%
38	Indiana	13	0.18%
38	Utah	13	0.18%
40	North Dakota	12	0.16%
40	Oregon	12	0.16%
42	Nevada	10	0.14%
43	New Mexico	8	0.11%
44	Ohio	4	0.05%
45	Idaho	3	0.04%
46	Hawaii	0	0.00%
46	Maine	0	0.00%
46	Mississippi	0	0.00%
46	Nebraska	0	0.00%
46	Washington	0	0.00%
	District of Columbia	3	0.04%

Source: U.S. Department of Health and Human Services, National Center for Health Statistics
"Morbidity and Mortality Weekly Report" (January 6, 1995, Vol. 43, Nos. 51 & 52)

Rabies (Animal) Rate in 1994

National Rate = 2.82 Cases Reported per 100,000 Human Population

ALPHA ORDER

RANK	STATE	RATE
18	Alabama	2.99
12	Alaska	4.95
29	Arizona	1.10
30	Arkansas	1.02
31	California	0.75
37	Colorado	0.41
2	Connecticut	22.72
9	Delaware	5.81
27	Florida	1.35
11	Georgia	5.19
46	Hawaii	0.00
41	Idaho	0.26
43	Illinois	0.16
42	Indiana	0.23
17	Iowa	3.22
25	Kansas	1.37
33	Kentucky	0.68
24	Louisiana	1.60
46	Maine	0.00
6	Maryland	10.39
5	Massachusetts	12.08
44	Michigan	0.15
39	Minnesota	0.37
46	Mississippi	0.00
35	Missouri	0.49
20	Montana	2.57
46	Nebraska	0.00
32	Nevada	0.69
3	New Hampshire	18.65
16	New Jersey	3.48
36	New Mexico	0.48
7	New York	7.22
21	North Carolina	2.50
23	North Dakota	1.88
45	Ohio	0.04
28	Oklahoma	1.32
38	Oregon	0.39
22	Pennsylvania	2.09
4	Rhode Island	12.94
13	South Carolina	4.83
10	South Dakota	5.41
25	Tennessee	1.37
19	Texas	2.76
33	Utah	0.68
1	Vermont	24.66
8	Virginia	6.53
46	Washington	0.00
14	West Virginia	4.50
40	Wisconsin	0.31
15	Wyoming	3.99

RANK ORDER

RANK	STATE	RATE
1	Vermont	24.66
2	Connecticut	22.72
3	New Hampshire	18.65
4	Rhode Island	12.94
5	Massachusetts	12.08
6	Maryland	10.39
7	New York	7.22
8	Virginia	6.53
9	Delaware	5.81
10	South Dakota	5.41
11	Georgia	5.19
12	Alaska	4.95
13	South Carolina	4.83
14	West Virginia	4.50
15	Wyoming	3.99
16	New Jersey	3.48
17	Iowa	3.22
18	Alabama	2.99
19	Texas	2.76
20	Montana	2.57
21	North Carolina	2.50
22	Pennsylvania	2.09
23	North Dakota	1.88
24	Louisiana	1.60
25	Kansas	1.37
25	Tennessee	1.37
27	Florida	1.35
28	Oklahoma	1.32
29	Arizona	1.10
30	Arkansas	1.02
31	California	0.75
32	Nevada	0.69
33	Kentucky	0.68
33	Utah	0.68
35	Missouri	0.49
36	New Mexico	0.48
37	Colorado	0.41
38	Oregon	0.39
39	Minnesota	0.37
40	Wisconsin	0.31
41	Idaho	0.26
42	Indiana	0.23
43	Illinois	0.16
44	Michigan	0.15
45	Ohio	0.04
46	Hawaii	0.00
46	Maine	0.00
46	Mississippi	0.00
46	Nebraska	0.00
46	Washington	0.00

District of Columbia 0.53

Source: Morgan Quitno Press using data from U.S. Dept of Health & Human Serv's, National Center for Health Statistics "Morbidity and Mortality Weekly Report" (January 6, 1995, Vol. 43, Nos. 51 & 52)

Salmonellosis Cases Reported in 1993

National Total = 41,641 Cases*

<u>ALPHA ORDER</u>

RANK	STATE	CASES	% of USA
21	Alabama	554	1.33%
49	Alaska	59	0.14%
26	Arizona	519	1.25%
29	Arkansas	402	0.97%
1	California	5,739	13.78%
23	Colorado	550	1.32%
17	Connecticut	811	1.95%
39	Delaware	185	0.44%
3	Florida	2,940	7.06%
8	Georgia	1,316	3.16%
31	Hawaii	345	0.83%
40	Idaho	173	0.42%
4	Illinois	2,232	5.36%
24	Indiana	543	1.30%
36	Iowa	241	0.58%
35	Kansas	299	0.72%
34	Kentucky	302	0.73%
19	Louisiana	650	1.56%
41	Maine	158	0.38%
14	Maryland	936	2.25%
5	Massachusetts	2,041	4.90%
16	Michigan	815	1.96%
22	Minnesota	551	1.32%
27	Mississippi	465	1.12%
25	Missouri	529	1.27%
46	Montana	106	0.25%
43	Nebraska	145	0.35%
44	Nevada	131	0.31%
38	New Hampshire	220	0.53%
9	New Jersey	1,215	2.92%
32	New Mexico	326	0.78%
2	New York	3,991	9.58%
11	North Carolina	1,121	2.69%
48	North Dakota	60	0.14%
10	Ohio	1,214	2.92%
33	Oklahoma	321	0.77%
30	Oregon	349	0.84%
7	Pennsylvania	1,799	4.32%
37	Rhode Island	231	0.55%
18	South Carolina	738	1.77%
47	South Dakota	99	0.24%
20	Tennessee	558	1.34%
6	Texas	1,924	4.62%
42	Utah	154	0.37%
28	Vermont	421	1.01%
12	Virginia	1,055	2.53%
15	Washington	832	2.00%
45	West Virginia	109	0.26%
13	Wisconsin	1,006	2.42%
49	Wyoming	59	0.14%

<u>RANK ORDER</u>

RANK	STATE	CASES	% of USA
1	California	5,739	13.78%
2	New York	3,991	9.58%
3	Florida	2,940	7.06%
4	Illinois	2,232	5.36%
5	Massachusetts	2,041	4.90%
6	Texas	1,924	4.62%
7	Pennsylvania	1,799	4.32%
8	Georgia	1,316	3.16%
9	New Jersey	1,215	2.92%
10	Ohio	1,214	2.92%
11	North Carolina	1,121	2.69%
12	Virginia	1,055	2.53%
13	Wisconsin	1,006	2.42%
14	Maryland	936	2.25%
15	Washington	832	2.00%
16	Michigan	815	1.96%
17	Connecticut	811	1.95%
18	South Carolina	738	1.77%
19	Louisiana	650	1.56%
20	Tennessee	558	1.34%
21	Alabama	554	1.33%
22	Minnesota	551	1.32%
23	Colorado	550	1.32%
24	Indiana	543	1.30%
25	Missouri	529	1.27%
26	Arizona	519	1.25%
27	Mississippi	465	1.12%
28	Vermont	421	1.01%
29	Arkansas	402	0.97%
30	Oregon	349	0.84%
31	Hawaii	345	0.83%
32	New Mexico	326	0.78%
33	Oklahoma	321	0.77%
34	Kentucky	302	0.73%
35	Kansas	299	0.72%
36	Iowa	241	0.58%
37	Rhode Island	231	0.55%
38	New Hampshire	220	0.53%
39	Delaware	185	0.44%
40	Idaho	173	0.42%
41	Maine	158	0.38%
42	Utah	154	0.37%
43	Nebraska	145	0.35%
44	Nevada	131	0.31%
45	West Virginia	109	0.26%
46	Montana	106	0.25%
47	South Dakota	99	0.24%
48	North Dakota	60	0.14%
49	Alaska	59	0.14%
49	Wyoming	59	0.14%
	District of Columbia	102	0.24%

Source: U.S. Department of Health and Human Services, National Center for Health Statistics
"Morbidity and Mortality Weekly Report" (October 21, 1994, Vol. 42, No. 53)
Any disease caused by a salmonellal infection, which may be manifested as food poisoning with acute gastroenteritis, vomiting and diarrhea.

Salmonellosis Rate in 1993

National Rate = 16.15 Cases Reported per 100,000 Population*

ALPHA ORDER			RANK ORDER		
RANK	**STATE**	**RATE**	**RANK**	**STATE**	**RATE**
28	Alabama	13.25	1	Vermont	73.09
41	Alaska	9.87	2	Massachusetts	33.91
29	Arizona	13.16	3	Hawaii	29.59
18	Arkansas	16.57	4	Delaware	26.50
16	California	18.38	5	Connecticut	24.74
24	Colorado	15.43	6	Rhode Island	23.10
5	Connecticut	24.74	7	New York	21.99
4	Delaware	26.50	8	Florida	21.42
8	Florida	21.42	9	South Carolina	20.33
14	Georgia	19.07	10	New Mexico	20.17
3	Hawaii	29.59	11	Wisconsin	19.94
22	Idaho	15.73	12	New Hampshire	19.57
13	Illinois	19.10	13	Illinois	19.10
42	Indiana	9.52	14	Georgia	19.07
47	Iowa	8.54	15	Maryland	18.88
34	Kansas	11.79	16	California	18.38
49	Kentucky	7.96	17	Mississippi	17.61
25	Louisiana	15.15	18	Arkansas	16.57
30	Maine	12.74	19	Virginia	16.30
15	Maryland	18.88	20	North Carolina	16.12
2	Massachusetts	33.91	21	Washington	15.82
46	Michigan	8.62	22	Idaho	15.73
33	Minnesota	12.18	23	New Jersey	15.46
17	Mississippi	17.61	24	Colorado	15.43
39	Missouri	10.11	25	Louisiana	15.15
31	Montana	12.60	26	Pennsylvania	14.95
45	Nebraska	8.99	27	South Dakota	13.83
43	Nevada	9.48	28	Alabama	13.25
12	New Hampshire	19.57	29	Arizona	13.16
23	New Jersey	15.46	30	Maine	12.74
10	New Mexico	20.17	31	Montana	12.60
7	New York	21.99	32	Wyoming	12.55
20	North Carolina	16.12	33	Minnesota	12.18
44	North Dakota	9.42	34	Kansas	11.79
36	Ohio	10.98	35	Oregon	11.50
40	Oklahoma	9.93	36	Ohio	10.98
35	Oregon	11.50	37	Tennessee	10.95
26	Pennsylvania	14.95	38	Texas	10.68
6	Rhode Island	23.10	39	Missouri	10.11
9	South Carolina	20.33	40	Oklahoma	9.93
27	South Dakota	13.83	41	Alaska	9.87
37	Tennessee	10.95	42	Indiana	9.52
38	Texas	10.68	43	Nevada	9.48
48	Utah	8.28	44	North Dakota	9.42
1	Vermont	73.09	45	Nebraska	8.99
19	Virginia	16.30	46	Michigan	8.62
21	Washington	15.82	47	Iowa	8.54
50	West Virginia	6.00	48	Utah	8.28
11	Wisconsin	19.94	49	Kentucky	7.96
32	Wyoming	12.55	50	West Virginia	6.00
				District of Columbia	17.62

Source: Morgan Quitno Press using data from U.S. Dept of Health & Human Serv's, National Center for Health Statistics "Morbidity and Mortality Weekly Report" (October 21, 1994, Vol. 42, No. 53)
Any disease caused by a salmonellal infection, which may be manifested as food poisoning with acute gastroenteritis, vomiting and diarrhea.

Shigellosis Cases Reported in 1993

National Total = 32,198 Cases*

<u>ALPHA ORDER</u>

RANK	STATE	CASES	% of USA
23	Alabama	375	1.16%
45	Alaska	30	0.09%
13	Arizona	693	2.15%
31	Arkansas	201	0.62%
1	California	5,093	15.82%
15	Colorado	611	1.90%
28	Connecticut	245	0.76%
33	Delaware	178	0.55%
3	Florida	2,393	7.43%
19	Georgia	474	1.47%
37	Hawaii	99	0.31%
40	Idaho	46	0.14%
5	Illinois	1,722	5.35%
10	Indiana	811	2.52%
38	Iowa	69	0.21%
30	Kansas	208	0.65%
34	Kentucky	171	0.53%
18	Louisiana	482	1.50%
48	Maine	8	0.02%
22	Maryland	384	1.19%
27	Massachusetts	285	0.89%
9	Michigan	829	2.57%
29	Minnesota	240	0.75%
24	Mississippi	365	1.13%
14	Missouri	674	2.09%
39	Montana	56	0.17%
32	Nebraska	200	0.62%
43	Nevada	40	0.12%
47	New Hampshire	17	0.05%
25	New Jersey	347	1.08%
21	New Mexico	411	1.28%
7	New York	1,344	4.17%
4	North Carolina	2,305	7.16%
50	North Dakota	7	0.02%
6	Ohio	1,411	4.38%
17	Oklahoma	484	1.50%
35	Oregon	169	0.52%
16	Pennsylvania	527	1.64%
41	Rhode Island	42	0.13%
20	South Carolina	414	1.29%
36	South Dakota	111	0.34%
8	Tennessee	938	2.91%
2	Texas	4,581	14.23%
41	Utah	42	0.13%
48	Vermont	8	0.02%
12	Virginia	776	2.41%
11	Washington	797	2.48%
44	West Virginia	38	0.12%
26	Wisconsin	338	1.05%
46	Wyoming	22	0.07%

<u>RANK ORDER</u>

RANK	STATE	CASES	% of USA
1	California	5,093	15.82%
2	Texas	4,581	14.23%
3	Florida	2,393	7.43%
4	North Carolina	2,305	7.16%
5	Illinois	1,722	5.35%
6	Ohio	1,411	4.38%
7	New York	1,344	4.17%
8	Tennessee	938	2.91%
9	Michigan	829	2.57%
10	Indiana	811	2.52%
11	Washington	797	2.48%
12	Virginia	776	2.41%
13	Arizona	693	2.15%
14	Missouri	674	2.09%
15	Colorado	611	1.90%
16	Pennsylvania	527	1.64%
17	Oklahoma	484	1.50%
18	Louisiana	482	1.50%
19	Georgia	474	1.47%
20	South Carolina	414	1.29%
21	New Mexico	411	1.28%
22	Maryland	384	1.19%
23	Alabama	375	1.16%
24	Mississippi	365	1.13%
25	New Jersey	347	1.08%
26	Wisconsin	338	1.05%
27	Massachusetts	285	0.89%
28	Connecticut	245	0.76%
29	Minnesota	240	0.75%
30	Kansas	208	0.65%
31	Arkansas	201	0.62%
32	Nebraska	200	0.62%
33	Delaware	178	0.55%
34	Kentucky	171	0.53%
35	Oregon	169	0.52%
36	South Dakota	111	0.34%
37	Hawaii	99	0.31%
38	Iowa	69	0.21%
39	Montana	56	0.17%
40	Idaho	46	0.14%
41	Rhode Island	42	0.13%
41	Utah	42	0.13%
43	Nevada	40	0.12%
44	West Virginia	38	0.12%
45	Alaska	30	0.09%
46	Wyoming	22	0.07%
47	New Hampshire	17	0.05%
48	Maine	8	0.02%
48	Vermont	8	0.02%
50	North Dakota	7	0.02%
	District of Columbia	87	0.27%

Source: U.S. Department of Health and Human Services, National Center for Health Statistics
"Morbidity and Mortality Weekly Report" (October 21, 1994, Vol. 42, No. 53)
*Produced by infection with Shigella organisms. These cause dysentery.

Shigellosis Rate in 1993

National Rate = 12.49 Cases Reported per 100,000 Population*

ALPHA ORDER				RANK ORDER		
RANK	STATE	RATE		RANK	STATE	RATE
22	Alabama	8.97		1	North Carolina	33.16
35	Alaska	5.02		2	Delaware	25.50
6	Arizona	17.57		3	New Mexico	25.43
25	Arkansas	8.29		4	Texas	25.42
9	California	16.31		5	Tennessee	18.41
8	Colorado	17.14		6	Arizona	17.57
28	Connecticut	7.47		7	Florida	17.43
2	Delaware	25.50		8	Colorado	17.14
7	Florida	17.43		9	California	16.31
30	Georgia	6.87		10	South Dakota	15.50
24	Hawaii	8.49		11	Washington	15.15
42	Idaho	4.18		12	Oklahoma	14.97
13	Illinois	14.74		13	Illinois	14.74
14	Indiana	14.21		14	Indiana	14.21
44	Iowa	2.45		15	Mississippi	13.83
26	Kansas	8.21		16	Missouri	12.87
38	Kentucky	4.51		17	Ohio	12.76
21	Louisiana	11.24		18	Nebraska	12.40
50	Maine	0.65		19	Virginia	11.99
27	Maryland	7.75		20	South Carolina	11.40
36	Massachusetts	4.74		21	Louisiana	11.24
23	Michigan	8.76		22	Alabama	8.97
34	Minnesota	5.31		23	Michigan	8.76
15	Mississippi	13.83		24	Hawaii	8.49
16	Missouri	12.87		25	Arkansas	8.29
32	Montana	6.66		26	Kansas	8.21
18	Nebraska	12.40		27	Maryland	7.75
43	Nevada	2.89		28	Connecticut	7.47
47	New Hampshire	1.51		29	New York	7.40
39	New Jersey	4.42		30	Georgia	6.87
3	New Mexico	25.43		31	Wisconsin	6.70
29	New York	7.40		32	Montana	6.66
1	North Carolina	33.16		33	Oregon	5.57
49	North Dakota	1.10		34	Minnesota	5.31
17	Ohio	12.76		35	Alaska	5.02
12	Oklahoma	14.97		36	Massachusetts	4.74
33	Oregon	5.57		37	Wyoming	4.68
40	Pennsylvania	4.38		38	Kentucky	4.51
41	Rhode Island	4.20		39	New Jersey	4.42
20	South Carolina	11.40		40	Pennsylvania	4.38
10	South Dakota	15.50		41	Rhode Island	4.20
5	Tennessee	18.41		42	Idaho	4.18
4	Texas	25.42		43	Nevada	2.89
45	Utah	2.26		44	Iowa	2.45
48	Vermont	1.39		45	Utah	2.26
19	Virginia	11.99		46	West Virginia	2.09
11	Washington	15.15		47	New Hampshire	1.51
46	West Virginia	2.09		48	Vermont	1.39
31	Wisconsin	6.70		49	North Dakota	1.10
37	Wyoming	4.68		50	Maine	0.65
					District of Columbia	15.03

Source: Morgan Quitno Press using data from U.S. Dept of Health & Human Serv's, National Center for Health Statistics "Morbidity and Mortality Weekly Report" (October 21, 1994, Vol. 42, No. 53)
*Produced by infection with Shigella organisms. These cause dysentery.

Syphilis Cases Reported in 1994

National Total = 20,183 Cases*

ALPHA ORDER

RANK	STATE	CASES	% of USA
15	Alabama	631	3.13%
41	Alaska	4	0.02%
31	Arizona	50	0.25%
16	Arkansas	465	2.30%
14	California	641	3.18%
24	Colorado	129	0.64%
26	Connecticut	101	0.50%
34	Delaware	27	0.13%
13	Florida	745	3.69%
10	Georgia	808	4.00%
45	Hawaii	3	0.01%
47	Idaho	2	0.01%
8	Illinois	845	4.19%
21	Indiana	259	1.28%
28	Iowa	71	0.35%
30	Kansas	52	0.26%
23	Kentucky	216	1.07%
3	Louisiana	1,653	8.19%
41	Maine	4	0.02%
18	Maryland	334	1.65%
27	Massachusetts	90	0.45%
20	Michigan	291	1.44%
29	Minnesota	55	0.27%
2	Mississippi	2,032	10.07%
7	Missouri	980	4.86%
41	Montana	4	0.02%
38	Nebraska	11	0.05%
33	Nevada	31	0.15%
41	New Hampshire	4	0.02%
22	New Jersey	234	1.16%
35	New Mexico	21	0.10%
12	New York	752	3.73%
4	North Carolina	1,640	8.13%
49	North Dakota	0	0.00%
5	Ohio	1,157	5.73%
25	Oklahoma	111	0.55%
35	Oregon	21	0.10%
17	Pennsylvania	404	2.00%
37	Rhode Island	16	0.08%
11	South Carolina	804	3.98%
48	South Dakota	1	0.00%
6	Tennessee	1,018	5.04%
1	Texas	2,074	10.28%
39	Utah	9	0.04%
49	Vermont	0	0.00%
9	Virginia	816	4.04%
32	Washington	35	0.17%
39	West Virginia	9	0.04%
19	Wisconsin	306	1.52%
45	Wyoming	3	0.01%

RANK ORDER

RANK	STATE	CASES	% of USA
1	Texas	2,074	10.28%
2	Mississippi	2,032	10.07%
3	Louisiana	1,653	8.19%
4	North Carolina	1,640	8.13%
5	Ohio	1,157	5.73%
6	Tennessee	1,018	5.04%
7	Missouri	980	4.86%
8	Illinois	845	4.19%
9	Virginia	816	4.04%
10	Georgia	808	4.00%
11	South Carolina	804	3.98%
12	New York	752	3.73%
13	Florida	745	3.69%
14	California	641	3.18%
15	Alabama	631	3.13%
16	Arkansas	465	2.30%
17	Pennsylvania	404	2.00%
18	Maryland	334	1.65%
19	Wisconsin	306	1.52%
20	Michigan	291	1.44%
21	Indiana	259	1.28%
22	New Jersey	234	1.16%
23	Kentucky	216	1.07%
24	Colorado	129	0.64%
25	Oklahoma	111	0.55%
26	Connecticut	101	0.50%
27	Massachusetts	90	0.45%
28	Iowa	71	0.35%
29	Minnesota	55	0.27%
30	Kansas	52	0.26%
31	Arizona	50	0.25%
32	Washington	35	0.17%
33	Nevada	31	0.15%
34	Delaware	27	0.13%
35	New Mexico	21	0.10%
35	Oregon	21	0.10%
37	Rhode Island	16	0.08%
38	Nebraska	11	0.05%
39	Utah	9	0.04%
39	West Virginia	9	0.04%
41	Alaska	4	0.02%
41	Maine	4	0.02%
41	Montana	4	0.02%
41	New Hampshire	4	0.02%
45	Hawaii	3	0.01%
45	Wyoming	3	0.01%
47	Idaho	2	0.01%
48	South Dakota	1	0.00%
49	North Dakota	0	0.00%
49	Vermont	0	0.00%
	District of Columbia	214	1.06%

Source: U.S. Department of Health and Human Services, National Center for Health Statistics
   "Morbidity and Mortality Weekly Report" (January 6, 1995, Vol. 43, Nos. 51 & 52)
*Includes primary and secondary cases.

Syphilis Rate in 1994

National Rate = 7.75 Cases Reported per 100,000 Population*

ALPHA ORDER			RANK ORDER		
RANK	STATE	RATE	RANK	STATE	RATE
8	Alabama	14.96	1	Mississippi	76.13
38	Alaska	0.66	2	Louisiana	38.31
34	Arizona	1.23	3	North Carolina	23.20
6	Arkansas	18.96	4	South Carolina	21.94
29	California	2.04	5	Tennessee	19.67
21	Colorado	3.53	6	Arkansas	18.96
24	Connecticut	3.08	7	Missouri	18.57
20	Delaware	3.82	8	Alabama	14.96
17	Florida	5.34	9	Virginia	12.45
10	Georgia	11.45	10	Georgia	11.45
46	Hawaii	0.25	11	Texas	11.29
47	Idaho	0.18	12	Ohio	10.42
13	Illinois	7.19	13	Illinois	7.19
18	Indiana	4.50	14	Maryland	6.67
27	Iowa	2.51	15	Wisconsin	6.02
29	Kansas	2.04	16	Kentucky	5.64
16	Kentucky	5.64	17	Florida	5.34
2	Louisiana	38.31	18	Indiana	4.50
45	Maine	0.32	19	New York	4.14
14	Maryland	6.67	20	Delaware	3.82
32	Massachusetts	1.49	21	Colorado	3.53
25	Michigan	3.06	22	Oklahoma	3.41
35	Minnesota	1.20	23	Pennsylvania	3.35
1	Mississippi	76.13	24	Connecticut	3.08
7	Missouri	18.57	25	Michigan	3.06
42	Montana	0.47	26	New Jersey	2.96
36	Nebraska	0.68	27	Iowa	2.51
28	Nevada	2.13	28	Nevada	2.13
44	New Hampshire	0.35	29	California	2.04
26	New Jersey	2.96	29	Kansas	2.04
33	New Mexico	1.27	31	Rhode Island	1.60
19	New York	4.14	32	Massachusetts	1.49
3	North Carolina	23.20	33	New Mexico	1.27
49	North Dakota	0.00	34	Arizona	1.23
12	Ohio	10.42	35	Minnesota	1.20
22	Oklahoma	3.41	36	Nebraska	0.68
36	Oregon	0.68	36	Oregon	0.68
23	Pennsylvania	3.35	38	Alaska	0.66
31	Rhode Island	1.60	38	Washington	0.66
4	South Carolina	21.94	40	Wyoming	0.63
48	South Dakota	0.14	41	West Virginia	0.49
5	Tennessee	19.67	42	Montana	0.47
11	Texas	11.29	42	Utah	0.47
42	Utah	0.47	44	New Hampshire	0.35
49	Vermont	0.00	45	Maine	0.32
9	Virginia	12.45	46	Hawaii	0.25
38	Washington	0.66	47	Idaho	0.18
41	West Virginia	0.49	48	South Dakota	0.14
15	Wisconsin	6.02	49	North Dakota	0.00
40	Wyoming	0.63	49	Vermont	0.00
				District of Columbia	37.54

Source: Morgan Quitno Press using data from U.S. Dept of Health & Human Serv's, National Center for Health Statistics "Morbidity and Mortality Weekly Report" (January 6, 1995, Vol. 43, Nos. 51 & 52)
*Includes primary and secondary cases.

Toxic Shock Syndrome Cases Reported in 1994

National Total = 183 Cases

<u>ALPHA ORDER</u>

RANK	STATE	CASES	% of USA
23	Alabama	1	0.55%
31	Alaska	0	0.00%
17	Arizona	2	1.09%
31	Arkansas	0	0.00%
1	California	48	26.23%
9	Colorado	6	3.28%
31	Connecticut	0	0.00%
31	Delaware	0	0.00%
10	Florida	5	2.73%
23	Georgia	1	0.55%
12	Hawaii	4	2.19%
14	Idaho	3	1.64%
5	Illinois	12	6.56%
17	Indiana	2	1.09%
7	Iowa	8	4.37%
10	Kansas	5	2.73%
17	Kentucky	2	1.09%
31	Louisiana	0	0.00%
23	Maine	1	0.55%
31	Maryland	0	0.00%
17	Massachusetts	2	1.09%
2	Michigan	15	8.20%
23	Minnesota	1	0.55%
31	Mississippi	0	0.00%
8	Missouri	7	3.83%
31	Montana	0	0.00%
12	Nebraska	4	2.19%
31	Nevada	0	0.00%
31	New Hampshire	0	0.00%
31	New Jersey	0	0.00%
31	New Mexico	0	0.00%
2	New York	15	8.20%
23	North Carolina	1	0.55%
23	North Dakota	1	0.55%
6	Ohio	11	6.01%
17	Oklahoma	2	1.09%
31	Oregon	0	0.00%
4	Pennsylvania	14	7.65%
31	Rhode Island	0	0.00%
31	South Carolina	0	0.00%
31	South Dakota	0	0.00%
14	Tennessee	3	1.64%
31	Texas	0	0.00%
17	Utah	2	1.09%
23	Vermont	1	0.55%
23	Virginia	1	0.55%
14	Washington	3	1.64%
31	West Virginia	0	0.00%
31	Wisconsin	0	0.00%
31	Wyoming	0	0.00%

<u>RANK ORDER</u>

RANK	STATE	CASES	% of USA
1	California	48	26.23%
2	Michigan	15	8.20%
2	New York	15	8.20%
4	Pennsylvania	14	7.65%
5	Illinois	12	6.56%
6	Ohio	11	6.01%
7	Iowa	8	4.37%
8	Missouri	7	3.83%
9	Colorado	6	3.28%
10	Florida	5	2.73%
10	Kansas	5	2.73%
12	Hawaii	4	2.19%
12	Nebraska	4	2.19%
14	Idaho	3	1.64%
14	Tennessee	3	1.64%
14	Washington	3	1.64%
17	Arizona	2	1.09%
17	Indiana	2	1.09%
17	Kentucky	2	1.09%
17	Massachusetts	2	1.09%
17	Oklahoma	2	1.09%
17	Utah	2	1.09%
23	Alabama	1	0.55%
23	Georgia	1	0.55%
23	Maine	1	0.55%
23	Minnesota	1	0.55%
23	North Carolina	1	0.55%
23	North Dakota	1	0.55%
23	Vermont	1	0.55%
23	Virginia	1	0.55%
31	Alaska	0	0.00%
31	Arkansas	0	0.00%
31	Connecticut	0	0.00%
31	Delaware	0	0.00%
31	Louisiana	0	0.00%
31	Maryland	0	0.00%
31	Mississippi	0	0.00%
31	Montana	0	0.00%
31	Nevada	0	0.00%
31	New Hampshire	0	0.00%
31	New Jersey	0	0.00%
31	New Mexico	0	0.00%
31	Oregon	0	0.00%
31	Rhode Island	0	0.00%
31	South Carolina	0	0.00%
31	South Dakota	0	0.00%
31	Texas	0	0.00%
31	West Virginia	0	0.00%
31	Wisconsin	0	0.00%
31	Wyoming	0	0.00%
	District of Columbia	0	0.00%

Source: U.S. Department of Health and Human Services, National Center for Health Statistics
"Morbidity and Mortality Weekly Report" (January 6, 1995, Vol. 43, Nos. 51 & 52)

Toxic Shock Syndrome Rate in 1994

National Rate = 0.07 Cases Reported per 100,000 Population

ALPHA ORDER

RANK ORDER

RANK	STATE	RATE	RANK	STATE	RATE
26	Alabama	0.02	1	Hawaii	0.34
31	Alaska	0.00	2	Iowa	0.28
21	Arizona	0.05	3	Idaho	0.26
31	Arkansas	0.00	4	Nebraska	0.25
10	California	0.15	5	Kansas	0.20
7	Colorado	0.16	6	Vermont	0.17
31	Connecticut	0.00	7	Colorado	0.16
31	Delaware	0.00	7	Michigan	0.16
23	Florida	0.04	7	North Dakota	0.16
29	Georgia	0.01	10	California	0.15
1	Hawaii	0.34	11	Missouri	0.13
3	Idaho	0.26	12	Pennsylvania	0.12
13	Illinois	0.10	13	Illinois	0.10
24	Indiana	0.03	13	Ohio	0.10
2	Iowa	0.28	13	Utah	0.10
5	Kansas	0.20	16	Maine	0.08
21	Kentucky	0.05	16	New York	0.08
31	Louisiana	0.00	18	Oklahoma	0.06
16	Maine	0.08	18	Tennessee	0.06
31	Maryland	0.00	18	Washington	0.06
24	Massachusetts	0.03	21	Arizona	0.05
7	Michigan	0.16	21	Kentucky	0.05
26	Minnesota	0.02	23	Florida	0.04
31	Mississippi	0.00	24	Indiana	0.03
11	Missouri	0.13	24	Massachusetts	0.03
31	Montana	0.00	26	Alabama	0.02
4	Nebraska	0.25	26	Minnesota	0.02
31	Nevada	0.00	26	Virginia	0.02
31	New Hampshire	0.00	29	Georgia	0.01
31	New Jersey	0.00	29	North Carolina	0.01
31	New Mexico	0.00	31	Alaska	0.00
16	New York	0.08	31	Arkansas	0.00
29	North Carolina	0.01	31	Connecticut	0.00
7	North Dakota	0.16	31	Delaware	0.00
13	Ohio	0.10	31	Louisiana	0.00
18	Oklahoma	0.06	31	Maryland	0.00
31	Oregon	0.00	31	Mississippi	0.00
12	Pennsylvania	0.12	31	Montana	0.00
31	Rhode Island	0.00	31	Nevada	0.00
31	South Carolina	0.00	31	New Hampshire	0.00
31	South Dakota	0.00	31	New Jersey	0.00
18	Tennessee	0.06	31	New Mexico	0.00
31	Texas	0.00	31	Oregon	0.00
13	Utah	0.10	31	Rhode Island	0.00
6	Vermont	0.17	31	South Carolina	0.00
26	Virginia	0.02	31	South Dakota	0.00
18	Washington	0.06	31	Texas	0.00
31	West Virginia	0.00	31	West Virginia	0.00
31	Wisconsin	0.00	31	Wisconsin	0.00
31	Wyoming	0.00	31	Wyoming	0.00
				District of Columbia	0.00

Source: Morgan Quitno Press using data from U.S. Dept of Health & Human Serv's, National Center for Health Statistics "Morbidity and Mortality Weekly Report" (January 6, 1995, Vol. 43, Nos. 51 & 52)

Tuberculosis Cases Reported in 1994

National Total = 22,152 Cases*

ALPHA ORDER

RANK	STATE	CASES	% of USA
11	Alabama	433	1.95%
37	Alaska	63	0.28%
22	Arizona	257	1.16%
21	Arkansas	258	1.16%
1	California	4,744	21.42%
44	Colorado	21	0.09%
28	Connecticut	142	0.64%
40	Delaware	40	0.18%
4	Florida	1,505	6.79%
7	Georgia	672	3.03%
23	Hawaii	253	1.14%
47	Idaho	13	0.06%
5	Illinois	1,108	5.00%
26	Indiana	193	0.87%
36	Iowa	66	0.30%
32	Kansas	83	0.37%
16	Kentucky	332	1.50%
26	Louisiana	193	0.87%
41	Maine	34	0.15%
14	Maryland	348	1.57%
18	Massachusetts	272	1.23%
10	Michigan	447	2.02%
30	Minnesota	130	0.59%
25	Mississippi	226	1.02%
24	Missouri	245	1.11%
43	Montana	24	0.11%
45	Nebraska	19	0.09%
29	Nevada	140	0.63%
46	New Hampshire	16	0.07%
6	New Jersey	820	3.70%
34	New Mexico	78	0.35%
2	New York	3,037	13.71%
9	North Carolina	567	2.56%
50	North Dakota	8	0.04%
15	Ohio	345	1.56%
20	Oklahoma	264	1.19%
31	Oregon	90	0.41%
8	Pennsylvania	612	2.76%
39	Rhode Island	54	0.24%
13	South Carolina	377	1.70%
42	South Dakota	27	0.12%
12	Tennessee	401	1.81%
3	Texas	2,299	10.38%
38	Utah	55	0.25%
49	Vermont	10	0.05%
17	Virginia	292	1.32%
19	Washington	266	1.20%
33	West Virginia	79	0.36%
35	Wisconsin	70	0.32%
48	Wyoming	12	0.05%

RANK ORDER

RANK	STATE	CASES	% of USA
1	California	4,744	21.42%
2	New York	3,037	13.71%
3	Texas	2,299	10.38%
4	Florida	1,505	6.79%
5	Illinois	1,108	5.00%
6	New Jersey	820	3.70%
7	Georgia	672	3.03%
8	Pennsylvania	612	2.76%
9	North Carolina	567	2.56%
10	Michigan	447	2.02%
11	Alabama	433	1.95%
12	Tennessee	401	1.81%
13	South Carolina	377	1.70%
14	Maryland	348	1.57%
15	Ohio	345	1.56%
16	Kentucky	332	1.50%
17	Virginia	292	1.32%
18	Massachusetts	272	1.23%
19	Washington	266	1.20%
20	Oklahoma	264	1.19%
21	Arkansas	258	1.16%
22	Arizona	257	1.16%
23	Hawaii	253	1.14%
24	Missouri	245	1.11%
25	Mississippi	226	1.02%
26	Indiana	193	0.87%
26	Louisiana	193	0.87%
28	Connecticut	142	0.64%
29	Nevada	140	0.63%
30	Minnesota	130	0.59%
31	Oregon	90	0.41%
32	Kansas	83	0.37%
33	West Virginia	79	0.36%
34	New Mexico	78	0.35%
35	Wisconsin	70	0.32%
36	Iowa	66	0.30%
37	Alaska	63	0.28%
38	Utah	55	0.25%
39	Rhode Island	54	0.24%
40	Delaware	40	0.18%
41	Maine	34	0.15%
42	South Dakota	27	0.12%
43	Montana	24	0.11%
44	Colorado	21	0.09%
45	Nebraska	19	0.09%
46	New Hampshire	16	0.07%
47	Idaho	13	0.06%
48	Wyoming	12	0.05%
49	Vermont	10	0.05%
50	North Dakota	8	0.04%
	District of Columbia	112	0.51%

Source: U.S. Department of Health and Human Services, National Center for Health Statistics
"Morbidity and Mortality Weekly Report" (January 6, 1995, Vol. 43, Nos. 51 & 52)
*Infectious disease usually centered in the lungs.

Tuberculosis Rate in 1994

National Rate = 8.51 Cases Reported per 100,000 Population*

ALPHA ORDER

RANK ORDER

RANK	STATE	RATE
10	Alabama	10.26
7	Alaska	10.40
20	Arizona	6.31
6	Arkansas	10.52
3	California	15.09
50	Colorado	0.57
31	Connecticut	4.34
21	Delaware	5.67
5	Florida	10.79
12	Georgia	9.53
1	Hawaii	21.46
49	Idaho	1.15
13	Illinois	9.43
34	Indiana	3.36
43	Iowa	2.33
35	Kansas	3.25
14	Kentucky	8.68
29	Louisiana	4.47
41	Maine	2.74
19	Maryland	6.95
28	Massachusetts	4.50
26	Michigan	4.71
39	Minnesota	2.85
15	Mississippi	8.47
27	Missouri	4.64
40	Montana	2.80
48	Nebraska	1.17
11	Nevada	9.61
45	New Hampshire	1.41
8	New Jersey	10.37
25	New Mexico	4.72
2	New York	16.72
17	North Carolina	8.02
47	North Dakota	1.25
36	Ohio	3.11
16	Oklahoma	8.10
37	Oregon	2.92
23	Pennsylvania	5.08
22	Rhode Island	5.42
9	South Carolina	10.29
33	South Dakota	3.74
18	Tennessee	7.75
4	Texas	12.51
38	Utah	2.88
44	Vermont	1.72
30	Virginia	4.46
24	Washington	4.98
31	West Virginia	4.34
46	Wisconsin	1.38
42	Wyoming	2.52

RANK	STATE	RATE
1	Hawaii	21.46
2	New York	16.72
3	California	15.09
4	Texas	12.51
5	Florida	10.79
6	Arkansas	10.52
7	Alaska	10.40
8	New Jersey	10.37
9	South Carolina	10.29
10	Alabama	10.26
11	Nevada	9.61
12	Georgia	9.53
13	Illinois	9.43
14	Kentucky	8.68
15	Mississippi	8.47
16	Oklahoma	8.10
17	North Carolina	8.02
18	Tennessee	7.75
19	Maryland	6.95
20	Arizona	6.31
21	Delaware	5.67
22	Rhode Island	5.42
23	Pennsylvania	5.08
24	Washington	4.98
25	New Mexico	4.72
26	Michigan	4.71
27	Missouri	4.64
28	Massachusetts	4.50
29	Louisiana	4.47
30	Virginia	4.46
31	Connecticut	4.34
31	West Virginia	4.34
33	South Dakota	3.74
34	Indiana	3.36
35	Kansas	3.25
36	Ohio	3.11
37	Oregon	2.92
38	Utah	2.88
39	Minnesota	2.85
40	Montana	2.80
41	Maine	2.74
42	Wyoming	2.52
43	Iowa	2.33
44	Vermont	1.72
45	New Hampshire	1.41
46	Wisconsin	1.38
47	North Dakota	1.25
48	Nebraska	1.17
49	Idaho	1.15
50	Colorado	0.57

District of Columbia   19.65

Source: Morgan Quitno Press using data from U.S. Dept of Health & Human Serv's, National Center for Health Statistics "Morbidity and Mortality Weekly Report" (January 6, 1995, Vol. 43, Nos. 51 & 52)
*Infectious disease usually centered in the lungs.

Typhoid Fever Cases Reported in 1994

National Total = 410 Cases*

ALPHA ORDER					RANK ORDER			
RANK	STATE		CASES	% of USA	RANK	STATE	CASES	% of USA
33	Alabama		0	0.00%	1	California	105	25.61%
33	Alaska		0	0.00%	2	New York	84	20.49%
18	Arizona		3	0.73%	3	Illinois	46	11.22%
33	Arkansas		0	0.00%	4	New Jersey	23	5.61%
1	California		105	25.61%	5	Florida	22	5.37%
18	Colorado		3	0.73%	6	Massachusetts	18	4.39%
18	Connecticut		3	0.73%	7	Maryland	14	3.41%
27	Delaware		1	0.24%	8	Texas	10	2.44%
5	Florida		22	5.37%	9	Virginia	9	2.20%
25	Georgia		2	0.49%	10	Indiana	7	1.71%
15	Hawaii		5	1.22%	10	Ohio	7	1.71%
33	Idaho		0	0.00%	10	Wisconsin	7	1.71%
3	Illinois		46	11.22%	13	Michigan	6	1.46%
10	Indiana		7	1.71%	13	Pennsylvania	6	1.46%
33	Iowa		0	0.00%	15	Hawaii	5	1.22%
33	Kansas		0	0.00%	15	Oregon	5	1.22%
27	Kentucky		1	0.24%	17	Washington	4	0.98%
18	Louisiana		3	0.73%	18	Arizona	3	0.73%
33	Maine		0	0.00%	18	Colorado	3	0.73%
7	Maryland		14	3.41%	18	Connecticut	3	0.73%
6	Massachusetts		18	4.39%	18	Louisiana	3	0.73%
13	Michigan		6	1.46%	18	Nevada	3	0.73%
33	Minnesota		0	0.00%	18	Oklahoma	3	0.73%
33	Mississippi		0	0.00%	18	Tennessee	3	0.73%
27	Missouri		1	0.24%	25	Georgia	2	0.49%
33	Montana		0	0.00%	25	Utah	2	0.49%
33	Nebraska		0	0.00%	27	Delaware	1	0.24%
18	Nevada		3	0.73%	27	Kentucky	1	0.24%
33	New Hampshire		0	0.00%	27	Missouri	1	0.24%
4	New Jersey		23	5.61%	27	New Mexico	1	0.24%
27	New Mexico		1	0.24%	27	North Carolina	1	0.24%
2	New York		84	20.49%	27	Rhode Island	1	0.24%
27	North Carolina		1	0.24%	33	Alabama	0	0.00%
33	North Dakota		0	0.00%	33	Alaska	0	0.00%
10	Ohio		7	1.71%	33	Arkansas	0	0.00%
18	Oklahoma		3	0.73%	33	Idaho	0	0.00%
15	Oregon		5	1.22%	33	Iowa	0	0.00%
13	Pennsylvania		6	1.46%	33	Kansas	0	0.00%
27	Rhode Island		1	0.24%	33	Maine	0	0.00%
33	South Carolina		0	0.00%	33	Minnesota	0	0.00%
33	South Dakota		0	0.00%	33	Mississippi	0	0.00%
18	Tennessee		3	0.73%	33	Montana	0	0.00%
8	Texas		10	2.44%	33	Nebraska	0	0.00%
25	Utah		2	0.49%	33	New Hampshire	0	0.00%
33	Vermont		0	0.00%	33	North Dakota	0	0.00%
9	Virginia		9	2.20%	33	South Carolina	0	0.00%
17	Washington		4	0.98%	33	South Dakota	0	0.00%
33	West Virginia		0	0.00%	33	Vermont	0	0.00%
10	Wisconsin		7	1.71%	33	West Virginia	0	0.00%
33	Wyoming		0	0.00%	33	Wyoming	0	0.00%
						District of Columbia	1	0.24%

Source: U.S. Department of Health and Human Services, National Center for Health Statistics
"Morbidity and Mortality Weekly Report" (January 6, 1995, Vol. 43, Nos. 51 & 52)
*An infectious, often fatal febrile disease characterized by intestinal inflammation and ulceration.

Typhoid Fever Rate in 1994

National Rate = 0.16 Cases Reported per 100,000 Population*

ALPHA ORDER				RANK ORDER		
RANK	STATE	RATE		RANK	STATE	RATE
33	Alabama	0.00		1	New York	0.46
33	Alaska	0.00		2	Hawaii	0.42
20	Arizona	0.07		3	Illinois	0.39
33	Arkansas	0.00		4	California	0.33
4	California	0.33		5	Massachusetts	0.30
19	Colorado	0.08		6	New Jersey	0.29
17	Connecticut	0.09		7	Maryland	0.28
11	Delaware	0.14		8	Nevada	0.21
9	Florida	0.16		9	Florida	0.16
29	Georgia	0.03		9	Oregon	0.16
2	Hawaii	0.42		11	Delaware	0.14
33	Idaho	0.00		11	Virginia	0.14
3	Illinois	0.39		11	Wisconsin	0.14
14	Indiana	0.12		14	Indiana	0.12
33	Iowa	0.00		15	Rhode Island	0.10
33	Kansas	0.00		15	Utah	0.10
29	Kentucky	0.03		17	Connecticut	0.09
20	Louisiana	0.07		17	Oklahoma	0.09
33	Maine	0.00		19	Colorado	0.08
7	Maryland	0.28		20	Arizona	0.07
5	Massachusetts	0.30		20	Louisiana	0.07
23	Michigan	0.06		20	Washington	0.07
33	Minnesota	0.00		23	Michigan	0.06
33	Mississippi	0.00		23	New Mexico	0.06
31	Missouri	0.02		23	Ohio	0.06
33	Montana	0.00		23	Tennessee	0.06
33	Nebraska	0.00		27	Pennsylvania	0.05
8	Nevada	0.21		27	Texas	0.05
33	New Hampshire	0.00		29	Georgia	0.03
6	New Jersey	0.29		29	Kentucky	0.03
23	New Mexico	0.06		31	Missouri	0.02
1	New York	0.46		32	North Carolina	0.01
32	North Carolina	0.01		33	Alabama	0.00
33	North Dakota	0.00		33	Alaska	0.00
23	Ohio	0.06		33	Arkansas	0.00
17	Oklahoma	0.09		33	Idaho	0.00
9	Oregon	0.16		33	Iowa	0.00
27	Pennsylvania	0.05		33	Kansas	0.00
15	Rhode Island	0.10		33	Maine	0.00
33	South Carolina	0.00		33	Minnesota	0.00
33	South Dakota	0.00		33	Mississippi	0.00
23	Tennessee	0.06		33	Montana	0.00
27	Texas	0.05		33	Nebraska	0.00
15	Utah	0.10		33	New Hampshire	0.00
33	Vermont	0.00		33	North Dakota	0.00
11	Virginia	0.14		33	South Carolina	0.00
20	Washington	0.07		33	South Dakota	0.00
33	West Virginia	0.00		33	Vermont	0.00
11	Wisconsin	0.14		33	West Virginia	0.00
33	Wyoming	0.00		33	Wyoming	0.00
					District of Columbia	0.18

Source: Morgan Quitno Press using data from U.S. Dept of Health & Human Serv's, National Center for Health Statistics "Morbidity and Mortality Weekly Report" (January 6, 1995, Vol. 43, Nos. 51 & 52)
An infectious, often fatal febrile disease characterized by intestinal inflammation and ulceration.

Typhus Fever Cases Reported in 1994

National Total = 441 Cases*

ALPHA ORDER

RANK	STATE	CASES	% of USA
26	Alabama	2	0.45%
35	Alaska	0	0.00%
31	Arizona	1	0.23%
11	Arkansas	11	2.49%
35	California	0	0.00%
22	Colorado	4	0.91%
14	Connecticut	8	1.81%
35	Delaware	0	0.00%
20	Florida	5	1.13%
2	Georgia	56	12.70%
35	Hawaii	0	0.00%
35	Idaho	0	0.00%
12	Illinois	10	2.27%
20	Indiana	5	1.13%
31	Iowa	1	0.23%
22	Kansas	4	0.91%
13	Kentucky	9	2.04%
35	Louisiana	0	0.00%
35	Maine	0	0.00%
5	Maryland	25	5.67%
16	Massachusetts	7	1.59%
26	Michigan	2	0.45%
35	Minnesota	0	0.00%
16	Mississippi	7	1.59%
7	Missouri	20	4.54%
22	Montana	4	0.91%
31	Nebraska	1	0.23%
31	Nevada	1	0.23%
35	New Hampshire	0	0.00%
22	New Jersey	4	0.91%
26	New Mexico	2	0.45%
14	New York	8	1.81%
1	North Carolina	88	19.95%
35	North Dakota	0	0.00%
6	Ohio	22	4.99%
3	Oklahoma	35	7.94%
35	Oregon	0	0.00%
16	Pennsylvania	7	1.59%
35	Rhode Island	0	0.00%
7	South Carolina	20	4.54%
10	South Dakota	13	2.95%
4	Tennessee	29	6.58%
16	Texas	7	1.59%
35	Utah	0	0.00%
35	Vermont	0	0.00%
9	Virginia	19	4.31%
35	Washington	0	0.00%
26	West Virginia	2	0.45%
35	Wisconsin	0	0.00%
26	Wyoming	2	0.45%

RANK ORDER

RANK	STATE	CASES	% of USA
1	North Carolina	88	19.95%
2	Georgia	56	12.70%
3	Oklahoma	35	7.94%
4	Tennessee	29	6.58%
5	Maryland	25	5.67%
6	Ohio	22	4.99%
7	Missouri	20	4.54%
7	South Carolina	20	4.54%
9	Virginia	19	4.31%
10	South Dakota	13	2.95%
11	Arkansas	11	2.49%
12	Illinois	10	2.27%
13	Kentucky	9	2.04%
14	Connecticut	8	1.81%
14	New York	8	1.81%
16	Massachusetts	7	1.59%
16	Mississippi	7	1.59%
16	Pennsylvania	7	1.59%
16	Texas	7	1.59%
20	Florida	5	1.13%
20	Indiana	5	1.13%
22	Colorado	4	0.91%
22	Kansas	4	0.91%
22	Montana	4	0.91%
22	New Jersey	4	0.91%
26	Alabama	2	0.45%
26	Michigan	2	0.45%
26	New Mexico	2	0.45%
26	West Virginia	2	0.45%
26	Wyoming	2	0.45%
31	Arizona	1	0.23%
31	Iowa	1	0.23%
31	Nebraska	1	0.23%
31	Nevada	1	0.23%
35	Alaska	0	0.00%
35	California	0	0.00%
35	Delaware	0	0.00%
35	Hawaii	0	0.00%
35	Idaho	0	0.00%
35	Louisiana	0	0.00%
35	Maine	0	0.00%
35	Minnesota	0	0.00%
35	New Hampshire	0	0.00%
35	North Dakota	0	0.00%
35	Oregon	0	0.00%
35	Rhode Island	0	0.00%
35	Utah	0	0.00%
35	Vermont	0	0.00%
35	Washington	0	0.00%
35	Wisconsin	0	0.00%
	District of Columbia	0	0.00%

Source: U.S. Department of Health and Human Services, National Center for Health Statistics
"Morbidity and Mortality Weekly Report" (January 6, 1995, Vol. 43, Nos. 51 & 52)
Tick-borne, RMSF. An acute, infectious disease characterized by great prostration, severe nervous symptoms, and a peculiar eruption of reddish spots on the body.

Typhus Fever Rate in 1994

National Rate = 0.17 Cases Reported per 100,000 Population*

<table>
<tr><th colspan="3">ALPHA ORDER</th><th colspan="3">RANK ORDER</th></tr>
<tr><th>RANK</th><th>STATE</th><th>RATE</th><th>RANK</th><th>STATE</th><th>RATE</th></tr>
<tr><td>27</td><td>Alabama</td><td>0.05</td><td>1</td><td>South Dakota</td><td>1.80</td></tr>
<tr><td>35</td><td>Alaska</td><td>0.00</td><td>2</td><td>North Carolina</td><td>1.24</td></tr>
<tr><td>33</td><td>Arizona</td><td>0.02</td><td>3</td><td>Oklahoma</td><td>1.07</td></tr>
<tr><td>9</td><td>Arkansas</td><td>0.45</td><td>4</td><td>Georgia</td><td>0.79</td></tr>
<tr><td>35</td><td>California</td><td>0.00</td><td>5</td><td>Tennessee</td><td>0.56</td></tr>
<tr><td>20</td><td>Colorado</td><td>0.11</td><td>6</td><td>South Carolina</td><td>0.55</td></tr>
<tr><td>14</td><td>Connecticut</td><td>0.24</td><td>7</td><td>Maryland</td><td>0.50</td></tr>
<tr><td>35</td><td>Delaware</td><td>0.00</td><td>8</td><td>Montana</td><td>0.47</td></tr>
<tr><td>29</td><td>Florida</td><td>0.04</td><td>9</td><td>Arkansas</td><td>0.45</td></tr>
<tr><td>4</td><td>Georgia</td><td>0.79</td><td>10</td><td>Wyoming</td><td>0.42</td></tr>
<tr><td>35</td><td>Hawaii</td><td>0.00</td><td>11</td><td>Missouri</td><td>0.38</td></tr>
<tr><td>35</td><td>Idaho</td><td>0.00</td><td>12</td><td>Virginia</td><td>0.29</td></tr>
<tr><td>22</td><td>Illinois</td><td>0.09</td><td>13</td><td>Mississippi</td><td>0.26</td></tr>
<tr><td>22</td><td>Indiana</td><td>0.09</td><td>14</td><td>Connecticut</td><td>0.24</td></tr>
<tr><td>29</td><td>Iowa</td><td>0.04</td><td>14</td><td>Kentucky</td><td>0.24</td></tr>
<tr><td>17</td><td>Kansas</td><td>0.16</td><td>16</td><td>Ohio</td><td>0.20</td></tr>
<tr><td>14</td><td>Kentucky</td><td>0.24</td><td>17</td><td>Kansas</td><td>0.16</td></tr>
<tr><td>35</td><td>Louisiana</td><td>0.00</td><td>18</td><td>Massachusetts</td><td>0.12</td></tr>
<tr><td>35</td><td>Maine</td><td>0.00</td><td>18</td><td>New Mexico</td><td>0.12</td></tr>
<tr><td>7</td><td>Maryland</td><td>0.50</td><td>20</td><td>Colorado</td><td>0.11</td></tr>
<tr><td>18</td><td>Massachusetts</td><td>0.12</td><td>20</td><td>West Virginia</td><td>0.11</td></tr>
<tr><td>33</td><td>Michigan</td><td>0.02</td><td>22</td><td>Illinois</td><td>0.09</td></tr>
<tr><td>35</td><td>Minnesota</td><td>0.00</td><td>22</td><td>Indiana</td><td>0.09</td></tr>
<tr><td>13</td><td>Mississippi</td><td>0.26</td><td>24</td><td>Nevada</td><td>0.07</td></tr>
<tr><td>11</td><td>Missouri</td><td>0.38</td><td>25</td><td>Nebraska</td><td>0.06</td></tr>
<tr><td>8</td><td>Montana</td><td>0.47</td><td>25</td><td>Pennsylvania</td><td>0.06</td></tr>
<tr><td>25</td><td>Nebraska</td><td>0.06</td><td>27</td><td>Alabama</td><td>0.05</td></tr>
<tr><td>24</td><td>Nevada</td><td>0.07</td><td>27</td><td>New Jersey</td><td>0.05</td></tr>
<tr><td>35</td><td>New Hampshire</td><td>0.00</td><td>29</td><td>Florida</td><td>0.04</td></tr>
<tr><td>27</td><td>New Jersey</td><td>0.05</td><td>29</td><td>Iowa</td><td>0.04</td></tr>
<tr><td>18</td><td>New Mexico</td><td>0.12</td><td>29</td><td>New York</td><td>0.04</td></tr>
<tr><td>29</td><td>New York</td><td>0.04</td><td>29</td><td>Texas</td><td>0.04</td></tr>
<tr><td>2</td><td>North Carolina</td><td>1.24</td><td>33</td><td>Arizona</td><td>0.02</td></tr>
<tr><td>35</td><td>North Dakota</td><td>0.00</td><td>33</td><td>Michigan</td><td>0.02</td></tr>
<tr><td>16</td><td>Ohio</td><td>0.20</td><td>35</td><td>Alaska</td><td>0.00</td></tr>
<tr><td>3</td><td>Oklahoma</td><td>1.07</td><td>35</td><td>California</td><td>0.00</td></tr>
<tr><td>35</td><td>Oregon</td><td>0.00</td><td>35</td><td>Delaware</td><td>0.00</td></tr>
<tr><td>25</td><td>Pennsylvania</td><td>0.06</td><td>35</td><td>Hawaii</td><td>0.00</td></tr>
<tr><td>35</td><td>Rhode Island</td><td>0.00</td><td>35</td><td>Idaho</td><td>0.00</td></tr>
<tr><td>6</td><td>South Carolina</td><td>0.55</td><td>35</td><td>Louisiana</td><td>0.00</td></tr>
<tr><td>1</td><td>South Dakota</td><td>1.80</td><td>35</td><td>Maine</td><td>0.00</td></tr>
<tr><td>5</td><td>Tennessee</td><td>0.56</td><td>35</td><td>Minnesota</td><td>0.00</td></tr>
<tr><td>29</td><td>Texas</td><td>0.04</td><td>35</td><td>New Hampshire</td><td>0.00</td></tr>
<tr><td>35</td><td>Utah</td><td>0.00</td><td>35</td><td>North Dakota</td><td>0.00</td></tr>
<tr><td>35</td><td>Vermont</td><td>0.00</td><td>35</td><td>Oregon</td><td>0.00</td></tr>
<tr><td>12</td><td>Virginia</td><td>0.29</td><td>35</td><td>Rhode Island</td><td>0.00</td></tr>
<tr><td>35</td><td>Washington</td><td>0.00</td><td>35</td><td>Utah</td><td>0.00</td></tr>
<tr><td>20</td><td>West Virginia</td><td>0.11</td><td>35</td><td>Vermont</td><td>0.00</td></tr>
<tr><td>35</td><td>Wisconsin</td><td>0.00</td><td>35</td><td>Washington</td><td>0.00</td></tr>
<tr><td>10</td><td>Wyoming</td><td>0.42</td><td>35</td><td>Wisconsin</td><td>0.00</td></tr>
<tr><td></td><td></td><td></td><td></td><td>District of Columbia</td><td>0.00</td></tr>
</table>

Source: Morgan Quitno Press using data from U.S. Dept of Health & Human Serv's, National Center for Health Statistics "Morbidity and Mortality Weekly Report" (January 6, 1995, Vol. 43, Nos. 51 & 52)

Tick-borne, RMSF. An acute, infectious disease characterized by great prostration, severe nervous symptoms, and a peculiar eruption of reddish spots on the body.

Whooping Cough (Pertussis) Cases Reported in 1994

National Total = 3,590 Cases*

ALPHA ORDER

RANK	STATE	CASES	% of USA
27	Alabama	35	0.97%
49	Alaska	1	0.03%
7	Arizona	148	4.12%
28	Arkansas	27	0.75%
1	California	573	15.96%
9	Colorado	125	3.48%
22	Connecticut	42	1.17%
46	Delaware	3	0.08%
18	Florida	47	1.31%
28	Georgia	27	0.75%
34	Hawaii	21	0.58%
5	Idaho	172	4.79%
11	Illinois	95	2.65%
13	Indiana	78	2.17%
32	Iowa	23	0.64%
36	Kansas	18	0.50%
15	Kentucky	59	1.64%
38	Louisiana	12	0.33%
34	Maine	21	0.58%
14	Maryland	75	2.09%
3	Massachusetts	316	8.80%
16	Michigan	50	1.39%
10	Minnesota	100	2.79%
42	Mississippi	7	0.19%
18	Missouri	47	1.31%
39	Montana	11	0.31%
39	Nebraska	11	0.31%
46	Nevada	3	0.08%
12	New Hampshire	84	2.34%
39	New Jersey	11	0.31%
24	New Mexico	36	1.00%
2	New York	442	12.31%
8	North Carolina	140	3.90%
45	North Dakota	5	0.14%
6	Ohio	162	4.51%
24	Oklahoma	36	1.00%
21	Oregon	43	1.20%
4	Pennsylvania	202	5.63%
42	Rhode Island	7	0.19%
37	South Carolina	14	0.39%
30	South Dakota	26	0.72%
33	Tennessee	22	0.61%
48	Texas	2	0.06%
30	Utah	26	0.72%
20	Vermont	45	1.25%
24	Virginia	36	1.00%
23	Washington	37	1.03%
44	West Virginia	6	0.17%
16	Wisconsin	50	1.39%
50	Wyoming	0	0.00%

RANK ORDER

RANK	STATE	CASES	% of USA
1	California	573	15.96%
2	New York	442	12.31%
3	Massachusetts	316	8.80%
4	Pennsylvania	202	5.63%
5	Idaho	172	4.79%
6	Ohio	162	4.51%
7	Arizona	148	4.12%
8	North Carolina	140	3.90%
9	Colorado	125	3.48%
10	Minnesota	100	2.79%
11	Illinois	95	2.65%
12	New Hampshire	84	2.34%
13	Indiana	78	2.17%
14	Maryland	75	2.09%
15	Kentucky	59	1.64%
16	Michigan	50	1.39%
16	Wisconsin	50	1.39%
18	Florida	47	1.31%
18	Missouri	47	1.31%
20	Vermont	45	1.25%
21	Oregon	43	1.20%
22	Connecticut	42	1.17%
23	Washington	37	1.03%
24	New Mexico	36	1.00%
24	Oklahoma	36	1.00%
24	Virginia	36	1.00%
27	Alabama	35	0.97%
28	Arkansas	27	0.75%
28	Georgia	27	0.75%
30	South Dakota	26	0.72%
30	Utah	26	0.72%
32	Iowa	23	0.64%
33	Tennessee	22	0.61%
34	Hawaii	21	0.58%
34	Maine	21	0.58%
36	Kansas	18	0.50%
37	South Carolina	14	0.39%
38	Louisiana	12	0.33%
39	Montana	11	0.31%
39	Nebraska	11	0.31%
39	New Jersey	11	0.31%
42	Mississippi	7	0.19%
42	Rhode Island	7	0.19%
44	West Virginia	6	0.17%
45	North Dakota	5	0.14%
46	Delaware	3	0.08%
46	Nevada	3	0.08%
48	Texas	2	0.06%
49	Alaska	1	0.03%
50	Wyoming	0	0.00%
	District of Columbia	11	0.31%

Source: U.S. Department of Health and Human Services, National Center for Health Statistics
"Morbidity and Mortality Weekly Report" (January 6, 1995, Vol. 43, Nos. 51 & 52)
*Acute, highly contagious infection of respiratory tract.

Whooping Cough (Pertussis) Rate in 1994

National Rate = 1.38 Cases Reported per 100,000 Population*

ALPHA ORDER				RANK ORDER		
RANK	STATE	RATE		RANK	STATE	RATE
28	Alabama	0.83		1	Idaho	15.18
47	Alaska	0.17		2	Vermont	7.76
5	Arizona	3.63		3	New Hampshire	7.39
24	Arkansas	1.10		4	Massachusetts	5.23
12	California	1.82		5	Arizona	3.63
7	Colorado	3.42		6	South Dakota	3.61
23	Connecticut	1.28		7	Colorado	3.42
39	Delaware	0.42		8	New York	2.43
42	Florida	0.34		9	Minnesota	2.19
40	Georgia	0.38		10	New Mexico	2.18
13	Hawaii	1.78		11	North Carolina	1.98
1	Idaho	15.18		12	California	1.82
29	Illinois	0.81		13	Hawaii	1.78
20	Indiana	1.36		14	Maine	1.69
29	Iowa	0.81		15	Pennsylvania	1.68
32	Kansas	0.70		16	Kentucky	1.54
16	Kentucky	1.54		17	Maryland	1.50
44	Louisiana	0.28		18	Ohio	1.46
14	Maine	1.69		19	Oregon	1.39
17	Maryland	1.50		20	Indiana	1.36
4	Massachusetts	5.23		20	Utah	1.36
37	Michigan	0.53		22	Montana	1.29
9	Minnesota	2.19		23	Connecticut	1.28
45	Mississippi	0.26		24	Arkansas	1.10
27	Missouri	0.89		24	Oklahoma	1.10
22	Montana	1.29		26	Wisconsin	0.98
35	Nebraska	0.68		27	Missouri	0.89
46	Nevada	0.21		28	Alabama	0.83
3	New Hampshire	7.39		29	Illinois	0.81
48	New Jersey	0.14		29	Iowa	0.81
10	New Mexico	2.18		31	North Dakota	0.78
8	New York	2.43		32	Kansas	0.70
11	North Carolina	1.98		32	Rhode Island	0.70
31	North Dakota	0.78		34	Washington	0.69
18	Ohio	1.46		35	Nebraska	0.68
24	Oklahoma	1.10		36	Virginia	0.55
19	Oregon	1.39		37	Michigan	0.53
15	Pennsylvania	1.68		38	Tennessee	0.43
32	Rhode Island	0.70		39	Delaware	0.42
40	South Carolina	0.38		40	Georgia	0.38
6	South Dakota	3.61		40	South Carolina	0.38
38	Tennessee	0.43		42	Florida	0.34
49	Texas	0.01		43	West Virginia	0.33
20	Utah	1.36		44	Louisiana	0.28
2	Vermont	7.76		45	Mississippi	0.26
36	Virginia	0.55		46	Nevada	0.21
34	Washington	0.69		47	Alaska	0.17
43	West Virginia	0.33		48	New Jersey	0.14
26	Wisconsin	0.98		49	Texas	0.01
50	Wyoming	0.00		50	Wyoming	0.00
					District of Columbia	1.93

Source: Morgan Quitno Press using data from U.S. Dept of Health & Human Serv's, National Center for Health Statistics
"Morbidity and Mortality Weekly Report" (January 6, 1995, Vol. 43, Nos. 51 & 52)
*Acute, highly contagious infection of respiratory tract.

Percent of Kindergarteners Entering School in 1993
Who Were Fully Immunized at Age Two
National Average Percent = 58.5%*

ALPHA ORDER

RANK ORDER

RANK	STATE	PERCENT		RANK	STATE	PERCENT
31	Alabama	56.5		1	Tennessee	72.0
16	Alaska	62.8		2	Illinois	71.3
33	Arizona	55.7		3	Maine	71.1
17	Arkansas	62.7		4	Massachusetts	70.8
30	California	57.2		5	Vermont	70.4
13	Colorado	63.3		6	Connecticut	70.3
6	Connecticut	70.3		7	Oklahoma	69.0
35	Delaware	54.2		8	Rhode Island	68.9
19	Florida	61.4		9	New Hampshire	68.4
22	Georgia	60.0		10	Mississippi	65.1
14	Hawaii	63.0		11	Wisconsin	64.0
NA	Idaho**	NA		12	Wyoming	63.9
2	Illinois	71.3		13	Colorado	63.3
37	Indiana	52.7		14	Hawaii	63.0
47	Iowa	30.9		14	Nebraska	63.0
34	Kansas	55.2		16	Alaska	62.8
23	Kentucky	59.4		17	Arkansas	62.7
29	Louisiana	58.0		18	Maryland	62.2
3	Maine	71.1		19	Florida	61.4
18	Maryland	62.2		20	South Dakota	60.3
4	Massachusetts	70.8		21	Virginia	60.1
46	Michigan	42.1		22	Georgia	60.0
NA	Minnesota**	NA		23	Kentucky	59.4
10	Mississippi	65.1		24	North Carolina	59.1
38	Missouri	52.0		25	South Carolina	58.7
39	Montana	51.9		26	New Mexico	58.2
14	Nebraska	63.0		26	Pennsylvania	58.2
41	Nevada	50.3		28	New York	58.1
9	New Hampshire	68.4		29	Louisiana	58.0
44	New Jersey	45.1		30	California	57.2
26	New Mexico	58.2		31	Alabama	56.5
28	New York	58.1		32	Washington	56.0
24	North Carolina	59.1		33	Arizona	55.7
NA	North Dakota**	NA		34	Kansas	55.2
43	Ohio	49.0		35	Delaware	54.2
7	Oklahoma	69.0		36	Oregon	53.0
36	Oregon	53.0		37	Indiana	52.7
26	Pennsylvania	58.2		38	Missouri	52.0
8	Rhode Island	68.9		39	Montana	51.9
25	South Carolina	58.7		40	West Virginia	50.8
20	South Dakota	60.3		41	Nevada	50.3
1	Tennessee	72.0		42	Utah	49.3
45	Texas	44.1		43	Ohio	49.0
42	Utah	49.3		44	New Jersey	45.1
5	Vermont	70.4		45	Texas	44.1
21	Virginia	60.1		46	Michigan	42.1
32	Washington	56.0		47	Iowa	30.9
40	West Virginia	50.8		NA	Idaho**	NA
11	Wisconsin	64.0		NA	Minnesota**	NA
12	Wyoming	63.9		NA	North Dakota**	NA

District of Columbia 48.0

*Source: US Dept of Health & Human Services, Cntrs for Disease Control & Prevention, National Immunization Program
"1990 Retrospective by State" (As of August 25, 1994) *National average calculated by the editors and is the average
of reporting states' percent. Fully immunized children received four doses of DTP (Diphtheria, Tetanus, Pertussis
(Whooping Cough)), three doses of OPV (Polio) and one dose of MMR (Measles, Mumps, Rubella) by their second birthday.
New York does not include New York City (50.4%), Texas does not include Houston (44.1%) or San Antonio (NA),
Wisconsin excludes Milwaukee. **Not reported.*   381

VI. PERSONNEL

Physicians in 1993

National Total = 659,654 Physicians*

RANK	STATE	PHYSICIANS	% of USA
25	Alabama	7,960	1.21%
49	Alaska	986	0.15%
23	Arizona	9,323	1.41%
32	Arkansas	4,519	0.69%
1	California	86,479	13.11%
24	Colorado	9,112	1.38%
18	Connecticut	11,747	1.78%
46	Delaware	1,661	0.25%
4	Florida	36,142	5.48%
14	Georgia	14,287	2.17%
38	Hawaii	3,340	0.51%
44	Idaho	1,696	0.26%
6	Illinois	29,652	4.50%
21	Indiana	10,713	1.62%
31	Iowa	5,116	0.78%
30	Kansas	5,394	0.82%
26	Kentucky	7,515	1.14%
22	Louisiana	9,559	1.45%
40	Maine	2,826	0.43%
11	Maryland	19,969	3.03%
8	Massachusetts	23,947	3.63%
10	Michigan	20,574	3.12%
19	Minnesota	11,726	1.78%
33	Mississippi	4,086	0.62%
17	Missouri	11,918	1.81%
45	Montana	1,687	0.26%
37	Nebraska	3,432	0.52%
42	Nevada	2,342	0.36%
41	New Hampshire	2,747	0.42%
9	New Jersey	22,883	3.47%
36	New Mexico	3,632	0.55%
2	New York	67,165	10.18%
13	North Carolina	15,548	2.36%
47	North Dakota	1,358	0.21%
7	Ohio	25,780	3.91%
29	Oklahoma	5,549	0.84%
27	Oregon	7,488	1.14%
5	Pennsylvania	34,224	5.19%
39	Rhode Island	3,045	0.46%
28	South Carolina	7,208	1.09%
48	South Dakota	1,325	0.20%
16	Tennessee	11,943	1.81%
3	Texas	36,487	5.53%
34	Utah	3,959	0.60%
43	Vermont	1,764	0.27%
12	Virginia	15,981	2.42%
15	Washington	13,618	2.06%
35	West Virginia	3,723	0.56%
20	Wisconsin	11,268	1.71%
50	Wyoming	780	0.12%

RANK	STATE	PHYSICIANS	% of USA
1	California	86,479	13.11%
2	New York	67,165	10.18%
3	Texas	36,487	5.53%
4	Florida	36,142	5.48%
5	Pennsylvania	34,224	5.19%
6	Illinois	29,652	4.50%
7	Ohio	25,780	3.91%
8	Massachusetts	23,947	3.63%
9	New Jersey	22,883	3.47%
10	Michigan	20,574	3.12%
11	Maryland	19,969	3.03%
12	Virginia	15,981	2.42%
13	North Carolina	15,548	2.36%
14	Georgia	14,287	2.17%
15	Washington	13,618	2.06%
16	Tennessee	11,943	1.81%
17	Missouri	11,918	1.81%
18	Connecticut	11,747	1.78%
19	Minnesota	11,726	1.78%
20	Wisconsin	11,268	1.71%
21	Indiana	10,713	1.62%
22	Louisiana	9,559	1.45%
23	Arizona	9,323	1.41%
24	Colorado	9,112	1.38%
25	Alabama	7,960	1.21%
26	Kentucky	7,515	1.14%
27	Oregon	7,488	1.14%
28	South Carolina	7,208	1.09%
29	Oklahoma	5,549	0.84%
30	Kansas	5,394	0.82%
31	Iowa	5,116	0.78%
32	Arkansas	4,519	0.69%
33	Mississippi	4,086	0.62%
34	Utah	3,959	0.60%
35	West Virginia	3,723	0.56%
36	New Mexico	3,632	0.55%
37	Nebraska	3,432	0.52%
38	Hawaii	3,340	0.51%
39	Rhode Island	3,045	0.46%
40	Maine	2,826	0.43%
41	New Hampshire	2,747	0.42%
42	Nevada	2,342	0.36%
43	Vermont	1,764	0.27%
44	Idaho	1,696	0.26%
45	Montana	1,687	0.26%
46	Delaware	1,661	0.25%
47	North Dakota	1,358	0.21%
48	South Dakota	1,325	0.20%
49	Alaska	986	0.15%
50	Wyoming	780	0.12%
	District of Columbia	4,471	0.68%

Source: American Medical Association (Chicago, Illinois)
"Physician Characteristics and Distribution in the U.S." (1994 Edition)
*As of January 1, 1993. Comprised of federal and nonfederal physicians. Total does not include 10,682 physicians in the U.S. territories and possessions, at APO's and FPO's and whose addresses are unknown.

Male Physicians in 1993

National Total = 536,140 Physicians*

ALPHA ORDER

ALPHA ORDER

RANK	STATE	PHYSICIANS	% of USA
25	Alabama	6,862	1.28%
49	Alaska	797	0.15%
23	Arizona	7,836	1.46%
32	Arkansas	3,921	0.73%
1	California	70,325	13.12%
24	Colorado	7,390	1.38%
19	Connecticut	9,408	1.75%
46	Delaware	1,314	0.25%
3	Florida	31,280	5.83%
14	Georgia	11,975	2.23%
38	Hawaii	2,741	0.51%
43	Idaho	1,536	0.29%
6	Illinois	23,018	4.29%
21	Indiana	9,038	1.69%
31	Iowa	4,374	0.82%
30	Kansas	4,496	0.84%
26	Kentucky	6,278	1.17%
22	Louisiana	8,074	1.51%
40	Maine	2,345	0.44%
11	Maryland	15,369	2.87%
8	Massachusetts	18,264	3.41%
10	Michigan	16,562	3.09%
18	Minnesota	9,518	1.78%
33	Mississippi	3,546	0.66%
17	Missouri	9,783	1.82%
44	Montana	1,487	0.28%
36	Nebraska	2,952	0.55%
42	Nevada	2,072	0.39%
41	New Hampshire	2,310	0.43%
9	New Jersey	17,862	3.33%
37	New Mexico	2,817	0.53%
2	New York	51,743	9.65%
13	North Carolina	12,895	2.41%
47	North Dakota	1,210	0.23%
7	Ohio	20,806	3.88%
29	Oklahoma	4,707	0.88%
27	Oregon	6,260	1.17%
5	Pennsylvania	27,346	5.10%
39	Rhode Island	2,405	0.45%
28	South Carolina	6,154	1.15%
48	South Dakota	1,169	0.22%
16	Tennessee	10,177	1.90%
4	Texas	30,213	5.64%
34	Utah	3,459	0.65%
45	Vermont	1,417	0.26%
12	Virginia	12,929	2.41%
15	Washington	11,182	2.09%
35	West Virginia	3,145	0.59%
20	Wisconsin	9,364	1.75%
50	Wyoming	700	0.13%

RANK ORDER

RANK	STATE	PHYSICIANS	% of USA
1	California	70,325	13.12%
2	New York	51,743	9.65%
3	Florida	31,280	5.83%
4	Texas	30,213	5.64%
5	Pennsylvania	27,346	5.10%
6	Illinois	23,018	4.29%
7	Ohio	20,806	3.88%
8	Massachusetts	18,264	3.41%
9	New Jersey	17,862	3.33%
10	Michigan	16,562	3.09%
11	Maryland	15,369	2.87%
12	Virginia	12,929	2.41%
13	North Carolina	12,895	2.41%
14	Georgia	11,975	2.23%
15	Washington	11,182	2.09%
16	Tennessee	10,177	1.90%
17	Missouri	9,783	1.82%
18	Minnesota	9,518	1.78%
19	Connecticut	9,408	1.75%
20	Wisconsin	9,364	1.75%
21	Indiana	9,038	1.69%
22	Louisiana	8,074	1.51%
23	Arizona	7,836	1.46%
24	Colorado	7,390	1.38%
25	Alabama	6,862	1.28%
26	Kentucky	6,278	1.17%
27	Oregon	6,260	1.17%
28	South Carolina	6,154	1.15%
29	Oklahoma	4,707	0.88%
30	Kansas	4,496	0.84%
31	Iowa	4,374	0.82%
32	Arkansas	3,921	0.73%
33	Mississippi	3,546	0.66%
34	Utah	3,459	0.65%
35	West Virginia	3,145	0.59%
36	Nebraska	2,952	0.55%
37	New Mexico	2,817	0.53%
38	Hawaii	2,741	0.51%
39	Rhode Island	2,405	0.45%
40	Maine	2,345	0.44%
41	New Hampshire	2,310	0.43%
42	Nevada	2,072	0.39%
43	Idaho	1,536	0.29%
44	Montana	1,487	0.28%
45	Vermont	1,417	0.26%
46	Delaware	1,314	0.25%
47	North Dakota	1,210	0.23%
48	South Dakota	1,169	0.22%
49	Alaska	797	0.15%
50	Wyoming	700	0.13%
	District of Columbia	3,309	0.62%

Source: American Medical Association (Chicago, Illinois)
"Physician Characteristics and Distribution in the U.S." (1994 Edition)
As of January 1, 1993. Comprised of federal and nonfederal physicians. Total does not include 8,297 male physicians in the U.S. territories and possessions, at APO's and FPO's and whose addresses are unknown.

Female Physicians in 1993

National Total = 123,514 Physicians*

ALPHA ORDER					RANK ORDER			
RANK	STATE	PHYSICIANS	% of USA		RANK	STATE	PHYSICIANS	% of USA
27	Alabama	1,098	0.89%		1	California	16,154	13.08%
46	Alaska	189	0.15%		2	New York	15,422	12.49%
23	Arizona	1,487	1.20%		3	Pennsylvania	6,878	5.57%
35	Arkansas	598	0.48%		4	Illinois	6,634	5.37%
1	California	16,154	13.08%		5	Texas	6,274	5.08%
21	Colorado	1,722	1.39%		6	Massachusetts	5,683	4.60%
15	Connecticut	2,339	1.89%		7	New Jersey	5,021	4.07%
42	Delaware	347	0.28%		8	Ohio	4,974	4.03%
9	Florida	4,862	3.94%		9	Florida	4,862	3.94%
16	Georgia	2,312	1.87%		10	Maryland	4,600	3.72%
34	Hawaii	599	0.48%		11	Michigan	4,012	3.25%
47	Idaho	160	0.13%		12	Virginia	3,052	2.47%
4	Illinois	6,634	5.37%		13	North Carolina	2,653	2.15%
22	Indiana	1,675	1.36%		14	Washington	2,436	1.97%
32	Iowa	742	0.60%		15	Connecticut	2,339	1.89%
29	Kansas	898	0.73%		16	Georgia	2,312	1.87%
25	Kentucky	1,237	1.00%		17	Minnesota	2,208	1.79%
24	Louisiana	1,485	1.20%		18	Missouri	2,135	1.73%
39	Maine	481	0.39%		19	Wisconsin	1,904	1.54%
10	Maryland	4,600	3.72%		20	Tennessee	1,766	1.43%
6	Massachusetts	5,683	4.60%		21	Colorado	1,722	1.39%
11	Michigan	4,012	3.25%		22	Indiana	1,675	1.36%
17	Minnesota	2,208	1.79%		23	Arizona	1,487	1.20%
37	Mississippi	540	0.44%		24	Louisiana	1,485	1.20%
18	Missouri	2,135	1.73%		25	Kentucky	1,237	1.00%
45	Montana	200	0.16%		26	Oregon	1,228	0.99%
40	Nebraska	480	0.39%		27	Alabama	1,098	0.89%
44	Nevada	270	0.22%		28	South Carolina	1,054	0.85%
41	New Hampshire	437	0.35%		29	Kansas	898	0.73%
7	New Jersey	5,021	4.07%		30	Oklahoma	842	0.68%
31	New Mexico	815	0.66%		31	New Mexico	815	0.66%
2	New York	15,422	12.49%		32	Iowa	742	0.60%
13	North Carolina	2,653	2.15%		33	Rhode Island	640	0.52%
49	North Dakota	148	0.12%		34	Hawaii	599	0.48%
8	Ohio	4,974	4.03%		35	Arkansas	598	0.48%
30	Oklahoma	842	0.68%		36	West Virginia	578	0.47%
26	Oregon	1,228	0.99%		37	Mississippi	540	0.44%
3	Pennsylvania	6,878	5.57%		38	Utah	500	0.40%
33	Rhode Island	640	0.52%		39	Maine	481	0.39%
28	South Carolina	1,054	0.85%		40	Nebraska	480	0.39%
48	South Dakota	156	0.13%		41	New Hampshire	437	0.35%
20	Tennessee	1,766	1.43%		42	Delaware	347	0.28%
5	Texas	6,274	5.08%		42	Vermont	347	0.28%
38	Utah	500	0.40%		44	Nevada	270	0.22%
42	Vermont	347	0.28%		45	Montana	200	0.16%
12	Virginia	3,052	2.47%		46	Alaska	189	0.15%
14	Washington	2,436	1.97%		47	Idaho	160	0.13%
36	West Virginia	578	0.47%		48	South Dakota	156	0.13%
19	Wisconsin	1,904	1.54%		49	North Dakota	148	0.12%
50	Wyoming	80	0.06%		50	Wyoming	80	0.06%
					District of Columbia		1,162	0.94%

Source: American Medical Association (Chicago, Illinois)
    "Physician Characteristics and Distribution in the U.S." (1994 Edition)
As of January 1, 1993. Comprised of federal and nonfederal physicians. Total does not include 2,385 female physicians in the U.S. territories and possessions, at APO's and FPO's and whose addresses are unknown.

Percent of Physicians Who Are Female in 1993

National Percent = 18.72% of Physicians*

ALPHA ORDER

RANK	STATE	PERCENT
40	Alabama	13.79
14	Alaska	19.17
30	Arizona	15.95
42	Arkansas	13.23
18	California	18.68
16	Colorado	18.90
10	Connecticut	19.91
8	Delaware	20.89
41	Florida	13.45
29	Georgia	16.18
19	Hawaii	17.93
50	Idaho	9.43
5	Illinois	22.37
32	Indiana	15.64
38	Iowa	14.50
26	Kansas	16.65
27	Kentucky	16.46
33	Louisiana	15.54
24	Maine	17.02
2	Maryland	23.04
1	Massachusetts	23.73
12	Michigan	19.50
17	Minnesota	18.83
43	Mississippi	13.22
20	Missouri	17.91
45	Montana	11.86
39	Nebraska	13.99
47	Nevada	11.53
31	New Hampshire	15.91
6	New Jersey	21.94
4	New Mexico	22.44
3	New York	22.96
23	North Carolina	17.06
48	North Dakota	10.90
13	Ohio	19.29
35	Oklahoma	15.17
28	Oregon	16.40
9	Pennsylvania	20.10
7	Rhode Island	21.02
37	South Carolina	14.62
46	South Dakota	11.77
36	Tennessee	14.79
22	Texas	17.20
44	Utah	12.63
11	Vermont	19.67
15	Virginia	19.10
21	Washington	17.89
34	West Virginia	15.53
25	Wisconsin	16.90
49	Wyoming	10.26

RANK ORDER

RANK	STATE	PERCENT
1	Massachusetts	23.73
2	Maryland	23.04
3	New York	22.96
4	New Mexico	22.44
5	Illinois	22.37
6	New Jersey	21.94
7	Rhode Island	21.02
8	Delaware	20.89
9	Pennsylvania	20.10
10	Connecticut	19.91
11	Vermont	19.67
12	Michigan	19.50
13	Ohio	19.29
14	Alaska	19.17
15	Virginia	19.10
16	Colorado	18.90
17	Minnesota	18.83
18	California	18.68
19	Hawaii	17.93
20	Missouri	17.91
21	Washington	17.89
22	Texas	17.20
23	North Carolina	17.06
24	Maine	17.02
25	Wisconsin	16.90
26	Kansas	16.65
27	Kentucky	16.46
28	Oregon	16.40
29	Georgia	16.18
30	Arizona	15.95
31	New Hampshire	15.91
32	Indiana	15.64
33	Louisiana	15.54
34	West Virginia	15.53
35	Oklahoma	15.17
36	Tennessee	14.79
37	South Carolina	14.62
38	Iowa	14.50
39	Nebraska	13.99
40	Alabama	13.79
41	Florida	13.45
42	Arkansas	13.23
43	Mississippi	13.22
44	Utah	12.63
45	Montana	11.86
46	South Dakota	11.77
47	Nevada	11.53
48	North Dakota	10.90
49	Wyoming	10.26
50	Idaho	9.43

District of Columbia   25.99

Source: Morgan Quitno Press using data from American Medical Association
"Physician Characteristics and Distribution in the U.S." (1994 Edition)
*As of January 1, 1993. Comprised of federal and nonfederal physicians. National rate does not include physicians in the U.S. territories and possessions, at APO's and FPO's and whose addresses are unknown.

Physicians Under 35 Years Old in 1993

National Total = 132,118 Physicians*

ALPHA ORDER

RANK	STATE	PHYSICIANS	% of USA
24	Alabama	1,579	1.18%
49	Alaska	109	0.08%
27	Arizona	1,486	1.11%
32	Arkansas	806	0.60%
2	California	13,836	10.32%
23	Colorado	1,609	1.20%
18	Connecticut	2,518	1.88%
43	Delaware	318	0.24%
8	Florida	4,869	3.63%
16	Georgia	2,745	2.05%
39	Hawaii	563	0.42%
47	Idaho	163	0.12%
5	Illinois	7,122	5.31%
22	Indiana	2,034	1.52%
28	Iowa	1,075	0.80%
29	Kansas	1,059	0.79%
26	Kentucky	1,502	1.12%
21	Louisiana	2,059	1.54%
42	Maine	323	0.24%
10	Maryland	4,459	3.33%
7	Massachusetts	5,902	4.40%
9	Michigan	4,850	3.62%
15	Minnesota	2,789	2.08%
35	Mississippi	713	0.53%
14	Missouri	2,905	2.17%
48	Montana	147	0.11%
34	Nebraska	734	0.55%
44	Nevada	239	0.18%
40	New Hampshire	385	0.29%
11	New Jersey	4,096	3.05%
38	New Mexico	574	0.43%
1	New York	15,811	11.79%
12	North Carolina	3,451	2.57%
46	North Dakota	202	0.15%
6	Ohio	6,039	4.50%
31	Oklahoma	948	0.71%
30	Oregon	973	0.73%
3	Pennsylvania	7,909	5.90%
36	Rhode Island	683	0.51%
25	South Carolina	1,567	1.17%
45	South Dakota	209	0.16%
17	Tennessee	2,529	1.89%
4	Texas	7,669	5.72%
33	Utah	770	0.57%
41	Vermont	338	0.25%
13	Virginia	3,293	2.46%
20	Washington	2,074	1.55%
37	West Virginia	634	0.47%
19	Wisconsin	2,297	1.71%
50	Wyoming	91	0.07%

RANK ORDER

RANK	STATE	PHYSICIANS	% of USA
1	New York	15,811	11.79%
2	California	13,836	10.32%
3	Pennsylvania	7,909	5.90%
4	Texas	7,669	5.72%
5	Illinois	7,122	5.31%
6	Ohio	6,039	4.50%
7	Massachusetts	5,902	4.40%
8	Florida	4,869	3.63%
9	Michigan	4,850	3.62%
10	Maryland	4,459	3.33%
11	New Jersey	4,096	3.05%
12	North Carolina	3,451	2.57%
13	Virginia	3,293	2.46%
14	Missouri	2,905	2.17%
15	Minnesota	2,789	2.08%
16	Georgia	2,745	2.05%
17	Tennessee	2,529	1.89%
18	Connecticut	2,518	1.88%
19	Wisconsin	2,297	1.71%
20	Washington	2,074	1.55%
21	Louisiana	2,059	1.54%
22	Indiana	2,034	1.52%
23	Colorado	1,609	1.20%
24	Alabama	1,579	1.18%
25	South Carolina	1,567	1.17%
26	Kentucky	1,502	1.12%
27	Arizona	1,486	1.11%
28	Iowa	1,075	0.80%
29	Kansas	1,059	0.79%
30	Oregon	973	0.73%
31	Oklahoma	948	0.71%
32	Arkansas	806	0.60%
33	Utah	770	0.57%
34	Nebraska	734	0.55%
35	Mississippi	713	0.53%
36	Rhode Island	683	0.51%
37	West Virginia	634	0.47%
38	New Mexico	574	0.43%
39	Hawaii	563	0.42%
40	New Hampshire	385	0.29%
41	Vermont	338	0.25%
42	Maine	323	0.24%
43	Delaware	318	0.24%
44	Nevada	239	0.18%
45	South Dakota	209	0.16%
46	North Dakota	202	0.15%
47	Idaho	163	0.12%
48	Montana	147	0.11%
49	Alaska	109	0.08%
50	Wyoming	91	0.07%
	District of Columbia	1,063	0.79%

Source: American Medical Association (Chicago, Illinois)
  "Physician Characteristics and Distribution in the U.S." (1994 Edition)
*As of January 1, 1993. Comprised of federal and nonfederal physicians. Total does not include 1,961 physicians in the U.S. territories and possessions, at APO's and FPO's and whose addresses are unknown.

Percent of Physicians Under 35 Years Old in 1993

National Percent = 20.03% of Physicians*

<table>
<tr><td colspan="3"><u>ALPHA ORDER</u></td><td colspan="3"><u>RANK ORDER</u></td></tr>
<tr><td>RANK</td><td>STATE</td><td>PERCENT</td><td>RANK</td><td>STATE</td><td>PERCENT</td></tr>
<tr><td>22</td><td>Alabama</td><td>19.84</td><td>1</td><td>Massachusetts</td><td>24.65</td></tr>
<tr><td>47</td><td>Alaska</td><td>11.05</td><td>2</td><td>Missouri</td><td>24.37</td></tr>
<tr><td>37</td><td>Arizona</td><td>15.94</td><td>3</td><td>Illinois</td><td>24.02</td></tr>
<tr><td>30</td><td>Arkansas</td><td>17.84</td><td>4</td><td>Minnesota</td><td>23.78</td></tr>
<tr><td>36</td><td>California</td><td>16.00</td><td>5</td><td>Michigan</td><td>23.57</td></tr>
<tr><td>31</td><td>Colorado</td><td>17.66</td><td>6</td><td>New York</td><td>23.54</td></tr>
<tr><td>14</td><td>Connecticut</td><td>21.44</td><td>7</td><td>Ohio</td><td>23.43</td></tr>
<tr><td>27</td><td>Delaware</td><td>19.15</td><td>8</td><td>Pennsylvania</td><td>23.11</td></tr>
<tr><td>43</td><td>Florida</td><td>13.47</td><td>9</td><td>Rhode Island</td><td>22.43</td></tr>
<tr><td>25</td><td>Georgia</td><td>19.21</td><td>10</td><td>Maryland</td><td>22.33</td></tr>
<tr><td>35</td><td>Hawaii</td><td>16.86</td><td>11</td><td>North Carolina</td><td>22.20</td></tr>
<tr><td>49</td><td>Idaho</td><td>9.61</td><td>12</td><td>South Carolina</td><td>21.74</td></tr>
<tr><td>3</td><td>Illinois</td><td>24.02</td><td>13</td><td>Louisiana</td><td>21.54</td></tr>
<tr><td>28</td><td>Indiana</td><td>18.99</td><td>14</td><td>Connecticut</td><td>21.44</td></tr>
<tr><td>18</td><td>Iowa</td><td>21.01</td><td>15</td><td>Nebraska</td><td>21.39</td></tr>
<tr><td>23</td><td>Kansas</td><td>19.63</td><td>16</td><td>Tennessee</td><td>21.18</td></tr>
<tr><td>21</td><td>Kentucky</td><td>19.99</td><td>17</td><td>Texas</td><td>21.02</td></tr>
<tr><td>13</td><td>Louisiana</td><td>21.54</td><td>18</td><td>Iowa</td><td>21.01</td></tr>
<tr><td>46</td><td>Maine</td><td>11.43</td><td>19</td><td>Virginia</td><td>20.61</td></tr>
<tr><td>10</td><td>Maryland</td><td>22.33</td><td>20</td><td>Wisconsin</td><td>20.39</td></tr>
<tr><td>1</td><td>Massachusetts</td><td>24.65</td><td>21</td><td>Kentucky</td><td>19.99</td></tr>
<tr><td>5</td><td>Michigan</td><td>23.57</td><td>22</td><td>Alabama</td><td>19.84</td></tr>
<tr><td>4</td><td>Minnesota</td><td>23.78</td><td>23</td><td>Kansas</td><td>19.63</td></tr>
<tr><td>32</td><td>Mississippi</td><td>17.45</td><td>24</td><td>Utah</td><td>19.45</td></tr>
<tr><td>2</td><td>Missouri</td><td>24.37</td><td>25</td><td>Georgia</td><td>19.21</td></tr>
<tr><td>50</td><td>Montana</td><td>8.71</td><td>26</td><td>Vermont</td><td>19.16</td></tr>
<tr><td>15</td><td>Nebraska</td><td>21.39</td><td>27</td><td>Delaware</td><td>19.15</td></tr>
<tr><td>48</td><td>Nevada</td><td>10.20</td><td>28</td><td>Indiana</td><td>18.99</td></tr>
<tr><td>42</td><td>New Hampshire</td><td>14.02</td><td>29</td><td>New Jersey</td><td>17.90</td></tr>
<tr><td>29</td><td>New Jersey</td><td>17.90</td><td>30</td><td>Arkansas</td><td>17.84</td></tr>
<tr><td>38</td><td>New Mexico</td><td>15.80</td><td>31</td><td>Colorado</td><td>17.66</td></tr>
<tr><td>6</td><td>New York</td><td>23.54</td><td>32</td><td>Mississippi</td><td>17.45</td></tr>
<tr><td>11</td><td>North Carolina</td><td>22.20</td><td>33</td><td>Oklahoma</td><td>17.08</td></tr>
<tr><td>41</td><td>North Dakota</td><td>14.87</td><td>34</td><td>West Virginia</td><td>17.03</td></tr>
<tr><td>7</td><td>Ohio</td><td>23.43</td><td>35</td><td>Hawaii</td><td>16.86</td></tr>
<tr><td>33</td><td>Oklahoma</td><td>17.08</td><td>36</td><td>California</td><td>16.00</td></tr>
<tr><td>44</td><td>Oregon</td><td>12.99</td><td>37</td><td>Arizona</td><td>15.94</td></tr>
<tr><td>8</td><td>Pennsylvania</td><td>23.11</td><td>38</td><td>New Mexico</td><td>15.80</td></tr>
<tr><td>9</td><td>Rhode Island</td><td>22.43</td><td>39</td><td>South Dakota</td><td>15.77</td></tr>
<tr><td>12</td><td>South Carolina</td><td>21.74</td><td>40</td><td>Washington</td><td>15.23</td></tr>
<tr><td>39</td><td>South Dakota</td><td>15.77</td><td>41</td><td>North Dakota</td><td>14.87</td></tr>
<tr><td>16</td><td>Tennessee</td><td>21.18</td><td>42</td><td>New Hampshire</td><td>14.02</td></tr>
<tr><td>17</td><td>Texas</td><td>21.02</td><td>43</td><td>Florida</td><td>13.47</td></tr>
<tr><td>24</td><td>Utah</td><td>19.45</td><td>44</td><td>Oregon</td><td>12.99</td></tr>
<tr><td>26</td><td>Vermont</td><td>19.16</td><td>45</td><td>Wyoming</td><td>11.67</td></tr>
<tr><td>19</td><td>Virginia</td><td>20.61</td><td>46</td><td>Maine</td><td>11.43</td></tr>
<tr><td>40</td><td>Washington</td><td>15.23</td><td>47</td><td>Alaska</td><td>11.05</td></tr>
<tr><td>34</td><td>West Virginia</td><td>17.03</td><td>48</td><td>Nevada</td><td>10.20</td></tr>
<tr><td>20</td><td>Wisconsin</td><td>20.39</td><td>49</td><td>Idaho</td><td>9.61</td></tr>
<tr><td>45</td><td>Wyoming</td><td>11.67</td><td>50</td><td>Montana</td><td>8.71</td></tr>
<tr><td></td><td></td><td></td><td></td><td>District of Columbia</td><td>23.78</td></tr>
</table>

Source: Morgan Quitno Press using data from American Medical Association
"Physician Characteristics and Distribution in the U.S." (1994 Edition)
As of January 1, 1993. Comprised of federal and nonfederal physicians. National rate does not include physicians in the U.S. territories and possessions, at APO's and FPO's and whose addresses are unknown.

Physicians 35 to 44 Years Old in 1993

National total = 199,048 Physicians*

ALPHA ORDER					RANK ORDER			
RANK	STATE	PHYSICIANS	% of USA		RANK	STATE	PHYSICIANS	% of USA
25	Alabama	2,648	1.33%		1	California	24,698	12.41%
49	Alaska	346	0.17%		2	New York	19,017	9.55%
24	Arizona	2,704	1.36%		3	Texas	11,188	5.62%
32	Arkansas	1,488	0.75%		4	Florida	10,361	5.21%
1	California	24,698	12.41%		5	Pennsylvania	10,302	5.18%
22	Colorado	3,005	1.51%		6	Illinois	8,521	4.28%
20	Connecticut	3,549	1.78%		7	Massachusetts	7,423	3.73%
48	Delaware	451	0.23%		8	Ohio	7,413	3.72%
4	Florida	10,361	5.21%		9	New Jersey	7,140	3.59%
14	Georgia	4,769	2.40%		10	Maryland	6,276	3.15%
38	Hawaii	1,060	0.53%		11	Michigan	5,814	2.92%
44	Idaho	529	0.27%		12	North Carolina	5,051	2.54%
6	Illinois	8,521	4.28%		13	Virginia	4,899	2.46%
21	Indiana	3,356	1.69%		14	Georgia	4,769	2.40%
31	Iowa	1,591	0.80%		15	Washington	4,561	2.29%
30	Kansas	1,599	0.80%		16	Tennessee	3,951	1.98%
26	Kentucky	2,358	1.18%		17	Minnesota	3,842	1.93%
23	Louisiana	2,874	1.44%		18	Missouri	3,642	1.83%
41	Maine	875	0.44%		19	Wisconsin	3,586	1.80%
10	Maryland	6,276	3.15%		20	Connecticut	3,549	1.78%
7	Massachusetts	7,423	3.73%		21	Indiana	3,356	1.69%
11	Michigan	5,814	2.92%		22	Colorado	3,005	1.51%
17	Minnesota	3,842	1.93%		23	Louisiana	2,874	1.44%
34	Mississippi	1,236	0.62%		24	Arizona	2,704	1.36%
18	Missouri	3,642	1.83%		25	Alabama	2,648	1.33%
45	Montana	523	0.26%		26	Kentucky	2,358	1.18%
36	Nebraska	1,099	0.55%		27	Oregon	2,315	1.16%
42	Nevada	809	0.41%		28	South Carolina	2,214	1.11%
39	New Hampshire	913	0.46%		29	Oklahoma	1,709	0.86%
9	New Jersey	7,140	3.59%		30	Kansas	1,599	0.80%
35	New Mexico	1,217	0.61%		31	Iowa	1,591	0.80%
2	New York	19,017	9.55%		32	Arkansas	1,488	0.75%
12	North Carolina	5,051	2.54%		33	Utah	1,282	0.64%
46	North Dakota	483	0.24%		34	Mississippi	1,236	0.62%
8	Ohio	7,413	3.72%		35	New Mexico	1,217	0.61%
29	Oklahoma	1,709	0.86%		36	Nebraska	1,099	0.55%
27	Oregon	2,315	1.16%		37	West Virginia	1,083	0.54%
5	Pennsylvania	10,302	5.18%		38	Hawaii	1,060	0.53%
40	Rhode Island	907	0.46%		39	New Hampshire	913	0.46%
28	South Carolina	2,214	1.11%		40	Rhode Island	907	0.46%
47	South Dakota	472	0.24%		41	Maine	875	0.44%
16	Tennessee	3,951	1.98%		42	Nevada	809	0.41%
3	Texas	11,188	5.62%		43	Vermont	541	0.27%
33	Utah	1,282	0.64%		44	Idaho	529	0.27%
43	Vermont	541	0.27%		45	Montana	523	0.26%
13	Virginia	4,899	2.46%		46	North Dakota	483	0.24%
15	Washington	4,561	2.29%		47	South Dakota	472	0.24%
37	West Virginia	1,083	0.54%		48	Delaware	451	0.23%
19	Wisconsin	3,586	1.80%		49	Alaska	346	0.17%
50	Wyoming	240	0.12%		50	Wyoming	240	0.12%
						District of Columbia	1,118	0.56%

Source: American Medical Association (Chicago, Illinois)
    "Physician Characteristics and Distribution in the U.S." (1994 Edition)
*As of January 1, 1993. Comprised of federal and nonfederal physicians. Total does not include 2,941 physicians in the U.S. territories and possessions, at APO's and FPO's and whose addresses are unknown.

Physicians 45 to 54 Years Old in 1993

National Total = 134,374 Physicians*

ALPHA ORDER

RANK	STATE	PHYSICIANS	% of USA
26	Alabama	1,592	1.18%
47	Alaska	303	0.23%
24	Arizona	1,892	1.41%
33	Arkansas	891	0.66%
1	California	19,431	14.46%
22	Colorado	2,013	1.50%
18	Connecticut	2,222	1.65%
45	Delaware	359	0.27%
4	Florida	7,118	5.30%
13	Georgia	3,030	2.25%
37	Hawaii	718	0.53%
44	Idaho	410	0.31%
6	Illinois	6,274	4.67%
21	Indiana	2,117	1.58%
31	Iowa	960	0.71%
30	Kansas	1,093	0.81%
27	Kentucky	1,514	1.13%
23	Louisiana	1,950	1.45%
39	Maine	624	0.46%
10	Maryland	4,173	3.11%
9	Massachusetts	4,584	3.41%
11	Michigan	4,136	3.08%
20	Minnesota	2,131	1.59%
36	Mississippi	802	0.60%
17	Missouri	2,300	1.71%
43	Montana	416	0.31%
38	Nebraska	666	0.50%
42	Nevada	532	0.40%
40	New Hampshire	568	0.42%
7	New Jersey	4,963	3.69%
35	New Mexico	820	0.61%
2	New York	12,537	9.33%
15	North Carolina	2,815	2.09%
48	North Dakota	294	0.22%
8	Ohio	4,879	3.63%
29	Oklahoma	1,161	0.86%
25	Oregon	1,824	1.36%
5	Pennsylvania	6,335	4.71%
41	Rhode Island	546	0.41%
28	South Carolina	1,384	1.03%
49	South Dakota	253	0.19%
16	Tennessee	2,322	1.73%
3	Texas	7,551	5.62%
34	Utah	871	0.65%
46	Vermont	334	0.25%
12	Virginia	3,324	2.47%
14	Washington	3,004	2.24%
32	West Virginia	920	0.68%
19	Wisconsin	2,207	1.64%
50	Wyoming	194	0.14%

RANK ORDER

RANK	STATE	PHYSICIANS	% of USA
1	California	19,431	14.46%
2	New York	12,537	9.33%
3	Texas	7,551	5.62%
4	Florida	7,118	5.30%
5	Pennsylvania	6,335	4.71%
6	Illinois	6,274	4.67%
7	New Jersey	4,963	3.69%
8	Ohio	4,879	3.63%
9	Massachusetts	4,584	3.41%
10	Maryland	4,173	3.11%
11	Michigan	4,136	3.08%
12	Virginia	3,324	2.47%
13	Georgia	3,030	2.25%
14	Washington	3,004	2.24%
15	North Carolina	2,815	2.09%
16	Tennessee	2,322	1.73%
17	Missouri	2,300	1.71%
18	Connecticut	2,222	1.65%
19	Wisconsin	2,207	1.64%
20	Minnesota	2,131	1.59%
21	Indiana	2,117	1.58%
22	Colorado	2,013	1.50%
23	Louisiana	1,950	1.45%
24	Arizona	1,892	1.41%
25	Oregon	1,824	1.36%
26	Alabama	1,592	1.18%
27	Kentucky	1,514	1.13%
28	South Carolina	1,384	1.03%
29	Oklahoma	1,161	0.86%
30	Kansas	1,093	0.81%
31	Iowa	960	0.71%
32	West Virginia	920	0.68%
33	Arkansas	891	0.66%
34	Utah	871	0.65%
35	New Mexico	820	0.61%
36	Mississippi	802	0.60%
37	Hawaii	718	0.53%
38	Nebraska	666	0.50%
39	Maine	624	0.46%
40	New Hampshire	568	0.42%
41	Rhode Island	546	0.41%
42	Nevada	532	0.40%
43	Montana	416	0.31%
44	Idaho	410	0.31%
45	Delaware	359	0.27%
46	Vermont	334	0.25%
47	Alaska	303	0.23%
48	North Dakota	294	0.22%
49	South Dakota	253	0.19%
50	Wyoming	194	0.14%
	District of Columbia	1,017	0.76%

Source: American Medical Association (Chicago, Illinois)
   "Physician Characteristics and Distribution in the U.S." (1994 Edition)
*As of January 1, 1993. Comprised of federal and nonfederal physicians. Total does not include 1,785 physicians in the U.S. territories and possessions, at APO's and FPO's and whose addresses are unknown.

Physicians 55 to 64 Years Old in 1993

National Total = 87,721 Physicians*

ALPHA ORDER					RANK ORDER			
RANK	STATE		PHYSICIANS	% of USA	RANK	STATE	PHYSICIANS	% of USA
26	Alabama		1,015	1.16%	1	California	12,443	14.18%
49	Alaska		149	0.17%	2	New York	9,250	10.54%
22	Arizona		1,339	1.53%	3	Florida	5,020	5.72%
33	Arkansas		599	0.68%	4	Texas	4,918	5.61%
1	California		12,443	14.18%	5	Pennsylvania	4,231	4.82%
24	Colorado		1,185	1.35%	6	Illinois	3,564	4.06%
16	Connecticut		1,517	1.73%	7	Ohio	3,360	3.83%
45	Delaware		253	0.29%	8	New Jersey	3,248	3.70%
3	Florida		5,020	5.72%	9	Michigan	2,808	3.20%
14	Georgia		1,866	2.13%	10	Massachusetts	2,714	3.09%
36	Hawaii		442	0.50%	11	Maryland	2,507	2.86%
43	Idaho		263	0.30%	12	Virginia	2,121	2.42%
6	Illinois		3,564	4.06%	13	North Carolina	1,880	2.14%
20	Indiana		1,445	1.65%	14	Georgia	1,866	2.13%
32	Iowa		643	0.73%	15	Washington	1,678	1.91%
30	Kansas		687	0.78%	16	Connecticut	1,517	1.73%
25	Kentucky		1,056	1.20%	17	Wisconsin	1,511	1.72%
23	Louisiana		1,300	1.48%	18	Missouri	1,493	1.70%
41	Maine		378	0.43%	19	Tennessee	1,483	1.69%
11	Maryland		2,507	2.86%	20	Indiana	1,445	1.65%
10	Massachusetts		2,714	3.09%	21	Minnesota	1,374	1.57%
9	Michigan		2,808	3.20%	22	Arizona	1,339	1.53%
21	Minnesota		1,374	1.57%	23	Louisiana	1,300	1.48%
31	Mississippi		644	0.73%	24	Colorado	1,185	1.35%
18	Missouri		1,493	1.70%	25	Kentucky	1,056	1.20%
44	Montana		261	0.30%	26	Alabama	1,015	1.16%
38	Nebraska		427	0.49%	27	Oregon	1,013	1.15%
40	Nevada		380	0.43%	28	South Carolina	894	1.02%
42	New Hampshire		356	0.41%	29	Oklahoma	854	0.97%
8	New Jersey		3,248	3.70%	30	Kansas	687	0.78%
37	New Mexico		438	0.50%	31	Mississippi	644	0.73%
2	New York		9,250	10.54%	32	Iowa	643	0.73%
13	North Carolina		1,880	2.14%	33	Arkansas	599	0.68%
47	North Dakota		208	0.24%	34	West Virginia	511	0.58%
7	Ohio		3,360	3.83%	35	Utah	448	0.51%
29	Oklahoma		854	0.97%	36	Hawaii	442	0.50%
27	Oregon		1,013	1.15%	37	New Mexico	438	0.50%
5	Pennsylvania		4,231	4.82%	38	Nebraska	427	0.49%
39	Rhode Island		398	0.45%	39	Rhode Island	398	0.45%
28	South Carolina		894	1.02%	40	Nevada	380	0.43%
48	South Dakota		180	0.21%	41	Maine	378	0.43%
19	Tennessee		1,483	1.69%	42	New Hampshire	356	0.41%
4	Texas		4,918	5.61%	43	Idaho	263	0.30%
35	Utah		448	0.51%	44	Montana	261	0.30%
46	Vermont		218	0.25%	45	Delaware	253	0.29%
12	Virginia		2,121	2.42%	46	Vermont	218	0.25%
15	Washington		1,678	1.91%	47	North Dakota	208	0.24%
34	West Virginia		511	0.58%	48	South Dakota	180	0.21%
17	Wisconsin		1,511	1.72%	49	Alaska	149	0.17%
50	Wyoming		119	0.14%	50	Wyoming	119	0.14%
						District of Columbia	632	0.72%

Source: American Medical Association (Chicago, Illinois)
"Physician Characteristics and Distribution in the U.S." (1994 Edition)
*As of January 1, 1993. Comprised of federal and nonfederal physicians. Total does not include 1,584 physicians in the U.S. territories and possessions, at APO's and FPO's and whose addresses are unknown.

Physicians 65 Years Old and Older in 1993

National Total = 106,393 Physicians*

ALPHA ORDER

RANK ORDER

RANK	STATE	PHYSICIANS	% of USA
27	Alabama	1,126	1.06%
50	Alaska	79	0.07%
16	Arizona	1,902	1.79%
32	Arkansas	735	0.69%
1	California	16,071	15.11%
25	Colorado	1,300	1.22%
15	Connecticut	1,941	1.82%
46	Delaware	280	0.26%
3	Florida	8,774	8.25%
17	Georgia	1,877	1.76%
38	Hawaii	557	0.52%
45	Idaho	331	0.31%
6	Illinois	4,171	3.92%
18	Indiana	1,761	1.66%
31	Iowa	847	0.80%
29	Kansas	956	0.90%
28	Kentucky	1,085	1.02%
23	Louisiana	1,376	1.29%
34	Maine	626	0.59%
11	Maryland	2,554	2.40%
9	Massachusetts	3,324	3.12%
10	Michigan	2,966	2.79%
21	Minnesota	1,590	1.49%
33	Mississippi	691	0.65%
22	Missouri	1,578	1.48%
43	Montana	340	0.32%
41	Nebraska	506	0.48%
42	Nevada	382	0.36%
39	New Hampshire	525	0.49%
8	New Jersey	3,436	3.23%
36	New Mexico	583	0.55%
2	New York	10,550	9.92%
12	North Carolina	2,351	2.21%
48	North Dakota	171	0.16%
7	Ohio	4,089	3.84%
30	Oklahoma	877	0.82%
24	Oregon	1,363	1.28%
4	Pennsylvania	5,447	5.12%
40	Rhode Island	511	0.48%
26	South Carolina	1,149	1.08%
47	South Dakota	211	0.20%
20	Tennessee	1,658	1.56%
5	Texas	5,161	4.85%
35	Utah	588	0.55%
44	Vermont	333	0.31%
13	Virginia	2,344	2.20%
14	Washington	2,301	2.16%
37	West Virginia	575	0.54%
19	Wisconsin	1,667	1.57%
49	Wyoming	136	0.13%

RANK	STATE	PHYSICIANS	% of USA
1	California	16,071	15.11%
2	New York	10,550	9.92%
3	Florida	8,774	8.25%
4	Pennsylvania	5,447	5.12%
5	Texas	5,161	4.85%
6	Illinois	4,171	3.92%
7	Ohio	4,089	3.84%
8	New Jersey	3,436	3.23%
9	Massachusetts	3,324	3.12%
10	Michigan	2,966	2.79%
11	Maryland	2,554	2.40%
12	North Carolina	2,351	2.21%
13	Virginia	2,344	2.20%
14	Washington	2,301	2.16%
15	Connecticut	1,941	1.82%
16	Arizona	1,902	1.79%
17	Georgia	1,877	1.76%
18	Indiana	1,761	1.66%
19	Wisconsin	1,667	1.57%
20	Tennessee	1,658	1.56%
21	Minnesota	1,590	1.49%
22	Missouri	1,578	1.48%
23	Louisiana	1,376	1.29%
24	Oregon	1,363	1.28%
25	Colorado	1,300	1.22%
26	South Carolina	1,149	1.08%
27	Alabama	1,126	1.06%
28	Kentucky	1,085	1.02%
29	Kansas	956	0.90%
30	Oklahoma	877	0.82%
31	Iowa	847	0.80%
32	Arkansas	735	0.69%
33	Mississippi	691	0.65%
34	Maine	626	0.59%
35	Utah	588	0.55%
36	New Mexico	583	0.55%
37	West Virginia	575	0.54%
38	Hawaii	557	0.52%
39	New Hampshire	525	0.49%
40	Rhode Island	511	0.48%
41	Nebraska	506	0.48%
42	Nevada	382	0.36%
43	Montana	340	0.32%
44	Vermont	333	0.31%
45	Idaho	331	0.31%
46	Delaware	280	0.26%
47	South Dakota	211	0.20%
48	North Dakota	171	0.16%
49	Wyoming	136	0.13%
50	Alaska	79	0.07%
	District of Columbia	641	0.60%

Source: American Medical Association (Chicago, Illinois)
"Physician Characteristics and Distribution in the U.S." (1994 Edition)
*As of January 1, 1993. Comprised of federal and nonfederal physicians. Total does not include 2,411 physicians in the U.S. territories and possessions, at APO's and FPO's and whose addresses are unknown.

Percent of Physicians 65 Years Old and Older in 1993

National Percent = 16.13% of Physicians*

ALPHA ORDER

RANK ORDER

RANK	STATE	PERCENT		RANK	STATE	PERCENT
40	Alabama	14.15		1	Florida	24.28
50	Alaska	8.01		2	Maine	22.15
3	Arizona	20.40		3	Arizona	20.40
21	Arkansas	16.26		4	Montana	20.15
8	California	18.58		5	Idaho	19.52
39	Colorado	14.27		6	New Hampshire	19.11
18	Connecticut	16.52		7	Vermont	18.88
14	Delaware	16.86		8	California	18.58
1	Florida	24.28		9	Oregon	18.20
47	Georgia	13.14		10	Kansas	17.72
16	Hawaii	16.68		11	Wyoming	17.44
5	Idaho	19.52		12	Mississippi	16.91
42	Illinois	14.07		13	Washington	16.90
19	Indiana	16.44		14	Delaware	16.86
17	Iowa	16.56		15	Rhode Island	16.78
10	Kansas	17.72		16	Hawaii	16.68
36	Kentucky	14.44		17	Iowa	16.56
38	Louisiana	14.39		18	Connecticut	16.52
2	Maine	22.15		19	Indiana	16.44
48	Maryland	12.79		20	Nevada	16.31
43	Massachusetts	13.88		21	Arkansas	16.26
37	Michigan	14.42		22	New Mexico	16.05
45	Minnesota	13.56		23	South Carolina	15.94
12	Mississippi	16.91		24	Pennsylvania	15.92
46	Missouri	13.24		24	South Dakota	15.92
4	Montana	20.15		26	Ohio	15.86
34	Nebraska	14.74		27	Oklahoma	15.80
20	Nevada	16.31		28	New York	15.71
6	New Hampshire	19.11		29	West Virginia	15.44
31	New Jersey	15.02		30	North Carolina	15.12
22	New Mexico	16.05		31	New Jersey	15.02
28	New York	15.71		32	Utah	14.85
30	North Carolina	15.12		33	Wisconsin	14.79
49	North Dakota	12.59		34	Nebraska	14.74
26	Ohio	15.86		35	Virginia	14.67
27	Oklahoma	15.80		36	Kentucky	14.44
9	Oregon	18.20		37	Michigan	14.42
24	Pennsylvania	15.92		38	Louisiana	14.39
15	Rhode Island	16.78		39	Colorado	14.27
23	South Carolina	15.94		40	Alabama	14.15
24	South Dakota	15.92		41	Texas	14.14
43	Tennessee	13.88		42	Illinois	14.07
41	Texas	14.14		43	Massachusetts	13.88
32	Utah	14.85		43	Tennessee	13.88
7	Vermont	18.88		45	Minnesota	13.56
35	Virginia	14.67		46	Missouri	13.24
13	Washington	16.90		47	Georgia	13.14
29	West Virginia	15.44		48	Maryland	12.79
33	Wisconsin	14.79		49	North Dakota	12.59
11	Wyoming	17.44		50	Alaska	8.01
					District of Columbia	14.34

Source: Morgan Quitno Press using data from American Medical Association
"Physician Characteristics and Distribution in the U.S." (1994 Edition)

*As of January 1, 1993. Comprised of federal and nonfederal physicians. National rate does not include physicians in the U.S. territories and possessions, at APO's and FPO's and whose addresses are unknown.

Federal Physicians in 1993

National Total = 20,439 Physicians*

<u>ALPHA ORDER</u>

RANK	STATE	PHYSICIANS	% of USA
22	Alabama	288	1.41%
37	Alaska	113	0.55%
15	Arizona	358	1.75%
33	Arkansas	166	0.81%
1	California	2,654	12.98%
13	Colorado	422	2.06%
32	Connecticut	167	0.82%
44	Delaware	62	0.30%
4	Florida	983	4.81%
7	Georgia	812	3.97%
24	Hawaii	266	1.30%
47	Idaho	54	0.26%
9	Illinois	578	2.83%
35	Indiana	141	0.69%
39	Iowa	98	0.48%
28	Kansas	187	0.91%
30	Kentucky	181	0.89%
20	Louisiana	293	1.43%
42	Maine	70	0.34%
3	Maryland	1,973	9.65%
14	Massachusetts	421	2.06%
23	Michigan	275	1.35%
25	Minnesota	233	1.14%
17	Mississippi	323	1.58%
19	Missouri	309	1.51%
46	Montana	58	0.28%
36	Nebraska	128	0.63%
43	Nevada	67	0.33%
49	New Hampshire	46	0.23%
21	New Jersey	290	1.42%
26	New Mexico	202	0.99%
6	New York	952	4.66%
11	North Carolina	512	2.51%
45	North Dakota	59	0.29%
10	Ohio	569	2.78%
27	Oklahoma	194	0.95%
29	Oregon	182	0.89%
12	Pennsylvania	498	2.44%
41	Rhode Island	79	0.39%
18	South Carolina	316	1.55%
40	South Dakota	82	0.40%
16	Tennessee	330	1.61%
2	Texas	1,981	9.69%
34	Utah	161	0.79%
50	Vermont	36	0.18%
5	Virginia	973	4.76%
8	Washington	597	2.92%
38	West Virginia	107	0.52%
31	Wisconsin	177	0.87%
48	Wyoming	52	0.25%

<u>RANK ORDER</u>

RANK	STATE	PHYSICIANS	% of USA
1	California	2,654	12.98%
2	Texas	1,981	9.69%
3	Maryland	1,973	9.65%
4	Florida	983	4.81%
5	Virginia	973	4.76%
6	New York	952	4.66%
7	Georgia	812	3.97%
8	Washington	597	2.92%
9	Illinois	578	2.83%
10	Ohio	569	2.78%
11	North Carolina	512	2.51%
12	Pennsylvania	498	2.44%
13	Colorado	422	2.06%
14	Massachusetts	421	2.06%
15	Arizona	358	1.75%
16	Tennessee	330	1.61%
17	Mississippi	323	1.58%
18	South Carolina	316	1.55%
19	Missouri	309	1.51%
20	Louisiana	293	1.43%
21	New Jersey	290	1.42%
22	Alabama	288	1.41%
23	Michigan	275	1.35%
24	Hawaii	266	1.30%
25	Minnesota	233	1.14%
26	New Mexico	202	0.99%
27	Oklahoma	194	0.95%
28	Kansas	187	0.91%
29	Oregon	182	0.89%
30	Kentucky	181	0.89%
31	Wisconsin	177	0.87%
32	Connecticut	167	0.82%
33	Arkansas	166	0.81%
34	Utah	161	0.79%
35	Indiana	141	0.69%
36	Nebraska	128	0.63%
37	Alaska	113	0.55%
38	West Virginia	107	0.52%
39	Iowa	98	0.48%
40	South Dakota	82	0.40%
41	Rhode Island	79	0.39%
42	Maine	70	0.34%
43	Nevada	67	0.33%
44	Delaware	62	0.30%
45	North Dakota	59	0.29%
46	Montana	58	0.28%
47	Idaho	54	0.26%
48	Wyoming	52	0.25%
49	New Hampshire	46	0.23%
50	Vermont	36	0.18%
	District of Columbia	364	1.78%

Source: American Medical Association (Chicago, Illinois)
"Physician Characteristics and Distribution in the U.S." (1994 Edition)
As of January 1, 1993. Total does not include 1,235 physicians in the U.S. territories and possessions, at APO's and FPO's.

Rate of Federal Physicians in 1993

National Rate = 7.93 Physicians per 100,000 Population*

ALPHA ORDER				RANK ORDER		
RANK	STATE	RATE		RANK	STATE	RATE
26	Alabama	6.89		1	Maryland	39.79
3	Alaska	18.90		2	Hawaii	22.81
14	Arizona	9.07		3	Alaska	18.90
27	Arkansas	6.84		4	Virginia	15.03
18	California	8.50		5	New Mexico	12.50
7	Colorado	11.84		6	Mississippi	12.23
39	Connecticut	5.09		7	Colorado	11.84
15	Delaware	8.88		8	Georgia	11.76
23	Florida	7.16		9	South Dakota	11.45
8	Georgia	11.76		10	Washington	11.35
2	Hawaii	22.81		11	Wyoming	11.06
41	Idaho	4.91		12	Texas	10.99
40	Illinois	4.95		13	North Dakota	9.26
50	Indiana	2.47		14	Arizona	9.07
48	Iowa	3.47		15	Delaware	8.88
21	Kansas	7.38		16	South Carolina	8.71
43	Kentucky	4.77		17	Utah	8.66
28	Louisiana	6.83		18	California	8.50
35	Maine	5.65		19	Nebraska	7.94
1	Maryland	39.79		20	Rhode Island	7.90
24	Massachusetts	7.00		21	Kansas	7.38
49	Michigan	2.91		22	North Carolina	7.36
37	Minnesota	5.15		23	Florida	7.16
6	Mississippi	12.23		24	Massachusetts	7.00
33	Missouri	5.90		25	Montana	6.90
25	Montana	6.90		26	Alabama	6.89
19	Nebraska	7.94		27	Arkansas	6.84
42	Nevada	4.85		28	Louisiana	6.83
45	New Hampshire	4.09		29	Tennessee	6.48
46	New Jersey	3.69		30	Vermont	6.25
5	New Mexico	12.50		31	Oklahoma	6.00
36	New York	5.24		31	Oregon	6.00
22	North Carolina	7.36		33	Missouri	5.90
13	North Dakota	9.26		34	West Virginia	5.89
38	Ohio	5.14		35	Maine	5.65
31	Oklahoma	6.00		36	New York	5.24
31	Oregon	6.00		37	Minnesota	5.15
44	Pennsylvania	4.14		38	Ohio	5.14
20	Rhode Island	7.90		39	Connecticut	5.09
16	South Carolina	8.71		40	Illinois	4.95
9	South Dakota	11.45		41	Idaho	4.91
29	Tennessee	6.48		42	Nevada	4.85
12	Texas	10.99		43	Kentucky	4.77
17	Utah	8.66		44	Pennsylvania	4.14
30	Vermont	6.25		45	New Hampshire	4.09
4	Virginia	15.03		46	New Jersey	3.69
10	Washington	11.35		47	Wisconsin	3.51
34	West Virginia	5.89		48	Iowa	3.47
47	Wisconsin	3.51		49	Michigan	2.91
11	Wyoming	11.06		50	Indiana	2.47
					District of Columbia	62.87

Source: Morgan Quitno Press using data from American Medical Association
  "Physician Characteristics and Distribution in the U.S." (1994 Edition)
As of January 1, 1993. National rate does not include physicians in the U.S. territories and possessions, at APO's and FPO's.

Nonfederal Physicians in 1993

National Total = 639,215 Physicians*

ALPHA ORDER

RANK	STATE	PHYSICIANS	% of USA
25	Alabama	7,672	1.20%
49	Alaska	873	0.14%
23	Arizona	8,965	1.40%
32	Arkansas	4,353	0.68%
1	California	83,825	13.11%
24	Colorado	8,690	1.36%
18	Connecticut	11,580	1.81%
46	Delaware	1,599	0.25%
3	Florida	35,159	5.50%
14	Georgia	13,475	2.11%
38	Hawaii	3,074	0.48%
44	Idaho	1,642	0.26%
6	Illinois	29,074	4.55%
21	Indiana	10,572	1.65%
31	Iowa	5,018	0.79%
30	Kansas	5,207	0.81%
26	Kentucky	7,334	1.15%
22	Louisiana	9,266	1.45%
40	Maine	2,756	0.43%
11	Maryland	17,996	2.82%
8	Massachusetts	23,526	3.68%
10	Michigan	20,299	3.18%
19	Minnesota	11,493	1.80%
34	Mississippi	3,763	0.59%
17	Missouri	11,609	1.82%
45	Montana	1,629	0.25%
37	Nebraska	3,304	0.52%
42	Nevada	2,275	0.36%
41	New Hampshire	2,701	0.42%
9	New Jersey	22,593	3.53%
36	New Mexico	3,430	0.54%
2	New York	66,213	10.36%
12	North Carolina	15,036	2.35%
47	North Dakota	1,299	0.20%
7	Ohio	25,211	3.94%
29	Oklahoma	5,355	0.84%
27	Oregon	7,306	1.14%
5	Pennsylvania	33,726	5.28%
39	Rhode Island	2,966	0.46%
28	South Carolina	6,892	1.08%
48	South Dakota	1,243	0.19%
16	Tennessee	11,613	1.82%
4	Texas	34,506	5.40%
33	Utah	3,798	0.59%
43	Vermont	1,728	0.27%
13	Virginia	15,008	2.35%
15	Washington	13,021	2.04%
35	West Virginia	3,616	0.57%
20	Wisconsin	11,091	1.74%
50	Wyoming	728	0.11%

RANK ORDER

RANK	STATE	PHYSICIANS	% of USA
1	California	83,825	13.11%
2	New York	66,213	10.36%
3	Florida	35,159	5.50%
4	Texas	34,506	5.40%
5	Pennsylvania	33,726	5.28%
6	Illinois	29,074	4.55%
7	Ohio	25,211	3.94%
8	Massachusetts	23,526	3.68%
9	New Jersey	22,593	3.53%
10	Michigan	20,299	3.18%
11	Maryland	17,996	2.82%
12	North Carolina	15,036	2.35%
13	Virginia	15,008	2.35%
14	Georgia	13,475	2.11%
15	Washington	13,021	2.04%
16	Tennessee	11,613	1.82%
17	Missouri	11,609	1.82%
18	Connecticut	11,580	1.81%
19	Minnesota	11,493	1.80%
20	Wisconsin	11,091	1.74%
21	Indiana	10,572	1.65%
22	Louisiana	9,266	1.45%
23	Arizona	8,965	1.40%
24	Colorado	8,690	1.36%
25	Alabama	7,672	1.20%
26	Kentucky	7,334	1.15%
27	Oregon	7,306	1.14%
28	South Carolina	6,892	1.08%
29	Oklahoma	5,355	0.84%
30	Kansas	5,207	0.81%
31	Iowa	5,018	0.79%
32	Arkansas	4,353	0.68%
33	Utah	3,798	0.59%
34	Mississippi	3,763	0.59%
35	West Virginia	3,616	0.57%
36	New Mexico	3,430	0.54%
37	Nebraska	3,304	0.52%
38	Hawaii	3,074	0.48%
39	Rhode Island	2,966	0.46%
40	Maine	2,756	0.43%
41	New Hampshire	2,701	0.42%
42	Nevada	2,275	0.36%
43	Vermont	1,728	0.27%
44	Idaho	1,642	0.26%
45	Montana	1,629	0.25%
46	Delaware	1,599	0.25%
47	North Dakota	1,299	0.20%
48	South Dakota	1,243	0.19%
49	Alaska	873	0.14%
50	Wyoming	728	0.11%
	District of Columbia	4,107	0.64%

Source: American Medical Association (Chicago, Illinois)
"Physician Characteristics and Distribution in the U.S." (1994 Edition)
*As of January 1, 1993. Total does not include 7,793 physicians in the U.S. territories and possessions.

Rate of Nonfederal Physicians in 1993

National Rate = 247.97 Physicians per 100,000 Population*

ALPHA ORDER				RANK ORDER		
RANK	STATE	RATE		RANK	STATE	RATE
41	Alabama	183.50		1	Massachusetts	390.93
49	Alaska	145.99		2	New York	364.75
22	Arizona	227.25		3	Maryland	362.97
42	Arkansas	179.43		4	Connecticut	353.26
9	California	268.52		5	Vermont	300.00
15	Colorado	243.83		6	Rhode Island	296.60
4	Connecticut	353.26		7	New Jersey	287.48
19	Delaware	229.08		8	Pennsylvania	280.35
11	Florida	256.15		9	California	268.52
35	Georgia	195.23		10	Hawaii	263.64
10	Hawaii	263.64		11	Florida	256.15
48	Idaho	149.27		12	Minnesota	254.05
13	Illinois	248.79		13	Illinois	248.79
40	Indiana	185.28		14	Washington	247.59
43	Iowa	177.88		15	Colorado	243.83
30	Kansas	205.40		16	Oregon	240.72
37	Kentucky	193.31		17	New Hampshire	240.30
27	Louisiana	215.99		18	Virginia	231.86
23	Maine	222.26		19	Delaware	229.08
3	Maryland	362.97		20	Tennessee	227.97
1	Massachusetts	390.93		21	Ohio	227.93
28	Michigan	214.58		22	Arizona	227.25
12	Minnesota	254.05		23	Maine	222.26
50	Mississippi	142.54		24	Missouri	221.76
24	Missouri	221.76		25	Wisconsin	219.89
36	Montana	193.70		26	North Carolina	216.28
31	Nebraska	204.84		27	Louisiana	215.99
46	Nevada	164.62		28	Michigan	214.58
17	New Hampshire	240.30		29	New Mexico	212.25
7	New Jersey	287.48		30	Kansas	205.40
29	New Mexico	212.25		31	Nebraska	204.84
2	New York	364.75		32	Utah	204.19
26	North Carolina	216.28		33	North Dakota	203.92
33	North Dakota	203.92		34	West Virginia	198.90
21	Ohio	227.93		35	Georgia	195.23
45	Oklahoma	165.64		36	Montana	193.70
16	Oregon	240.72		37	Kentucky	193.31
8	Pennsylvania	280.35		38	Texas	191.47
6	Rhode Island	296.60		39	South Carolina	189.86
39	South Carolina	189.86		40	Indiana	185.28
44	South Dakota	173.60		41	Alabama	183.50
20	Tennessee	227.97		42	Arkansas	179.43
38	Texas	191.47		43	Iowa	177.88
32	Utah	204.19		44	South Dakota	173.60
5	Vermont	300.00		45	Oklahoma	165.64
18	Virginia	231.86		46	Nevada	164.62
14	Washington	247.59		47	Wyoming	154.89
34	West Virginia	198.90		48	Idaho	149.27
25	Wisconsin	219.89		49	Alaska	145.99
47	Wyoming	154.89		50	Mississippi	142.54
					District of Columbia	709.33

Source: Morgan Quitno Press using data from American Medical Association
"Physician Characteristics and Distribution in the U.S." (1994 Edition)
*As of January 1, 1993. National rate does not include physicians in the U.S. territories and possessions.

Nonfederal Physicians in Patient Care in 1993

National Total = 525,131 Physicians*

<table>
<tr><td colspan="4"><u>ALPHA ORDER</u></td><td colspan="4"><u>RANK ORDER</u></td></tr>
<tr><td>RANK</td><td>STATE</td><td>PHYSICIANS</td><td>% of USA</td><td>RANK</td><td>STATE</td><td>PHYSICIANS</td><td>% of USA</td></tr>
<tr><td>25</td><td>Alabama</td><td>6,538</td><td>1.25%</td><td>1</td><td>California</td><td>67,022</td><td>12.76%</td></tr>
<tr><td>49</td><td>Alaska</td><td>770</td><td>0.15%</td><td>2</td><td>New York</td><td>54,399</td><td>10.36%</td></tr>
<tr><td>24</td><td>Arizona</td><td>7,013</td><td>1.34%</td><td>3</td><td>Texas</td><td>29,170</td><td>5.55%</td></tr>
<tr><td>32</td><td>Arkansas</td><td>3,684</td><td>0.70%</td><td>4</td><td>Pennsylvania</td><td>27,848</td><td>5.30%</td></tr>
<tr><td>1</td><td>California</td><td>67,022</td><td>12.76%</td><td>5</td><td>Florida</td><td>26,927</td><td>5.13%</td></tr>
<tr><td>23</td><td>Colorado</td><td>7,148</td><td>1.36%</td><td>6</td><td>Illinois</td><td>24,515</td><td>4.67%</td></tr>
<tr><td>19</td><td>Connecticut</td><td>9,355</td><td>1.78%</td><td>7</td><td>Ohio</td><td>21,127</td><td>4.02%</td></tr>
<tr><td>46</td><td>Delaware</td><td>1,323</td><td>0.25%</td><td>8</td><td>New Jersey</td><td>18,866</td><td>3.59%</td></tr>
<tr><td>5</td><td>Florida</td><td>26,927</td><td>5.13%</td><td>9</td><td>Massachusetts</td><td>18,786</td><td>3.58%</td></tr>
<tr><td>14</td><td>Georgia</td><td>11,541</td><td>2.20%</td><td>10</td><td>Michigan</td><td>16,990</td><td>3.24%</td></tr>
<tr><td>38</td><td>Hawaii</td><td>2,516</td><td>0.48%</td><td>11</td><td>Maryland</td><td>14,123</td><td>2.69%</td></tr>
<tr><td>43</td><td>Idaho</td><td>1,349</td><td>0.26%</td><td>12</td><td>Virginia</td><td>12,506</td><td>2.38%</td></tr>
<tr><td>6</td><td>Illinois</td><td>24,515</td><td>4.67%</td><td>13</td><td>North Carolina</td><td>12,349</td><td>2.35%</td></tr>
<tr><td>21</td><td>Indiana</td><td>8,917</td><td>1.70%</td><td>14</td><td>Georgia</td><td>11,541</td><td>2.20%</td></tr>
<tr><td>31</td><td>Iowa</td><td>4,042</td><td>0.77%</td><td>15</td><td>Washington</td><td>10,451</td><td>1.99%</td></tr>
<tr><td>30</td><td>Kansas</td><td>4,301</td><td>0.82%</td><td>16</td><td>Tennessee</td><td>9,947</td><td>1.89%</td></tr>
<tr><td>26</td><td>Kentucky</td><td>6,308</td><td>1.20%</td><td>17</td><td>Missouri</td><td>9,887</td><td>1.88%</td></tr>
<tr><td>22</td><td>Louisiana</td><td>7,970</td><td>1.52%</td><td>18</td><td>Minnesota</td><td>9,665</td><td>1.84%</td></tr>
<tr><td>41</td><td>Maine</td><td>2,158</td><td>0.41%</td><td>19</td><td>Connecticut</td><td>9,355</td><td>1.78%</td></tr>
<tr><td>11</td><td>Maryland</td><td>14,123</td><td>2.69%</td><td>20</td><td>Wisconsin</td><td>9,267</td><td>1.76%</td></tr>
<tr><td>9</td><td>Massachusetts</td><td>18,786</td><td>3.58%</td><td>21</td><td>Indiana</td><td>8,917</td><td>1.70%</td></tr>
<tr><td>10</td><td>Michigan</td><td>16,990</td><td>3.24%</td><td>22</td><td>Louisiana</td><td>7,970</td><td>1.52%</td></tr>
<tr><td>18</td><td>Minnesota</td><td>9,665</td><td>1.84%</td><td>23</td><td>Colorado</td><td>7,148</td><td>1.36%</td></tr>
<tr><td>33</td><td>Mississippi</td><td>3,228</td><td>0.61%</td><td>24</td><td>Arizona</td><td>7,013</td><td>1.34%</td></tr>
<tr><td>17</td><td>Missouri</td><td>9,887</td><td>1.88%</td><td>25</td><td>Alabama</td><td>6,538</td><td>1.25%</td></tr>
<tr><td>45</td><td>Montana</td><td>1,335</td><td>0.25%</td><td>26</td><td>Kentucky</td><td>6,308</td><td>1.20%</td></tr>
<tr><td>36</td><td>Nebraska</td><td>2,801</td><td>0.53%</td><td>27</td><td>Oregon</td><td>5,857</td><td>1.12%</td></tr>
<tr><td>42</td><td>Nevada</td><td>1,917</td><td>0.37%</td><td>28</td><td>South Carolina</td><td>5,804</td><td>1.11%</td></tr>
<tr><td>40</td><td>New Hampshire</td><td>2,190</td><td>0.42%</td><td>29</td><td>Oklahoma</td><td>4,537</td><td>0.86%</td></tr>
<tr><td>8</td><td>New Jersey</td><td>18,866</td><td>3.59%</td><td>30</td><td>Kansas</td><td>4,301</td><td>0.82%</td></tr>
<tr><td>37</td><td>New Mexico</td><td>2,765</td><td>0.53%</td><td>31</td><td>Iowa</td><td>4,042</td><td>0.77%</td></tr>
<tr><td>2</td><td>New York</td><td>54,399</td><td>10.36%</td><td>32</td><td>Arkansas</td><td>3,684</td><td>0.70%</td></tr>
<tr><td>13</td><td>North Carolina</td><td>12,349</td><td>2.35%</td><td>33</td><td>Mississippi</td><td>3,228</td><td>0.61%</td></tr>
<tr><td>47</td><td>North Dakota</td><td>1,114</td><td>0.21%</td><td>34</td><td>Utah</td><td>3,177</td><td>0.60%</td></tr>
<tr><td>7</td><td>Ohio</td><td>21,127</td><td>4.02%</td><td>35</td><td>West Virginia</td><td>3,068</td><td>0.58%</td></tr>
<tr><td>29</td><td>Oklahoma</td><td>4,537</td><td>0.86%</td><td>36</td><td>Nebraska</td><td>2,801</td><td>0.53%</td></tr>
<tr><td>27</td><td>Oregon</td><td>5,857</td><td>1.12%</td><td>37</td><td>New Mexico</td><td>2,765</td><td>0.53%</td></tr>
<tr><td>4</td><td>Pennsylvania</td><td>27,848</td><td>5.30%</td><td>38</td><td>Hawaii</td><td>2,516</td><td>0.48%</td></tr>
<tr><td>39</td><td>Rhode Island</td><td>2,444</td><td>0.47%</td><td>39</td><td>Rhode Island</td><td>2,444</td><td>0.47%</td></tr>
<tr><td>28</td><td>South Carolina</td><td>5,804</td><td>1.11%</td><td>40</td><td>New Hampshire</td><td>2,190</td><td>0.42%</td></tr>
<tr><td>48</td><td>South Dakota</td><td>1,042</td><td>0.20%</td><td>41</td><td>Maine</td><td>2,158</td><td>0.41%</td></tr>
<tr><td>16</td><td>Tennessee</td><td>9,947</td><td>1.89%</td><td>42</td><td>Nevada</td><td>1,917</td><td>0.37%</td></tr>
<tr><td>3</td><td>Texas</td><td>29,170</td><td>5.55%</td><td>43</td><td>Idaho</td><td>1,349</td><td>0.26%</td></tr>
<tr><td>34</td><td>Utah</td><td>3,177</td><td>0.60%</td><td>44</td><td>Vermont</td><td>1,344</td><td>0.26%</td></tr>
<tr><td>44</td><td>Vermont</td><td>1,344</td><td>0.26%</td><td>45</td><td>Montana</td><td>1,335</td><td>0.25%</td></tr>
<tr><td>12</td><td>Virginia</td><td>12,506</td><td>2.38%</td><td>46</td><td>Delaware</td><td>1,323</td><td>0.25%</td></tr>
<tr><td>15</td><td>Washington</td><td>10,451</td><td>1.99%</td><td>47</td><td>North Dakota</td><td>1,114</td><td>0.21%</td></tr>
<tr><td>35</td><td>West Virginia</td><td>3,068</td><td>0.58%</td><td>48</td><td>South Dakota</td><td>1,042</td><td>0.20%</td></tr>
<tr><td>20</td><td>Wisconsin</td><td>9,267</td><td>1.76%</td><td>49</td><td>Alaska</td><td>770</td><td>0.15%</td></tr>
<tr><td>50</td><td>Wyoming</td><td>605</td><td>0.12%</td><td>50</td><td>Wyoming</td><td>605</td><td>0.12%</td></tr>
<tr><td></td><td></td><td></td><td></td><td></td><td>District of Columbia</td><td>3,125</td><td>0.60%</td></tr>
</table>

Source: American Medical Association (Chicago, Illinois)
   "Physician Characteristics and Distribution in the U.S." (1994 Edition)
As of January 1, 1993. Total does not include 6,528 physicians in the U.S. territories and possessions.

Rate of Nonfederal Physicians in Patient Care in 1993

National Rate = 203.71 Physicians Per 100,000 Population*

ALPHA ORDER				RANK ORDER		
RANK	STATE	RATE		RANK	STATE	RATE
40	Alabama	156.37		1	Massachusetts	312.16
47	Alaska	128.76		2	New York	299.67
26	Arizona	177.77		3	Connecticut	285.39
42	Arkansas	151.85		4	Maryland	284.85
10	California	214.70		5	Rhode Island	244.40
13	Colorado	200.56		6	New Jersey	240.06
3	Connecticut	285.39		7	Vermont	233.33
21	Delaware	189.54		8	Pennsylvania	231.49
15	Florida	196.18		9	Hawaii	215.78
35	Georgia	167.21		10	California	214.70
9	Hawaii	215.78		11	Minnesota	213.64
49	Idaho	122.64		12	Illinois	209.78
12	Illinois	209.78		13	Colorado	200.56
41	Indiana	156.27		14	Washington	198.73
44	Iowa	143.28		15	Florida	196.18
33	Kansas	169.66		16	Tennessee	195.27
36	Kentucky	166.26		17	New Hampshire	194.84
23	Louisiana	185.78		18	Virginia	193.20
29	Maine	174.03		19	Oregon	192.98
4	Maryland	284.85		20	Ohio	191.00
1	Massachusetts	312.16		21	Delaware	189.54
25	Michigan	179.60		22	Missouri	188.86
11	Minnesota	213.64		23	Louisiana	185.78
50	Mississippi	122.27		24	Wisconsin	183.72
22	Missouri	188.86		25	Michigan	179.60
39	Montana	158.74		26	Arizona	177.77
30	Nebraska	173.65		27	North Carolina	177.63
46	Nevada	138.71		28	North Dakota	174.88
17	New Hampshire	194.84		29	Maine	174.03
6	New Jersey	240.06		30	Nebraska	173.65
31	New Mexico	171.10		31	New Mexico	171.10
2	New York	299.67		32	Utah	170.81
27	North Carolina	177.63		33	Kansas	169.66
28	North Dakota	174.88		34	West Virginia	168.76
20	Ohio	191.00		35	Georgia	167.21
45	Oklahoma	140.33		36	Kentucky	166.26
19	Oregon	192.98		37	Texas	161.86
8	Pennsylvania	231.49		38	South Carolina	159.89
5	Rhode Island	244.40		39	Montana	158.74
38	South Carolina	159.89		40	Alabama	156.37
43	South Dakota	145.53		41	Indiana	156.27
16	Tennessee	195.27		42	Arkansas	151.85
37	Texas	161.86		43	South Dakota	145.53
32	Utah	170.81		44	Iowa	143.28
7	Vermont	233.33		45	Oklahoma	140.33
18	Virginia	193.20		46	Nevada	138.71
14	Washington	198.73		47	Alaska	128.76
34	West Virginia	168.76		48	Wyoming	128.72
24	Wisconsin	183.72		49	Idaho	122.64
48	Wyoming	128.72		50	Mississippi	122.27
					District of Columbia	539.72

Source: Morgan Quitno Press using data from American Medical Association
"Physician Characteristics and Distribution in the U.S." (1994 Edition)
*As of January 1, 1993. National rate does not include physicians in the U.S. territories and possessions.

Nonfederal Physicians in Primary Care Specialties in 1993

National Total = 226,406 Physicians*

<table>
<tr><td colspan="4"><u>ALPHA ORDER</u></td><td colspan="4"><u>RANK ORDER</u></td></tr>
<tr><th>RANK</th><th>STATE</th><th>PHYSICIANS</th><th>% of USA</th><th>RANK</th><th>STATE</th><th>PHYSICIANS</th><th>% of USA</th></tr>
<tr><td>24</td><td>Alabama</td><td>2,984</td><td>1.32%</td><td>1</td><td>California</td><td>28,497</td><td>12.59%</td></tr>
<tr><td>49</td><td>Alaska</td><td>434</td><td>0.19%</td><td>2</td><td>New York</td><td>23,541</td><td>10.40%</td></tr>
<tr><td>25</td><td>Arizona</td><td>2,970</td><td>1.31%</td><td>3</td><td>Texas</td><td>12,339</td><td>5.45%</td></tr>
<tr><td>32</td><td>Arkansas</td><td>1,725</td><td>0.76%</td><td>4</td><td>Illinois</td><td>11,390</td><td>5.03%</td></tr>
<tr><td>1</td><td>California</td><td>28,497</td><td>12.59%</td><td>5</td><td>Pennsylvania</td><td>11,189</td><td>4.94%</td></tr>
<tr><td>23</td><td>Colorado</td><td>3,075</td><td>1.36%</td><td>6</td><td>Florida</td><td>10,581</td><td>4.67%</td></tr>
<tr><td>21</td><td>Connecticut</td><td>3,895</td><td>1.72%</td><td>7</td><td>Ohio</td><td>8,951</td><td>3.95%</td></tr>
<tr><td>46</td><td>Delaware</td><td>562</td><td>0.25%</td><td>8</td><td>New Jersey</td><td>8,372</td><td>3.70%</td></tr>
<tr><td>6</td><td>Florida</td><td>10,581</td><td>4.67%</td><td>9</td><td>Massachusetts</td><td>7,514</td><td>3.32%</td></tr>
<tr><td>14</td><td>Georgia</td><td>5,005</td><td>2.21%</td><td>10</td><td>Michigan</td><td>7,265</td><td>3.21%</td></tr>
<tr><td>38</td><td>Hawaii</td><td>1,234</td><td>0.55%</td><td>11</td><td>Maryland</td><td>6,447</td><td>2.85%</td></tr>
<tr><td>43</td><td>Idaho</td><td>634</td><td>0.28%</td><td>12</td><td>Virginia</td><td>5,641</td><td>2.49%</td></tr>
<tr><td>4</td><td>Illinois</td><td>11,390</td><td>5.03%</td><td>13</td><td>North Carolina</td><td>5,380</td><td>2.38%</td></tr>
<tr><td>20</td><td>Indiana</td><td>3,941</td><td>1.74%</td><td>14</td><td>Georgia</td><td>5,005</td><td>2.21%</td></tr>
<tr><td>31</td><td>Iowa</td><td>1,805</td><td>0.80%</td><td>15</td><td>Washington</td><td>4,682</td><td>2.07%</td></tr>
<tr><td>30</td><td>Kansas</td><td>1,950</td><td>0.86%</td><td>16</td><td>Minnesota</td><td>4,479</td><td>1.98%</td></tr>
<tr><td>26</td><td>Kentucky</td><td>2,775</td><td>1.23%</td><td>17</td><td>Tennessee</td><td>4,188</td><td>1.85%</td></tr>
<tr><td>22</td><td>Louisiana</td><td>3,203</td><td>1.41%</td><td>18</td><td>Wisconsin</td><td>4,042</td><td>1.79%</td></tr>
<tr><td>40</td><td>Maine</td><td>987</td><td>0.44%</td><td>19</td><td>Missouri</td><td>3,992</td><td>1.76%</td></tr>
<tr><td>11</td><td>Maryland</td><td>6,447</td><td>2.85%</td><td>20</td><td>Indiana</td><td>3,941</td><td>1.74%</td></tr>
<tr><td>9</td><td>Massachusetts</td><td>7,514</td><td>3.32%</td><td>21</td><td>Connecticut</td><td>3,895</td><td>1.72%</td></tr>
<tr><td>10</td><td>Michigan</td><td>7,265</td><td>3.21%</td><td>22</td><td>Louisiana</td><td>3,203</td><td>1.41%</td></tr>
<tr><td>16</td><td>Minnesota</td><td>4,479</td><td>1.98%</td><td>23</td><td>Colorado</td><td>3,075</td><td>1.36%</td></tr>
<tr><td>33</td><td>Mississippi</td><td>1,558</td><td>0.69%</td><td>24</td><td>Alabama</td><td>2,984</td><td>1.32%</td></tr>
<tr><td>19</td><td>Missouri</td><td>3,992</td><td>1.76%</td><td>25</td><td>Arizona</td><td>2,970</td><td>1.31%</td></tr>
<tr><td>45</td><td>Montana</td><td>580</td><td>0.26%</td><td>26</td><td>Kentucky</td><td>2,775</td><td>1.23%</td></tr>
<tr><td>36</td><td>Nebraska</td><td>1,306</td><td>0.58%</td><td>27</td><td>South Carolina</td><td>2,620</td><td>1.16%</td></tr>
<tr><td>42</td><td>Nevada</td><td>797</td><td>0.35%</td><td>28</td><td>Oregon</td><td>2,514</td><td>1.11%</td></tr>
<tr><td>41</td><td>New Hampshire</td><td>902</td><td>0.40%</td><td>29</td><td>Oklahoma</td><td>2,012</td><td>0.89%</td></tr>
<tr><td>8</td><td>New Jersey</td><td>8,372</td><td>3.70%</td><td>30</td><td>Kansas</td><td>1,950</td><td>0.86%</td></tr>
<tr><td>37</td><td>New Mexico</td><td>1,287</td><td>0.57%</td><td>31</td><td>Iowa</td><td>1,805</td><td>0.80%</td></tr>
<tr><td>2</td><td>New York</td><td>23,541</td><td>10.40%</td><td>32</td><td>Arkansas</td><td>1,725</td><td>0.76%</td></tr>
<tr><td>13</td><td>North Carolina</td><td>5,380</td><td>2.38%</td><td>33</td><td>Mississippi</td><td>1,558</td><td>0.69%</td></tr>
<tr><td>47</td><td>North Dakota</td><td>548</td><td>0.24%</td><td>34</td><td>West Virginia</td><td>1,382</td><td>0.61%</td></tr>
<tr><td>7</td><td>Ohio</td><td>8,951</td><td>3.95%</td><td>35</td><td>Utah</td><td>1,318</td><td>0.58%</td></tr>
<tr><td>29</td><td>Oklahoma</td><td>2,012</td><td>0.89%</td><td>36</td><td>Nebraska</td><td>1,306</td><td>0.58%</td></tr>
<tr><td>28</td><td>Oregon</td><td>2,514</td><td>1.11%</td><td>37</td><td>New Mexico</td><td>1,287</td><td>0.57%</td></tr>
<tr><td>5</td><td>Pennsylvania</td><td>11,189</td><td>4.94%</td><td>38</td><td>Hawaii</td><td>1,234</td><td>0.55%</td></tr>
<tr><td>39</td><td>Rhode Island</td><td>1,065</td><td>0.47%</td><td>39</td><td>Rhode Island</td><td>1,065</td><td>0.47%</td></tr>
<tr><td>27</td><td>South Carolina</td><td>2,620</td><td>1.16%</td><td>40</td><td>Maine</td><td>987</td><td>0.44%</td></tr>
<tr><td>48</td><td>South Dakota</td><td>541</td><td>0.24%</td><td>41</td><td>New Hampshire</td><td>902</td><td>0.40%</td></tr>
<tr><td>17</td><td>Tennessee</td><td>4,188</td><td>1.85%</td><td>42</td><td>Nevada</td><td>797</td><td>0.35%</td></tr>
<tr><td>3</td><td>Texas</td><td>12,339</td><td>5.45%</td><td>43</td><td>Idaho</td><td>634</td><td>0.28%</td></tr>
<tr><td>35</td><td>Utah</td><td>1,318</td><td>0.58%</td><td>44</td><td>Vermont</td><td>622</td><td>0.27%</td></tr>
<tr><td>44</td><td>Vermont</td><td>622</td><td>0.27%</td><td>45</td><td>Montana</td><td>580</td><td>0.26%</td></tr>
<tr><td>12</td><td>Virginia</td><td>5,641</td><td>2.49%</td><td>46</td><td>Delaware</td><td>562</td><td>0.25%</td></tr>
<tr><td>15</td><td>Washington</td><td>4,682</td><td>2.07%</td><td>47</td><td>North Dakota</td><td>548</td><td>0.24%</td></tr>
<tr><td>34</td><td>West Virginia</td><td>1,382</td><td>0.61%</td><td>48</td><td>South Dakota</td><td>541</td><td>0.24%</td></tr>
<tr><td>18</td><td>Wisconsin</td><td>4,042</td><td>1.79%</td><td>49</td><td>Alaska</td><td>434</td><td>0.19%</td></tr>
<tr><td>50</td><td>Wyoming</td><td>332</td><td>0.15%</td><td>50</td><td>Wyoming</td><td>332</td><td>0.15%</td></tr>
<tr><td></td><td></td><td></td><td></td><td></td><td>District of Columbia</td><td>1,353</td><td>0.60%</td></tr>
</table>

Source: American Medical Association (Chicago, Illinois)
    "Physician Characteristics and Distribution in the U.S." (1994 Edition)
As of January 1, 1993. National total does not include 4,026 physicians in the U.S. territories and possessions. Primary Care Specialties include Family Practice, General Practice, Internal Medicine, Obstetrics/Gynecology and Pediatrics.

Rate of Nonfederal Physicians in Primary Care Specialties in 1993

National Rate = 87.83 Physicians per 100,000 Population*

<u>ALPHA ORDER</u>

RANK	STATE	RATE
39	Alabama	71.37
36	Alaska	72.58
33	Arizona	75.29
40	Arkansas	71.10
12	California	91.29
15	Colorado	86.28
4	Connecticut	118.82
21	Delaware	80.52
27	Florida	77.09
37	Georgia	72.52
8	Hawaii	105.83
50	Idaho	57.64
10	Illinois	97.47
43	Indiana	69.07
46	Iowa	63.98
28	Kansas	76.92
35	Kentucky	73.14
34	Louisiana	74.66
25	Maine	79.60
1	Maryland	130.03
3	Massachusetts	124.86
29	Michigan	76.80
9	Minnesota	99.01
48	Mississippi	59.02
30	Missouri	76.26
44	Montana	68.97
19	Nebraska	80.97
49	Nevada	57.67
22	New Hampshire	80.25
6	New Jersey	106.53
24	New Mexico	79.64
2	New York	129.68
26	North Carolina	77.39
16	North Dakota	86.03
20	Ohio	80.92
47	Oklahoma	62.23
17	Oregon	82.83
11	Pennsylvania	93.01
7	Rhode Island	106.50
38	South Carolina	72.18
32	South Dakota	75.56
18	Tennessee	82.21
45	Texas	68.47
41	Utah	70.86
5	Vermont	107.99
14	Virginia	87.15
13	Washington	89.03
31	West Virginia	76.02
23	Wisconsin	80.13
42	Wyoming	70.64

<u>RANK ORDER</u>

RANK	STATE	RATE
1	Maryland	130.03
2	New York	129.68
3	Massachusetts	124.86
4	Connecticut	118.82
5	Vermont	107.99
6	New Jersey	106.53
7	Rhode Island	106.50
8	Hawaii	105.83
9	Minnesota	99.01
10	Illinois	97.47
11	Pennsylvania	93.01
12	California	91.29
13	Washington	89.03
14	Virginia	87.15
15	Colorado	86.28
16	North Dakota	86.03
17	Oregon	82.83
18	Tennessee	82.21
19	Nebraska	80.97
20	Ohio	80.92
21	Delaware	80.52
22	New Hampshire	80.25
23	Wisconsin	80.13
24	New Mexico	79.64
25	Maine	79.60
26	North Carolina	77.39
27	Florida	77.09
28	Kansas	76.92
29	Michigan	76.80
30	Missouri	76.26
31	West Virginia	76.02
32	South Dakota	75.56
33	Arizona	75.29
34	Louisiana	74.66
35	Kentucky	73.14
36	Alaska	72.58
37	Georgia	72.52
38	South Carolina	72.18
39	Alabama	71.37
40	Arkansas	71.10
41	Utah	70.86
42	Wyoming	70.64
43	Indiana	69.07
44	Montana	68.97
45	Texas	68.47
46	Iowa	63.98
47	Oklahoma	62.23
48	Mississippi	59.02
49	Nevada	57.67
50	Idaho	57.64

	District of Columbia	233.68

Source: Morgan Quitno Press using data from American Medical Association
"Physician Characteristics and Distribution in the U.S." (1994 Edition)
As of January 1, 1993. National rate does not include physicians in the U.S. territories and possessions. Primary Care Specialties include Family Practice, General Practice, Internal Medicine, Obstetrics/Gynecology and Pediatrics.

Percent of Nonfederal Physicians in Primary Care Specialties in 1993

National Percent = 35.42% of Physicians*

ALPHA ORDER		
RANK	STATE	PERCENT
11	Alabama	38.89
1	Alaska	49.71
48	Arizona	33.13
7	Arkansas	39.63
44	California	34.00
37	Colorado	35.39
45	Connecticut	33.64
38	Delaware	35.15
50	Florida	30.09
21	Georgia	37.14
6	Hawaii	40.14
12	Idaho	38.61
9	Illinois	39.18
20	Indiana	37.28
26	Iowa	35.97
19	Kansas	37.45
15	Kentucky	37.84
41	Louisiana	34.57
30	Maine	35.81
29	Maryland	35.82
49	Massachusetts	31.94
31	Michigan	35.79
10	Minnesota	38.97
5	Mississippi	41.40
43	Missouri	34.39
34	Montana	35.60
8	Nebraska	39.53
39	Nevada	35.03
46	New Hampshire	33.40
22	New Jersey	37.06
18	New Mexico	37.52
35	New York	35.55
32	North Carolina	35.78
4	North Dakota	42.19
36	Ohio	35.50
17	Oklahoma	37.57
42	Oregon	34.41
47	Pennsylvania	33.18
28	Rhode Island	35.91
14	South Carolina	38.02
3	South Dakota	43.52
24	Tennessee	36.06
33	Texas	35.76
40	Utah	34.70
25	Vermont	36.00
16	Virginia	37.59
27	Washington	35.96
13	West Virginia	38.22
23	Wisconsin	36.44
2	Wyoming	45.60

RANK ORDER		
RANK	STATE	PERCENT
1	Alaska	49.71
2	Wyoming	45.60
3	South Dakota	43.52
4	North Dakota	42.19
5	Mississippi	41.40
6	Hawaii	40.14
7	Arkansas	39.63
8	Nebraska	39.53
9	Illinois	39.18
10	Minnesota	38.97
11	Alabama	38.89
12	Idaho	38.61
13	West Virginia	38.22
14	South Carolina	38.02
15	Kentucky	37.84
16	Virginia	37.59
17	Oklahoma	37.57
18	New Mexico	37.52
19	Kansas	37.45
20	Indiana	37.28
21	Georgia	37.14
22	New Jersey	37.06
23	Wisconsin	36.44
24	Tennessee	36.06
25	Vermont	36.00
26	Iowa	35.97
27	Washington	35.96
28	Rhode Island	35.91
29	Maryland	35.82
30	Maine	35.81
31	Michigan	35.79
32	North Carolina	35.78
33	Texas	35.76
34	Montana	35.60
35	New York	35.55
36	Ohio	35.50
37	Colorado	35.39
38	Delaware	35.15
39	Nevada	35.03
40	Utah	34.70
41	Louisiana	34.57
42	Oregon	34.41
43	Missouri	34.39
44	California	34.00
45	Connecticut	33.64
46	New Hampshire	33.40
47	Pennsylvania	33.18
48	Arizona	33.13
49	Massachusetts	31.94
50	Florida	30.09
	District of Columbia	32.94

Source: Morgan Quitno Press using data from American Medical Association
   "Physician Characteristics and Distribution in the U.S." (1994 Edition)
*As of January 1, 1993. National percent does not include physicians in the U.S. territories and possessions. Primary Care Specialties include Family Practice, General Practice, Internal Medicine, Obstetrics/Gynecology and Pediatrics.

Percent of Population Lacking Access to Primary Care in 1993

National Percent = 9.5% of Population*

<u>ALPHA ORDER</u>

<u>RANK ORDER</u>

RANK	STATE	PERCENT	RANK	STATE	PERCENT
9	Alabama	16.4	1	Mississippi	24.9
10	Alaska	16.3	2	South Dakota	22.0
35	Arizona	6.4	3	Louisiana	20.2
12	Arkansas	13.8	4	New Mexico	19.6
26	California	8.0	5	North Dakota	19.3
43	Colorado	4.8	6	South Carolina	19.0
46	Connecticut	4.2	7	Wyoming	18.9
46	Delaware	4.2	8	West Virginia	18.4
36	Florida	6.2	9	Alabama	16.4
13	Georgia	13.3	10	Alaska	16.3
50	Hawaii	2.5	11	Idaho	16.1
11	Idaho	16.1	12	Arkansas	13.8
32	Illinois	7.5	13	Georgia	13.3
30	Indiana	7.6	14	Montana	12.6
29	Iowa	7.8	15	North Carolina	11.3
40	Kansas	5.6	16	Kentucky	10.9
16	Kentucky	10.9	16	New York	10.9
3	Louisiana	20.2	18	Missouri	10.3
38	Maine	6.1	19	Tennessee	10.1
48	Maryland	3.9	20	Rhode Island	9.9
36	Massachusetts	6.2	21	Nebraska	9.7
25	Michigan	8.4	22	Wisconsin	9.3
44	Minnesota	4.3	23	Oklahoma	9.1
1	Mississippi	24.9	24	Washington	8.6
18	Missouri	10.3	25	Michigan	8.4
14	Montana	12.6	26	California	8.0
21	Nebraska	9.7	26	Nevada	8.0
26	Nevada	8.0	26	Texas	8.0
48	New Hampshire	3.9	29	Iowa	7.8
44	New Jersey	4.3	30	Indiana	7.6
4	New Mexico	19.6	30	Utah	7.6
16	New York	10.9	32	Illinois	7.5
15	North Carolina	11.3	33	Ohio	7.0
5	North Dakota	19.3	34	Oregon	6.9
33	Ohio	7.0	35	Arizona	6.4
23	Oklahoma	9.1	36	Florida	6.2
34	Oregon	6.9	36	Massachusetts	6.2
42	Pennsylvania	5.2	38	Maine	6.1
20	Rhode Island	9.9	39	Virginia	5.7
6	South Carolina	19.0	40	Kansas	5.6
2	South Dakota	22.0	41	Vermont	5.4
19	Tennessee	10.1	42	Pennsylvania	5.2
26	Texas	8.0	43	Colorado	4.8
30	Utah	7.6	44	Minnesota	4.3
41	Vermont	5.4	44	New Jersey	4.3
39	Virginia	5.7	46	Connecticut	4.2
24	Washington	8.6	46	Delaware	4.2
8	West Virginia	18.4	48	Maryland	3.9
22	Wisconsin	9.3	48	New Hampshire	3.9
7	Wyoming	18.9	50	Hawaii	2.5
				District of Columbia**	NA

Source: U.S. Department of Health and Human Services, Division of Shortage Designation

Percent of population considered under-served by primary medical practitioners (Family & General Practice doctors, Internists, Ob/Gyns and Pediatricians). An under-served population does not have primary medical care within reasonable economic and geographic bounds.

Nonfederal Physicians in General/Family Practice in 1993

National Total = 68,089 Physicians*

ALPHA ORDER

RANK ORDER

RANK	STATE	PHYSICIANS	% of USA
21	Alabama	1,046	1.54%
47	Alaska	188	0.28%
23	Arizona	1,012	1.49%
28	Arkansas	905	1.33%
1	California	8,887	13.05%
20	Colorado	1,148	1.69%
35	Connecticut	568	0.83%
48	Delaware	185	0.27%
3	Florida	3,604	5.29%
15	Georgia	1,470	2.16%
45	Hawaii	255	0.37%
39	Idaho	369	0.54%
6	Illinois	3,121	4.58%
11	Indiana	1,925	2.83%
26	Iowa	956	1.40%
29	Kansas	886	1.30%
19	Kentucky	1,158	1.70%
24	Louisiana	977	1.43%
38	Maine	422	0.62%
22	Maryland	1,035	1.52%
27	Massachusetts	917	1.35%
10	Michigan	1,987	2.92%
9	Minnesota	2,046	3.00%
32	Mississippi	703	1.03%
24	Missouri	977	1.43%
44	Montana	279	0.41%
33	Nebraska	640	0.94%
43	Nevada	282	0.41%
42	New Hampshire	293	0.43%
16	New Jersey	1,409	2.07%
36	New Mexico	489	0.72%
5	New York	3,297	4.84%
12	North Carolina	1,830	2.69%
40	North Dakota	303	0.45%
7	Ohio	2,775	4.08%
31	Oklahoma	828	1.22%
29	Oregon	886	1.30%
4	Pennsylvania	3,458	5.08%
50	Rhode Island	174	0.26%
18	South Carolina	1,160	1.70%
40	South Dakota	303	0.45%
17	Tennessee	1,303	1.91%
2	Texas	4,462	6.55%
37	Utah	444	0.65%
46	Vermont	195	0.29%
13	Virginia	1,791	2.63%
8	Washington	2,097	3.08%
34	West Virginia	587	0.86%
14	Wisconsin	1,707	2.51%
49	Wyoming	181	0.27%

RANK	STATE	PHYSICIANS	% of USA
1	California	8,887	13.05%
2	Texas	4,462	6.55%
3	Florida	3,604	5.29%
4	Pennsylvania	3,458	5.08%
5	New York	3,297	4.84%
6	Illinois	3,121	4.58%
7	Ohio	2,775	4.08%
8	Washington	2,097	3.08%
9	Minnesota	2,046	3.00%
10	Michigan	1,987	2.92%
11	Indiana	1,925	2.83%
12	North Carolina	1,830	2.69%
13	Virginia	1,791	2.63%
14	Wisconsin	1,707	2.51%
15	Georgia	1,470	2.16%
16	New Jersey	1,409	2.07%
17	Tennessee	1,303	1.91%
18	South Carolina	1,160	1.70%
19	Kentucky	1,158	1.70%
20	Colorado	1,148	1.69%
21	Alabama	1,046	1.54%
22	Maryland	1,035	1.52%
23	Arizona	1,012	1.49%
24	Louisiana	977	1.43%
24	Missouri	977	1.43%
26	Iowa	956	1.40%
27	Massachusetts	917	1.35%
28	Arkansas	905	1.33%
29	Kansas	886	1.30%
29	Oregon	886	1.30%
31	Oklahoma	828	1.22%
32	Mississippi	703	1.03%
33	Nebraska	640	0.94%
34	West Virginia	587	0.86%
35	Connecticut	568	0.83%
36	New Mexico	489	0.72%
37	Utah	444	0.65%
38	Maine	422	0.62%
39	Idaho	369	0.54%
40	North Dakota	303	0.45%
40	South Dakota	303	0.45%
42	New Hampshire	293	0.43%
43	Nevada	282	0.41%
44	Montana	279	0.41%
45	Hawaii	255	0.37%
46	Vermont	195	0.29%
47	Alaska	188	0.28%
48	Delaware	185	0.27%
49	Wyoming	181	0.27%
50	Rhode Island	174	0.26%
	District of Columbia	169	0.25%

Source: American Medical Association (Chicago, Illinois)
"Physician Characteristics and Distribution in the U.S." (1994 Edition)
*As of January 1, 1993. Total does not include 1,402 physicians in the U.S. territories and possessions.

Rate of Nonfederal Physicians in General/Family Practice in 1993

National Rate = 26.41 Physicians per 100,000 Population*

ALPHA ORDER			RANK ORDER		
RANK	STATE	RATE	RANK	STATE	RATE
36	Alabama	25.02	1	North Dakota	47.57
19	Alaska	31.44	2	Minnesota	45.23
32	Arizona	25.65	3	South Dakota	42.32
7	Arkansas	37.30	4	Washington	39.87
24	California	28.47	5	Nebraska	39.68
17	Colorado	32.21	6	Wyoming	38.51
49	Connecticut	17.33	7	Arkansas	37.30
28	Delaware	26.50	8	Kansas	34.95
30	Florida	26.26	9	Maine	34.03
41	Georgia	21.30	10	Iowa	33.89
40	Hawaii	21.87	11	Vermont	33.85
14	Idaho	33.55	12	Wisconsin	33.84
26	Illinois	26.71	13	Indiana	33.74
13	Indiana	33.74	14	Idaho	33.55
10	Iowa	33.89	15	Montana	33.17
8	Kansas	34.95	16	West Virginia	32.29
20	Kentucky	30.52	17	Colorado	32.21
39	Louisiana	22.77	18	South Carolina	31.96
9	Maine	34.03	19	Alaska	31.44
43	Maryland	20.88	20	Kentucky	30.52
50	Massachusetts	15.24	21	New Mexico	30.26
42	Michigan	21.00	22	Oregon	29.19
2	Minnesota	45.23	23	Pennsylvania	28.74
27	Mississippi	26.63	24	California	28.47
45	Missouri	18.66	25	Virginia	27.67
15	Montana	33.17	26	Illinois	26.71
5	Nebraska	39.68	27	Mississippi	26.63
44	Nevada	20.41	28	Delaware	26.50
31	New Hampshire	26.07	29	North Carolina	26.32
47	New Jersey	17.93	30	Florida	26.26
21	New Mexico	30.26	31	New Hampshire	26.07
46	New York	18.16	32	Arizona	25.65
29	North Carolina	26.32	33	Oklahoma	25.61
1	North Dakota	47.57	34	Tennessee	25.58
35	Ohio	25.09	35	Ohio	25.09
33	Oklahoma	25.61	36	Alabama	25.02
22	Oregon	29.19	37	Texas	24.76
23	Pennsylvania	28.74	38	Utah	23.87
48	Rhode Island	17.40	39	Louisiana	22.77
18	South Carolina	31.96	40	Hawaii	21.87
3	South Dakota	42.32	41	Georgia	21.30
34	Tennessee	25.58	42	Michigan	21.00
37	Texas	24.76	43	Maryland	20.88
38	Utah	23.87	44	Nevada	20.41
11	Vermont	33.85	45	Missouri	18.66
25	Virginia	27.67	46	New York	18.16
4	Washington	39.87	47	New Jersey	17.93
16	West Virginia	32.29	48	Rhode Island	17.40
12	Wisconsin	33.84	49	Connecticut	17.33
6	Wyoming	38.51	50	Massachusetts	15.24
				District of Columbia	29.19

*Source: Morgan Quitno Press using data from American Medical Association
"Physician Characteristics and Distribution in the U.S." (1994 Edition)*
As of January 1, 1993. National rate does not include physicians in the U.S. territories and possessions.

Nonfederal Physicians in Medical Specialties in 1993

National Total = 192,281 Physicians*

ALPHA ORDER

RANK	STATE	PHYSICIANS	% of USA
25	Alabama	2,227	1.16%
49	Alaska	193	0.10%
24	Arizona	2,277	1.18%
34	Arkansas	994	0.52%
2	California	23,821	12.39%
23	Colorado	2,360	1.23%
14	Connecticut	4,132	2.15%
44	Delaware	456	0.24%
5	Florida	9,361	4.87%
16	Georgia	3,763	1.96%
35	Hawaii	960	0.50%
47	Idaho	289	0.15%
4	Illinois	9,619	5.00%
22	Indiana	2,562	1.33%
31	Iowa	1,157	0.60%
30	Kansas	1,227	0.64%
26	Kentucky	1,922	1.00%
21	Louisiana	2,563	1.33%
41	Maine	640	0.33%
10	Maryland	6,381	3.32%
7	Massachusetts	8,811	4.58%
11	Michigan	6,181	3.21%
18	Minnesota	3,275	1.70%
38	Mississippi	846	0.44%
15	Missouri	3,869	2.01%
45	Montana	345	0.18%
39	Nebraska	822	0.43%
42	Nevada	600	0.31%
40	New Hampshire	730	0.38%
8	New Jersey	8,583	4.46%
37	New Mexico	860	0.45%
1	New York	24,854	12.93%
13	North Carolina	4,272	2.22%
46	North Dakota	290	0.15%
9	Ohio	7,466	3.88%
29	Oklahoma	1,405	0.73%
27	Oregon	1,883	0.98%
3	Pennsylvania	10,187	5.30%
32	Rhode Island	1,145	0.60%
28	South Carolina	1,594	0.83%
48	South Dakota	260	0.14%
17	Tennessee	3,462	1.80%
6	Texas	9,307	4.84%
33	Utah	1,051	0.55%
43	Vermont	479	0.25%
12	Virginia	4,283	2.23%
19	Washington	3,138	1.63%
36	West Virginia	929	0.48%
20	Wisconsin	2,929	1.52%
50	Wyoming	120	0.06%

RANK ORDER

RANK	STATE	PHYSICIANS	% of USA
1	New York	24,854	12.93%
2	California	23,821	12.39%
3	Pennsylvania	10,187	5.30%
4	Illinois	9,619	5.00%
5	Florida	9,361	4.87%
6	Texas	9,307	4.84%
7	Massachusetts	8,811	4.58%
8	New Jersey	8,583	4.46%
9	Ohio	7,466	3.88%
10	Maryland	6,381	3.32%
11	Michigan	6,181	3.21%
12	Virginia	4,283	2.23%
13	North Carolina	4,272	2.22%
14	Connecticut	4,132	2.15%
15	Missouri	3,869	2.01%
16	Georgia	3,763	1.96%
17	Tennessee	3,462	1.80%
18	Minnesota	3,275	1.70%
19	Washington	3,138	1.63%
20	Wisconsin	2,929	1.52%
21	Louisiana	2,563	1.33%
22	Indiana	2,562	1.33%
23	Colorado	2,360	1.23%
24	Arizona	2,277	1.18%
25	Alabama	2,227	1.16%
26	Kentucky	1,922	1.00%
27	Oregon	1,883	0.98%
28	South Carolina	1,594	0.83%
29	Oklahoma	1,405	0.73%
30	Kansas	1,227	0.64%
31	Iowa	1,157	0.60%
32	Rhode Island	1,145	0.60%
33	Utah	1,051	0.55%
34	Arkansas	994	0.52%
35	Hawaii	960	0.50%
36	West Virginia	929	0.48%
37	New Mexico	860	0.45%
38	Mississippi	846	0.44%
39	Nebraska	822	0.43%
40	New Hampshire	730	0.38%
41	Maine	640	0.33%
42	Nevada	600	0.31%
43	Vermont	479	0.25%
44	Delaware	456	0.24%
45	Montana	345	0.18%
46	North Dakota	290	0.15%
47	Idaho	289	0.15%
48	South Dakota	260	0.14%
49	Alaska	193	0.10%
50	Wyoming	120	0.06%
	District of Columbia	1,401	0.73%

Source: American Medical Association (Chicago, Illinois)
  "Physician Characteristics and Distribution in the U.S." (1994 Edition)
As of January 1, 1993. Total does not include 2,336 physicians in the U.S. territories and possessions. Medical Specialties are Allergy/Immunology, Cardiovascular Diseases, Dermatology, Gastroenterology, Internal Medicine, Pediatrics, Pediatric Cardiology and Pulmonary Diseases.

Rate of Nonfederal Physicians in Medical Specialties in 1993

National Rate = 74.59 Physicians per 100,000 Population*

ALPHA ORDER				RANK ORDER		
RANK	STATE	RATE		RANK	STATE	RATE
30	Alabama	53.26		1	Massachusetts	146.41
47	Alaska	32.27		2	New York	136.91
27	Arizona	57.72		3	Maryland	128.70
45	Arkansas	40.97		4	Connecticut	126.05
11	California	76.31		5	Rhode Island	114.50
17	Colorado	66.22		6	New Jersey	109.21
4	Connecticut	126.05		7	Pennsylvania	84.68
20	Delaware	65.33		8	Vermont	83.16
14	Florida	68.20		9	Hawaii	82.33
29	Georgia	54.52		10	Illinois	82.31
9	Hawaii	82.33		11	California	76.31
49	Idaho	26.27		12	Missouri	73.91
10	Illinois	82.31		13	Minnesota	72.39
39	Indiana	44.90		14	Florida	68.20
44	Iowa	41.01		15	Tennessee	67.96
37	Kansas	48.40		16	Ohio	67.50
36	Kentucky	50.66		17	Colorado	66.22
24	Louisiana	59.74		18	Virginia	66.17
33	Maine	51.61		19	Michigan	65.34
3	Maryland	128.70		20	Delaware	65.33
1	Massachusetts	146.41		21	New Hampshire	64.95
19	Michigan	65.34		22	Oregon	62.04
13	Minnesota	72.39		23	North Carolina	61.45
48	Mississippi	32.05		24	Louisiana	59.74
12	Missouri	73.91		25	Washington	59.67
43	Montana	41.02		26	Wisconsin	58.07
35	Nebraska	50.96		27	Arizona	57.72
42	Nevada	43.42		28	Utah	56.51
21	New Hampshire	64.95		29	Georgia	54.52
6	New Jersey	109.21		30	Alabama	53.26
31	New Mexico	53.22		31	New Mexico	53.22
2	New York	136.91		32	Texas	51.64
23	North Carolina	61.45		33	Maine	51.61
38	North Dakota	45.53		34	West Virginia	51.10
16	Ohio	67.50		35	Nebraska	50.96
41	Oklahoma	43.46		36	Kentucky	50.66
22	Oregon	62.04		37	Kansas	48.40
7	Pennsylvania	84.68		38	North Dakota	45.53
5	Rhode Island	114.50		39	Indiana	44.90
40	South Carolina	43.91		40	South Carolina	43.91
46	South Dakota	36.31		41	Oklahoma	43.46
15	Tennessee	67.96		42	Nevada	43.42
32	Texas	51.64		43	Montana	41.02
28	Utah	56.51		44	Iowa	41.01
8	Vermont	83.16		45	Arkansas	40.97
18	Virginia	66.17		46	South Dakota	36.31
25	Washington	59.67		47	Alaska	32.27
34	West Virginia	51.10		48	Mississippi	32.05
26	Wisconsin	58.07		49	Idaho	26.27
50	Wyoming	25.53		50	Wyoming	25.53
					District of Columbia	241.97

Source: Morgan Quitno Press using data from American Medical Association
"Physician Characteristics and Distribution in the U.S." (1994 Edition)
As of January 1, 1993. National rate does not include physicians in the U.S. territories and possessions. Medical Specialties are Allergy/Immunology, Cardiovascular Diseases, Dermatology, Gastroenterology, Internal Medicine, Pediatrics, Pediatric Cardiology and Pulmonary Diseases.

Nonfederal Physicians in Internal Medicine in 1993

National Total = 104,973 Physicians*

<u>ALPHA ORDER</u>

RANK	STATE	PHYSICIANS	% of USA
23	Alabama	1,250	1.19%
49	Alaska	92	0.09%
26	Arizona	1,127	1.07%
36	Arkansas	445	0.42%
2	California	12,387	11.80%
24	Colorado	1,224	1.17%
12	Connecticut	2,449	2.33%
44	Delaware	236	0.22%
8	Florida	4,398	4.19%
16	Georgia	1,972	1.88%
33	Hawaii	539	0.51%
47	Idaho	150	0.14%
4	Illinois	5,701	5.43%
21	Indiana	1,298	1.24%
32	Iowa	575	0.55%
30	Kansas	691	0.66%
27	Kentucky	959	0.91%
22	Louisiana	1,268	1.21%
41	Maine	343	0.33%
10	Maryland	3,583	3.41%
5	Massachusetts	5,400	5.14%
11	Michigan	3,557	3.39%
18	Minnesota	1,860	1.77%
39	Mississippi	412	0.39%
15	Missouri	2,131	2.03%
45	Montana	185	0.18%
38	Nebraska	413	0.39%
42	Nevada	334	0.32%
40	New Hampshire	390	0.37%
6	New Jersey	4,729	4.50%
37	New Mexico	433	0.41%
1	New York	14,727	14.03%
14	North Carolina	2,208	2.10%
46	North Dakota	160	0.15%
9	Ohio	4,009	3.82%
29	Oklahoma	736	0.70%
25	Oregon	1,138	1.08%
3	Pennsylvania	5,766	5.49%
31	Rhode Island	667	0.64%
28	South Carolina	805	0.77%
47	South Dakota	150	0.14%
17	Tennessee	1,875	1.79%
7	Texas	4,517	4.30%
35	Utah	486	0.46%
43	Vermont	284	0.27%
13	Virginia	2,240	2.13%
19	Washington	1,665	1.59%
34	West Virginia	518	0.49%
20	Wisconsin	1,623	1.55%
50	Wyoming	64	0.06%

<u>RANK ORDER</u>

RANK	STATE	PHYSICIANS	% of USA
1	New York	14,727	14.03%
2	California	12,387	11.80%
3	Pennsylvania	5,766	5.49%
4	Illinois	5,701	5.43%
5	Massachusetts	5,400	5.14%
6	New Jersey	4,729	4.50%
7	Texas	4,517	4.30%
8	Florida	4,398	4.19%
9	Ohio	4,009	3.82%
10	Maryland	3,583	3.41%
11	Michigan	3,557	3.39%
12	Connecticut	2,449	2.33%
13	Virginia	2,240	2.13%
14	North Carolina	2,208	2.10%
15	Missouri	2,131	2.03%
16	Georgia	1,972	1.88%
17	Tennessee	1,875	1.79%
18	Minnesota	1,860	1.77%
19	Washington	1,665	1.59%
20	Wisconsin	1,623	1.55%
21	Indiana	1,298	1.24%
22	Louisiana	1,268	1.21%
23	Alabama	1,250	1.19%
24	Colorado	1,224	1.17%
25	Oregon	1,138	1.08%
26	Arizona	1,127	1.07%
27	Kentucky	959	0.91%
28	South Carolina	805	0.77%
29	Oklahoma	736	0.70%
30	Kansas	691	0.66%
31	Rhode Island	667	0.64%
32	Iowa	575	0.55%
33	Hawaii	539	0.51%
34	West Virginia	518	0.49%
35	Utah	486	0.46%
36	Arkansas	445	0.42%
37	New Mexico	433	0.41%
38	Nebraska	413	0.39%
39	Mississippi	412	0.39%
40	New Hampshire	390	0.37%
41	Maine	343	0.33%
42	Nevada	334	0.32%
43	Vermont	284	0.27%
44	Delaware	236	0.22%
45	Montana	185	0.18%
46	North Dakota	160	0.15%
47	Idaho	150	0.14%
47	South Dakota	150	0.14%
49	Alaska	92	0.09%
50	Wyoming	64	0.06%
	District of Columbia	804	0.77%

Source: American Medical Association (Chicago, Illinois)
    "Physician Characteristics and Distribution in the U.S." (1994 Edition)
*As of January 1, 1993. Total does not include 1,064 physicians in the U.S. territories and possessions. Internal Medicine includes Diabetes, Endocrinology, Geriatrics, Hematology, Infectious Diseases, Nephrology, Nutrition, Medical Oncology and Rheumatology.

Rate of Nonfederal Physicians in Internal Medicine in 1993

National Rate = 40.72 Physicians per 100,000 Population*

ALPHA ORDER			RANK ORDER		
RANK	STATE	RATE	RANK	STATE	RATE
26	Alabama	29.90	1	Massachusetts	89.73
48	Alaska	15.38	2	New York	81.13
28	Arizona	28.57	3	Connecticut	74.71
46	Arkansas	18.34	4	Maryland	72.27
13	California	39.68	5	Rhode Island	66.70
20	Colorado	34.34	6	New Jersey	60.17
3	Connecticut	74.71	7	Vermont	49.31
21	Delaware	33.81	8	Illinois	48.78
23	Florida	32.04	9	Pennsylvania	47.93
28	Georgia	28.57	10	Hawaii	46.23
10	Hawaii	46.23	11	Minnesota	41.11
49	Idaho	13.64	12	Missouri	40.71
8	Illinois	48.78	13	California	39.68
41	Indiana	22.75	14	Michigan	37.60
45	Iowa	20.38	15	Oregon	37.50
32	Kansas	27.26	16	Tennessee	36.81
36	Kentucky	25.28	17	Ohio	36.24
27	Louisiana	29.56	18	New Hampshire	34.70
31	Maine	27.66	19	Virginia	34.61
4	Maryland	72.27	20	Colorado	34.34
1	Massachusetts	89.73	21	Delaware	33.81
14	Michigan	37.60	22	Wisconsin	32.18
11	Minnesota	41.11	23	Florida	32.04
47	Mississippi	15.61	24	North Carolina	31.76
12	Missouri	40.71	25	Washington	31.66
43	Montana	22.00	26	Alabama	29.90
35	Nebraska	25.60	27	Louisiana	29.56
39	Nevada	24.17	28	Arizona	28.57
18	New Hampshire	34.70	28	Georgia	28.57
6	New Jersey	60.17	30	West Virginia	28.49
33	New Mexico	26.79	31	Maine	27.66
2	New York	81.13	32	Kansas	27.26
24	North Carolina	31.76	33	New Mexico	26.79
37	North Dakota	25.12	34	Utah	26.13
17	Ohio	36.24	35	Nebraska	25.60
40	Oklahoma	22.77	36	Kentucky	25.28
15	Oregon	37.50	37	North Dakota	25.12
9	Pennsylvania	47.93	38	Texas	25.06
5	Rhode Island	66.70	39	Nevada	24.17
42	South Carolina	22.18	40	Oklahoma	22.77
44	South Dakota	20.95	41	Indiana	22.75
16	Tennessee	36.81	42	South Carolina	22.18
38	Texas	25.06	43	Montana	22.00
34	Utah	26.13	44	South Dakota	20.95
7	Vermont	49.31	45	Iowa	20.38
19	Virginia	34.61	46	Arkansas	18.34
25	Washington	31.66	47	Mississippi	15.61
30	West Virginia	28.49	48	Alaska	15.38
22	Wisconsin	32.18	49	Idaho	13.64
50	Wyoming	13.62	50	Wyoming	13.62
				District of Columbia	138.86

Source: Morgan Quitno Press using data from American Medical Association
   "Physician Characteristics and Distribution in the U.S." (1994 Edition)
*As of January 1, 1993. National rate does not include physicians in the U.S. territories and possessions. Internal Medicine includes Diabetes, Endocrinology, Geriatrics, Hematology, Infectious Diseases, Nephrology, Nutrition, Medical Oncology and Rheumatology.

Nonfederal Physicians in Pediatrics in 1993

National Total = 44,114 Physicians*

<table>
<tr><td colspan="4">ALPHA ORDER</td><td colspan="4">RANK ORDER</td></tr>
<tr><th>RANK</th><th>STATE</th><th>PHYSICIANS</th><th>% of USA</th><th>RANK</th><th>STATE</th><th>PHYSICIANS</th><th>% of USA</th></tr>
<tr><td>26</td><td>Alabama</td><td>485</td><td>1.10%</td><td>1</td><td>California</td><td>5,831</td><td>13.22%</td></tr>
<tr><td>46</td><td>Alaska</td><td>69</td><td>0.16%</td><td>2</td><td>New York</td><td>5,525</td><td>12.52%</td></tr>
<tr><td>24</td><td>Arizona</td><td>552</td><td>1.25%</td><td>3</td><td>Texas</td><td>2,409</td><td>5.46%</td></tr>
<tr><td>31</td><td>Arkansas</td><td>271</td><td>0.61%</td><td>4</td><td>Florida</td><td>2,181</td><td>4.94%</td></tr>
<tr><td>1</td><td>California</td><td>5,831</td><td>13.22%</td><td>5</td><td>Illinois</td><td>2,082</td><td>4.72%</td></tr>
<tr><td>23</td><td>Colorado</td><td>565</td><td>1.28%</td><td>6</td><td>New Jersey</td><td>2,049</td><td>4.64%</td></tr>
<tr><td>15</td><td>Connecticut</td><td>840</td><td>1.90%</td><td>7</td><td>Pennsylvania</td><td>1,947</td><td>4.41%</td></tr>
<tr><td>42</td><td>Delaware</td><td>124</td><td>0.28%</td><td>8</td><td>Ohio</td><td>1,817</td><td>4.12%</td></tr>
<tr><td>4</td><td>Florida</td><td>2,181</td><td>4.94%</td><td>9</td><td>Massachusetts</td><td>1,669</td><td>3.78%</td></tr>
<tr><td>14</td><td>Georgia</td><td>911</td><td>2.07%</td><td>10</td><td>Maryland</td><td>1,518</td><td>3.44%</td></tr>
<tr><td>34</td><td>Hawaii</td><td>258</td><td>0.58%</td><td>11</td><td>Michigan</td><td>1,346</td><td>3.05%</td></tr>
<tr><td>47</td><td>Idaho</td><td>62</td><td>0.14%</td><td>12</td><td>Virginia</td><td>1,060</td><td>2.40%</td></tr>
<tr><td>5</td><td>Illinois</td><td>2,082</td><td>4.72%</td><td>13</td><td>North Carolina</td><td>1,052</td><td>2.38%</td></tr>
<tr><td>22</td><td>Indiana</td><td>584</td><td>1.32%</td><td>14</td><td>Georgia</td><td>911</td><td>2.07%</td></tr>
<tr><td>33</td><td>Iowa</td><td>260</td><td>0.59%</td><td>15</td><td>Connecticut</td><td>840</td><td>1.90%</td></tr>
<tr><td>32</td><td>Kansas</td><td>266</td><td>0.60%</td><td>16</td><td>Tennessee</td><td>820</td><td>1.86%</td></tr>
<tr><td>25</td><td>Kentucky</td><td>499</td><td>1.13%</td><td>17</td><td>Missouri</td><td>815</td><td>1.85%</td></tr>
<tr><td>21</td><td>Louisiana</td><td>626</td><td>1.42%</td><td>18</td><td>Washington</td><td>751</td><td>1.70%</td></tr>
<tr><td>41</td><td>Maine</td><td>152</td><td>0.34%</td><td>19</td><td>Wisconsin</td><td>661</td><td>1.50%</td></tr>
<tr><td>10</td><td>Maryland</td><td>1,518</td><td>3.44%</td><td>20</td><td>Minnesota</td><td>655</td><td>1.48%</td></tr>
<tr><td>9</td><td>Massachusetts</td><td>1,669</td><td>3.78%</td><td>21</td><td>Louisiana</td><td>626</td><td>1.42%</td></tr>
<tr><td>11</td><td>Michigan</td><td>1,346</td><td>3.05%</td><td>22</td><td>Indiana</td><td>584</td><td>1.32%</td></tr>
<tr><td>20</td><td>Minnesota</td><td>655</td><td>1.48%</td><td>23</td><td>Colorado</td><td>565</td><td>1.28%</td></tr>
<tr><td>37</td><td>Mississippi</td><td>225</td><td>0.51%</td><td>24</td><td>Arizona</td><td>552</td><td>1.25%</td></tr>
<tr><td>17</td><td>Missouri</td><td>815</td><td>1.85%</td><td>25</td><td>Kentucky</td><td>499</td><td>1.13%</td></tr>
<tr><td>45</td><td>Montana</td><td>71</td><td>0.16%</td><td>26</td><td>Alabama</td><td>485</td><td>1.10%</td></tr>
<tr><td>39</td><td>Nebraska</td><td>191</td><td>0.43%</td><td>27</td><td>South Carolina</td><td>406</td><td>0.92%</td></tr>
<tr><td>44</td><td>Nevada</td><td>108</td><td>0.24%</td><td>28</td><td>Oregon</td><td>345</td><td>0.78%</td></tr>
<tr><td>40</td><td>New Hampshire</td><td>169</td><td>0.38%</td><td>29</td><td>Oklahoma</td><td>315</td><td>0.71%</td></tr>
<tr><td>6</td><td>New Jersey</td><td>2,049</td><td>4.64%</td><td>30</td><td>Utah</td><td>302</td><td>0.68%</td></tr>
<tr><td>35</td><td>New Mexico</td><td>235</td><td>0.53%</td><td>31</td><td>Arkansas</td><td>271</td><td>0.61%</td></tr>
<tr><td>2</td><td>New York</td><td>5,525</td><td>12.52%</td><td>32</td><td>Kansas</td><td>266</td><td>0.60%</td></tr>
<tr><td>13</td><td>North Carolina</td><td>1,052</td><td>2.38%</td><td>33</td><td>Iowa</td><td>260</td><td>0.59%</td></tr>
<tr><td>48</td><td>North Dakota</td><td>58</td><td>0.13%</td><td>34</td><td>Hawaii</td><td>258</td><td>0.58%</td></tr>
<tr><td>8</td><td>Ohio</td><td>1,817</td><td>4.12%</td><td>35</td><td>New Mexico</td><td>235</td><td>0.53%</td></tr>
<tr><td>29</td><td>Oklahoma</td><td>315</td><td>0.71%</td><td>36</td><td>Rhode Island</td><td>233</td><td>0.53%</td></tr>
<tr><td>28</td><td>Oregon</td><td>345</td><td>0.78%</td><td>37</td><td>Mississippi</td><td>225</td><td>0.51%</td></tr>
<tr><td>7</td><td>Pennsylvania</td><td>1,947</td><td>4.41%</td><td>38</td><td>West Virginia</td><td>203</td><td>0.46%</td></tr>
<tr><td>36</td><td>Rhode Island</td><td>233</td><td>0.53%</td><td>39</td><td>Nebraska</td><td>191</td><td>0.43%</td></tr>
<tr><td>27</td><td>South Carolina</td><td>406</td><td>0.92%</td><td>40</td><td>New Hampshire</td><td>169</td><td>0.38%</td></tr>
<tr><td>49</td><td>South Dakota</td><td>47</td><td>0.11%</td><td>41</td><td>Maine</td><td>152</td><td>0.34%</td></tr>
<tr><td>16</td><td>Tennessee</td><td>820</td><td>1.86%</td><td>42</td><td>Delaware</td><td>124</td><td>0.28%</td></tr>
<tr><td>3</td><td>Texas</td><td>2,409</td><td>5.46%</td><td>43</td><td>Vermont</td><td>122</td><td>0.28%</td></tr>
<tr><td>30</td><td>Utah</td><td>302</td><td>0.68%</td><td>44</td><td>Nevada</td><td>108</td><td>0.24%</td></tr>
<tr><td>43</td><td>Vermont</td><td>122</td><td>0.28%</td><td>45</td><td>Montana</td><td>71</td><td>0.16%</td></tr>
<tr><td>12</td><td>Virginia</td><td>1,060</td><td>2.40%</td><td>46</td><td>Alaska</td><td>69</td><td>0.16%</td></tr>
<tr><td>18</td><td>Washington</td><td>751</td><td>1.70%</td><td>47</td><td>Idaho</td><td>62</td><td>0.14%</td></tr>
<tr><td>38</td><td>West Virginia</td><td>203</td><td>0.46%</td><td>48</td><td>North Dakota</td><td>58</td><td>0.13%</td></tr>
<tr><td>19</td><td>Wisconsin</td><td>661</td><td>1.50%</td><td>49</td><td>South Dakota</td><td>47</td><td>0.11%</td></tr>
<tr><td>50</td><td>Wyoming</td><td>35</td><td>0.08%</td><td>50</td><td>Wyoming</td><td>35</td><td>0.08%</td></tr>
<tr><td></td><td></td><td></td><td></td><td></td><td>District of Columbia</td><td>337</td><td>0.76%</td></tr>
</table>

Source: American Medical Association (Chicago, Illinois)
   "Physician Characteristics and Distribution in the U.S." (1994 Edition)
*As of January 1, 1993. Total does not include 846 physicians in the U.S. territories and possessions. Pediatrics includes Adolescent Medicine, Neonatal-Perinatal, Pediatric Allergy, Pediatric Endocrinology, Pediatric Pulmonology, Pediatric Hematology-Oncology and Pediatric Nephrology.

Rate of Nonfederal Physicians in Pediatrics in 1993

National Rate = 65.73 Physicians per 100,000 Population 17 Years and Younger*

ALPHA ORDER

RANK	STATE	RATE
34	Alabama	45.30
41	Alaska	36.65
26	Arizona	50.25
38	Arkansas	42.57
11	California	68.27
19	Colorado	59.74
4	Connecticut	107.65
9	Delaware	71.55
10	Florida	68.42
29	Georgia	49.20
7	Hawaii	86.26
50	Idaho	18.71
12	Illinois	68.17
39	Indiana	39.91
43	Iowa	35.84
40	Kansas	38.94
24	Kentucky	51.70
25	Louisiana	50.87
27	Maine	49.55
2	Maryland	121.99
3	Massachusetts	118.78
22	Michigan	53.68
23	Minnesota	53.51
47	Mississippi	29.96
18	Missouri	59.87
45	Montana	30.44
36	Nebraska	43.63
46	Nevada	30.27
20	New Hampshire	58.70
5	New Jersey	107.48
30	New Mexico	48.59
1	New York	123.47
17	North Carolina	61.08
44	North Dakota	33.87
16	Ohio	64.01
42	Oklahoma	36.26
35	Oregon	44.54
13	Pennsylvania	67.71
6	Rhode Island	98.73
37	South Carolina	42.91
49	South Dakota	22.74
15	Tennessee	64.33
32	Texas	46.37
33	Utah	45.69
8	Vermont	84.34
14	Virginia	66.88
21	Washington	54.29
31	West Virginia	47.12
28	Wisconsin	49.53
48	Wyoming	25.64

RANK ORDER

RANK	STATE	RATE
1	New York	123.47
2	Maryland	121.99
3	Massachusetts	118.78
4	Connecticut	107.65
5	New Jersey	107.48
6	Rhode Island	98.73
7	Hawaii	86.26
8	Vermont	84.34
9	Delaware	71.55
10	Florida	68.42
11	California	68.27
12	Illinois	68.17
13	Pennsylvania	67.71
14	Virginia	66.88
15	Tennessee	64.33
16	Ohio	64.01
17	North Carolina	61.08
18	Missouri	59.87
19	Colorado	59.74
20	New Hampshire	58.70
21	Washington	54.29
22	Michigan	53.68
23	Minnesota	53.51
24	Kentucky	51.70
25	Louisiana	50.87
26	Arizona	50.25
27	Maine	49.55
28	Wisconsin	49.53
29	Georgia	49.20
30	New Mexico	48.59
31	West Virginia	47.12
32	Texas	46.37
33	Utah	45.69
34	Alabama	45.30
35	Oregon	44.54
36	Nebraska	43.63
37	South Carolina	42.91
38	Arkansas	42.57
39	Indiana	39.91
40	Kansas	38.94
41	Alaska	36.65
42	Oklahoma	36.26
43	Iowa	35.84
44	North Dakota	33.87
45	Montana	30.44
46	Nevada	30.27
47	Mississippi	29.96
48	Wyoming	25.64
49	South Dakota	22.74
50	Idaho	18.71
	District of Columbia	288.39

Source: Morgan Quitno Press using data from American Medical Association
"Physician Characteristics and Distribution in the U.S." (1994 Edition)
As of January 1, 1993. National rate does not include physicians in the U.S. territories and possessions. Pediatrics includes Adolescent Medicine, Neonatal-Perinatal, Pediatric Allergy, Pediatric Endocrinology, Pediatric Pulmonology, Pediatric Hematology-Oncology and Pediatric Nephrology.

Nonfederal Physicians in Surgical Specialties in 1993

National Total = 136,378 Physicians*

ALPHA ORDER					RANK ORDER			
RANK	STATE	PHYSICIANS	% of USA		RANK	STATE	PHYSICIANS	% of USA
23	Alabama	1,886	1.38%		1	California	17,094	12.53%
49	Alaska	195	0.14%		2	New York	13,205	9.68%
24	Arizona	1,873	1.37%		3	Texas	8,173	5.99%
33	Arkansas	940	0.69%		4	Florida	7,354	5.39%
1	California	17,094	12.53%		5	Pennsylvania	6,985	5.12%
25	Colorado	1,836	1.35%		6	Illinois	5,961	4.37%
19	Connecticut	2,340	1.72%		7	Ohio	5,596	4.10%
45	Delaware	340	0.25%		8	New Jersey	4,688	3.44%
4	Florida	7,354	5.39%		9	Michigan	4,468	3.28%
13	Georgia	3,404	2.50%		10	Massachusetts	4,328	3.17%
38	Hawaii	675	0.49%		11	Maryland	3,595	2.64%
43	Idaho	379	0.28%		12	North Carolina	3,412	2.50%
6	Illinois	5,961	4.37%		13	Georgia	3,404	2.50%
22	Indiana	2,204	1.62%		14	Virginia	3,401	2.49%
30	Iowa	1,089	0.80%		15	Tennessee	2,830	2.08%
31	Kansas	1,056	0.77%		16	Missouri	2,716	1.99%
26	Kentucky	1,685	1.24%		17	Louisiana	2,555	1.87%
17	Louisiana	2,555	1.87%		18	Washington	2,536	1.86%
41	Maine	554	0.41%		19	Connecticut	2,340	1.72%
11	Maryland	3,595	2.64%		20	Minnesota	2,262	1.66%
10	Massachusetts	4,328	3.17%		21	Wisconsin	2,254	1.65%
9	Michigan	4,468	3.28%		22	Indiana	2,204	1.62%
20	Minnesota	2,262	1.66%		23	Alabama	1,886	1.38%
32	Mississippi	973	0.71%		24	Arizona	1,873	1.37%
16	Missouri	2,716	1.99%		25	Colorado	1,836	1.35%
44	Montana	355	0.26%		26	Kentucky	1,685	1.24%
36	Nebraska	739	0.54%		27	South Carolina	1,631	1.20%
42	Nevada	533	0.39%		28	Oregon	1,595	1.17%
40	New Hampshire	568	0.42%		29	Oklahoma	1,201	0.88%
8	New Jersey	4,688	3.44%		30	Iowa	1,089	0.80%
37	New Mexico	697	0.51%		31	Kansas	1,056	0.77%
2	New York	13,205	9.68%		32	Mississippi	973	0.71%
12	North Carolina	3,412	2.50%		33	Arkansas	940	0.69%
47	North Dakota	262	0.19%		34	Utah	858	0.63%
7	Ohio	5,596	4.10%		35	West Virginia	846	0.62%
29	Oklahoma	1,201	0.88%		36	Nebraska	739	0.54%
28	Oregon	1,595	1.17%		37	New Mexico	697	0.51%
5	Pennsylvania	6,985	5.12%		38	Hawaii	675	0.49%
39	Rhode Island	621	0.46%		39	Rhode Island	621	0.46%
27	South Carolina	1,631	1.20%		40	New Hampshire	568	0.42%
48	South Dakota	248	0.18%		41	Maine	554	0.41%
15	Tennessee	2,830	2.08%		42	Nevada	533	0.39%
3	Texas	8,173	5.99%		43	Idaho	379	0.28%
34	Utah	858	0.63%		44	Montana	355	0.26%
46	Vermont	336	0.25%		45	Delaware	340	0.25%
14	Virginia	3,401	2.49%		46	Vermont	336	0.25%
18	Washington	2,536	1.86%		47	North Dakota	262	0.19%
35	West Virginia	846	0.62%		48	South Dakota	248	0.18%
21	Wisconsin	2,254	1.65%		49	Alaska	195	0.14%
50	Wyoming	162	0.12%		50	Wyoming	162	0.12%
						District of Columbia	884	0.65%

Source: American Medical Association
   "Physician Characteristics and Distribution in the U.S." (1994 Edition)
*As of January 1, 1993. Total does not include 1,448 physicians in the U.S. territories and possessions. Surgical Specialties include Colon and Rectal, General, Neurological, Obstetrics & Gynecology, Ophthalmology, Orthopedic, Otolaryngology, Plastic, Thoracic and Urological Surgeries.

Rate of Nonfederal Physicians in Surgical Specialties in 1993

National Rate = 52.90 Physicians per 100,000 Population*

ALPHA ORDER				RANK ORDER		
RANK	STATE	RATE		RANK	STATE	RATE
32	Alabama	45.11		1	New York	72.74
50	Alaska	32.61		2	Maryland	72.51
26	Arizona	47.48		3	Massachusetts	71.92
41	Arkansas	38.75		4	Connecticut	71.38
12	California	54.76		5	Rhode Island	62.10
17	Colorado	51.52		6	New Jersey	59.65
4	Connecticut	71.38		7	Louisiana	59.56
24	Delaware	48.71		8	Vermont	58.33
13	Florida	53.58		9	Pennsylvania	58.06
22	Georgia	49.32		10	Hawaii	57.89
10	Hawaii	57.89		11	Tennessee	55.56
49	Idaho	34.45		12	California	54.76
18	Illinois	51.01		13	Florida	53.58
42	Indiana	38.63		14	Oregon	52.55
43	Iowa	38.60		15	Virginia	52.54
39	Kansas	41.66		16	Missouri	51.88
36	Kentucky	44.41		17	Colorado	51.52
7	Louisiana	59.56		18	Illinois	51.01
35	Maine	44.68		19	Ohio	50.59
2	Maryland	72.51		20	New Hampshire	50.53
3	Massachusetts	71.92		21	Minnesota	50.00
27	Michigan	47.23		22	Georgia	49.32
21	Minnesota	50.00		23	North Carolina	49.08
46	Mississippi	36.86		24	Delaware	48.71
16	Missouri	51.88		25	Washington	48.22
38	Montana	42.21		26	Arizona	47.48
30	Nebraska	45.82		27	Michigan	47.23
44	Nevada	38.57		28	West Virginia	46.53
20	New Hampshire	50.53		29	Utah	46.13
6	New Jersey	59.65		30	Nebraska	45.82
37	New Mexico	43.13		31	Texas	45.35
1	New York	72.74		32	Alabama	45.11
23	North Carolina	49.08		33	South Carolina	44.93
40	North Dakota	41.13		34	Wisconsin	44.69
19	Ohio	50.59		35	Maine	44.68
45	Oklahoma	37.15		36	Kentucky	44.41
14	Oregon	52.55		37	New Mexico	43.13
9	Pennsylvania	58.06		38	Montana	42.21
5	Rhode Island	62.10		39	Kansas	41.66
33	South Carolina	44.93		40	North Dakota	41.13
47	South Dakota	34.64		41	Arkansas	38.75
11	Tennessee	55.56		42	Indiana	38.63
31	Texas	45.35		43	Iowa	38.60
29	Utah	46.13		44	Nevada	38.57
8	Vermont	58.33		45	Oklahoma	37.15
15	Virginia	52.54		46	Mississippi	36.86
25	Washington	48.22		47	South Dakota	34.64
28	West Virginia	46.53		48	Wyoming	34.47
34	Wisconsin	44.69		49	Idaho	34.45
48	Wyoming	34.47		50	Alaska	32.61
					District of Columbia	152.68

Source: Morgan Quitno Press using data from American Medical Association
  "Physician Characteristics and Distribution in the U.S." (1994 Edition)
*As of January 1, 1993. National rate does not include physicians in the U.S. territories and possessions. Surgical Specialties include Colon and Rectal, General, Neurological, Obstetrics & Gynecology, Ophthalmology, Orthopedic, Otolaryngology, Plastic, Thoracic and Urological Surgeries.

Nonfederal Physicians in General Surgery in 1993

National Total = 36,263 Physicians*

ALPHA ORDER					RANK ORDER			
RANK	STATE	PHYSICIANS	% of USA		RANK	STATE	PHYSICIANS	% of USA
23	Alabama	546	1.51%		1	New York	3,963	10.93%
50	Alaska	39	0.11%		2	California	3,916	10.80%
25	Arizona	457	1.26%		3	Texas	2,055	5.67%
34	Arkansas	249	0.69%		4	Pennsylvania	2,029	5.60%
2	California	3,916	10.80%		5	Florida	1,693	4.67%
27	Colorado	437	1.21%		6	Illinois	1,686	4.65%
19	Connecticut	605	1.67%		7	Ohio	1,598	4.41%
44	Delaware	98	0.27%		8	Massachusetts	1,303	3.59%
5	Florida	1,693	4.67%		9	Michigan	1,280	3.53%
12	Georgia	875	2.41%		10	New Jersey	1,259	3.47%
39	Hawaii	172	0.47%		11	Maryland	915	2.52%
45	Idaho	91	0.25%		12	Georgia	875	2.41%
6	Illinois	1,686	4.65%		12	North Carolina	875	2.41%
20	Indiana	602	1.66%		14	Virginia	864	2.38%
30	Iowa	311	0.86%		15	Tennessee	821	2.26%
29	Kansas	317	0.87%		16	Missouri	715	1.97%
24	Kentucky	492	1.36%		17	Louisiana	660	1.82%
17	Louisiana	660	1.82%		18	Minnesota	607	1.67%
40	Maine	158	0.44%		19	Connecticut	605	1.67%
11	Maryland	915	2.52%		20	Indiana	602	1.66%
8	Massachusetts	1,303	3.59%		21	Washington	595	1.64%
9	Michigan	1,280	3.53%		22	Wisconsin	580	1.60%
18	Minnesota	607	1.67%		23	Alabama	546	1.51%
33	Mississippi	253	0.70%		24	Kentucky	492	1.36%
16	Missouri	715	1.97%		25	Arizona	457	1.26%
45	Montana	91	0.25%		26	South Carolina	447	1.23%
35	Nebraska	235	0.65%		27	Colorado	437	1.21%
42	Nevada	134	0.37%		28	Oregon	391	1.08%
40	New Hampshire	158	0.44%		29	Kansas	317	0.87%
10	New Jersey	1,259	3.47%		30	Iowa	311	0.86%
38	New Mexico	178	0.49%		31	Oklahoma	309	0.85%
1	New York	3,963	10.93%		32	West Virginia	260	0.72%
12	North Carolina	875	2.41%		33	Mississippi	253	0.70%
47	North Dakota	89	0.25%		34	Arkansas	249	0.69%
7	Ohio	1,598	4.41%		35	Nebraska	235	0.65%
31	Oklahoma	309	0.85%		36	Rhode Island	186	0.51%
28	Oregon	391	1.08%		37	Utah	181	0.50%
4	Pennsylvania	2,029	5.60%		38	New Mexico	178	0.49%
36	Rhode Island	186	0.51%		39	Hawaii	172	0.47%
26	South Carolina	447	1.23%		40	Maine	158	0.44%
48	South Dakota	72	0.20%		40	New Hampshire	158	0.44%
15	Tennessee	821	2.26%		42	Nevada	134	0.37%
3	Texas	2,055	5.67%		43	Vermont	100	0.28%
37	Utah	181	0.50%		44	Delaware	98	0.27%
43	Vermont	100	0.28%		45	Idaho	91	0.25%
14	Virginia	864	2.38%		45	Montana	91	0.25%
21	Washington	595	1.64%		47	North Dakota	89	0.25%
32	West Virginia	260	0.72%		48	South Dakota	72	0.20%
22	Wisconsin	580	1.60%		49	Wyoming	45	0.12%
49	Wyoming	45	0.12%		50	Alaska	39	0.11%
					District of Columbia		271	0.75%

Source: American Medical Association (Chicago, Illinois)
   "Physician Characteristics and Distribution in the U.S." (1994 Edition)
*As of January 1, 1993. Total does not include 398 physicians in the U.S. territories and possessions. General Surgery
includes Abdominal, Cardiovascular, Hand, Head and Neck, Pediatric, Traumatic and Vascular Surgeries.

Rate of Nonfederal Physicians in General Surgery in 1993

National Rate = 14.07 Physicians per 100,000 Population*

ALPHA ORDER

RANK ORDER

RANK	STATE	RATE
23	Alabama	13.06
50	Alaska	6.52
34	Arizona	11.58
42	Arkansas	10.26
29	California	12.54
33	Colorado	12.26
4	Connecticut	18.46
17	Delaware	14.04
31	Florida	12.33
27	Georgia	12.68
11	Hawaii	14.75
49	Idaho	8.27
14	Illinois	14.43
41	Indiana	10.55
38	Iowa	11.02
30	Kansas	12.50
24	Kentucky	12.97
10	Louisiana	15.38
26	Maine	12.74
4	Maryland	18.46
2	Massachusetts	21.65
20	Michigan	13.53
21	Minnesota	13.42
46	Mississippi	9.58
19	Missouri	13.66
40	Montana	10.82
12	Nebraska	14.57
45	Nevada	9.70
16	New Hampshire	14.06
9	New Jersey	16.02
39	New Mexico	11.01
1	New York	21.83
28	North Carolina	12.59
18	North Dakota	13.97
13	Ohio	14.45
48	Oklahoma	9.56
25	Oregon	12.88
7	Pennsylvania	16.87
3	Rhode Island	18.60
32	South Carolina	12.31
43	South Dakota	10.06
8	Tennessee	16.12
36	Texas	11.40
44	Utah	9.73
6	Vermont	17.36
22	Virginia	13.35
37	Washington	11.31
15	West Virginia	14.30
35	Wisconsin	11.50
47	Wyoming	9.57

RANK	STATE	RATE
1	New York	21.83
2	Massachusetts	21.65
3	Rhode Island	18.60
4	Connecticut	18.46
4	Maryland	18.46
6	Vermont	17.36
7	Pennsylvania	16.87
8	Tennessee	16.12
9	New Jersey	16.02
10	Louisiana	15.38
11	Hawaii	14.75
12	Nebraska	14.57
13	Ohio	14.45
14	Illinois	14.43
15	West Virginia	14.30
16	New Hampshire	14.06
17	Delaware	14.04
18	North Dakota	13.97
19	Missouri	13.66
20	Michigan	13.53
21	Minnesota	13.42
22	Virginia	13.35
23	Alabama	13.06
24	Kentucky	12.97
25	Oregon	12.88
26	Maine	12.74
27	Georgia	12.68
28	North Carolina	12.59
29	California	12.54
30	Kansas	12.50
31	Florida	12.33
32	South Carolina	12.31
33	Colorado	12.26
34	Arizona	11.58
35	Wisconsin	11.50
36	Texas	11.40
37	Washington	11.31
38	Iowa	11.02
39	New Mexico	11.01
40	Montana	10.82
41	Indiana	10.55
42	Arkansas	10.26
43	South Dakota	10.06
44	Utah	9.73
45	Nevada	9.70
46	Mississippi	9.58
47	Wyoming	9.57
48	Oklahoma	9.56
49	Idaho	8.27
50	Alaska	6.52

| | District of Columbia | 46.80 |

Source: Morgan Quitno Press using data from American Medical Association
    "Physician Characteristics and Distribution in the U.S." (1994 Edition)
*As of January 1, 1993. National rate does not include physicians in the U.S. territories and possessions. General Surgery
includes Abdominal, Cardiovascular, Hand, Head and Neck, Pediatric, Traumatic and Vascular Surgeries.

Nonfederal Physicians in Obstetrics and Gynecology in 1993

National Total = 34,389 Physicians*

ALPHA ORDER

RANK	STATE	PHYSICIANS	% of USA
22	Alabama	471	1.37%
47	Alaska	51	0.15%
21	Arizona	503	1.46%
34	Arkansas	202	0.59%
1	California	4,489	13.05%
24	Colorado	466	1.36%
18	Connecticut	636	1.85%
44	Delaware	77	0.22%
4	Florida	1,735	5.05%
12	Georgia	997	2.90%
33	Hawaii	203	0.59%
43	Idaho	82	0.24%
6	Illinois	1,597	4.64%
20	Indiana	509	1.48%
35	Iowa	201	0.58%
31	Kansas	236	0.69%
27	Kentucky	396	1.15%
17	Louisiana	652	1.90%
42	Maine	130	0.38%
10	Maryland	1,041	3.03%
11	Massachusetts	1,014	2.95%
9	Michigan	1,214	3.53%
25	Minnesota	458	1.33%
30	Mississippi	239	0.69%
16	Missouri	665	1.93%
46	Montana	73	0.21%
38	Nebraska	151	0.44%
39	Nevada	149	0.43%
41	New Hampshire	135	0.39%
8	New Jersey	1,283	3.73%
36	New Mexico	184	0.54%
2	New York	3,371	9.80%
14	North Carolina	890	2.59%
49	North Dakota	45	0.13%
7	Ohio	1,356	3.94%
29	Oklahoma	282	0.82%
28	Oregon	365	1.06%
5	Pennsylvania	1,600	4.65%
39	Rhode Island	149	0.43%
26	South Carolina	418	1.22%
48	South Dakota	46	0.13%
15	Tennessee	685	1.99%
3	Texas	2,180	6.34%
32	Utah	220	0.64%
45	Vermont	75	0.22%
13	Virginia	943	2.74%
19	Washington	590	1.72%
36	West Virginia	184	0.54%
23	Wisconsin	469	1.36%
50	Wyoming	33	0.10%

RANK ORDER

RANK	STATE	PHYSICIANS	% of USA
1	California	4,489	13.05%
2	New York	3,371	9.80%
3	Texas	2,180	6.34%
4	Florida	1,735	5.05%
5	Pennsylvania	1,600	4.65%
6	Illinois	1,597	4.64%
7	Ohio	1,356	3.94%
8	New Jersey	1,283	3.73%
9	Michigan	1,214	3.53%
10	Maryland	1,041	3.03%
11	Massachusetts	1,014	2.95%
12	Georgia	997	2.90%
13	Virginia	943	2.74%
14	North Carolina	890	2.59%
15	Tennessee	685	1.99%
16	Missouri	665	1.93%
17	Louisiana	652	1.90%
18	Connecticut	636	1.85%
19	Washington	590	1.72%
20	Indiana	509	1.48%
21	Arizona	503	1.46%
22	Alabama	471	1.37%
23	Wisconsin	469	1.36%
24	Colorado	466	1.36%
25	Minnesota	458	1.33%
26	South Carolina	418	1.22%
27	Kentucky	396	1.15%
28	Oregon	365	1.06%
29	Oklahoma	282	0.82%
30	Mississippi	239	0.69%
31	Kansas	236	0.69%
32	Utah	220	0.64%
33	Hawaii	203	0.59%
34	Arkansas	202	0.59%
35	Iowa	201	0.58%
36	New Mexico	184	0.54%
36	West Virginia	184	0.54%
38	Nebraska	151	0.44%
39	Nevada	149	0.43%
39	Rhode Island	149	0.43%
41	New Hampshire	135	0.39%
42	Maine	130	0.38%
43	Idaho	82	0.24%
44	Delaware	77	0.22%
45	Vermont	75	0.22%
46	Montana	73	0.21%
47	Alaska	51	0.15%
48	South Dakota	46	0.13%
49	North Dakota	45	0.13%
50	Wyoming	33	0.10%
	District of Columbia	249	0.72%

Source: American Medical Association (Chicago, Illinois)
   "Physician Characteristics and Distribution in the U.S." (1994 Edition)
*As of January 1, 1993. Total does not include 519 physicians in the U.S. territories and possessions. Obstetrics and Gynecology includes Gynecology and Oncology, Maternal and Fetal Medicine and Reproductive Endocrinology.

Rate of Nonfederal Physicians in Obstetrics and Gynecology in 1993

National Rate = 27.34 Physicians per 100,000 Female Population*

ALPHA ORDER				RANK ORDER		
RANK	**STATE**	**RATE**		**RANK**	**STATE**	**RATE**
28	Alabama	23.49		1	Maryland	43.25
45	Alaska	16.16		2	Connecticut	40.05
21	Arizona	25.82		3	New York	38.65
44	Arkansas	17.27		4	Massachusetts	35.03
11	California	28.73		5	Hawaii	34.37
18	Colorado	26.38		6	New Jersey	33.76
2	Connecticut	40.05		7	Louisiana	31.59
30	Delaware	22.68		8	Rhode Island	31.03
20	Florida	26.10		9	Georgia	29.73
9	Georgia	29.73		10	Virginia	29.72
5	Hawaii	34.37		11	California	28.73
46	Idaho	14.95		12	Illinois	28.10
12	Illinois	28.10		13	Tennessee	27.91
41	Indiana	18.37		14	Pennsylvania	27.71
47	Iowa	14.67		15	Vermont	26.55
39	Kansas	18.95		16	Michigan	26.41
32	Kentucky	21.54		17	North Carolina	26.39
7	Louisiana	31.59		18	Colorado	26.38
33	Maine	21.52		19	Missouri	26.32
1	Maryland	43.25		20	Florida	26.10
4	Massachusetts	35.03		21	Arizona	25.82
16	Michigan	26.41		22	Ohio	25.41
36	Minnesota	20.60		23	Texas	24.55
40	Mississippi	18.90		24	New Hampshire	24.50
19	Missouri	26.32		25	Oregon	24.42
43	Montana	17.48		26	South Carolina	23.83
37	Nebraska	19.18		27	Utah	23.80
34	Nevada	21.19		28	Alabama	23.49
24	New Hampshire	24.50		29	New Mexico	23.14
6	New Jersey	33.76		30	Delaware	22.68
29	New Mexico	23.14		31	Washington	22.60
3	New York	38.65		32	Kentucky	21.54
17	North Carolina	26.39		33	Maine	21.52
48	North Dakota	14.19		34	Nevada	21.19
22	Ohio	25.41		35	West Virginia	21.03
42	Oklahoma	17.89		36	Minnesota	20.60
25	Oregon	24.42		37	Nebraska	19.18
14	Pennsylvania	27.71		38	Wisconsin	18.97
8	Rhode Island	31.03		39	Kansas	18.95
26	South Carolina	23.83		40	Mississippi	18.90
50	South Dakota	13.04		41	Indiana	18.37
13	Tennessee	27.91		42	Oklahoma	17.89
23	Texas	24.55		43	Montana	17.48
27	Utah	23.80		44	Arkansas	17.27
15	Vermont	26.55		45	Alaska	16.16
10	Virginia	29.72		46	Idaho	14.95
31	Washington	22.60		47	Iowa	14.67
35	West Virginia	21.03		48	North Dakota	14.19
38	Wisconsin	18.97		49	Wyoming	14.00
49	Wyoming	14.00		50	South Dakota	13.04
					District of Columbia	92.08

Source: Morgan Quitno Press using data from American Medical Association
"Physician Characteristics and Distribution in the U.S." (1994 Edition)
*As of January 1, 1993. National rate does not include physicians in the U.S. territories and possessions. Obstetrics and Gynecology includes Gynecology and Oncology, Maternal and Fetal Medicine and Reproductive Endocrinology.

Nonfederal Physicians in Ophthalmology in 1993

National Total = 16,128 Physicians*

<u>ALPHA ORDER</u>

RANK	STATE	PHYSICIANS	% of USA
27	Alabama	182	1.13%
49	Alaska	23	0.14%
23	Arizona	233	1.44%
30	Arkansas	128	0.79%
1	California	2,028	12.57%
24	Colorado	226	1.40%
21	Connecticut	283	1.75%
44	Delaware	43	0.27%
3	Florida	1,018	6.31%
15	Georgia	330	2.05%
37	Hawaii	81	0.50%
43	Idaho	49	0.30%
6	Illinois	688	4.27%
22	Indiana	251	1.56%
29	Iowa	155	0.96%
30	Kansas	128	0.79%
28	Kentucky	175	1.09%
16	Louisiana	315	1.95%
40	Maine	58	0.36%
11	Maryland	441	2.73%
9	Massachusetts	526	3.26%
10	Michigan	504	3.13%
19	Minnesota	291	1.80%
33	Mississippi	121	0.75%
14	Missouri	342	2.12%
45	Montana	42	0.26%
36	Nebraska	87	0.54%
42	Nevada	50	0.31%
41	New Hampshire	55	0.34%
8	New Jersey	557	3.45%
38	New Mexico	67	0.42%
2	New York	1,647	10.21%
12	North Carolina	367	2.28%
48	North Dakota	29	0.18%
7	Ohio	603	3.74%
32	Oklahoma	127	0.79%
25	Oregon	211	1.31%
5	Pennsylvania	867	5.38%
39	Rhode Island	64	0.40%
26	South Carolina	187	1.16%
47	South Dakota	33	0.20%
20	Tennessee	288	1.79%
4	Texas	926	5.74%
34	Utah	95	0.59%
46	Vermont	34	0.21%
13	Virginia	361	2.24%
18	Washington	295	1.83%
35	West Virginia	89	0.55%
17	Wisconsin	310	1.92%
50	Wyoming	18	0.11%

<u>RANK ORDER</u>

RANK	STATE	PHYSICIANS	% of USA
1	California	2,028	12.57%
2	New York	1,647	10.21%
3	Florida	1,018	6.31%
4	Texas	926	5.74%
5	Pennsylvania	867	5.38%
6	Illinois	688	4.27%
7	Ohio	603	3.74%
8	New Jersey	557	3.45%
9	Massachusetts	526	3.26%
10	Michigan	504	3.13%
11	Maryland	441	2.73%
12	North Carolina	367	2.28%
13	Virginia	361	2.24%
14	Missouri	342	2.12%
15	Georgia	330	2.05%
16	Louisiana	315	1.95%
17	Wisconsin	310	1.92%
18	Washington	295	1.83%
19	Minnesota	291	1.80%
20	Tennessee	288	1.79%
21	Connecticut	283	1.75%
22	Indiana	251	1.56%
23	Arizona	233	1.44%
24	Colorado	226	1.40%
25	Oregon	211	1.31%
26	South Carolina	187	1.16%
27	Alabama	182	1.13%
28	Kentucky	175	1.09%
29	Iowa	155	0.96%
30	Arkansas	128	0.79%
30	Kansas	128	0.79%
32	Oklahoma	127	0.79%
33	Mississippi	121	0.75%
34	Utah	95	0.59%
35	West Virginia	89	0.55%
36	Nebraska	87	0.54%
37	Hawaii	81	0.50%
38	New Mexico	67	0.42%
39	Rhode Island	64	0.40%
40	Maine	58	0.36%
41	New Hampshire	55	0.34%
42	Nevada	50	0.31%
43	Idaho	49	0.30%
44	Delaware	43	0.27%
45	Montana	42	0.26%
46	Vermont	34	0.21%
47	South Dakota	33	0.20%
48	North Dakota	29	0.18%
49	Alaska	23	0.14%
50	Wyoming	18	0.11%
	District of Columbia	100	0.62%

Source: American Medical Association (Chicago, Illinois)
"Physician Characteristics and Distribution in the U.S." (1994 Edition)
*As of January 1, 1993. Total does not include 155 physicians in the U.S. territories and possessions.

Rate of Nonfederal Physicians in Ophthalmology in 1993

National Rate = 6.26 Physicians per 100,000 Population*

<u>ALPHA ORDER</u>

RANK	STATE	RATE
45	Alabama	4.35
48	Alaska	3.85
18	Arizona	5.91
28	Arkansas	5.28
12	California	6.50
15	Colorado	6.34
4	Connecticut	8.63
16	Delaware	6.16
5	Florida	7.42
37	Georgia	4.78
9	Hawaii	6.95
43	Idaho	4.45
20	Illinois	5.89
44	Indiana	4.40
24	Iowa	5.49
33	Kansas	5.05
39	Kentucky	4.61
6	Louisiana	7.34
38	Maine	4.68
2	Maryland	8.89
3	Massachusetts	8.74
27	Michigan	5.33
13	Minnesota	6.43
41	Mississippi	4.58
11	Missouri	6.53
34	Montana	4.99
26	Nebraska	5.39
50	Nevada	3.62
36	New Hampshire	4.89
8	New Jersey	7.09
46	New Mexico	4.15
1	New York	9.07
28	North Carolina	5.28
42	North Dakota	4.55
25	Ohio	5.45
47	Oklahoma	3.93
9	Oregon	6.95
7	Pennsylvania	7.21
14	Rhode Island	6.40
30	South Carolina	5.15
39	South Dakota	4.61
21	Tennessee	5.65
31	Texas	5.14
32	Utah	5.11
19	Vermont	5.90
23	Virginia	5.58
22	Washington	5.61
35	West Virginia	4.90
17	Wisconsin	6.15
49	Wyoming	3.83

<u>RANK ORDER</u>

RANK	STATE	RATE
1	New York	9.07
2	Maryland	8.89
3	Massachusetts	8.74
4	Connecticut	8.63
5	Florida	7.42
6	Louisiana	7.34
7	Pennsylvania	7.21
8	New Jersey	7.09
9	Hawaii	6.95
9	Oregon	6.95
11	Missouri	6.53
12	California	6.50
13	Minnesota	6.43
14	Rhode Island	6.40
15	Colorado	6.34
16	Delaware	6.16
17	Wisconsin	6.15
18	Arizona	5.91
19	Vermont	5.90
20	Illinois	5.89
21	Tennessee	5.65
22	Washington	5.61
23	Virginia	5.58
24	Iowa	5.49
25	Ohio	5.45
26	Nebraska	5.39
27	Michigan	5.33
28	Arkansas	5.28
28	North Carolina	5.28
30	South Carolina	5.15
31	Texas	5.14
32	Utah	5.11
33	Kansas	5.05
34	Montana	4.99
35	West Virginia	4.90
36	New Hampshire	4.89
37	Georgia	4.78
38	Maine	4.68
39	Kentucky	4.61
39	South Dakota	4.61
41	Mississippi	4.58
42	North Dakota	4.55
43	Idaho	4.45
44	Indiana	4.40
45	Alabama	4.35
46	New Mexico	4.15
47	Oklahoma	3.93
48	Alaska	3.85
49	Wyoming	3.83
50	Nevada	3.62
	District of Columbia	17.27

Source: Morgan Quitno Press using data from American Medical Association
"Physician Characteristics and Distribution in the U.S." (1994 Edition)
*As of January 1, 1993. National rate does not include physicians in the U.S. territories and possessions.

Nonfederal Physicians in Orthopedic Surgery in 1993

National Total = 20,259 Physicians*

ALPHA ORDER

RANK	STATE	PHYSICIANS	% of USA
26	Alabama	257	1.27%
47	Alaska	49	0.24%
24	Arizona	301	1.49%
33	Arkansas	150	0.74%
1	California	2,858	14.11%
23	Colorado	332	1.64%
22	Connecticut	351	1.73%
46	Delaware	51	0.25%
4	Florida	1,086	5.36%
13	Georgia	471	2.32%
41	Hawaii	88	0.43%
42	Idaho	76	0.38%
7	Illinois	793	3.91%
21	Indiana	353	1.74%
31	Iowa	167	0.82%
30	Kansas	174	0.86%
28	Kentucky	236	1.16%
20	Louisiana	360	1.78%
39	Maine	99	0.49%
15	Maryland	466	2.30%
8	Massachusetts	663	3.27%
10	Michigan	573	2.83%
17	Minnesota	396	1.95%
34	Mississippi	135	0.67%
19	Missouri	381	1.88%
44	Montana	74	0.37%
36	Nebraska	114	0.56%
43	Nevada	75	0.37%
38	New Hampshire	105	0.52%
9	New Jersey	640	3.16%
35	New Mexico	130	0.64%
2	New York	1,629	8.04%
11	North Carolina	517	2.55%
49	North Dakota	39	0.19%
6	Ohio	842	4.16%
29	Oklahoma	191	0.94%
25	Oregon	278	1.37%
5	Pennsylvania	996	4.92%
40	Rhode Island	97	0.48%
27	South Carolina	245	1.21%
48	South Dakota	41	0.20%
18	Tennessee	387	1.91%
3	Texas	1,188	5.86%
32	Utah	151	0.75%
45	Vermont	64	0.32%
12	Virginia	494	2.44%
14	Washington	469	2.32%
37	West Virginia	109	0.54%
16	Wisconsin	400	1.97%
50	Wyoming	35	0.17%

RANK ORDER

RANK	STATE	PHYSICIANS	% of USA
1	California	2,858	14.11%
2	New York	1,629	8.04%
3	Texas	1,188	5.86%
4	Florida	1,086	5.36%
5	Pennsylvania	996	4.92%
6	Ohio	842	4.16%
7	Illinois	793	3.91%
8	Massachusetts	663	3.27%
9	New Jersey	640	3.16%
10	Michigan	573	2.83%
11	North Carolina	517	2.55%
12	Virginia	494	2.44%
13	Georgia	471	2.32%
14	Washington	469	2.32%
15	Maryland	466	2.30%
16	Wisconsin	400	1.97%
17	Minnesota	396	1.95%
18	Tennessee	387	1.91%
19	Missouri	381	1.88%
20	Louisiana	360	1.78%
21	Indiana	353	1.74%
22	Connecticut	351	1.73%
23	Colorado	332	1.64%
24	Arizona	301	1.49%
25	Oregon	278	1.37%
26	Alabama	257	1.27%
27	South Carolina	245	1.21%
28	Kentucky	236	1.16%
29	Oklahoma	191	0.94%
30	Kansas	174	0.86%
31	Iowa	167	0.82%
32	Utah	151	0.75%
33	Arkansas	150	0.74%
34	Mississippi	135	0.67%
35	New Mexico	130	0.64%
36	Nebraska	114	0.56%
37	West Virginia	109	0.54%
38	New Hampshire	105	0.52%
39	Maine	99	0.49%
40	Rhode Island	97	0.48%
41	Hawaii	88	0.43%
42	Idaho	76	0.38%
43	Nevada	75	0.37%
44	Montana	74	0.37%
45	Vermont	64	0.32%
46	Delaware	51	0.25%
47	Alaska	49	0.24%
48	South Dakota	41	0.20%
49	North Dakota	39	0.19%
50	Wyoming	35	0.17%
	District of Columbia	83	0.41%

Source: American Medical Association (Chicago, Illinois)
"Physician Characteristics and Distribution in the U.S." (1994 Edition)
*As of January 1, 1993. Total does not include 115 physicians in the U.S. territories and possessions.

Rate of Nonfederal Physicians in Orthopedic Surgery in 1993

National Rate = 7.86 Physicians per 100,000 Population*

ALPHA ORDER

RANK ORDER

RANK	STATE	RATE
42	Alabama	6.15
16	Alaska	8.19
23	Arizona	7.63
41	Arkansas	6.18
8	California	9.16
7	Colorado	9.32
3	Connecticut	10.71
30	Delaware	7.31
22	Florida	7.91
35	Georgia	6.82
27	Hawaii	7.55
33	Idaho	6.91
36	Illinois	6.79
40	Indiana	6.19
46	Iowa	5.92
34	Kansas	6.86
39	Kentucky	6.22
14	Louisiana	8.39
20	Maine	7.98
5	Maryland	9.40
2	Massachusetts	11.02
44	Michigan	6.06
13	Minnesota	8.75
50	Mississippi	5.11
31	Missouri	7.28
12	Montana	8.80
32	Nebraska	7.07
49	Nevada	5.43
6	New Hampshire	9.34
17	New Jersey	8.14
19	New Mexico	8.04
10	New York	8.97
29	North Carolina	7.44
43	North Dakota	6.12
25	Ohio	7.61
47	Oklahoma	5.91
8	Oregon	9.16
15	Pennsylvania	8.28
4	Rhode Island	9.70
37	South Carolina	6.75
48	South Dakota	5.73
26	Tennessee	7.60
38	Texas	6.59
18	Utah	8.12
1	Vermont	11.11
23	Virginia	7.63
11	Washington	8.92
45	West Virginia	6.00
21	Wisconsin	7.93
28	Wyoming	7.45

RANK	STATE	RATE
1	Vermont	11.11
2	Massachusetts	11.02
3	Connecticut	10.71
4	Rhode Island	9.70
5	Maryland	9.40
6	New Hampshire	9.34
7	Colorado	9.32
8	California	9.16
8	Oregon	9.16
10	New York	8.97
11	Washington	8.92
12	Montana	8.80
13	Minnesota	8.75
14	Louisiana	8.39
15	Pennsylvania	8.28
16	Alaska	8.19
17	New Jersey	8.14
18	Utah	8.12
19	New Mexico	8.04
20	Maine	7.98
21	Wisconsin	7.93
22	Florida	7.91
23	Arizona	7.63
23	Virginia	7.63
25	Ohio	7.61
26	Tennessee	7.60
27	Hawaii	7.55
28	Wyoming	7.45
29	North Carolina	7.44
30	Delaware	7.31
31	Missouri	7.28
32	Nebraska	7.07
33	Idaho	6.91
34	Kansas	6.86
35	Georgia	6.82
36	Illinois	6.79
37	South Carolina	6.75
38	Texas	6.59
39	Kentucky	6.22
40	Indiana	6.19
41	Arkansas	6.18
42	Alabama	6.15
43	North Dakota	6.12
44	Michigan	6.06
45	West Virginia	6.00
46	Iowa	5.92
47	Oklahoma	5.91
48	South Dakota	5.73
49	Nevada	5.43
50	Mississippi	5.11

District of Columbia 14.34

Source: Morgan Quitno Press using data from American Medical Association
"Physician Characteristics and Distribution in the U.S." (1994 Edition)
*As of January 1, 1993. National rate does not include physicians in the U.S. territories and possessions.

Nonfederal Physicians in Plastic Surgery in 1993

National Total = 4,772 Physicians*

RANK	STATE	PHYSICIANS	% of USA
26	Alabama	52	1.09%
49	Alaska	5	0.10%
18	Arizona	85	1.78%
37	Arkansas	19	0.40%
1	California	743	15.57%
19	Colorado	72	1.51%
21	Connecticut	68	1.42%
44	Delaware	11	0.23%
4	Florida	334	7.00%
13	Georgia	118	2.47%
33	Hawaii	27	0.57%
42	Idaho	14	0.29%
7	Illinois	176	3.69%
23	Indiana	60	1.26%
39	Iowa	17	0.36%
31	Kansas	31	0.65%
24	Kentucky	59	1.24%
20	Louisiana	70	1.47%
43	Maine	12	0.25%
12	Maryland	131	2.75%
10	Massachusetts	140	2.93%
9	Michigan	145	3.04%
24	Minnesota	59	1.24%
34	Mississippi	24	0.50%
14	Missouri	108	2.26%
45	Montana	7	0.15%
39	Nebraska	17	0.36%
32	Nevada	28	0.59%
37	New Hampshire	19	0.40%
8	New Jersey	163	3.42%
35	New Mexico	22	0.46%
2	New York	469	9.83%
15	North Carolina	106	2.22%
47	North Dakota	6	0.13%
6	Ohio	181	3.79%
30	Oklahoma	37	0.78%
29	Oregon	43	0.90%
5	Pennsylvania	204	4.27%
41	Rhode Island	15	0.31%
28	South Carolina	44	0.92%
47	South Dakota	6	0.13%
16	Tennessee	101	2.12%
3	Texas	338	7.08%
27	Utah	45	0.94%
45	Vermont	7	0.15%
11	Virginia	132	2.77%
17	Washington	88	1.84%
36	West Virginia	21	0.44%
22	Wisconsin	64	1.34%
50	Wyoming	3	0.06%

RANK	STATE	PHYSICIANS	% of USA
1	California	743	15.57%
2	New York	469	9.83%
3	Texas	338	7.08%
4	Florida	334	7.00%
5	Pennsylvania	204	4.27%
6	Ohio	181	3.79%
7	Illinois	176	3.69%
8	New Jersey	163	3.42%
9	Michigan	145	3.04%
10	Massachusetts	140	2.93%
11	Virginia	132	2.77%
12	Maryland	131	2.75%
13	Georgia	118	2.47%
14	Missouri	108	2.26%
15	North Carolina	106	2.22%
16	Tennessee	101	2.12%
17	Washington	88	1.84%
18	Arizona	85	1.78%
19	Colorado	72	1.51%
20	Louisiana	70	1.47%
21	Connecticut	68	1.42%
22	Wisconsin	64	1.34%
23	Indiana	60	1.26%
24	Kentucky	59	1.24%
24	Minnesota	59	1.24%
26	Alabama	52	1.09%
27	Utah	45	0.94%
28	South Carolina	44	0.92%
29	Oregon	43	0.90%
30	Oklahoma	37	0.78%
31	Kansas	31	0.65%
32	Nevada	28	0.59%
33	Hawaii	27	0.57%
34	Mississippi	24	0.50%
35	New Mexico	22	0.46%
36	West Virginia	21	0.44%
37	Arkansas	19	0.40%
37	New Hampshire	19	0.40%
39	Iowa	17	0.36%
39	Nebraska	17	0.36%
41	Rhode Island	15	0.31%
42	Idaho	14	0.29%
43	Maine	12	0.25%
44	Delaware	11	0.23%
45	Montana	7	0.15%
45	Vermont	7	0.15%
47	North Dakota	6	0.13%
47	South Dakota	6	0.13%
49	Alaska	5	0.10%
50	Wyoming	3	0.06%
	District of Columbia	26	0.54%

Source: American Medical Association (Chicago, Illinois)
    "Physician Characteristics and Distribution in the U.S." (1994 Edition)
*As of January 1, 1993. Total does not include 25 physicians in the U.S. territories and possessions.

Rate of Nonfederal Physicians in Plastic Surgery in 1993

National Rate = 1.85 Physicians per 100,000 Population*

ALPHA ORDER				RANK ORDER		
RANK	STATE	RATE		RANK	STATE	RATE
34	Alabama	1.24		1	Maryland	2.64
45	Alaska	0.84		2	New York	2.58
8	Arizona	2.15		3	Florida	2.43
48	Arkansas	0.78		4	Utah	2.42
5	California	2.38		5	California	2.38
14	Colorado	2.02		6	Massachusetts	2.33
9	Connecticut	2.07		7	Hawaii	2.32
23	Delaware	1.58		8	Arizona	2.15
3	Florida	2.43		9	Connecticut	2.07
17	Georgia	1.71		9	New Jersey	2.07
7	Hawaii	2.32		11	Missouri	2.06
32	Idaho	1.27		12	Virginia	2.04
27	Illinois	1.51		13	Nevada	2.03
40	Indiana	1.05		14	Colorado	2.02
50	Iowa	0.60		15	Tennessee	1.98
35	Kansas	1.22		16	Texas	1.88
24	Kentucky	1.56		17	Georgia	1.71
22	Louisiana	1.63		18	Pennsylvania	1.70
42	Maine	0.97		19	New Hampshire	1.69
1	Maryland	2.64		20	Washington	1.67
6	Massachusetts	2.33		21	Ohio	1.64
25	Michigan	1.53		22	Louisiana	1.63
31	Minnesota	1.30		23	Delaware	1.58
44	Mississippi	0.91		24	Kentucky	1.56
11	Missouri	2.06		25	Michigan	1.53
47	Montana	0.83		26	North Carolina	1.52
40	Nebraska	1.05		27	Illinois	1.51
13	Nevada	2.03		28	Rhode Island	1.50
19	New Hampshire	1.69		29	Oregon	1.42
9	New Jersey	2.07		30	New Mexico	1.36
30	New Mexico	1.36		31	Minnesota	1.30
2	New York	2.58		32	Idaho	1.27
26	North Carolina	1.52		32	Wisconsin	1.27
43	North Dakota	0.94		34	Alabama	1.24
21	Ohio	1.64		35	Kansas	1.22
39	Oklahoma	1.14		35	Vermont	1.22
29	Oregon	1.42		37	South Carolina	1.21
18	Pennsylvania	1.70		38	West Virginia	1.16
28	Rhode Island	1.50		39	Oklahoma	1.14
37	South Carolina	1.21		40	Indiana	1.05
45	South Dakota	0.84		40	Nebraska	1.05
15	Tennessee	1.98		42	Maine	0.97
16	Texas	1.88		43	North Dakota	0.94
4	Utah	2.42		44	Mississippi	0.91
35	Vermont	1.22		45	Alaska	0.84
12	Virginia	2.04		45	South Dakota	0.84
20	Washington	1.67		47	Montana	0.83
38	West Virginia	1.16		48	Arkansas	0.78
32	Wisconsin	1.27		49	Wyoming	0.64
49	Wyoming	0.64		50	Iowa	0.60
					District of Columbia	4.49

Source: Morgan Quitno Press using data from American Medical Association
"Physician Characteristics and Distribution in the U.S." (1994 Edition)
As of January 1, 1993. National rate does not include physicians in the U.S. territories and possessions.

Nonfederal Physicians in Other Specialties in 1993

National Total = 165,718 Physicians*

ALPHA ORDER

RANK	STATE	PHYSICIANS	% of USA
27	Alabama	1,754	1.06%
49	Alaska	227	0.14%
24	Arizona	2,248	1.36%
33	Arkansas	1,015	0.61%
1	California	21,867	13.20%
22	Colorado	2,334	1.41%
16	Connecticut	3,218	1.94%
44	Delaware	436	0.26%
5	Florida	7,910	4.77%
14	Georgia	3,601	2.17%
37	Hawaii	796	0.48%
46	Idaho	350	0.21%
6	Illinois	7,506	4.53%
20	Indiana	2,739	1.65%
31	Iowa	1,164	0.70%
29	Kansas	1,362	0.82%
25	Kentucky	1,838	1.11%
23	Louisiana	2,319	1.40%
41	Maine	654	0.39%
11	Maryland	5,051	3.05%
7	Massachusetts	6,818	4.11%
10	Michigan	5,475	3.30%
21	Minnesota	2,695	1.63%
36	Mississippi	826	0.50%
17	Missouri	3,027	1.83%
45	Montana	390	0.24%
38	Nebraska	763	0.46%
42	Nevada	580	0.35%
39	New Hampshire	724	0.44%
9	New Jersey	5,480	3.31%
34	New Mexico	917	0.55%
2	New York	17,694	10.68%
13	North Carolina	3,821	2.31%
47	North Dakota	305	0.18%
8	Ohio	6,599	3.98%
30	Oklahoma	1,357	0.82%
26	Oregon	1,821	1.10%
3	Pennsylvania	9,386	5.66%
40	Rhode Island	688	0.42%
28	South Carolina	1,729	1.04%
48	South Dakota	271	0.16%
19	Tennessee	2,918	1.76%
4	Texas	9,088	5.48%
32	Utah	1,060	0.64%
43	Vermont	446	0.27%
12	Virginia	3,840	2.32%
15	Washington	3,381	2.04%
35	West Virginia	875	0.53%
18	Wisconsin	2,944	1.78%
50	Wyoming	165	0.10%

RANK ORDER

RANK	STATE	PHYSICIANS	% of USA
1	California	21,867	13.20%
2	New York	17,694	10.68%
3	Pennsylvania	9,386	5.66%
4	Texas	9,088	5.48%
5	Florida	7,910	4.77%
6	Illinois	7,506	4.53%
7	Massachusetts	6,818	4.11%
8	Ohio	6,599	3.98%
9	New Jersey	5,480	3.31%
10	Michigan	5,475	3.30%
11	Maryland	5,051	3.05%
12	Virginia	3,840	2.32%
13	North Carolina	3,821	2.31%
14	Georgia	3,601	2.17%
15	Washington	3,381	2.04%
16	Connecticut	3,218	1.94%
17	Missouri	3,027	1.83%
18	Wisconsin	2,944	1.78%
19	Tennessee	2,918	1.76%
20	Indiana	2,739	1.65%
21	Minnesota	2,695	1.63%
22	Colorado	2,334	1.41%
23	Louisiana	2,319	1.40%
24	Arizona	2,248	1.36%
25	Kentucky	1,838	1.11%
26	Oregon	1,821	1.10%
27	Alabama	1,754	1.06%
28	South Carolina	1,729	1.04%
29	Kansas	1,362	0.82%
30	Oklahoma	1,357	0.82%
31	Iowa	1,164	0.70%
32	Utah	1,060	0.64%
33	Arkansas	1,015	0.61%
34	New Mexico	917	0.55%
35	West Virginia	875	0.53%
36	Mississippi	826	0.50%
37	Hawaii	796	0.48%
38	Nebraska	763	0.46%
39	New Hampshire	724	0.44%
40	Rhode Island	688	0.42%
41	Maine	654	0.39%
42	Nevada	580	0.35%
43	Vermont	446	0.27%
44	Delaware	436	0.26%
45	Montana	390	0.24%
46	Idaho	350	0.21%
47	North Dakota	305	0.18%
48	South Dakota	271	0.16%
49	Alaska	227	0.14%
50	Wyoming	165	0.10%
	District of Columbia	1,246	0.75%

Source: American Medical Association (Chicago, Illinois)
"Physician Characteristics and Distribution in the U.S." (1994 Edition)
As of January 1, 1993. Total does not include 1,691 physicians in the U.S. territories and possessions. Other Specialties include Aerospace Medicine, Anesthesiology, Child Psychiatry, Diagnostic Radiology, Emergency Medicine, Forensic Pathology, Nuclear Medicine, Occupational Medicine, Neurology, Psychiatry, Public Health, Anatomic/Clinical Pathology, Radiology, Radiation Oncology and other specialties.   423

Rate of Nonfederal Physicians in Other Specialties in 1993

National Rate = 64.29 Physicians per 100,000 Population*

ALPHA ORDER

RANK	STATE	RATE
43	Alabama	41.95
46	Alaska	37.96
26	Arizona	56.98
44	Arkansas	41.84
7	California	70.05
11	Colorado	65.49
3	Connecticut	98.17
15	Delaware	62.46
23	Florida	57.63
32	Georgia	52.17
10	Hawaii	68.27
49	Idaho	31.82
14	Illinois	64.23
36	Indiana	48.00
45	Iowa	41.26
30	Kansas	53.73
34	Kentucky	48.44
29	Louisiana	54.06
31	Maine	52.74
2	Maryland	101.88
1	Massachusetts	113.29
21	Michigan	57.88
18	Minnesota	59.57
50	Mississippi	31.29
22	Missouri	57.82
40	Montana	46.37
39	Nebraska	47.30
41	Nevada	41.97
12	New Hampshire	64.41
8	New Jersey	69.73
27	New Mexico	56.75
4	New York	97.47
28	North Carolina	54.96
37	North Dakota	47.88
17	Ohio	59.66
41	Oklahoma	41.97
16	Oregon	60.00
5	Pennsylvania	78.02
9	Rhode Island	68.80
38	South Carolina	47.63
47	South Dakota	37.85
24	Tennessee	57.28
33	Texas	50.43
25	Utah	56.99
6	Vermont	77.43
19	Virginia	59.32
13	Washington	64.29
35	West Virginia	48.13
20	Wisconsin	58.37
48	Wyoming	35.11

RANK ORDER

RANK	STATE	RATE
1	Massachusetts	113.29
2	Maryland	101.88
3	Connecticut	98.17
4	New York	97.47
5	Pennsylvania	78.02
6	Vermont	77.43
7	California	70.05
8	New Jersey	69.73
9	Rhode Island	68.80
10	Hawaii	68.27
11	Colorado	65.49
12	New Hampshire	64.41
13	Washington	64.29
14	Illinois	64.23
15	Delaware	62.46
16	Oregon	60.00
17	Ohio	59.66
18	Minnesota	59.57
19	Virginia	59.32
20	Wisconsin	58.37
21	Michigan	57.88
22	Missouri	57.82
23	Florida	57.63
24	Tennessee	57.28
25	Utah	56.99
26	Arizona	56.98
27	New Mexico	56.75
28	North Carolina	54.96
29	Louisiana	54.06
30	Kansas	53.73
31	Maine	52.74
32	Georgia	52.17
33	Texas	50.43
34	Kentucky	48.44
35	West Virginia	48.13
36	Indiana	48.00
37	North Dakota	47.88
38	South Carolina	47.63
39	Nebraska	47.30
40	Montana	46.37
41	Nevada	41.97
41	Oklahoma	41.97
43	Alabama	41.95
44	Arkansas	41.84
45	Iowa	41.26
46	Alaska	37.96
47	South Dakota	37.85
48	Wyoming	35.11
49	Idaho	31.82
50	Mississippi	31.29

District of Columbia   215.20

Source: Morgan Quitno Press using data from American Medical Association
    "Physician Characteristics and Distribution in the U.S." (1994 Edition)
*As of January 1, 1993. Nat'l rate does not include physicians in the U.S. territories and possessions. Other Specialties include Aerospace Medicine, Anesthesiology, Child Psychiatry, Diagnostic Radiology, Emergency Medicine, Forensic Pathology, Nuclear Medicine, Occupational Medicine, Neurology, Psychiatry, Public Health, Anatomic/Clinical Pathology, Radiology, Radiation Oncology and other specialties.   424

Nonfederal Physicians in Anesthesiology in 1993

National Total = 28,837 Physicians*

ALPHA ORDER

RANK	STATE	PHYSICIANS	% of USA
27	Alabama	346	1.20%
49	Alaska	32	0.11%
20	Arizona	479	1.66%
33	Arkansas	182	0.63%
1	California	3,793	13.15%
24	Colorado	402	1.39%
21	Connecticut	473	1.64%
47	Delaware	48	0.17%
4	Florida	1,628	5.65%
13	Georgia	677	2.35%
41	Hawaii	108	0.37%
44	Idaho	60	0.21%
6	Illinois	1,348	4.67%
15	Indiana	601	2.08%
29	Iowa	245	0.85%
32	Kansas	229	0.79%
25	Kentucky	372	1.29%
23	Louisiana	414	1.44%
39	Maine	118	0.41%
10	Maryland	737	2.56%
8	Massachusetts	1,042	3.61%
11	Michigan	729	2.53%
22	Minnesota	431	1.49%
34	Mississippi	161	0.56%
19	Missouri	508	1.76%
42	Montana	87	0.30%
36	Nebraska	136	0.47%
37	Nevada	134	0.46%
40	New Hampshire	111	0.38%
9	New Jersey	1,022	3.54%
35	New Mexico	146	0.51%
2	New York	2,693	9.34%
16	North Carolina	587	2.04%
46	North Dakota	50	0.17%
7	Ohio	1,230	4.27%
30	Oklahoma	244	0.85%
26	Oregon	360	1.25%
5	Pennsylvania	1,489	5.16%
43	Rhode Island	79	0.27%
28	South Carolina	329	1.14%
48	South Dakota	36	0.12%
17	Tennessee	565	1.96%
3	Texas	1,907	6.61%
30	Utah	244	0.85%
45	Vermont	56	0.19%
14	Virginia	608	2.11%
12	Washington	727	2.52%
38	West Virginia	124	0.43%
18	Wisconsin	560	1.94%
49	Wyoming	32	0.11%

RANK ORDER

RANK	STATE	PHYSICIANS	% of USA
1	California	3,793	13.15%
2	New York	2,693	9.34%
3	Texas	1,907	6.61%
4	Florida	1,628	5.65%
5	Pennsylvania	1,489	5.16%
6	Illinois	1,348	4.67%
7	Ohio	1,230	4.27%
8	Massachusetts	1,042	3.61%
9	New Jersey	1,022	3.54%
10	Maryland	737	2.56%
11	Michigan	729	2.53%
12	Washington	727	2.52%
13	Georgia	677	2.35%
14	Virginia	608	2.11%
15	Indiana	601	2.08%
16	North Carolina	587	2.04%
17	Tennessee	565	1.96%
18	Wisconsin	560	1.94%
19	Missouri	508	1.76%
20	Arizona	479	1.66%
21	Connecticut	473	1.64%
22	Minnesota	431	1.49%
23	Louisiana	414	1.44%
24	Colorado	402	1.39%
25	Kentucky	372	1.29%
26	Oregon	360	1.25%
27	Alabama	346	1.20%
28	South Carolina	329	1.14%
29	Iowa	245	0.85%
30	Oklahoma	244	0.85%
30	Utah	244	0.85%
32	Kansas	229	0.79%
33	Arkansas	182	0.63%
34	Mississippi	161	0.56%
35	New Mexico	146	0.51%
36	Nebraska	136	0.47%
37	Nevada	134	0.46%
38	West Virginia	124	0.43%
39	Maine	118	0.41%
40	New Hampshire	111	0.38%
41	Hawaii	108	0.37%
42	Montana	87	0.30%
43	Rhode Island	79	0.27%
44	Idaho	60	0.21%
45	Vermont	56	0.19%
46	North Dakota	50	0.17%
47	Delaware	48	0.17%
48	South Dakota	36	0.12%
49	Alaska	32	0.11%
49	Wyoming	32	0.11%
	District of Columbia	118	0.41%

Source: American Medical Association (Chicago, Illinois)
"Physician Characteristics and Distribution in the U.S." (1994 Edition)
As of January 1, 1993. Total does not include 205 physicians in the U.S. territories and possessions.

Rate of Nonfederal Physicians in Anesthesiology in 1993

National Total = 11.19 Physicians per 100,000 Population*

<u>ALPHA ORDER</u>

RANK	STATE	RATE
38	Alabama	8.28
49	Alaska	5.35
10	Arizona	12.14
43	Arkansas	7.50
9	California	12.15
14	Colorado	11.28
4	Connecticut	14.43
44	Delaware	6.88
11	Florida	11.86
22	Georgia	9.81
31	Hawaii	9.26
48	Idaho	5.45
13	Illinois	11.54
19	Indiana	10.53
35	Iowa	8.68
33	Kansas	9.03
23	Kentucky	9.80
27	Louisiana	9.65
29	Maine	9.52
2	Maryland	14.86
1	Massachusetts	17.31
41	Michigan	7.71
28	Minnesota	9.53
47	Mississippi	6.10
25	Missouri	9.70
20	Montana	10.34
37	Nebraska	8.43
25	Nevada	9.70
21	New Hampshire	9.88
7	New Jersey	13.00
33	New Mexico	9.03
3	New York	14.84
36	North Carolina	8.44
40	North Dakota	7.85
15	Ohio	11.12
42	Oklahoma	7.55
11	Oregon	11.86
8	Pennsylvania	12.38
39	Rhode Island	7.90
32	South Carolina	9.06
50	South Dakota	5.03
17	Tennessee	11.09
18	Texas	10.58
6	Utah	13.12
24	Vermont	9.72
30	Virginia	9.39
5	Washington	13.82
45	West Virginia	6.82
16	Wisconsin	11.10
46	Wyoming	6.81

<u>RANK ORDER</u>

RANK	STATE	RATE
1	Massachusetts	17.31
2	Maryland	14.86
3	New York	14.84
4	Connecticut	14.43
5	Washington	13.82
6	Utah	13.12
7	New Jersey	13.00
8	Pennsylvania	12.38
9	California	12.15
10	Arizona	12.14
11	Florida	11.86
11	Oregon	11.86
13	Illinois	11.54
14	Colorado	11.28
15	Ohio	11.12
16	Wisconsin	11.10
17	Tennessee	11.09
18	Texas	10.58
19	Indiana	10.53
20	Montana	10.34
21	New Hampshire	9.88
22	Georgia	9.81
23	Kentucky	9.80
24	Vermont	9.72
25	Missouri	9.70
25	Nevada	9.70
27	Louisiana	9.65
28	Minnesota	9.53
29	Maine	9.52
30	Virginia	9.39
31	Hawaii	9.26
32	South Carolina	9.06
33	Kansas	9.03
33	New Mexico	9.03
35	Iowa	8.68
36	North Carolina	8.44
37	Nebraska	8.43
38	Alabama	8.28
39	Rhode Island	7.90
40	North Dakota	7.85
41	Michigan	7.71
42	Oklahoma	7.55
43	Arkansas	7.50
44	Delaware	6.88
45	West Virginia	6.82
46	Wyoming	6.81
47	Mississippi	6.10
48	Idaho	5.45
49	Alaska	5.35
50	South Dakota	5.03

District of Columbia 20.38

Source: Morgan Quitno Press using data from American Medical Association
"Physician Characteristics and Distribution in the U.S." (1994 Edition)
*As of January 1, 1993. National rate does not include physicians in the U.S. territories and possessions.

Nonfederal Physicians in Psychiatry in 1993

National Total = 34,766 Psychiatrists*

ALPHA ORDER

RANK	STATE	PHYSICIANS	% of USA
30	Alabama	243	0.70%
49	Alaska	45	0.13%
23	Arizona	391	1.12%
34	Arkansas	168	0.48%
2	California	4,814	13.85%
17	Colorado	529	1.52%
12	Connecticut	943	2.71%
43	Delaware	89	0.26%
7	Florida	1,315	3.78%
15	Georgia	679	1.95%
33	Hawaii	174	0.50%
47	Idaho	65	0.19%
6	Illinois	1,407	4.05%
24	Indiana	388	1.12%
34	Iowa	168	0.48%
27	Kansas	318	0.91%
28	Kentucky	312	0.90%
21	Louisiana	426	1.23%
38	Maine	147	0.42%
9	Maryland	1,193	3.43%
3	Massachusetts	1,849	5.32%
11	Michigan	1,039	2.99%
22	Minnesota	422	1.21%
42	Mississippi	113	0.33%
18	Missouri	526	1.51%
45	Montana	67	0.19%
40	Nebraska	136	0.39%
44	Nevada	72	0.21%
32	New Hampshire	193	0.56%
8	New Jersey	1,204	3.46%
31	New Mexico	200	0.58%
1	New York	5,424	15.60%
13	North Carolina	795	2.29%
45	North Dakota	67	0.19%
10	Ohio	1,060	3.05%
29	Oklahoma	251	0.72%
26	Oregon	329	0.95%
4	Pennsylvania	1,813	5.21%
36	Rhode Island	162	0.47%
25	South Carolina	375	1.08%
48	South Dakota	46	0.13%
20	Tennessee	453	1.30%
5	Texas	1,635	4.70%
37	Utah	161	0.46%
41	Vermont	126	0.36%
14	Virginia	792	2.28%
16	Washington	598	1.72%
39	West Virginia	144	0.41%
19	Wisconsin	510	1.47%
50	Wyoming	27	0.08%

RANK ORDER

RANK	STATE	PHYSICIANS	% of USA
1	New York	5,424	15.60%
2	California	4,814	13.85%
3	Massachusetts	1,849	5.32%
4	Pennsylvania	1,813	5.21%
5	Texas	1,635	4.70%
6	Illinois	1,407	4.05%
7	Florida	1,315	3.78%
8	New Jersey	1,204	3.46%
9	Maryland	1,193	3.43%
10	Ohio	1,060	3.05%
11	Michigan	1,039	2.99%
12	Connecticut	943	2.71%
13	North Carolina	795	2.29%
14	Virginia	792	2.28%
15	Georgia	679	1.95%
16	Washington	598	1.72%
17	Colorado	529	1.52%
18	Missouri	526	1.51%
19	Wisconsin	510	1.47%
20	Tennessee	453	1.30%
21	Louisiana	426	1.23%
22	Minnesota	422	1.21%
23	Arizona	391	1.12%
24	Indiana	388	1.12%
25	South Carolina	375	1.08%
26	Oregon	329	0.95%
27	Kansas	318	0.91%
28	Kentucky	312	0.90%
29	Oklahoma	251	0.72%
30	Alabama	243	0.70%
31	New Mexico	200	0.58%
32	New Hampshire	193	0.56%
33	Hawaii	174	0.50%
34	Arkansas	168	0.48%
34	Iowa	168	0.48%
36	Rhode Island	162	0.47%
37	Utah	161	0.46%
38	Maine	147	0.42%
39	West Virginia	144	0.41%
40	Nebraska	136	0.39%
41	Vermont	126	0.36%
42	Mississippi	113	0.33%
43	Delaware	89	0.26%
44	Nevada	72	0.21%
45	Montana	67	0.19%
45	North Dakota	67	0.19%
47	Idaho	65	0.19%
48	South Dakota	46	0.13%
49	Alaska	45	0.13%
50	Wyoming	27	0.08%
	District of Columbia	363	1.04%

Source: American Medical Association (Chicago, Illinois)
"Physician Characteristics and Distribution in the U.S." (1994 Edition)
*As of January 1, 1993. Total does not include 1,402 physicians in the U.S. territories and possessions. Psychiatry includes psychoanalysis.

Rate of Nonfederal Physicians in Psychiatry in 1993

National Rate = 13.49 Psychiatrists per 100,000 Population*

<table>
<tr><td colspan="3">ALPHA ORDER</td><td colspan="3">RANK ORDER</td></tr>
<tr><td>RANK</td><td>STATE</td><td>RATE</td><td>RANK</td><td>STATE</td><td>RATE</td></tr>
<tr><td>47</td><td>Alabama</td><td>5.81</td><td>1</td><td>Massachusetts</td><td>30.72</td></tr>
<tr><td>41</td><td>Alaska</td><td>7.53</td><td>2</td><td>New York</td><td>29.88</td></tr>
<tr><td>28</td><td>Arizona</td><td>9.91</td><td>3</td><td>Connecticut</td><td>28.77</td></tr>
<tr><td>42</td><td>Arkansas</td><td>6.92</td><td>4</td><td>Maryland</td><td>24.06</td></tr>
<tr><td>8</td><td>California</td><td>15.42</td><td>5</td><td>Vermont</td><td>21.88</td></tr>
<tr><td>12</td><td>Colorado</td><td>14.84</td><td>6</td><td>New Hampshire</td><td>17.17</td></tr>
<tr><td>3</td><td>Connecticut</td><td>28.77</td><td>7</td><td>Rhode Island</td><td>16.20</td></tr>
<tr><td>13</td><td>Delaware</td><td>12.75</td><td>8</td><td>California</td><td>15.42</td></tr>
<tr><td>30</td><td>Florida</td><td>9.58</td><td>9</td><td>New Jersey</td><td>15.32</td></tr>
<tr><td>29</td><td>Georgia</td><td>9.84</td><td>10</td><td>Pennsylvania</td><td>15.07</td></tr>
<tr><td>11</td><td>Hawaii</td><td>14.92</td><td>11</td><td>Hawaii</td><td>14.92</td></tr>
<tr><td>46</td><td>Idaho</td><td>5.91</td><td>12</td><td>Colorado</td><td>14.84</td></tr>
<tr><td>17</td><td>Illinois</td><td>12.04</td><td>13</td><td>Delaware</td><td>12.75</td></tr>
<tr><td>43</td><td>Indiana</td><td>6.80</td><td>14</td><td>Kansas</td><td>12.54</td></tr>
<tr><td>45</td><td>Iowa</td><td>5.96</td><td>15</td><td>New Mexico</td><td>12.38</td></tr>
<tr><td>14</td><td>Kansas</td><td>12.54</td><td>16</td><td>Virginia</td><td>12.24</td></tr>
<tr><td>37</td><td>Kentucky</td><td>8.22</td><td>17</td><td>Illinois</td><td>12.04</td></tr>
<tr><td>27</td><td>Louisiana</td><td>9.93</td><td>18</td><td>Maine</td><td>11.85</td></tr>
<tr><td>18</td><td>Maine</td><td>11.85</td><td>19</td><td>North Carolina</td><td>11.44</td></tr>
<tr><td>4</td><td>Maryland</td><td>24.06</td><td>20</td><td>Washington</td><td>11.37</td></tr>
<tr><td>1</td><td>Massachusetts</td><td>30.72</td><td>21</td><td>Michigan</td><td>10.98</td></tr>
<tr><td>21</td><td>Michigan</td><td>10.98</td><td>22</td><td>Oregon</td><td>10.84</td></tr>
<tr><td>32</td><td>Minnesota</td><td>9.33</td><td>23</td><td>North Dakota</td><td>10.52</td></tr>
<tr><td>50</td><td>Mississippi</td><td>4.28</td><td>24</td><td>South Carolina</td><td>10.33</td></tr>
<tr><td>26</td><td>Missouri</td><td>10.05</td><td>25</td><td>Wisconsin</td><td>10.11</td></tr>
<tr><td>38</td><td>Montana</td><td>7.97</td><td>26</td><td>Missouri</td><td>10.05</td></tr>
<tr><td>36</td><td>Nebraska</td><td>8.43</td><td>27</td><td>Louisiana</td><td>9.93</td></tr>
<tr><td>49</td><td>Nevada</td><td>5.21</td><td>28</td><td>Arizona</td><td>9.91</td></tr>
<tr><td>6</td><td>New Hampshire</td><td>17.17</td><td>29</td><td>Georgia</td><td>9.84</td></tr>
<tr><td>9</td><td>New Jersey</td><td>15.32</td><td>30</td><td>Florida</td><td>9.58</td></tr>
<tr><td>15</td><td>New Mexico</td><td>12.38</td><td>30</td><td>Ohio</td><td>9.58</td></tr>
<tr><td>2</td><td>New York</td><td>29.88</td><td>32</td><td>Minnesota</td><td>9.33</td></tr>
<tr><td>19</td><td>North Carolina</td><td>11.44</td><td>33</td><td>Texas</td><td>9.07</td></tr>
<tr><td>23</td><td>North Dakota</td><td>10.52</td><td>34</td><td>Tennessee</td><td>8.89</td></tr>
<tr><td>30</td><td>Ohio</td><td>9.58</td><td>35</td><td>Utah</td><td>8.66</td></tr>
<tr><td>40</td><td>Oklahoma</td><td>7.76</td><td>36</td><td>Nebraska</td><td>8.43</td></tr>
<tr><td>22</td><td>Oregon</td><td>10.84</td><td>37</td><td>Kentucky</td><td>8.22</td></tr>
<tr><td>10</td><td>Pennsylvania</td><td>15.07</td><td>38</td><td>Montana</td><td>7.97</td></tr>
<tr><td>7</td><td>Rhode Island</td><td>16.20</td><td>39</td><td>West Virginia</td><td>7.92</td></tr>
<tr><td>24</td><td>South Carolina</td><td>10.33</td><td>40</td><td>Oklahoma</td><td>7.76</td></tr>
<tr><td>44</td><td>South Dakota</td><td>6.42</td><td>41</td><td>Alaska</td><td>7.53</td></tr>
<tr><td>34</td><td>Tennessee</td><td>8.89</td><td>42</td><td>Arkansas</td><td>6.92</td></tr>
<tr><td>33</td><td>Texas</td><td>9.07</td><td>43</td><td>Indiana</td><td>6.80</td></tr>
<tr><td>35</td><td>Utah</td><td>8.66</td><td>44</td><td>South Dakota</td><td>6.42</td></tr>
<tr><td>5</td><td>Vermont</td><td>21.88</td><td>45</td><td>Iowa</td><td>5.96</td></tr>
<tr><td>16</td><td>Virginia</td><td>12.24</td><td>46</td><td>Idaho</td><td>5.91</td></tr>
<tr><td>20</td><td>Washington</td><td>11.37</td><td>47</td><td>Alabama</td><td>5.81</td></tr>
<tr><td>39</td><td>West Virginia</td><td>7.92</td><td>48</td><td>Wyoming</td><td>5.74</td></tr>
<tr><td>25</td><td>Wisconsin</td><td>10.11</td><td>49</td><td>Nevada</td><td>5.21</td></tr>
<tr><td>48</td><td>Wyoming</td><td>5.74</td><td>50</td><td>Mississippi</td><td>4.28</td></tr>
<tr><td></td><td></td><td></td><td></td><td>District of Columbia</td><td>62.69</td></tr>
</table>

Source: Morgan Quitno Press using data from American Medical Association
   "Physician Characteristics and Distribution in the U.S." (1994 Edition)
As of January 1, 1993. National rate does not include physicians in the U.S. territories and possessions. Psychiatry includes psychoanalysis.

International Medical School Graduates Practicing in U.S. in 1993

National Total = 141,359 Nonfederal Physicians*

ALPHA ORDER

RANK	STATE	PHYSICIANS	% of USA
27	Alabama	768	0.54%
48	Alaska	51	0.04%
20	Arizona	1,267	0.90%
42	Arkansas	258	0.18%
2	California	16,031	11.34%
32	Colorado	485	0.34%
12	Connecticut	2,790	1.97%
35	Delaware	418	0.30%
3	Florida	11,299	7.99%
15	Georgia	1,974	1.40%
31	Hawaii	487	0.34%
49	Idaho	46	0.03%
5	Illinois	9,890	7.00%
16	Indiana	1,703	1.20%
30	Iowa	652	0.46%
28	Kansas	764	0.54%
24	Kentucky	1,069	0.76%
25	Louisiana	1,030	0.73%
40	Maine	276	0.20%
10	Maryland	4,893	3.46%
11	Massachusetts	4,170	2.95%
9	Michigan	5,882	4.16%
22	Minnesota	1,155	0.82%
43	Mississippi	234	0.17%
14	Missouri	2,153	1.52%
47	Montana	70	0.05%
39	Nebraska	280	0.20%
37	Nevada	372	0.26%
38	New Hampshire	354	0.25%
4	New Jersey	10,002	7.08%
36	New Mexico	381	0.27%
1	New York	26,717	18.90%
18	North Carolina	1,324	0.94%
41	North Dakota	271	0.19%
8	Ohio	6,394	4.52%
29	Oklahoma	697	0.49%
34	Oregon	435	0.31%
6	Pennsylvania	7,005	4.96%
26	Rhode Island	790	0.56%
33	South Carolina	477	0.34%
45	South Dakota	123	0.09%
19	Tennessee	1,314	0.93%
7	Texas	6,788	4.80%
44	Utah	201	0.14%
46	Vermont	114	0.08%
13	Virginia	2,779	1.97%
23	Washington	1,114	0.79%
21	West Virginia	1,229	0.87%
17	Wisconsin	1,628	1.15%
50	Wyoming	41	0.03%

RANK ORDER

RANK	STATE	PHYSICIANS	% of USA
1	New York	26,717	18.90%
2	California	16,031	11.34%
3	Florida	11,299	7.99%
4	New Jersey	10,002	7.08%
5	Illinois	9,890	7.00%
6	Pennsylvania	7,005	4.96%
7	Texas	6,788	4.80%
8	Ohio	6,394	4.52%
9	Michigan	5,882	4.16%
10	Maryland	4,893	3.46%
11	Massachusetts	4,170	2.95%
12	Connecticut	2,790	1.97%
13	Virginia	2,779	1.97%
14	Missouri	2,153	1.52%
15	Georgia	1,974	1.40%
16	Indiana	1,703	1.20%
17	Wisconsin	1,628	1.15%
18	North Carolina	1,324	0.94%
19	Tennessee	1,314	0.93%
20	Arizona	1,267	0.90%
21	West Virginia	1,229	0.87%
22	Minnesota	1,155	0.82%
23	Washington	1,114	0.79%
24	Kentucky	1,069	0.76%
25	Louisiana	1,030	0.73%
26	Rhode Island	790	0.56%
27	Alabama	768	0.54%
28	Kansas	764	0.54%
29	Oklahoma	697	0.49%
30	Iowa	652	0.46%
31	Hawaii	487	0.34%
32	Colorado	485	0.34%
33	South Carolina	477	0.34%
34	Oregon	435	0.31%
35	Delaware	418	0.30%
36	New Mexico	381	0.27%
37	Nevada	372	0.26%
38	New Hampshire	354	0.25%
39	Nebraska	280	0.20%
40	Maine	276	0.20%
41	North Dakota	271	0.19%
42	Arkansas	258	0.18%
43	Mississippi	234	0.17%
44	Utah	201	0.14%
45	South Dakota	123	0.09%
46	Vermont	114	0.08%
47	Montana	70	0.05%
48	Alaska	51	0.04%
49	Idaho	46	0.03%
50	Wyoming	41	0.03%
	District of Columbia	714	0.51%

Source: American Medical Association (Chicago, Illinois)
  "Physician Characteristics and Distribution in the U.S." (1994 Edition)
As of January 1, 1993. Total does not include 4,142 physicians in the U.S. territories and possessions.

Rate of International Medical School Graduates Practicing in the U.S. in 1993

National Rate = 54.84 Nonfederal Physicians per 100,000 Population*

ALPHA ORDER

RANK	STATE	RATE
38	Alabama	18.37
48	Alaska	8.53
21	Arizona	32.12
45	Arkansas	10.63
14	California	51.35
42	Colorado	13.61
4	Connecticut	85.11
11	Delaware	59.89
6	Florida	82.32
25	Georgia	28.60
17	Hawaii	41.77
50	Idaho	4.18
5	Illinois	84.63
24	Indiana	29.85
32	Iowa	23.11
23	Kansas	30.14
26	Kentucky	28.18
30	Louisiana	24.01
33	Maine	22.26
3	Maryland	98.69
8	Massachusetts	69.29
10	Michigan	62.18
29	Minnesota	25.53
46	Mississippi	8.86
18	Missouri	41.13
49	Montana	8.32
39	Nebraska	17.36
27	Nevada	26.92
22	New Hampshire	31.49
2	New Jersey	127.27
31	New Mexico	23.58
1	New York	147.18
37	North Carolina	19.04
16	North Dakota	42.54
13	Ohio	57.81
34	Oklahoma	21.56
41	Oregon	14.33
12	Pennsylvania	58.23
7	Rhode Island	79.00
43	South Carolina	13.14
40	South Dakota	17.18
28	Tennessee	25.80
19	Texas	37.67
44	Utah	10.81
36	Vermont	19.79
15	Virginia	42.93
35	Washington	21.18
9	West Virginia	67.60
20	Wisconsin	32.28
47	Wyoming	8.72

RANK ORDER

RANK	STATE	RATE
1	New York	147.18
2	New Jersey	127.27
3	Maryland	98.69
4	Connecticut	85.11
5	Illinois	84.63
6	Florida	82.32
7	Rhode Island	79.00
8	Massachusetts	69.29
9	West Virginia	67.60
10	Michigan	62.18
11	Delaware	59.89
12	Pennsylvania	58.23
13	Ohio	57.81
14	California	51.35
15	Virginia	42.93
16	North Dakota	42.54
17	Hawaii	41.77
18	Missouri	41.13
19	Texas	37.67
20	Wisconsin	32.28
21	Arizona	32.12
22	New Hampshire	31.49
23	Kansas	30.14
24	Indiana	29.85
25	Georgia	28.60
26	Kentucky	28.18
27	Nevada	26.92
28	Tennessee	25.80
29	Minnesota	25.53
30	Louisiana	24.01
31	New Mexico	23.58
32	Iowa	23.11
33	Maine	22.26
34	Oklahoma	21.56
35	Washington	21.18
36	Vermont	19.79
37	North Carolina	19.04
38	Alabama	18.37
39	Nebraska	17.36
40	South Dakota	17.18
41	Oregon	14.33
42	Colorado	13.61
43	South Carolina	13.14
44	Utah	10.81
45	Arkansas	10.63
46	Mississippi	8.86
47	Wyoming	8.72
48	Alaska	8.53
49	Montana	8.32
50	Idaho	4.18

	District of Columbia	123.32

Source: Morgan Quitno Press using data from American Medical Association
"Physician Characteristics and Distribution in the U.S." (1994 Edition)
*As of January 1, 1993. National rate does not include physicians in the U.S. territories and possessions.

International Medical School Graduates as a Percent of Nonfederal Physicians in 1993

National Percent = 22.11% of Nonfederal Physicians*

ALPHA ORDER			RANK ORDER		
RANK	STATE	PERCENT	RANK	STATE	PERCENT
34	Alabama	10.01	1	New Jersey	44.27
45	Alaska	5.84	2	New York	40.35
26	Arizona	14.13	3	Illinois	34.02
44	Arkansas	5.93	4	West Virginia	33.99
15	California	19.12	5	Florida	32.14
47	Colorado	5.58	6	Michigan	28.98
11	Connecticut	24.09	7	Maryland	27.19
9	Delaware	26.14	8	Rhode Island	26.64
5	Florida	32.14	9	Delaware	26.14
24	Georgia	14.65	10	Ohio	25.36
21	Hawaii	15.84	11	Connecticut	24.09
50	Idaho	2.80	12	North Dakota	20.86
3	Illinois	34.02	13	Pennsylvania	20.77
20	Indiana	16.11	14	Texas	19.67
29	Iowa	12.99	15	California	19.12
23	Kansas	14.67	16	Missouri	18.55
25	Kentucky	14.58	17	Virginia	18.52
31	Louisiana	11.12	18	Massachusetts	17.73
34	Maine	10.01	19	Nevada	16.35
7	Maryland	27.19	20	Indiana	16.11
18	Massachusetts	17.73	21	Hawaii	15.84
6	Michigan	28.98	22	Wisconsin	14.68
33	Minnesota	10.05	23	Kansas	14.67
42	Mississippi	6.22	24	Georgia	14.65
16	Missouri	18.55	25	Kentucky	14.58
49	Montana	4.30	26	Arizona	14.13
39	Nebraska	8.47	27	New Hampshire	13.11
19	Nevada	16.35	28	Oklahoma	13.02
27	New Hampshire	13.11	29	Iowa	12.99
1	New Jersey	44.27	30	Tennessee	11.31
32	New Mexico	11.11	31	Louisiana	11.12
2	New York	40.35	32	New Mexico	11.11
37	North Carolina	8.81	33	Minnesota	10.05
12	North Dakota	20.86	34	Alabama	10.01
10	Ohio	25.36	34	Maine	10.01
28	Oklahoma	13.02	36	South Dakota	9.90
43	Oregon	5.95	37	North Carolina	8.81
13	Pennsylvania	20.77	38	Washington	8.56
8	Rhode Island	26.64	39	Nebraska	8.47
40	South Carolina	6.92	40	South Carolina	6.92
36	South Dakota	9.90	41	Vermont	6.60
30	Tennessee	11.31	42	Mississippi	6.22
14	Texas	19.67	43	Oregon	5.95
48	Utah	5.29	44	Arkansas	5.93
41	Vermont	6.60	45	Alaska	5.84
17	Virginia	18.52	46	Wyoming	5.63
38	Washington	8.56	47	Colorado	5.58
4	West Virginia	33.99	48	Utah	5.29
22	Wisconsin	14.68	49	Montana	4.30
46	Wyoming	5.63	50	Idaho	2.80
				District of Columbia	17.38

Source: Morgan Quitno Press using data from American Medical Association
"Physician Characteristics and Distribution in the U.S." (1994 Edition)
*As of January 1, 1993. National rate does not include physicians in the U.S. territories and possessions.

Osteopathic Physicians in 1993

National Total = 33,514 Osteopathic Physicians*

	ALPHA ORDER				RANK ORDER		
RANK	STATE	OSTEOPATHS	% of USA	RANK	STATE	OSTEOPATHS	% of USA
31	Alabama	154	0.46%	1	Michigan	4,319	12.89%
48	Alaska	41	0.12%	2	Pennsylvania	4,187	12.49%
12	Arizona	885	2.64%	3	Ohio	2,832	8.45%
36	Arkansas	118	0.35%	4	Florida	2,275	6.79%
9	California	1,429	4.26%	5	New Jersey	2,046	6.10%
14	Colorado	562	1.68%	6	Texas	2,039	6.08%
34	Connecticut	130	0.39%	7	New York	1,688	5.04%
32	Delaware	152	0.45%	8	Missouri	1,551	4.63%
4	Florida	2,275	6.79%	9	California	1,429	4.26%
20	Georgia	353	1.05%	10	Illinois	1,352	4.03%
41	Hawaii	62	0.18%	11	Oklahoma	1,026	3.06%
40	Idaho	74	0.22%	12	Arizona	885	2.64%
10	Illinois	1,352	4.03%	13	Iowa	848	2.53%
15	Indiana	455	1.36%	14	Colorado	562	1.68%
13	Iowa	848	2.53%	15	Indiana	455	1.36%
16	Kansas	453	1.35%	16	Kansas	453	1.35%
33	Kentucky	138	0.41%	17	Washington	436	1.30%
39	Louisiana	93	0.28%	18	Maine	398	1.19%
18	Maine	398	1.19%	19	Wisconsin	355	1.06%
27	Maryland	181	0.54%	20	Georgia	353	1.05%
23	Massachusetts	295	0.88%	21	West Virginia	350	1.04%
1	Michigan	4,319	12.89%	22	Oregon	344	1.03%
29	Minnesota	167	0.50%	23	Massachusetts	295	0.88%
37	Mississippi	108	0.32%	24	Virginia	251	0.75%
8	Missouri	1,551	4.63%	25	Tennessee	215	0.64%
42	Montana	60	0.18%	26	Nevada	189	0.56%
44	Nebraska	55	0.16%	27	Maryland	181	0.54%
26	Nevada	189	0.56%	28	New Mexico	172	0.51%
43	New Hampshire	59	0.18%	29	Minnesota	167	0.50%
5	New Jersey	2,046	6.10%	30	Rhode Island	162	0.48%
28	New Mexico	172	0.51%	31	Alabama	154	0.46%
7	New York	1,688	5.04%	32	Delaware	152	0.45%
35	North Carolina	123	0.37%	33	Kentucky	138	0.41%
49	North Dakota	34	0.10%	34	Connecticut	130	0.39%
3	Ohio	2,832	8.45%	35	North Carolina	123	0.37%
11	Oklahoma	1,026	3.06%	36	Arkansas	118	0.35%
22	Oregon	344	1.03%	37	Mississippi	108	0.32%
2	Pennsylvania	4,187	12.49%	37	South Carolina	108	0.32%
30	Rhode Island	162	0.48%	39	Louisiana	93	0.28%
37	South Carolina	108	0.32%	40	Idaho	74	0.22%
47	South Dakota	42	0.13%	41	Hawaii	62	0.18%
25	Tennessee	215	0.64%	42	Montana	60	0.18%
6	Texas	2,039	6.08%	43	New Hampshire	59	0.18%
44	Utah	55	0.16%	44	Nebraska	55	0.16%
46	Vermont	45	0.13%	44	Utah	55	0.16%
24	Virginia	251	0.75%	46	Vermont	45	0.13%
17	Washington	436	1.30%	47	South Dakota	42	0.13%
21	West Virginia	350	1.04%	48	Alaska	41	0.12%
19	Wisconsin	355	1.06%	49	North Dakota	34	0.10%
50	Wyoming	32	0.10%	50	Wyoming	32	0.10%
					District of Columbia	16	0.05%

Source: American Osteopathic Association
unpublished data (October 14, 1993)
*Active, retired and disabled osteopaths. Total does not include 1,391 osteopathic physicians not shown separately (1,173 in military service, 115 in U.S. Public Health Service, 81 in U.S. territories or foreign countries and 22 in APO/FPOs).

Rate of Osteopathic Physicians in 1993

National Rate = 12.99 Osteopaths per 100,000 Population*

ALPHA ORDER

RANK	STATE	RATE
43	Alabama	3.68
27	Alaska	6.84
9	Arizona	22.48
36	Arkansas	4.87
37	California	4.58
15	Colorado	15.76
40	Connecticut	3.97
10	Delaware	21.71
13	Florida	16.63
34	Georgia	5.10
32	Hawaii	5.29
29	Idaho	6.73
17	Illinois	11.56
23	Indiana	7.96
5	Iowa	30.14
12	Kansas	17.90
45	Kentucky	3.64
49	Louisiana	2.17
3	Maine	32.12
44	Maryland	3.65
35	Massachusetts	4.91
1	Michigan	45.57
42	Minnesota	3.70
39	Mississippi	4.09
6	Missouri	29.63
25	Montana	7.15
46	Nebraska	3.42
16	Nevada	13.61
33	New Hampshire	5.24
7	New Jersey	25.97
20	New Mexico	10.64
21	New York	9.28
50	North Carolina	1.77
31	North Dakota	5.35
8	Ohio	25.53
4	Oklahoma	31.75
18	Oregon	11.35
2	Pennsylvania	34.75
14	Rhode Island	16.20
47	South Carolina	2.96
30	South Dakota	5.87
38	Tennessee	4.22
19	Texas	11.31
47	Utah	2.96
24	Vermont	7.81
41	Virginia	3.87
22	Washington	8.30
11	West Virginia	19.23
26	Wisconsin	7.05
28	Wyoming	6.81

RANK ORDER

RANK	STATE	RATE
1	Michigan	45.57
2	Pennsylvania	34.75
3	Maine	32.12
4	Oklahoma	31.75
5	Iowa	30.14
6	Missouri	29.63
7	New Jersey	25.97
8	Ohio	25.53
9	Arizona	22.48
10	Delaware	21.71
11	West Virginia	19.23
12	Kansas	17.90
13	Florida	16.63
14	Rhode Island	16.20
15	Colorado	15.76
16	Nevada	13.61
17	Illinois	11.56
18	Oregon	11.35
19	Texas	11.31
20	New Mexico	10.64
21	New York	9.28
22	Washington	8.30
23	Indiana	7.96
24	Vermont	7.81
25	Montana	7.15
26	Wisconsin	7.05
27	Alaska	6.84
28	Wyoming	6.81
29	Idaho	6.73
30	South Dakota	5.87
31	North Dakota	5.35
32	Hawaii	5.29
33	New Hampshire	5.24
34	Georgia	5.10
35	Massachusetts	4.91
36	Arkansas	4.87
37	California	4.58
38	Tennessee	4.22
39	Mississippi	4.09
40	Connecticut	3.97
41	Virginia	3.87
42	Minnesota	3.70
43	Alabama	3.68
44	Maryland	3.65
45	Kentucky	3.64
46	Nebraska	3.42
47	South Carolina	2.96
47	Utah	2.96
49	Louisiana	2.17
50	North Carolina	1.77
	District of Columbia	2.77

*Source: Morgan Quitno Press using data from American Osteopathic Association
unpublished data (October 14, 1993)*

Active, retired and disabled osteopaths. Total does not include 1,391 osteopathic physicians not shown separately (1,173 in military service, 115 in U.S. Public Health Service, 81 in U.S. territories or foreign countries and 22 in APO/FPOs).

Podiatric Physicians in 1991

National Total = 12,786 Podiatric Physicians*

ALPHA ORDER					RANK ORDER			
RANK	STATE	PODIATRISTS	% of USA		RANK	STATE	PODIATRISTS	% of USA
35	Alabama	49	0.38%		1	New York	1,896	14.83%
50	Alaska	7	0.05%		2	California	1,610	12.59%
17	Arizona	161	1.26%		3	Pennsylvania	1,124	8.79%
40	Arkansas	33	0.26%		4	Illinois	947	7.41%
2	California	1,610	12.59%		5	New Jersey	753	5.89%
21	Colorado	118	0.92%		6	Florida	717	5.61%
13	Connecticut	244	1.91%		7	Ohio	634	4.96%
40	Delaware	33	0.26%		8	Michigan	562	4.40%
6	Florida	717	5.61%		9	Texas	503	3.93%
20	Georgia	132	1.03%		10	Massachusetts	420	3.28%
46	Hawaii	15	0.12%		11	Maryland	272	2.13%
42	Idaho	28	0.22%		12	Indiana	269	2.10%
4	Illinois	947	7.41%		13	Connecticut	244	1.91%
12	Indiana	269	2.10%		14	Virginia	239	1.87%
23	Iowa	109	0.85%		15	Washington	176	1.38%
27	Kansas	77	0.60%		16	Wisconsin	173	1.35%
31	Kentucky	63	0.49%		17	Arizona	161	1.26%
29	Louisiana	68	0.53%		18	North Carolina	155	1.21%
34	Maine	52	0.41%		19	Missouri	144	1.13%
11	Maryland	272	2.13%		20	Georgia	132	1.03%
10	Massachusetts	420	3.28%		21	Colorado	118	0.92%
8	Michigan	562	4.40%		22	Tennessee	114	0.89%
24	Minnesota	106	0.83%		23	Iowa	109	0.85%
44	Mississippi	26	0.20%		24	Minnesota	106	0.83%
19	Missouri	144	1.13%		25	Utah	94	0.74%
42	Montana	28	0.22%		26	Oregon	85	0.66%
38	Nebraska	41	0.32%		27	Kansas	77	0.60%
39	Nevada	36	0.28%		28	Oklahoma	73	0.57%
35	New Hampshire	49	0.38%		29	Louisiana	68	0.53%
5	New Jersey	753	5.89%		30	Rhode Island	66	0.52%
32	New Mexico	56	0.44%		31	Kentucky	63	0.49%
1	New York	1,896	14.83%		32	New Mexico	56	0.44%
18	North Carolina	155	1.21%		33	South Carolina	53	0.41%
49	North Dakota	12	0.09%		34	Maine	52	0.41%
7	Ohio	634	4.96%		35	Alabama	49	0.38%
28	Oklahoma	73	0.57%		35	New Hampshire	49	0.38%
26	Oregon	85	0.66%		37	West Virginia	45	0.35%
3	Pennsylvania	1,124	8.79%		38	Nebraska	41	0.32%
30	Rhode Island	66	0.52%		39	Nevada	36	0.28%
33	South Carolina	53	0.41%		40	Arkansas	33	0.26%
45	South Dakota	18	0.14%		40	Delaware	33	0.26%
22	Tennessee	114	0.89%		42	Idaho	28	0.22%
9	Texas	503	3.93%		42	Montana	28	0.22%
25	Utah	94	0.74%		44	Mississippi	26	0.20%
47	Vermont	14	0.11%		45	South Dakota	18	0.14%
14	Virginia	239	1.87%		46	Hawaii	15	0.12%
15	Washington	176	1.38%		47	Vermont	14	0.11%
37	West Virginia	45	0.35%		47	Wyoming	14	0.11%
16	Wisconsin	173	1.35%		49	North Dakota	12	0.09%
47	Wyoming	14	0.11%		50	Alaska	7	0.05%
						District of Columbia	73	0.57%

Source: Morgan Quitno Press

*Calculated by the editors using American Podiatric Medical Association, Inc. "Podiatric Physicians per 100,000 Population in 1991" and Census 1991 population figures.

Rate of Podiatric Physicians in 1991

National Rate = 5.0 Podiatrists per 100,000 Population*

ALPHA ORDER

RANK	STATE	RATE
48	Alabama	1.2
48	Alaska	1.2
17	Arizona	4.3
46	Arkansas	1.4
12	California	5.3
22	Colorado	3.5
5	Connecticut	7.4
14	Delaware	4.9
11	Florida	5.4
41	Georgia	2.0
47	Hawaii	1.3
32	Idaho	2.7
4	Illinois	8.2
15	Indiana	4.8
19	Iowa	3.9
26	Kansas	3.1
43	Kentucky	1.7
44	Louisiana	1.6
18	Maine	4.2
10	Maryland	5.6
6	Massachusetts	7.0
8	Michigan	6.0
37	Minnesota	2.4
50	Mississippi	1.0
30	Missouri	2.8
22	Montana	3.5
33	Nebraska	2.6
30	Nevada	2.8
16	New Hampshire	4.4
2	New Jersey	9.7
21	New Mexico	3.6
1	New York	10.5
38	North Carolina	2.3
42	North Dakota	1.9
9	Ohio	5.8
38	Oklahoma	2.3
28	Oregon	2.9
3	Pennsylvania	9.4
7	Rhode Island	6.6
45	South Carolina	1.5
33	South Dakota	2.6
38	Tennessee	2.3
28	Texas	2.9
12	Utah	5.3
35	Vermont	2.5
20	Virginia	3.8
22	Washington	3.5
35	West Virginia	2.5
22	Wisconsin	3.5
27	Wyoming	3.0

RANK ORDER

RANK	STATE	RATE
1	New York	10.5
2	New Jersey	9.7
3	Pennsylvania	9.4
4	Illinois	8.2
5	Connecticut	7.4
6	Massachusetts	7.0
7	Rhode Island	6.6
8	Michigan	6.0
9	Ohio	5.8
10	Maryland	5.6
11	Florida	5.4
12	California	5.3
12	Utah	5.3
14	Delaware	4.9
15	Indiana	4.8
16	New Hampshire	4.4
17	Arizona	4.3
18	Maine	4.2
19	Iowa	3.9
20	Virginia	3.8
21	New Mexico	3.6
22	Colorado	3.5
22	Montana	3.5
22	Washington	3.5
22	Wisconsin	3.5
26	Kansas	3.1
27	Wyoming	3.0
28	Oregon	2.9
28	Texas	2.9
30	Missouri	2.8
30	Nevada	2.8
32	Idaho	2.7
33	Nebraska	2.6
33	South Dakota	2.6
35	Vermont	2.5
35	West Virginia	2.5
37	Minnesota	2.4
38	North Carolina	2.3
38	Oklahoma	2.3
38	Tennessee	2.3
41	Georgia	2.0
42	North Dakota	1.9
43	Kentucky	1.7
44	Louisiana	1.6
45	South Carolina	1.5
46	Arkansas	1.4
47	Hawaii	1.3
48	Alabama	1.2
48	Alaska	1.2
50	Mississippi	1.0

	District of Columbia	12.2

Source: American Podiatric Medical Association, Inc.
"Podiatric Physicians per 100,000 Population, 1991"

435

Doctors of Chiropractic in 1993

National Total = 73,579 Chiropractors*

ALPHA ORDER					RANK ORDER			
RANK	STATE	CHIROPRACTORS	% of USA		RANK	STATE	CHIROPRACTORS	% of USA
27	Alabama	661	0.90%		1	California	10,692	14.53%
49	Alaska	162	0.22%		2	New York	7,558	10.27%
9	Arizona	2,167	2.95%		3	Pennsylvania	5,127	6.97%
32	Arkansas	493	0.67%		4	Florida*	3,896	5.29%
1	California	10,692	14.53%		5	Texas	3,347	4.55%
15	Colorado	1,566	2.13%		6	New Jersey	2,850	3.87%
25	Connecticut	893	1.21%		7	Illinois	2,399	3.26%
46	Delaware	200	0.27%		8	Michigan	2,390	3.25%
4	Florida*	3,896	5.29%		9	Arizona	2,167	2.95%
10	Georgia	2,026	2.75%		10	Georgia	2,026	2.75%
34	Hawaii	486	0.66%		11	Missouri	1,864	2.53%
42	Idaho	301	0.41%		12	Wisconsin	1,661	2.26%
7	Illinois	2,399	3.26%		13	Washington	1,593	2.17%
24	Indiana	919	1.25%		14	Minnesota	1,582	2.15%
18	Iowa	1,270	1.73%		15	Colorado	1,566	2.13%
28	Kansas	614	0.83%		16	Ohio	1,563	2.12%
19	Kentucky	1,162	1.58%		17	Massachusetts	1,422	1.93%
30	Louisiana	566	0.77%		18	Iowa	1,270	1.73%
38	Maine	358	0.49%		19	Kentucky	1,162	1.58%
33	Maryland	489	0.66%		20	North Carolina	1,101	1.50%
17	Massachusetts	1,422	1.93%		21	South Carolina	1,015	1.38%
8	Michigan	2,390	3.25%		22	Oklahoma	960	1.30%
14	Minnesota	1,582	2.15%		23	Virginia	950	1.29%
39	Mississippi	335	0.46%		24	Indiana	919	1.25%
11	Missouri	1,864	2.53%		25	Connecticut	893	1.21%
37	Montana	364	0.49%		26	Oregon	785	1.07%
44	Nebraska	263	0.36%		27	Alabama	661	0.90%
41	Nevada	308	0.42%		28	Kansas	614	0.83%
36	New Hampshire	401	0.54%		29	Tennessee	600	0.82%
6	New Jersey	2,850	3.87%		30	Louisiana	566	0.77%
31	New Mexico	558	0.76%		31	New Mexico	558	0.76%
2	New York	7,558	10.27%		32	Arkansas	493	0.67%
20	North Carolina	1,101	1.50%		33	Maryland	489	0.66%
45	North Dakota	205	0.28%		34	Hawaii	486	0.66%
16	Ohio	1,563	2.12%		35	Utah	425	0.58%
22	Oklahoma	960	1.30%		36	New Hampshire	401	0.54%
26	Oregon	785	1.07%		37	Montana	364	0.49%
3	Pennsylvania	5,127	6.97%		38	Maine	358	0.49%
50	Rhode Island	161	0.22%		39	Mississippi	335	0.46%
21	South Carolina	1,015	1.38%		40	Vermont	330	0.45%
48	South Dakota	188	0.26%		41	Nevada	308	0.42%
29	Tennessee	600	0.82%		42	Idaho	301	0.41%
5	Texas	3,347	4.55%		43	West Virginia	280	0.38%
35	Utah	425	0.58%		44	Nebraska	263	0.36%
40	Vermont	330	0.45%		45	North Dakota	205	0.28%
23	Virginia	950	1.29%		46	Delaware	200	0.27%
13	Washington	1,593	2.17%		47	Wyoming	198	0.27%
43	West Virginia	280	0.38%		48	South Dakota	188	0.26%
12	Wisconsin	1,661	2.26%		49	Alaska	162	0.22%
47	Wyoming	198	0.27%		50	Rhode Island	161	0.22%
						District of Columbia	93	0.13%

Source: Federation of Chiropractic Licensing Boards
   "1994–95 Official Directory"

Licensed active doctors. National total and Florida's total are not considered precise due to incomplete information.
There is some duplication as some doctors are licensed in more than one state.

Rate of Doctors of Chiropractic in 1993

National Rate = 28.54 Chiropractors per 100,000 Population*

ALPHA ORDER

RANK	STATE	RATE
43	Alabama	15.81
28	Alaska	27.09
2	Arizona	54.93
37	Arkansas	20.32
15	California	34.25
4	Colorado	43.94
27	Connecticut	27.24
23	Delaware	28.65
24	Florida	28.38
21	Georgia	29.35
8	Hawaii	41.68
26	Idaho	27.36
36	Illinois	20.53
40	Indiana	16.11
3	Iowa	45.02
32	Kansas	24.22
18	Kentucky	30.63
47	Louisiana	13.19
22	Maine	28.87
50	Maryland	9.86
33	Massachusetts	23.63
31	Michigan	25.26
13	Minnesota	34.97
48	Mississippi	12.69
12	Missouri	35.61
5	Montana	43.28
39	Nebraska	16.31
35	Nevada	22.29
11	New Hampshire	35.68
10	New Jersey	36.26
14	New Mexico	34.53
9	New York	41.63
42	North Carolina	15.84
17	North Dakota	32.18
46	Ohio	14.13
20	Oklahoma	29.69
30	Oregon	25.86
6	Pennsylvania	42.62
41	Rhode Island	16.10
25	South Carolina	27.96
29	South Dakota	26.26
49	Tennessee	11.78
38	Texas	18.57
34	Utah	22.85
1	Vermont	57.29
45	Virginia	14.68
19	Washington	30.29
44	West Virginia	15.40
16	Wisconsin	32.93
7	Wyoming	42.13

RANK ORDER

RANK	STATE	RATE
1	Vermont	57.29
2	Arizona	54.93
3	Iowa	45.02
4	Colorado	43.94
5	Montana	43.28
6	Pennsylvania	42.62
7	Wyoming	42.13
8	Hawaii	41.68
9	New York	41.63
10	New Jersey	36.26
11	New Hampshire	35.68
12	Missouri	35.61
13	Minnesota	34.97
14	New Mexico	34.53
15	California	34.25
16	Wisconsin	32.93
17	North Dakota	32.18
18	Kentucky	30.63
19	Washington	30.29
20	Oklahoma	29.69
21	Georgia	29.35
22	Maine	28.87
23	Delaware	28.65
24	Florida	28.38
25	South Carolina	27.96
26	Idaho	27.36
27	Connecticut	27.24
28	Alaska	27.09
29	South Dakota	26.26
30	Oregon	25.86
31	Michigan	25.26
32	Kansas	24.22
33	Massachusetts	23.63
34	Utah	22.85
35	Nevada	22.29
36	Illinois	20.53
37	Arkansas	20.32
38	Texas	18.57
39	Nebraska	16.31
40	Indiana	16.11
41	Rhode Island	16.10
42	North Carolina	15.84
43	Alabama	15.81
44	West Virginia	15.40
45	Virginia	14.68
46	Ohio	14.13
47	Louisiana	13.19
48	Mississippi	12.69
49	Tennessee	11.78
50	Maryland	9.86

District of Columbia — 16.06

Source: Morgan Quitno Press using data from Federation of Chiropractic Licensing Boards
"1994–95 Official Directory"
*Licensed active doctors. National rate and Florida's rate are not considered precise due to incomplete information. There is some duplication as some doctors are licensed in more than one state. Calculated using updated 1993 Census population estimates.

Registered Nurses in 1992

National Total = 1,853,024 Registered Nurses*

ALPHA ORDER				RANK ORDER			
RANK	STATE	NURSES	% of USA	RANK	STATE	NURSES	% of USA
22	Alabama	27,717	1.50%	1	California	173,973	9.39%
49	Alaska	3,583	0.19%	2	New York	159,297	8.60%
23	Arizona	27,093	1.46%	3	Pennsylvania	108,663	5.86%
32	Arkansas	14,001	0.76%	4	Florida	94,591	5.10%
1	California	173,973	9.39%	5	Illinois	93,069	5.02%
24	Colorado	26,697	1.44%	6	Texas	92,810	5.01%
21	Connecticut	30,918	1.67%	7	Ohio	89,799	4.85%
45	Delaware	6,137	0.33%	8	Michigan	65,441	3.53%
4	Florida	94,591	5.10%	9	New Jersey	64,519	3.48%
12	Georgia	43,386	2.34%	10	Massachusetts	63,751	3.44%
41	Hawaii	7,674	0.41%	11	North Carolina	47,602	2.57%
47	Idaho	5,702	0.31%	12	Georgia	43,386	2.34%
5	Illinois	93,069	5.02%	13	Virginia	42,519	2.29%
17	Indiana	39,602	2.14%	14	Missouri	42,035	2.27%
25	Iowa	25,838	1.39%	15	Wisconsin	39,883	2.15%
30	Kansas	19,773	1.07%	16	Minnesota	39,876	2.15%
26	Kentucky	24,552	1.32%	17	Indiana	39,602	2.14%
27	Louisiana	24,233	1.31%	18	Washington	38,698	2.09%
37	Maine	10,584	0.57%	19	Maryland	38,170	2.06%
19	Maryland	38,170	2.06%	20	Tennessee	35,318	1.91%
10	Massachusetts	63,751	3.44%	21	Connecticut	30,918	1.67%
8	Michigan	65,441	3.53%	22	Alabama	27,717	1.50%
16	Minnesota	39,876	2.15%	23	Arizona	27,093	1.46%
33	Mississippi	13,415	0.72%	24	Colorado	26,697	1.44%
14	Missouri	42,035	2.27%	25	Iowa	25,838	1.39%
46	Montana	5,848	0.32%	26	Kentucky	24,552	1.32%
34	Nebraska	13,257	0.72%	27	Louisiana	24,233	1.31%
42	Nevada	7,135	0.39%	28	Oregon	23,992	1.29%
36	New Hampshire	10,743	0.58%	29	South Carolina	20,684	1.12%
9	New Jersey	64,519	3.48%	30	Kansas	19,773	1.07%
40	New Mexico	9,393	0.51%	31	Oklahoma	16,972	0.92%
2	New York	159,297	8.60%	32	Arkansas	14,001	0.76%
11	North Carolina	47,602	2.57%	33	Mississippi	13,415	0.72%
44	North Dakota	6,300	0.34%	34	Nebraska	13,257	0.72%
7	Ohio	89,799	4.85%	35	West Virginia	11,875	0.64%
31	Oklahoma	16,972	0.92%	36	New Hampshire	10,743	0.58%
28	Oregon	23,992	1.29%	37	Maine	10,584	0.57%
3	Pennsylvania	108,663	5.86%	38	Utah	9,831	0.53%
39	Rhode Island	9,665	0.52%	39	Rhode Island	9,665	0.52%
29	South Carolina	20,684	1.12%	40	New Mexico	9,393	0.51%
43	South Dakota	6,828	0.37%	41	Hawaii	7,674	0.41%
20	Tennessee	35,318	1.91%	42	Nevada	7,135	0.39%
6	Texas	92,810	5.01%	43	South Dakota	6,828	0.37%
38	Utah	9,831	0.53%	44	North Dakota	6,300	0.34%
48	Vermont	5,199	0.28%	45	Delaware	6,137	0.33%
13	Virginia	42,519	2.29%	46	Montana	5,848	0.32%
18	Washington	38,698	2.09%	47	Idaho	5,702	0.31%
35	West Virginia	11,875	0.64%	48	Vermont	5,199	0.28%
15	Wisconsin	39,883	2.15%	49	Alaska	3,583	0.19%
50	Wyoming	3,032	0.16%	50	Wyoming	3,032	0.16%
					District of Columbia	11,352	0.61%

Source: U.S. Department of Health and Human Services, Bureau of Health Professionals, Division of Nursing
   unpublished data
*As of March, 1992.

Rate of Registered Nurses in 1992

National Rate = 726.60 Nurses per 100,000 Population*

ALPHA ORDER			RANK ORDER		
RANK	STATE	RATE	RANK	STATE	RATE
32	Alabama	670.95	1	Massachusetts	1,062.69
39	Alaska	610.39	2	North Dakota	992.13
26	Arizona	706.47	3	Rhode Island	964.57
41	Arkansas	584.59	4	New Hampshire	964.36
44	California	562.86	5	South Dakota	963.05
23	Colorado	770.92	6	Connecticut	942.91
6	Connecticut	942.91	7	Iowa	920.16
11	Delaware	889.42	8	Vermont	910.51
29	Florida	700.16	9	Pennsylvania	906.28
38	Georgia	641.33	10	Minnesota	891.28
33	Hawaii	665.57	11	Delaware	889.42
47	Idaho	534.90	12	New York	880.34
19	Illinois	801.63	13	Maine	855.62
28	Indiana	700.67	14	Nebraska	826.50
7	Iowa	920.16	15	New Jersey	825.79
21	Kansas	785.27	16	Ohio	815.98
36	Kentucky	654.20	17	Missouri	809.46
43	Louisiana	567.12	18	Oregon	806.45
13	Maine	855.62	19	Illinois	801.63
22	Maryland	776.76	20	Wisconsin	798.14
1	Massachusetts	1,062.69	21	Kansas	785.27
31	Michigan	694.48	22	Maryland	776.76
10	Minnesota	891.28	23	Colorado	770.92
50	Mississippi	513.39	24	Washington	752.00
17	Missouri	809.46	25	Montana	710.57
25	Montana	710.57	26	Arizona	706.47
14	Nebraska	826.50	27	Tennessee	703.41
46	Nevada	536.06	28	Indiana	700.67
4	New Hampshire	964.36	29	Florida	700.16
15	New Jersey	825.79	30	North Carolina	696.14
40	New Mexico	594.12	31	Michigan	694.48
12	New York	880.34	32	Alabama	670.95
30	North Carolina	696.14	33	Hawaii	665.57
2	North Dakota	992.13	34	Virginia	665.50
16	Ohio	815.98	35	West Virginia	657.17
48	Oklahoma	529.38	36	Kentucky	654.20
18	Oregon	806.45	37	Wyoming	653.45
9	Pennsylvania	906.28	38	Georgia	641.33
3	Rhode Island	964.57	39	Alaska	610.39
42	South Carolina	575.35	40	New Mexico	594.12
5	South Dakota	963.05	41	Arkansas	584.59
27	Tennessee	703.41	42	South Carolina	575.35
49	Texas	525.33	43	Louisiana	567.12
45	Utah	542.85	44	California	562.86
8	Vermont	910.51	45	Utah	542.85
34	Virginia	665.50	46	Nevada	536.06
24	Washington	752.00	47	Idaho	534.90
35	West Virginia	657.17	48	Oklahoma	529.38
20	Wisconsin	798.14	49	Texas	525.33
37	Wyoming	653.45	50	Mississippi	513.39

	District of Columbia	1,937.20

Source: Morgan Quitno Press using data from U.S. Dept of Health and Human Services, Bureau of Health Professionals
   unpublished data

*As of March, 1992.

Active Civilian Dentists in 1992

National Total = 155,058 Active Civilian Dentists

ALPHA ORDER				RANK ORDER			
RANK	STATE	DENTISTS	% of USA	RANK	STATE	DENTISTS	% of USA
27	Alabama	1,776	1.15%	1	California	20,751	13.38%
47	Alaska	317	0.20%	2	New York	14,859	9.58%
26	Arizona	1,918	1.24%	3	Texas	8,688	5.60%
35	Arkansas	989	0.64%	4	Pennsylvania	8,097	5.22%
1	California	20,751	13.38%	5	Illinois	8,066	5.20%
22	Colorado	2,451	1.58%	6	Florida	7,079	4.57%
21	Connecticut	2,635	1.70%	7	New Jersey	6,418	4.14%
46	Delaware	320	0.21%	8	Ohio	6,090	3.93%
6	Florida	7,079	4.57%	9	Michigan	5,955	3.84%
14	Georgia	3,165	2.04%	10	Massachusetts	4,765	3.07%
36	Hawaii	920	0.59%	11	Maryland	3,669	2.37%
41	Idaho	567	0.37%	12	Virginia	3,502	2.26%
5	Illinois	8,066	5.20%	13	Washington	3,179	2.05%
18	Indiana	2,798	1.80%	14	Georgia	3,165	2.04%
29	Iowa	1,528	0.99%	15	Wisconsin	3,101	2.00%
31	Kansas	1,322	0.85%	16	Minnesota	2,913	1.88%
23	Kentucky	2,113	1.36%	17	North Carolina	2,895	1.87%
25	Louisiana	2,005	1.29%	18	Indiana	2,798	1.80%
40	Maine	590	0.38%	19	Tennessee	2,767	1.78%
11	Maryland	3,669	2.37%	20	Missouri	2,756	1.78%
10	Massachusetts	4,765	3.07%	21	Connecticut	2,635	1.70%
9	Michigan	5,955	3.84%	22	Colorado	2,451	1.58%
16	Minnesota	2,913	1.88%	23	Kentucky	2,113	1.36%
34	Mississippi	1,019	0.66%	24	Oregon	2,050	1.32%
20	Missouri	2,756	1.78%	25	Louisiana	2,005	1.29%
44	Montana	468	0.30%	26	Arizona	1,918	1.24%
33	Nebraska	1,079	0.70%	27	Alabama	1,776	1.15%
43	Nevada	553	0.36%	28	Oklahoma	1,556	1.00%
38	New Hampshire	673	0.43%	29	Iowa	1,528	0.99%
7	New Jersey	6,418	4.14%	30	South Carolina	1,521	0.98%
39	New Mexico	662	0.43%	31	Kansas	1,322	0.85%
2	New York	14,859	9.58%	32	Utah	1,167	0.75%
17	North Carolina	2,895	1.87%	33	Nebraska	1,079	0.70%
49	North Dakota	299	0.19%	34	Mississippi	1,019	0.66%
8	Ohio	6,090	3.93%	35	Arkansas	989	0.64%
28	Oklahoma	1,556	1.00%	36	Hawaii	920	0.59%
24	Oregon	2,050	1.32%	37	West Virginia	867	0.56%
4	Pennsylvania	8,097	5.22%	38	New Hampshire	673	0.43%
42	Rhode Island	556	0.36%	39	New Mexico	662	0.43%
30	South Carolina	1,521	0.98%	40	Maine	590	0.38%
48	South Dakota	308	0.20%	41	Idaho	567	0.37%
19	Tennessee	2,767	1.78%	42	Rhode Island	556	0.36%
3	Texas	8,688	5.60%	43	Nevada	553	0.36%
32	Utah	1,167	0.75%	44	Montana	468	0.30%
45	Vermont	326	0.21%	45	Vermont	326	0.21%
12	Virginia	3,502	2.26%	46	Delaware	320	0.21%
13	Washington	3,179	2.05%	47	Alaska	317	0.20%
37	West Virginia	867	0.56%	48	South Dakota	308	0.20%
15	Wisconsin	3,101	2.00%	49	North Dakota	299	0.19%
50	Wyoming	240	0.15%	50	Wyoming	240	0.15%
					District of Columbia	750	0.48%

Source: U.S. Department of Health and Human Services, Health Resources and Services Administration unpublished data

Rate of Active Civilian Dentists in 1992

National Rate = 61 Dentists per 100,000 Population

<table>
<tr><td colspan="3">ALPHA ORDER</td><td colspan="3">RANK ORDER</td></tr>
<tr><td>RANK</td><td>STATE</td><td>RATE</td><td>RANK</td><td>STATE</td><td>RATE</td></tr>
<tr><td>44</td><td>Alabama</td><td>43</td><td>1</td><td>Hawaii</td><td>83</td></tr>
<tr><td>23</td><td>Alaska</td><td>56</td><td>1</td><td>New Jersey</td><td>83</td></tr>
<tr><td>33</td><td>Arizona</td><td>50</td><td>3</td><td>New York</td><td>82</td></tr>
<tr><td>49</td><td>Arkansas</td><td>41</td><td>4</td><td>Connecticut</td><td>81</td></tr>
<tr><td>10</td><td>California</td><td>68</td><td>5</td><td>Massachusetts</td><td>80</td></tr>
<tr><td>7</td><td>Colorado</td><td>71</td><td>6</td><td>Maryland</td><td>75</td></tr>
<tr><td>4</td><td>Connecticut</td><td>81</td><td>7</td><td>Colorado</td><td>71</td></tr>
<tr><td>40</td><td>Delaware</td><td>47</td><td>8</td><td>Illinois</td><td>70</td></tr>
<tr><td>28</td><td>Florida</td><td>53</td><td>9</td><td>Oregon</td><td>69</td></tr>
<tr><td>40</td><td>Georgia</td><td>47</td><td>10</td><td>California</td><td>68</td></tr>
<tr><td>1</td><td>Hawaii</td><td>83</td><td>10</td><td>Nebraska</td><td>68</td></tr>
<tr><td>28</td><td>Idaho</td><td>53</td><td>12</td><td>Pennsylvania</td><td>67</td></tr>
<tr><td>8</td><td>Illinois</td><td>70</td><td>13</td><td>Minnesota</td><td>65</td></tr>
<tr><td>35</td><td>Indiana</td><td>49</td><td>13</td><td>Utah</td><td>65</td></tr>
<tr><td>27</td><td>Iowa</td><td>54</td><td>15</td><td>Michigan</td><td>63</td></tr>
<tr><td>28</td><td>Kansas</td><td>53</td><td>15</td><td>Washington</td><td>63</td></tr>
<tr><td>19</td><td>Kentucky</td><td>57</td><td>17</td><td>Wisconsin</td><td>62</td></tr>
<tr><td>40</td><td>Louisiana</td><td>47</td><td>18</td><td>New Hampshire</td><td>61</td></tr>
<tr><td>37</td><td>Maine</td><td>48</td><td>19</td><td>Kentucky</td><td>57</td></tr>
<tr><td>6</td><td>Maryland</td><td>75</td><td>19</td><td>Montana</td><td>57</td></tr>
<tr><td>5</td><td>Massachusetts</td><td>80</td><td>19</td><td>Vermont</td><td>57</td></tr>
<tr><td>15</td><td>Michigan</td><td>63</td><td>19</td><td>Virginia</td><td>57</td></tr>
<tr><td>13</td><td>Minnesota</td><td>65</td><td>23</td><td>Alaska</td><td>56</td></tr>
<tr><td>50</td><td>Mississippi</td><td>39</td><td>23</td><td>Rhode Island</td><td>56</td></tr>
<tr><td>28</td><td>Missouri</td><td>53</td><td>25</td><td>Ohio</td><td>55</td></tr>
<tr><td>19</td><td>Montana</td><td>57</td><td>25</td><td>Tennessee</td><td>55</td></tr>
<tr><td>10</td><td>Nebraska</td><td>68</td><td>27</td><td>Iowa</td><td>54</td></tr>
<tr><td>47</td><td>Nevada</td><td>42</td><td>28</td><td>Florida</td><td>53</td></tr>
<tr><td>18</td><td>New Hampshire</td><td>61</td><td>28</td><td>Idaho</td><td>53</td></tr>
<tr><td>1</td><td>New Jersey</td><td>83</td><td>28</td><td>Kansas</td><td>53</td></tr>
<tr><td>47</td><td>New Mexico</td><td>42</td><td>28</td><td>Missouri</td><td>53</td></tr>
<tr><td>3</td><td>New York</td><td>82</td><td>32</td><td>Wyoming</td><td>52</td></tr>
<tr><td>44</td><td>North Carolina</td><td>43</td><td>33</td><td>Arizona</td><td>50</td></tr>
<tr><td>37</td><td>North Dakota</td><td>48</td><td>33</td><td>Texas</td><td>50</td></tr>
<tr><td>25</td><td>Ohio</td><td>55</td><td>35</td><td>Indiana</td><td>49</td></tr>
<tr><td>35</td><td>Oklahoma</td><td>49</td><td>35</td><td>Oklahoma</td><td>49</td></tr>
<tr><td>9</td><td>Oregon</td><td>69</td><td>37</td><td>Maine</td><td>48</td></tr>
<tr><td>12</td><td>Pennsylvania</td><td>67</td><td>37</td><td>North Dakota</td><td>48</td></tr>
<tr><td>23</td><td>Rhode Island</td><td>56</td><td>37</td><td>West Virginia</td><td>48</td></tr>
<tr><td>44</td><td>South Carolina</td><td>43</td><td>40</td><td>Delaware</td><td>47</td></tr>
<tr><td>43</td><td>South Dakota</td><td>44</td><td>40</td><td>Georgia</td><td>47</td></tr>
<tr><td>25</td><td>Tennessee</td><td>55</td><td>40</td><td>Louisiana</td><td>47</td></tr>
<tr><td>33</td><td>Texas</td><td>50</td><td>43</td><td>South Dakota</td><td>44</td></tr>
<tr><td>13</td><td>Utah</td><td>65</td><td>44</td><td>Alabama</td><td>43</td></tr>
<tr><td>19</td><td>Vermont</td><td>57</td><td>44</td><td>North Carolina</td><td>43</td></tr>
<tr><td>19</td><td>Virginia</td><td>57</td><td>44</td><td>South Carolina</td><td>43</td></tr>
<tr><td>15</td><td>Washington</td><td>63</td><td>47</td><td>Nevada</td><td>42</td></tr>
<tr><td>37</td><td>West Virginia</td><td>48</td><td>47</td><td>New Mexico</td><td>42</td></tr>
<tr><td>17</td><td>Wisconsin</td><td>62</td><td>49</td><td>Arkansas</td><td>41</td></tr>
<tr><td>32</td><td>Wyoming</td><td>52</td><td>50</td><td>Mississippi</td><td>39</td></tr>
<tr><td></td><td></td><td></td><td></td><td>District of Columbia</td><td>129</td></tr>
</table>

Source: U.S. Department of Health and Human Services, Health Resources and Services Administration unpublished data

441

Hospital Personnel in 1993

National Total = 4,289,379 Personnel*

ALPHA ORDER					RANK ORDER			
RANK	**STATE**	**PERSONNEL**	**% of USA**		**RANK**	**STATE**	**PERSONNEL**	**% of USA**
19	Alabama	75,683	1.76%		1	New York	380,016	8.86%
49	Alaska	8,442	0.20%		2	California	377,752	8.81%
28	Arizona	50,529	1.18%		3	Texas	276,590	6.45%
32	Arkansas	42,645	0.99%		4	Pennsylvania	258,051	6.02%
2	California	377,752	8.81%		5	Florida	220,052	5.13%
27	Colorado	52,090	1.21%		6	Illinois	204,250	4.76%
24	Connecticut	54,878	1.28%		7	Ohio	191,786	4.47%
47	Delaware	12,761	0.30%		8	Michigan	154,004	3.59%
5	Florida	220,052	5.13%		9	New Jersey	134,923	3.15%
11	Georgia	119,445	2.78%		10	Massachusetts	125,930	2.94%
40	Hawaii	17,763	0.41%		11	Georgia	119,445	2.78%
45	Idaho	13,461	0.31%		12	North Carolina	114,814	2.68%
6	Illinois	204,250	4.76%		13	Missouri	108,714	2.53%
14	Indiana	98,507	2.30%		14	Indiana	98,507	2.30%
29	Iowa	49,642	1.16%		15	Tennessee	98,123	2.29%
31	Kansas	46,150	1.08%		16	Virginia	97,130	2.26%
21	Kentucky	66,522	1.55%		17	Louisiana	84,371	1.97%
17	Louisiana	84,371	1.97%		18	Maryland	80,990	1.89%
38	Maine	21,431	0.50%		19	Alabama	75,683	1.76%
18	Maryland	80,990	1.89%		20	Wisconsin	73,565	1.72%
10	Massachusetts	125,930	2.94%		21	Kentucky	66,522	1.55%
8	Michigan	154,004	3.59%		22	Washington	64,576	1.51%
23	Minnesota	63,869	1.49%		23	Minnesota	63,869	1.49%
30	Mississippi	46,811	1.09%		24	Connecticut	54,878	1.28%
13	Missouri	108,714	2.53%		25	South Carolina	54,205	1.26%
46	Montana	13,238	0.31%		26	Oklahoma	52,217	1.22%
35	Nebraska	30,854	0.72%		27	Colorado	52,090	1.21%
43	Nevada	14,989	0.35%		28	Arizona	50,529	1.18%
41	New Hampshire	16,330	0.38%		29	Iowa	49,642	1.16%
9	New Jersey	134,923	3.15%		30	Mississippi	46,811	1.09%
36	New Mexico	27,112	0.63%		31	Kansas	46,150	1.08%
1	New York	380,016	8.86%		32	Arkansas	42,645	0.99%
12	North Carolina	114,814	2.68%		33	Oregon	38,326	0.89%
44	North Dakota	14,596	0.34%		34	West Virginia	34,228	0.80%
7	Ohio	191,786	4.47%		35	Nebraska	30,854	0.72%
26	Oklahoma	52,217	1.22%		36	New Mexico	27,112	0.63%
33	Oregon	38,326	0.89%		37	Utah	23,890	0.56%
4	Pennsylvania	258,051	6.02%		38	Maine	21,431	0.50%
39	Rhode Island	17,881	0.42%		39	Rhode Island	17,881	0.42%
25	South Carolina	54,205	1.26%		40	Hawaii	17,763	0.41%
42	South Dakota	15,265	0.36%		41	New Hampshire	16,330	0.38%
15	Tennessee	98,123	2.29%		42	South Dakota	15,265	0.36%
3	Texas	276,590	6.45%		43	Nevada	14,989	0.35%
37	Utah	23,890	0.56%		44	North Dakota	14,596	0.34%
50	Vermont	8,431	0.20%		45	Idaho	13,461	0.31%
16	Virginia	97,130	2.26%		46	Montana	13,238	0.31%
22	Washington	64,576	1.51%		47	Delaware	12,761	0.30%
34	West Virginia	34,228	0.80%		48	Wyoming	10,311	0.24%
20	Wisconsin	73,565	1.72%		49	Alaska	8,442	0.20%
48	Wyoming	10,311	0.24%		50	Vermont	8,431	0.20%
						District of Columbia	31,240	0.73%

Source: American Hospital Association (Chicago, Illinois)
   "Hospital Statistics" (1994–95 edition)
*Includes physicians, dentists, nurses and other salaried personnel in federal and nonfederal hospitals.

Employment in Health Service Industries in 1992

National Total = 9,726,647 Employees*

ALPHA ORDER

RANK ORDER

RANK	STATE	EMPLOYEES	% of USA		RANK	STATE	EMPLOYEES	% of USA
23	Alabama	141,408	1.45%		1	California	979,419	10.07%
49	Alaska	14,926	0.15%		2	New York	861,326	8.86%
26	Arizona	124,056	1.28%		3	Texas	590,256	6.07%
32	Arkansas	82,364	0.85%		4	Pennsylvania	549,627	5.65%
1	California	979,419	10.07%		5	Florida	520,805	5.35%
25	Colorado	126,052	1.30%		6	Ohio	463,622	4.77%
21	Connecticut	158,976	1.63%		7	Illinois	458,390	4.71%
46	Delaware	28,910	0.30%		8	Michigan	356,311	3.66%
5	Florida	520,805	5.35%		9	Massachusetts	323,333	3.32%
13	Georgia	224,197	2.30%		10	New Jersey	308,423	3.17%
41	Hawaii	37,758	0.39%		11	North Carolina	228,049	2.34%
47	Idaho	26,980	0.28%		12	Missouri	227,692	2.34%
7	Illinois	458,390	4.71%		13	Georgia	224,197	2.30%
15	Indiana	218,448	2.25%		14	Wisconsin	219,112	2.25%
27	Iowa	118,311	1.22%		15	Indiana	218,448	2.25%
29	Kansas	105,030	1.08%		16	Minnesota	205,889	2.12%
24	Kentucky	136,211	1.40%		17	Tennessee	204,145	2.10%
22	Louisiana	142,136	1.46%		18	Virginia	199,486	2.05%
37	Maine	52,411	0.54%		19	Maryland	186,808	1.92%
19	Maryland	186,808	1.92%		20	Washington	183,695	1.89%
9	Massachusetts	323,333	3.32%		21	Connecticut	158,976	1.63%
8	Michigan	356,311	3.66%		22	Louisiana	142,136	1.46%
16	Minnesota	205,889	2.12%		23	Alabama	141,408	1.45%
33	Mississippi	70,493	0.72%		24	Kentucky	136,211	1.40%
12	Missouri	227,692	2.34%		25	Colorado	126,052	1.30%
45	Montana	29,345	0.30%		26	Arizona	124,056	1.28%
35	Nebraska	64,846	0.67%		27	Iowa	118,311	1.22%
44	Nevada	32,323	0.33%		28	Oklahoma	107,398	1.10%
40	New Hampshire	43,279	0.44%		29	Kansas	105,030	1.08%
10	New Jersey	308,423	3.17%		30	Oregon	100,606	1.03%
39	New Mexico	45,303	0.47%		31	South Carolina	100,369	1.03%
2	New York	861,326	8.86%		32	Arkansas	82,364	0.85%
11	North Carolina	228,049	2.34%		33	Mississippi	70,493	0.72%
42	North Dakota	34,320	0.35%		34	West Virginia	65,275	0.67%
6	Ohio	463,622	4.77%		35	Nebraska	64,846	0.67%
28	Oklahoma	107,398	1.10%		36	Utah	56,898	0.58%
30	Oregon	100,606	1.03%		37	Maine	52,411	0.54%
4	Pennsylvania	549,627	5.65%		38	Rhode Island	47,120	0.48%
38	Rhode Island	47,120	0.48%		39	New Mexico	45,303	0.47%
31	South Carolina	100,369	1.03%		40	New Hampshire	43,279	0.44%
43	South Dakota	32,959	0.34%		41	Hawaii	37,758	0.39%
17	Tennessee	204,145	2.10%		42	North Dakota	34,320	0.35%
3	Texas	590,256	6.07%		43	South Dakota	32,959	0.34%
36	Utah	56,898	0.58%		44	Nevada	32,323	0.33%
48	Vermont	20,165	0.21%		45	Montana	29,345	0.30%
18	Virginia	199,486	2.05%		46	Delaware	28,910	0.30%
20	Washington	183,695	1.89%		47	Idaho	26,980	0.28%
34	West Virginia	65,275	0.67%		48	Vermont	20,165	0.21%
14	Wisconsin	219,112	2.25%		49	Alaska	14,926	0.15%
50	Wyoming	9,658	0.10%		50	Wyoming	9,658	0.10%
						District of Columbia	61,728	0.63%

Source: U.S. Bureau of the Census
"County Business Patterns"

*Total of employment in March 1992 at establishments classified in Standard Industrial Classification (S.I.C.) code 8000.
An establishment is a single physical location at which business is conducted or where services or industrial operations are performed. It is not necessarily identical with a company or enterprise, which may consist of one establishment or more.

VII. PHYSICAL FITNESS

Users of Exercising Equipment in 1993

National Total = 37,130,000 Participants

ALPHA ORDER					RANK ORDER			
RANK	STATE	PARTICIPANTS	% of USA		RANK	STATE	PARTICIPANTS	% of USA
22	Alabama	654,000	1.76%		1	California	4,363,000	11.75%
NA	Alaska*	NA	NA		2	New York	2,658,000	7.16%
21	Arizona	661,000	1.78%		3	Texas	2,276,000	6.13%
34	Arkansas	357,000	0.96%		4	Florida	2,115,000	5.70%
1	California	4,363,000	11.75%		5	Pennsylvania	1,794,000	4.83%
24	Colorado	647,000	1.74%		6	Illinois	1,484,000	4.00%
19	Connecticut	673,000	1.81%		7	Ohio	1,480,000	3.99%
46	Delaware	86,000	0.23%		8	Michigan	1,363,000	3.67%
4	Florida	2,115,000	5.70%		9	New Jersey	1,360,000	3.66%
10	Georgia	1,063,000	2.86%		10	Georgia	1,063,000	2.86%
NA	Hawaii*	NA	NA		11	North Carolina	982,000	2.64%
44	Idaho	131,000	0.35%		12	Missouri	908,000	2.45%
6	Illinois	1,484,000	4.00%		13	Maryland	841,000	2.27%
17	Indiana	678,000	1.83%		14	Minnesota	805,000	2.17%
32	Iowa	372,000	1.00%		15	Massachusetts	795,000	2.14%
35	Kansas	354,000	0.95%		16	Wisconsin	709,000	1.91%
28	Kentucky	489,000	1.32%		17	Indiana	678,000	1.83%
20	Louisiana	666,000	1.79%		18	Virginia	674,000	1.82%
38	Maine	242,000	0.65%		19	Connecticut	673,000	1.81%
13	Maryland	841,000	2.27%		20	Louisiana	666,000	1.79%
15	Massachusetts	795,000	2.14%		21	Arizona	661,000	1.78%
8	Michigan	1,363,000	3.67%		22	Alabama	654,000	1.76%
14	Minnesota	805,000	2.17%		23	Washington	651,000	1.75%
33	Mississippi	358,000	0.96%		24	Colorado	647,000	1.74%
12	Missouri	908,000	2.45%		25	Tennessee	632,000	1.70%
37	Montana	252,000	0.68%		26	Oklahoma	502,000	1.35%
36	Nebraska	293,000	0.79%		27	Oregon	492,000	1.33%
41	Nevada	171,000	0.46%		28	Kentucky	489,000	1.32%
45	New Hampshire	105,000	0.28%		29	South Carolina	425,000	1.14%
9	New Jersey	1,360,000	3.66%		30	Utah	380,000	1.02%
43	New Mexico	141,000	0.38%		31	West Virginia	375,000	1.01%
2	New York	2,658,000	7.16%		32	Iowa	372,000	1.00%
11	North Carolina	982,000	2.64%		33	Mississippi	358,000	0.96%
48	North Dakota	59,000	0.16%		34	Arkansas	357,000	0.96%
7	Ohio	1,480,000	3.99%		35	Kansas	354,000	0.95%
26	Oklahoma	502,000	1.35%		36	Nebraska	293,000	0.79%
27	Oregon	492,000	1.33%		37	Montana	252,000	0.68%
5	Pennsylvania	1,794,000	4.83%		38	Maine	242,000	0.65%
39	Rhode Island	186,000	0.50%		39	Rhode Island	186,000	0.50%
29	South Carolina	425,000	1.14%		40	Wyoming	174,000	0.47%
47	South Dakota	65,000	0.18%		41	Nevada	171,000	0.46%
25	Tennessee	632,000	1.70%		42	Vermont	149,000	0.40%
3	Texas	2,276,000	6.13%		43	New Mexico	141,000	0.38%
30	Utah	380,000	1.02%		44	Idaho	131,000	0.35%
42	Vermont	149,000	0.40%		45	New Hampshire	105,000	0.28%
18	Virginia	674,000	1.82%		46	Delaware	86,000	0.23%
23	Washington	651,000	1.75%		47	South Dakota	65,000	0.18%
31	West Virginia	375,000	1.01%		48	North Dakota	59,000	0.16%
16	Wisconsin	709,000	1.91%		NA	Alaska*	NA	NA
40	Wyoming	174,000	0.47%		NA	Hawaii*	NA	NA
						District of Columbia*	NA	NA

Source: The National Sporting Goods Association
*NSGA Sports Participation Survey, January-December 1993 (Copyright 1994, reprinted with permission)
*Not available.

Participants in Golf in 1993

National Total = 23,327,000 Golfers

ALPHA ORDER				RANK ORDER			
RANK	STATE	GOLFERS	% of USA	RANK	STATE	GOLFERS	% of USA
31	Alabama	266,000	1.14%	1	California	2,520,000	10.80%
NA	Alaska*	NA	NA	2	New York	1,565,000	6.71%
24	Arizona	308,000	1.32%	3	Michigan	1,320,000	5.66%
40	Arkansas	116,000	0.50%	4	Ohio	1,311,000	5.62%
1	California	2,520,000	10.80%	5	Illinois	1,247,000	5.35%
17	Colorado	405,000	1.74%	6	Florida	1,214,000	5.20%
22	Connecticut	359,000	1.54%	7	Texas	1,160,000	4.97%
48	Delaware	17,000	0.07%	8	Pennsylvania	1,096,000	4.70%
6	Florida	1,214,000	5.20%	9	New Jersey	795,000	3.41%
11	Georgia	642,000	2.75%	10	Wisconsin	751,000	3.22%
NA	Hawaii*	NA	NA	11	Georgia	642,000	2.75%
37	Idaho	161,000	0.69%	12	Indiana	618,000	2.65%
5	Illinois	1,247,000	5.35%	13	Minnesota	565,000	2.42%
12	Indiana	618,000	2.65%	14	North Carolina	539,000	2.31%
18	Iowa	394,000	1.69%	15	Missouri	522,000	2.24%
34	Kansas	216,000	0.93%	16	Maryland	424,000	1.82%
27	Kentucky	293,000	1.26%	17	Colorado	405,000	1.74%
23	Louisiana	329,000	1.41%	18	Iowa	394,000	1.69%
36	Maine	179,000	0.77%	19	Virginia	390,000	1.67%
16	Maryland	424,000	1.82%	20	Oklahoma	383,000	1.64%
21	Massachusetts	369,000	1.58%	21	Massachusetts	369,000	1.58%
3	Michigan	1,320,000	5.66%	22	Connecticut	359,000	1.54%
13	Minnesota	565,000	2.42%	23	Louisiana	329,000	1.41%
33	Mississippi	232,000	0.99%	24	Arizona	308,000	1.32%
15	Missouri	522,000	2.24%	25	South Carolina	306,000	1.31%
35	Montana	186,000	0.80%	26	Nebraska	294,000	1.26%
26	Nebraska	294,000	1.26%	27	Kentucky	293,000	1.26%
39	Nevada	117,000	0.50%	28	Utah	290,000	1.24%
45	New Hampshire	55,000	0.24%	29	Oregon	285,000	1.22%
9	New Jersey	795,000	3.41%	30	Tennessee	275,000	1.18%
43	New Mexico	63,000	0.27%	31	Alabama	266,000	1.14%
2	New York	1,565,000	6.71%	31	Washington	266,000	1.14%
14	North Carolina	539,000	2.31%	33	Mississippi	232,000	0.99%
41	North Dakota	108,000	0.46%	34	Kansas	216,000	0.93%
4	Ohio	1,311,000	5.62%	35	Montana	186,000	0.80%
20	Oklahoma	383,000	1.64%	36	Maine	179,000	0.77%
29	Oregon	285,000	1.22%	37	Idaho	161,000	0.69%
8	Pennsylvania	1,096,000	4.70%	38	West Virginia	152,000	0.65%
42	Rhode Island	80,000	0.34%	39	Nevada	117,000	0.50%
25	South Carolina	306,000	1.31%	40	Arkansas	116,000	0.50%
44	South Dakota	60,000	0.26%	41	North Dakota	108,000	0.46%
30	Tennessee	275,000	1.18%	42	Rhode Island	80,000	0.34%
7	Texas	1,160,000	4.97%	43	New Mexico	63,000	0.27%
28	Utah	290,000	1.24%	44	South Dakota	60,000	0.26%
46	Vermont	37,000	0.16%	45	New Hampshire	55,000	0.24%
19	Virginia	390,000	1.67%	46	Vermont	37,000	0.16%
31	Washington	266,000	1.14%	46	Wyoming	37,000	0.16%
38	West Virginia	152,000	0.65%	48	Delaware	17,000	0.07%
10	Wisconsin	751,000	3.22%	NA	Alaska*	NA	NA
46	Wyoming	37,000	0.16%	NA	Hawaii*	NA	NA
					District of Columbia*	NA	NA

Source: The National Sporting Goods Association
    "NSGA Sports Participation Survey, January-December 1993 (Copyright 1994, reprinted with permission)
*Not available.

Participants in Running/Jogging in 1993

National Total = 21,108,000 Runners/Joggers

ALPHA ORDER					RANK ORDER			
RANK	**STATE**	**RUNNERS**	**% of USA**		**RANK**	**STATE**	**RUNNERS**	**% of USA**
23	Alabama	326,000	1.54%		1	California	2,926,000	13.86%
NA	Alaska*	NA	NA		2	Texas	1,672,000	7.92%
20	Arizona	348,000	1.65%		3	Florida	1,267,000	6.00%
41	Arkansas	64,000	0.30%		4	New York	1,236,000	5.86%
1	California	2,926,000	13.86%		5	Pennsylvania	873,000	4.14%
13	Colorado	498,000	2.36%		6	Illinois	849,000	4.02%
22	Connecticut	334,000	1.58%		7	Georgia	739,000	3.50%
40	Delaware	81,000	0.38%		8	New Jersey	707,000	3.35%
3	Florida	1,267,000	6.00%		9	Ohio	692,000	3.28%
7	Georgia	739,000	3.50%		10	Michigan	690,000	3.27%
NA	Hawaii*	NA	NA		11	North Carolina	652,000	3.09%
38	Idaho	99,000	0.47%		12	Virginia	542,000	2.57%
6	Illinois	849,000	4.02%		13	Colorado	498,000	2.36%
16	Indiana	438,000	2.08%		14	Maryland	491,000	2.33%
29	Iowa	244,000	1.16%		15	Louisiana	444,000	2.10%
30	Kansas	234,000	1.11%		16	Indiana	438,000	2.08%
26	Kentucky	295,000	1.40%		17	Massachusetts	436,000	2.07%
15	Louisiana	444,000	2.10%		18	Missouri	371,000	1.76%
39	Maine	89,000	0.42%		19	Wisconsin	357,000	1.69%
14	Maryland	491,000	2.33%		20	Arizona	348,000	1.65%
17	Massachusetts	436,000	2.07%		21	Minnesota	342,000	1.62%
10	Michigan	690,000	3.27%		22	Connecticut	334,000	1.58%
21	Minnesota	342,000	1.62%		23	Alabama	326,000	1.54%
24	Mississippi	314,000	1.49%		24	Mississippi	314,000	1.49%
18	Missouri	371,000	1.76%		25	Tennessee	310,000	1.47%
36	Montana	115,000	0.54%		26	Kentucky	295,000	1.40%
35	Nebraska	148,000	0.70%		27	Oregon	290,000	1.37%
43	Nevada	61,000	0.29%		28	Washington	289,000	1.37%
47	New Hampshire	21,000	0.10%		29	Iowa	244,000	1.16%
8	New Jersey	707,000	3.35%		30	Kansas	234,000	1.11%
43	New Mexico	61,000	0.29%		31	Oklahoma	232,000	1.10%
4	New York	1,236,000	5.86%		32	South Carolina	218,000	1.03%
11	North Carolina	652,000	3.09%		33	Utah	196,000	0.93%
42	North Dakota	63,000	0.30%		34	West Virginia	168,000	0.80%
9	Ohio	692,000	3.28%		35	Nebraska	148,000	0.70%
31	Oklahoma	232,000	1.10%		36	Montana	115,000	0.54%
27	Oregon	290,000	1.37%		37	Vermont	107,000	0.51%
5	Pennsylvania	873,000	4.14%		38	Idaho	99,000	0.47%
45	Rhode Island	58,000	0.27%		39	Maine	89,000	0.42%
32	South Carolina	218,000	1.03%		40	Delaware	81,000	0.38%
48	South Dakota	17,000	0.08%		41	Arkansas	64,000	0.30%
25	Tennessee	310,000	1.47%		42	North Dakota	63,000	0.30%
2	Texas	1,672,000	7.92%		43	Nevada	61,000	0.29%
33	Utah	196,000	0.93%		43	New Mexico	61,000	0.29%
37	Vermont	107,000	0.51%		45	Rhode Island	58,000	0.27%
12	Virginia	542,000	2.57%		46	Wyoming	54,000	0.26%
28	Washington	289,000	1.37%		47	New Hampshire	21,000	0.10%
34	West Virginia	168,000	0.80%		48	South Dakota	17,000	0.08%
19	Wisconsin	357,000	1.69%		NA	Alaska*	NA	NA
46	Wyoming	54,000	0.26%		NA	Hawaii*	NA	NA
						District of Columbia*	NA	NA

Source: The National Sporting Goods Association
"NSGA Sports Participation Survey, January–December 1993 (Copyright 1994, reprinted with permission)
Not available.

Participants in Softball in 1993

National Total = 18,565,000 Softball Players

ALPHA ORDER

RANK	STATE	PLAYERS	% of USA
22	Alabama	309,000	1.66%
NA	Alaska*	NA	NA
23	Arizona	286,000	1.54%
37	Arkansas	114,000	0.61%
1	California	1,964,000	10.58%
21	Colorado	314,000	1.69%
13	Connecticut	495,000	2.67%
45	Delaware	38,000	0.20%
7	Florida	784,000	4.22%
11	Georgia	502,000	2.70%
NA	Hawaii*	NA	NA
38	Idaho	98,000	0.53%
4	Illinois	1,019,000	5.49%
16	Indiana	396,000	2.13%
33	Iowa	175,000	0.94%
34	Kansas	168,000	0.90%
27	Kentucky	249,000	1.34%
20	Louisiana	331,000	1.78%
39	Maine	92,000	0.50%
17	Maryland	390,000	2.10%
24	Massachusetts	263,000	1.42%
5	Michigan	822,000	4.43%
15	Minnesota	428,000	2.31%
25	Mississippi	261,000	1.41%
12	Missouri	500,000	2.69%
40	Montana	73,000	0.39%
30	Nebraska	223,000	1.20%
43	Nevada	52,000	0.28%
47	New Hampshire	17,000	0.09%
9	New Jersey	617,000	3.32%
44	New Mexico	40,000	0.22%
2	New York	1,569,000	8.45%
10	North Carolina	566,000	3.05%
40	North Dakota	73,000	0.39%
6	Ohio	808,000	4.35%
31	Oklahoma	219,000	1.18%
32	Oregon	209,000	1.13%
8	Pennsylvania	689,000	3.71%
NA	Rhode Island*	NA	NA
28	South Carolina	248,000	1.34%
46	South Dakota	35,000	0.19%
18	Tennessee	384,000	2.07%
3	Texas	1,022,000	5.50%
29	Utah	246,000	1.33%
36	Vermont	147,000	0.79%
19	Virginia	366,000	1.97%
26	Washington	254,000	1.37%
35	West Virginia	154,000	0.83%
14	Wisconsin	478,000	2.57%
42	Wyoming	57,000	0.31%

RANK ORDER

RANK	STATE	PLAYERS	% of USA
1	California	1,964,000	10.58%
2	New York	1,569,000	8.45%
3	Texas	1,022,000	5.50%
4	Illinois	1,019,000	5.49%
5	Michigan	822,000	4.43%
6	Ohio	808,000	4.35%
7	Florida	784,000	4.22%
8	Pennsylvania	689,000	3.71%
9	New Jersey	617,000	3.32%
10	North Carolina	566,000	3.05%
11	Georgia	502,000	2.70%
12	Missouri	500,000	2.69%
13	Connecticut	495,000	2.67%
14	Wisconsin	478,000	2.57%
15	Minnesota	428,000	2.31%
16	Indiana	396,000	2.13%
17	Maryland	390,000	2.10%
18	Tennessee	384,000	2.07%
19	Virginia	366,000	1.97%
20	Louisiana	331,000	1.78%
21	Colorado	314,000	1.69%
22	Alabama	309,000	1.66%
23	Arizona	286,000	1.54%
24	Massachusetts	263,000	1.42%
25	Mississippi	261,000	1.41%
26	Washington	254,000	1.37%
27	Kentucky	249,000	1.34%
28	South Carolina	248,000	1.34%
29	Utah	246,000	1.33%
30	Nebraska	223,000	1.20%
31	Oklahoma	219,000	1.18%
32	Oregon	209,000	1.13%
33	Iowa	175,000	0.94%
34	Kansas	168,000	0.90%
35	West Virginia	154,000	0.83%
36	Vermont	147,000	0.79%
37	Arkansas	114,000	0.61%
38	Idaho	98,000	0.53%
39	Maine	92,000	0.50%
40	Montana	73,000	0.39%
40	North Dakota	73,000	0.39%
42	Wyoming	57,000	0.31%
43	Nevada	52,000	0.28%
44	New Mexico	40,000	0.22%
45	Delaware	38,000	0.20%
46	South Dakota	35,000	0.19%
47	New Hampshire	17,000	0.09%
NA	Alaska*	NA	NA
NA	Hawaii*	NA	NA
NA	Rhode Island*	NA	NA
	District of Columbia*	NA	NA

Source: The National Sporting Goods Association

"NSGA Sports Participation Survey, January–December 1993 (Copyright 1994, reprinted with permission)

*Not available.

Participants in Swimming in 1993

National Total = 62,250,000 Swimmers

ALPHA ORDER					RANK ORDER			
RANK	STATE	SWIMMERS	% of USA		RANK	STATE	SWIMMERS	% of USA
25	Alabama	868,000	1.39%		1	California	6,906,000	11.09%
NA	Alaska*	NA	NA		2	New York	4,943,000	7.94%
15	Arizona	1,276,000	2.05%		3	Florida	4,460,000	7.16%
36	Arkansas	379,000	0.61%		4	Texas	4,040,000	6.49%
1	California	6,906,000	11.09%		5	Pennsylvania	3,219,000	5.17%
29	Colorado	704,000	1.13%		6	Ohio	2,567,000	4.12%
17	Connecticut	1,172,000	1.88%		7	Illinois	2,530,000	4.06%
47	Delaware	85,000	0.14%		8	New Jersey	2,447,000	3.93%
3	Florida	4,460,000	7.16%		9	Michigan	2,148,000	3.45%
10	Georgia	1,882,000	3.02%		10	Georgia	1,882,000	3.02%
NA	Hawaii*	NA	NA		11	Indiana	1,453,000	2.33%
39	Idaho	250,000	0.40%		12	North Carolina	1,390,000	2.23%
7	Illinois	2,530,000	4.06%		13	Massachusetts	1,307,000	2.10%
11	Indiana	1,453,000	2.33%		14	Missouri	1,303,000	2.09%
32	Iowa	620,000	1.00%		15	Arizona	1,276,000	2.05%
34	Kansas	536,000	0.86%		16	Washington	1,267,000	2.04%
26	Kentucky	863,000	1.39%		17	Connecticut	1,172,000	1.88%
20	Louisiana	1,143,000	1.84%		18	Tennessee	1,145,000	1.84%
35	Maine	472,000	0.76%		19	Wisconsin	1,144,000	1.84%
21	Maryland	1,139,000	1.83%		20	Louisiana	1,143,000	1.84%
13	Massachusetts	1,307,000	2.10%		21	Maryland	1,139,000	1.83%
9	Michigan	2,148,000	3.45%		22	Virginia	1,137,000	1.83%
23	Minnesota	1,051,000	1.69%		23	Minnesota	1,051,000	1.69%
24	Mississippi	981,000	1.58%		24	Mississippi	981,000	1.58%
14	Missouri	1,303,000	2.09%		25	Alabama	868,000	1.39%
38	Montana	275,000	0.44%		26	Kentucky	863,000	1.39%
37	Nebraska	336,000	0.54%		27	South Carolina	843,000	1.35%
42	Nevada	212,000	0.34%		28	Oregon	705,000	1.13%
43	New Hampshire	161,000	0.26%		29	Colorado	704,000	1.13%
8	New Jersey	2,447,000	3.93%		30	Oklahoma	700,000	1.12%
44	New Mexico	156,000	0.25%		31	West Virginia	638,000	1.02%
2	New York	4,943,000	7.94%		32	Iowa	620,000	1.00%
12	North Carolina	1,390,000	2.23%		33	Utah	572,000	0.92%
48	North Dakota	66,000	0.11%		34	Kansas	536,000	0.86%
6	Ohio	2,567,000	4.12%		35	Maine	472,000	0.76%
30	Oklahoma	700,000	1.12%		36	Arkansas	379,000	0.61%
28	Oregon	705,000	1.13%		37	Nebraska	336,000	0.54%
5	Pennsylvania	3,219,000	5.17%		38	Montana	275,000	0.44%
45	Rhode Island	138,000	0.22%		39	Idaho	250,000	0.40%
27	South Carolina	843,000	1.35%		40	Vermont	229,000	0.37%
46	South Dakota	111,000	0.18%		41	Wyoming	215,000	0.35%
18	Tennessee	1,145,000	1.84%		42	Nevada	212,000	0.34%
4	Texas	4,040,000	6.49%		43	New Hampshire	161,000	0.26%
33	Utah	572,000	0.92%		44	New Mexico	156,000	0.25%
40	Vermont	229,000	0.37%		45	Rhode Island	138,000	0.22%
22	Virginia	1,137,000	1.83%		46	South Dakota	111,000	0.18%
16	Washington	1,267,000	2.04%		47	Delaware	85,000	0.14%
31	West Virginia	638,000	1.02%		48	North Dakota	66,000	0.11%
19	Wisconsin	1,144,000	1.84%		NA	Alaska*	NA	NA
41	Wyoming	215,000	0.35%		NA	Hawaii*	NA	NA
						District of Columbia*	NA	NA

Source: The National Sporting Goods Association

"NSGA Sports Participation Survey, January–December 1993 (Copyright 1994, reprinted with permission)

*Not available.

Participants in Tennis in 1993

National Total = 15,760,000 Tennis Players

ALPHA ORDER

RANK	STATE	PLAYERS	% of USA
17	Alabama	309,000	1.96%
NA	Alaska*	NA	NA
26	Arizona	207,000	1.31%
36	Arkansas	103,000	0.65%
1	California	1,567,000	9.94%
24	Colorado	241,000	1.53%
13	Connecticut	441,000	2.80%
46	Delaware	17,000	0.11%
4	Florida	794,000	5.04%
6	Georgia	648,000	4.11%
NA	Hawaii*	NA	NA
41	Idaho	38,000	0.24%
9	Illinois	628,000	3.98%
19	Indiana	284,000	1.80%
35	Iowa	108,000	0.69%
34	Kansas	126,000	0.80%
33	Kentucky	135,000	0.86%
16	Louisiana	360,000	2.28%
32	Maine	139,000	0.88%
14	Maryland	391,000	2.48%
25	Massachusetts	233,000	1.48%
7	Michigan	639,000	4.05%
22	Minnesota	252,000	1.60%
21	Mississippi	279,000	1.77%
15	Missouri	381,000	2.42%
39	Montana	65,000	0.41%
37	Nebraska	90,000	0.57%
40	Nevada	57,000	0.36%
43	New Hampshire	28,000	0.18%
5	New Jersey	731,000	4.64%
42	New Mexico	35,000	0.22%
2	New York	1,344,000	8.53%
11	North Carolina	518,000	3.29%
44	North Dakota	27,000	0.17%
10	Ohio	554,000	3.52%
31	Oklahoma	147,000	0.93%
30	Oregon	165,000	1.05%
8	Pennsylvania	632,000	4.01%
45	Rhode Island	19,000	0.12%
27	South Carolina	186,000	1.18%
48	South Dakota	4,000	0.03%
29	Tennessee	176,000	1.12%
3	Texas	1,052,000	6.68%
22	Utah	252,000	1.60%
38	Vermont	75,000	0.48%
12	Virginia	467,000	2.96%
20	Washington	283,000	1.80%
28	West Virginia	177,000	1.12%
18	Wisconsin	305,000	1.94%
47	Wyoming	10,000	0.06%

RANK ORDER

RANK	STATE	PLAYERS	% of USA
1	California	1,567,000	9.94%
2	New York	1,344,000	8.53%
3	Texas	1,052,000	6.68%
4	Florida	794,000	5.04%
5	New Jersey	731,000	4.64%
6	Georgia	648,000	4.11%
7	Michigan	639,000	4.05%
8	Pennsylvania	632,000	4.01%
9	Illinois	628,000	3.98%
10	Ohio	554,000	3.52%
11	North Carolina	518,000	3.29%
12	Virginia	467,000	2.96%
13	Connecticut	441,000	2.80%
14	Maryland	391,000	2.48%
15	Missouri	381,000	2.42%
16	Louisiana	360,000	2.28%
17	Alabama	309,000	1.96%
18	Wisconsin	305,000	1.94%
19	Indiana	284,000	1.80%
20	Washington	283,000	1.80%
21	Mississippi	279,000	1.77%
22	Minnesota	252,000	1.60%
22	Utah	252,000	1.60%
24	Colorado	241,000	1.53%
25	Massachusetts	233,000	1.48%
26	Arizona	207,000	1.31%
27	South Carolina	186,000	1.18%
28	West Virginia	177,000	1.12%
29	Tennessee	176,000	1.12%
30	Oregon	165,000	1.05%
31	Oklahoma	147,000	0.93%
32	Maine	139,000	0.88%
33	Kentucky	135,000	0.86%
34	Kansas	126,000	0.80%
35	Iowa	108,000	0.69%
36	Arkansas	103,000	0.65%
37	Nebraska	90,000	0.57%
38	Vermont	75,000	0.48%
39	Montana	65,000	0.41%
40	Nevada	57,000	0.36%
41	Idaho	38,000	0.24%
42	New Mexico	35,000	0.22%
43	New Hampshire	28,000	0.18%
44	North Dakota	27,000	0.17%
45	Rhode Island	19,000	0.12%
46	Delaware	17,000	0.11%
47	Wyoming	10,000	0.06%
48	South Dakota	4,000	0.03%
NA	Alaska*	NA	NA
NA	Hawaii*	NA	NA
	District of Columbia*	NA	NA

Source: The National Sporting Goods Association

"NSGA Sports Participation Survey, January–December 1993 (Copyright 1994, reprinted with permission)
Not available.

Apparent Alcohol Consumption in 1993

National Total = 447,223,000 Gallons*

ALPHA ORDER					RANK ORDER			
RANK	STATE	GALLONS	% of USA		RANK	STATE	GALLONS	% of USA
25	Alabama	6,143,000	1.37%		1	California	55,418,000	12.39%
48	Alaska	1,177,000	0.26%		2	Texas	32,579,000	7.28%
21	Arizona	8,099,000	1.81%		3	Florida	29,417,000	6.58%
35	Arkansas	3,450,000	0.77%		4	New York	28,203,000	6.31%
1	California	55,418,000	12.39%		5	Illinois	21,603,000	4.83%
23	Colorado	7,014,000	1.57%		6	Pennsylvania	18,865,000	4.22%
26	Connecticut	5,709,000	1.28%		7	Ohio	16,717,000	3.74%
45	Delaware	1,518,000	0.34%		8	Michigan	15,928,000	3.56%
3	Florida	29,417,000	6.58%		9	New Jersey	14,127,000	3.16%
10	Georgia	11,836,000	2.65%		10	Georgia	11,836,000	2.65%
39	Hawaii	2,272,000	0.51%		11	Massachusetts	11,369,000	2.54%
42	Idaho	1,747,000	0.39%		12	Wisconsin	10,698,000	2.39%
5	Illinois	21,603,000	4.83%		13	Virginia	10,418,000	2.33%
17	Indiana	8,676,000	1.94%		14	North Carolina	10,397,000	2.32%
32	Iowa	4,108,000	0.92%		15	Washington	9,316,000	2.08%
34	Kansas	3,457,000	0.77%		16	Missouri	8,772,000	1.96%
28	Kentucky	5,225,000	1.17%		17	Indiana	8,676,000	1.94%
19	Louisiana	8,173,000	1.83%		18	Maryland	8,397,000	1.88%
40	Maine	2,131,000	0.48%		19	Louisiana	8,173,000	1.83%
18	Maryland	8,397,000	1.88%		20	Minnesota	8,131,000	1.82%
11	Massachusetts	11,369,000	2.54%		21	Arizona	8,099,000	1.81%
8	Michigan	15,928,000	3.56%		22	Tennessee	7,611,000	1.70%
20	Minnesota	8,131,000	1.82%		23	Colorado	7,014,000	1.57%
31	Mississippi	4,276,000	0.96%		24	South Carolina	6,576,000	1.47%
16	Missouri	8,772,000	1.96%		25	Alabama	6,143,000	1.37%
44	Montana	1,600,000	0.36%		26	Connecticut	5,709,000	1.28%
37	Nebraska	2,691,000	0.60%		27	Oregon	5,466,000	1.22%
30	Nevada	4,434,000	0.99%		28	Kentucky	5,225,000	1.17%
33	New Hampshire	3,769,000	0.84%		29	Oklahoma	4,530,000	1.01%
9	New Jersey	14,127,000	3.16%		30	Nevada	4,434,000	0.99%
36	New Mexico	2,939,000	0.66%		31	Mississippi	4,276,000	0.96%
4	New York	28,203,000	6.31%		32	Iowa	4,108,000	0.92%
14	North Carolina	10,397,000	2.32%		33	New Hampshire	3,769,000	0.84%
47	North Dakota	1,210,000	0.27%		34	Kansas	3,457,000	0.77%
7	Ohio	16,717,000	3.74%		35	Arkansas	3,450,000	0.77%
29	Oklahoma	4,530,000	1.01%		36	New Mexico	2,939,000	0.66%
27	Oregon	5,466,000	1.22%		37	Nebraska	2,691,000	0.60%
6	Pennsylvania	18,865,000	4.22%		38	West Virginia	2,462,000	0.55%
41	Rhode Island	1,812,000	0.41%		39	Hawaii	2,272,000	0.51%
24	South Carolina	6,576,000	1.47%		40	Maine	2,131,000	0.48%
46	South Dakota	1,213,000	0.27%		41	Rhode Island	1,812,000	0.41%
22	Tennessee	7,611,000	1.70%		42	Idaho	1,747,000	0.39%
2	Texas	32,579,000	7.28%		43	Utah	1,741,000	0.39%
43	Utah	1,741,000	0.39%		44	Montana	1,600,000	0.36%
49	Vermont	1,120,000	0.25%		45	Delaware	1,518,000	0.34%
13	Virginia	10,418,000	2.33%		46	South Dakota	1,213,000	0.27%
15	Washington	9,316,000	2.08%		47	North Dakota	1,210,000	0.27%
38	West Virginia	2,462,000	0.55%		48	Alaska	1,177,000	0.26%
12	Wisconsin	10,698,000	2.39%		49	Vermont	1,120,000	0.25%
50	Wyoming	880,000	0.20%		50	Wyoming	880,000	0.20%
						District of Columbia	1,806,000	0.40%

Source: Wine Institute & Beer Institute as published by the Distilled Spirits Council of the United States, Inc.
"1993 Statistical Information for the Distilled Spirits Industry" (August 31, 1994)
*This is apparent consumption of actual alcohol, not entire volume of an alcoholic beverage (e.g. wine is roughly 11% absolute alcohol content). Apparent consumption is based on several sources which together approximate sales but do not actually measure consumption. Reported state volumes reflect only in-state purchases. Accordingly, figures for some states may be skewed by purchases by nonresidents.   450

Adult Per Capita Apparent Alcohol Consumption in 1993

National Per Capita = 2.48 Gallons Consumed per Adult Age 21 Years and Older *

<u>ALPHA ORDER</u>

RANK	STATE	PER CAPITA
42	Alabama	2.10
3	Alaska	3.07
6	Arizona	2.99
45	Arkansas	2.05
20	California	2.59
10	Colorado	2.82
34	Connecticut	2.39
5	Delaware	3.04
7	Florida	2.93
26	Georgia	2.48
13	Hawaii	2.76
28	Idaho	2.45
17	Illinois	2.65
37	Indiana	2.17
44	Iowa	2.09
47	Kansas	1.98
48	Kentucky	1.97
8	Louisiana	2.86
31	Maine	2.42
35	Maryland	2.37
21	Massachusetts	2.58
31	Michigan	2.42
18	Minnesota	2.61
30	Mississippi	2.44
33	Missouri	2.40
11	Montana	2.80
28	Nebraska	2.45
2	Nevada	4.48
1	New Hampshire	4.72
26	New Jersey	2.48
13	New Mexico	2.76
38	New York	2.16
42	North Carolina	2.10
12	North Dakota	2.78
40	Ohio	2.15
46	Oklahoma	2.04
22	Oregon	2.56
38	Pennsylvania	2.16
25	Rhode Island	2.49
19	South Carolina	2.60
23	South Dakota	2.55
41	Tennessee	2.11
16	Texas	2.70
50	Utah	1.59
15	Vermont	2.74
36	Virginia	2.25
23	Washington	2.55
49	West Virginia	1.89
4	Wisconsin	3.06
9	Wyoming	2.84

<u>RANK ORDER</u>

RANK	STATE	PER CAPITA
1	New Hampshire	4.72
2	Nevada	4.48
3	Alaska	3.07
4	Wisconsin	3.06
5	Delaware	3.04
6	Arizona	2.99
7	Florida	2.93
8	Louisiana	2.86
9	Wyoming	2.84
10	Colorado	2.82
11	Montana	2.80
12	North Dakota	2.78
13	Hawaii	2.76
13	New Mexico	2.76
15	Vermont	2.74
16	Texas	2.70
17	Illinois	2.65
18	Minnesota	2.61
19	South Carolina	2.60
20	California	2.59
21	Massachusetts	2.58
22	Oregon	2.56
23	South Dakota	2.55
23	Washington	2.55
25	Rhode Island	2.49
26	Georgia	2.48
26	New Jersey	2.48
28	Idaho	2.45
28	Nebraska	2.45
30	Mississippi	2.44
31	Maine	2.42
31	Michigan	2.42
33	Missouri	2.40
34	Connecticut	2.39
35	Maryland	2.37
36	Virginia	2.25
37	Indiana	2.17
38	New York	2.16
38	Pennsylvania	2.16
40	Ohio	2.15
41	Tennessee	2.11
42	Alabama	2.10
42	North Carolina	2.10
44	Iowa	2.09
45	Arkansas	2.05
46	Oklahoma	2.04
47	Kansas	1.98
48	Kentucky	1.97
49	West Virginia	1.89
50	Utah	1.59

	District of Columbia	4.07

Source: Morgan Quitno Press using data from Wine Institute & Beer Institute as published by the Distilled Spirits Council of the United States, Inc. "1993 Statistical Information for the Distilled Spirits Industry" (August 31, 1994) and Census
*This is apparent consumption of actual alcohol, not entire volume of an alcoholic beverage (e.g. wine is roughly 11% absolute alcohol content). Apparent consumption is based on several sources which together approximate sales but do not actually measure consumption. Reported state volumes reflect only in-state purchases. Accordingly, figures for some states may be skewed by purchases by nonresidents.

Apparent Beer Consumption in 1993

National Total = 5,818,122,000 Gallons of Beer Consumed*

ALPHA ORDER

ALPHA ORDER

RANK ORDER

RANK	STATE	GALLONS	% of USA
24	Alabama	85,155,000	1.46%
48	Alaska	13,987,000	0.24%
18	Arizona	110,720,000	1.90%
34	Arkansas	47,873,000	0.82%
1	California	648,435,000	11.15%
25	Colorado	83,661,000	1.44%
31	Connecticut	58,516,000	1.01%
45	Delaware	18,324,000	0.31%
3	Florida	357,347,000	6.14%
10	Georgia	150,381,000	2.58%
39	Hawaii	30,845,000	0.53%
42	Idaho	23,913,000	0.41%
6	Illinois	275,365,000	4.73%
16	Indiana	116,929,000	2.01%
28	Iowa	64,734,000	1.11%
32	Kansas	48,989,000	0.84%
26	Kentucky	73,290,000	1.26%
17	Louisiana	113,850,000	1.96%
40	Maine	25,478,000	0.44%
22	Maryland	96,952,000	1.67%
14	Massachusetts	126,936,000	2.18%
8	Michigan	210,621,000	3.62%
21	Minnesota	99,065,000	1.70%
30	Mississippi	63,281,000	1.09%
15	Missouri	123,669,000	2.13%
44	Montana	22,015,000	0.38%
37	Nebraska	39,105,000	0.67%
33	Nevada	48,813,000	0.84%
38	New Hampshire	36,412,000	0.63%
9	New Jersey	152,645,000	2.62%
35	New Mexico	42,591,000	0.73%
4	New York	328,600,000	5.65%
11	North Carolina	144,898,000	2.49%
47	North Dakota	16,234,000	0.28%
7	Ohio	254,701,000	4.38%
29	Oklahoma	64,700,000	1.11%
27	Oregon	67,415,000	1.16%
5	Pennsylvania	285,850,000	4.91%
43	Rhode Island	22,328,000	0.38%
23	South Carolina	88,229,000	1.52%
46	South Dakota	16,809,000	0.29%
19	Tennessee	110,246,000	1.89%
2	Texas	506,485,000	8.71%
41	Utah	24,018,000	0.41%
49	Vermont	13,674,000	0.24%
12	Virginia	143,868,000	2.47%
20	Washington	110,142,000	1.89%
36	West Virginia	39,348,000	0.68%
13	Wisconsin	142,560,000	2.45%
50	Wyoming	11,401,000	0.20%

RANK	STATE	GALLONS	% of USA
1	California	648,435,000	11.15%
2	Texas	506,485,000	8.71%
3	Florida	357,347,000	6.14%
4	New York	328,600,000	5.65%
5	Pennsylvania	285,850,000	4.91%
6	Illinois	275,365,000	4.73%
7	Ohio	254,701,000	4.38%
8	Michigan	210,621,000	3.62%
9	New Jersey	152,645,000	2.62%
10	Georgia	150,381,000	2.58%
11	North Carolina	144,898,000	2.49%
12	Virginia	143,868,000	2.47%
13	Wisconsin	142,560,000	2.45%
14	Massachusetts	126,936,000	2.18%
15	Missouri	123,669,000	2.13%
16	Indiana	116,929,000	2.01%
17	Louisiana	113,850,000	1.96%
18	Arizona	110,720,000	1.90%
19	Tennessee	110,246,000	1.89%
20	Washington	110,142,000	1.89%
21	Minnesota	99,065,000	1.70%
22	Maryland	96,952,000	1.67%
23	South Carolina	88,229,000	1.52%
24	Alabama	85,155,000	1.46%
25	Colorado	83,661,000	1.44%
26	Kentucky	73,290,000	1.26%
27	Oregon	67,415,000	1.16%
28	Iowa	64,734,000	1.11%
29	Oklahoma	64,700,000	1.11%
30	Mississippi	63,281,000	1.09%
31	Connecticut	58,516,000	1.01%
32	Kansas	48,989,000	0.84%
33	Nevada	48,813,000	0.84%
34	Arkansas	47,873,000	0.82%
35	New Mexico	42,591,000	0.73%
36	West Virginia	39,348,000	0.68%
37	Nebraska	39,105,000	0.67%
38	New Hampshire	36,412,000	0.63%
39	Hawaii	30,845,000	0.53%
40	Maine	25,478,000	0.44%
41	Utah	24,018,000	0.41%
42	Idaho	23,913,000	0.41%
43	Rhode Island	22,328,000	0.38%
44	Montana	22,015,000	0.38%
45	Delaware	18,324,000	0.31%
46	South Dakota	16,809,000	0.29%
47	North Dakota	16,234,000	0.28%
48	Alaska	13,987,000	0.24%
49	Vermont	13,674,000	0.24%
50	Wyoming	11,401,000	0.20%
	District of Columbia	16,721,000	0.29%

Source: Beer Institute as published by the Distilled Spirits Council of the United States, Inc.
"1993 Statistical Information for the Distilled Spirits Industry" (August 31, 1994)
*Apparent consumption is based on several sources which together approximate sales but do not actually measure consumption. Reported state volumes reflect only in-state purchases. Accordingly, figures for some states may be skewed by purchases by nonresidents.

Adult Per Capita Apparent Beer Consumption in 1993

National Per Capita = 32.27 Gallons Consumed per Adult Age 21 Years and Older*

ALPHA ORDER				RANK ORDER		
RANK	STATE	PER CAPITA		RANK	STATE	PER CAPITA
39	Alabama	29.16		1	Nevada	49.38
13	Alaska	36.46		2	New Hampshire	45.55
4	Arizona	40.89		3	Texas	42.03
43	Arkansas	28.48		4	Arizona	40.89
34	California	30.30		5	Wisconsin	40.81
21	Colorado	33.64		6	New Mexico	40.00
49	Connecticut	24.51		7	Louisiana	39.83
12	Delaware	36.72		8	Montana	38.52
15	Florida	35.62		9	Hawaii	37.51
30	Georgia	31.51		10	North Dakota	37.29
9	Hawaii	37.51		11	Wyoming	36.81
22	Idaho	33.49		12	Delaware	36.72
20	Illinois	33.76		13	Alaska	36.46
38	Indiana	29.27		14	Mississippi	36.04
24	Iowa	32.92		15	Florida	35.62
44	Kansas	28.10		16	Nebraska	35.54
45	Kentucky	27.69		17	South Dakota	35.30
7	Louisiana	39.83		18	South Carolina	34.94
41	Maine	28.89		19	Missouri	33.79
46	Maryland	27.37		20	Illinois	33.76
42	Massachusetts	28.83		21	Colorado	33.64
27	Michigan	32.05		22	Idaho	33.49
28	Minnesota	31.80		23	Vermont	33.47
14	Mississippi	36.04		24	Iowa	32.92
19	Missouri	33.79		25	Pennsylvania	32.80
8	Montana	38.52		26	Ohio	32.76
16	Nebraska	35.54		27	Michigan	32.05
1	Nevada	49.38		28	Minnesota	31.80
2	New Hampshire	45.55		29	Oregon	31.61
47	New Jersey	26.83		30	Georgia	31.51
6	New Mexico	40.00		31	Virginia	31.05
48	New York	25.21		32	Rhode Island	30.66
37	North Carolina	29.30		33	Tennessee	30.52
10	North Dakota	37.29		34	California	30.30
26	Ohio	32.76		35	West Virginia	30.23
40	Oklahoma	29.13		36	Washington	30.11
29	Oregon	31.61		37	North Carolina	29.30
25	Pennsylvania	32.80		38	Indiana	29.27
32	Rhode Island	30.66		39	Alabama	29.16
18	South Carolina	34.94		40	Oklahoma	29.13
17	South Dakota	35.30		41	Maine	28.89
33	Tennessee	30.52		42	Massachusetts	28.83
3	Texas	42.03		43	Arkansas	28.48
50	Utah	21.94		44	Kansas	28.10
23	Vermont	33.47		45	Kentucky	27.69
31	Virginia	31.05		46	Maryland	27.37
36	Washington	30.11		47	New Jersey	26.83
35	West Virginia	30.23		48	New York	25.21
5	Wisconsin	40.81		49	Connecticut	24.51
11	Wyoming	36.81		50	Utah	21.94
					District of Columbia	37.63

Source: Morgan Quitno Press using data from Beer Institute as published by the Distilled Spirits Council of the U.S.
"1993 Statistical Information for the Distilled Spirits Industry" (August 31, 1994) and Census
*Apparent consumption is based on several sources which together approximate sales but do not actually measure consumption. Reported state volumes reflect only in-state purchases. Accordingly, figures for some states may be skewed by purchases by nonresidents.

Apparent Wine Consumption in 1993

National Total = 453,961,000 Gallons of Wine Consumed*

ALPHA ORDER					RANK ORDER			
RANK	STATE	GALLONS	% of USA		RANK	STATE	GALLONS	% of USA
28	Alabama	4,342,000	0.96%		1	California	90,987,000	20.04%
46	Alaska	1,172,000	0.26%		2	New York	40,680,000	8.96%
19	Arizona	6,997,000	1.54%		3	Florida	28,761,000	6.34%
40	Arkansas	1,747,000	0.38%		4	Illinois	24,360,000	5.37%
1	California	90,987,000	20.04%		5	Texas	23,195,000	5.11%
17	Colorado	7,689,000	1.69%		6	New Jersey	20,864,000	4.60%
13	Connecticut	8,686,000	1.91%		7	Massachusetts	16,657,000	3.67%
41	Delaware	1,592,000	0.35%		8	Washington	13,999,000	3.08%
3	Florida	28,761,000	6.34%		9	Pennsylvania	12,800,000	2.82%
14	Georgia	8,659,000	1.91%		10	Michigan	11,965,000	2.64%
30	Hawaii	2,701,000	0.59%		11	Ohio	10,991,000	2.42%
37	Idaho	1,918,000	0.42%		12	Virginia	10,772,000	2.37%
4	Illinois	24,360,000	5.37%		13	Connecticut	8,686,000	1.91%
21	Indiana	6,881,000	1.52%		14	Georgia	8,659,000	1.91%
38	Iowa	1,873,000	0.41%		15	Maryland	8,541,000	1.88%
36	Kansas	2,141,000	0.47%		16	Oregon	8,192,000	1.80%
32	Kentucky	2,473,000	0.54%		17	Colorado	7,689,000	1.69%
24	Louisiana	5,557,000	1.22%		18	Wisconsin	7,031,000	1.55%
34	Maine	2,215,000	0.49%		19	Arizona	6,997,000	1.54%
15	Maryland	8,541,000	1.88%		20	North Carolina	6,920,000	1.52%
7	Massachusetts	16,657,000	3.67%		21	Indiana	6,881,000	1.52%
10	Michigan	11,965,000	2.64%		22	Minnesota	6,785,000	1.49%
22	Minnesota	6,785,000	1.49%		23	Missouri	6,626,000	1.46%
43	Mississippi	1,417,000	0.31%		24	Louisiana	5,557,000	1.22%
23	Missouri	6,626,000	1.46%		25	Nevada	5,029,000	1.11%
44	Montana	1,274,000	0.28%		26	South Carolina	4,425,000	0.97%
39	Nebraska	1,755,000	0.39%		27	Tennessee	4,393,000	0.97%
25	Nevada	5,029,000	1.11%		28	Alabama	4,342,000	0.96%
29	New Hampshire	3,649,000	0.80%		29	New Hampshire	3,649,000	0.80%
6	New Jersey	20,864,000	4.60%		30	Hawaii	2,701,000	0.59%
35	New Mexico	2,191,000	0.48%		31	Oklahoma	2,514,000	0.55%
2	New York	40,680,000	8.96%		32	Kentucky	2,473,000	0.54%
20	North Carolina	6,920,000	1.52%		33	Rhode Island	2,331,000	0.51%
48	North Dakota	604,000	0.13%		34	Maine	2,215,000	0.49%
11	Ohio	10,991,000	2.42%		35	New Mexico	2,191,000	0.48%
31	Oklahoma	2,514,000	0.55%		36	Kansas	2,141,000	0.47%
16	Oregon	8,192,000	1.80%		37	Idaho	1,918,000	0.42%
9	Pennsylvania	12,800,000	2.82%		38	Iowa	1,873,000	0.41%
33	Rhode Island	2,331,000	0.51%		39	Nebraska	1,755,000	0.39%
26	South Carolina	4,425,000	0.97%		40	Arkansas	1,747,000	0.38%
49	South Dakota	544,000	0.12%		41	Delaware	1,592,000	0.35%
27	Tennessee	4,393,000	0.97%		42	Vermont	1,565,000	0.34%
5	Texas	23,195,000	5.11%		43	Mississippi	1,417,000	0.31%
45	Utah	1,184,000	0.26%		44	Montana	1,274,000	0.28%
42	Vermont	1,565,000	0.34%		45	Utah	1,184,000	0.26%
12	Virginia	10,772,000	2.37%		46	Alaska	1,172,000	0.26%
8	Washington	13,999,000	3.08%		47	West Virginia	968,000	0.21%
47	West Virginia	968,000	0.21%		48	North Dakota	604,000	0.13%
18	Wisconsin	7,031,000	1.55%		49	South Dakota	544,000	0.12%
49	Wyoming	544,000	0.12%		49	Wyoming	544,000	0.12%
						District of Columbia	2,805,000	0.62%

Source: Wine Institute as published by the Distilled Spirits Council of the United States, Inc.
"1993 Statistical Information for the Distilled Spirits Industry" (August 31, 1994)
*Apparent consumption is based on several sources which together approximate sales but do not actually measure consumption. Reported state volumes reflect only in-state purchases. Accordingly, figures for some states may be skewed by purchases by nonresidents.

Adult Per Capita Apparent Wine Consumption in 1993

National Per Capita = 2.52 Gallons Consumed per Adult Age 21 Years and Older*

ALPHA ORDER

RANK ORDER

RANK	STATE	PER CAPITA	RANK	STATE	PER CAPITA
36	Alabama	1.49	1	Nevada	5.09
15	Alaska	3.06	2	New Hampshire	4.56
19	Arizona	2.58	3	California	4.25
46	Arkansas	1.04	4	Oregon	3.84
3	California	4.25	5	Vermont	3.83
14	Colorado	3.09	5	Washington	3.83
9	Connecticut	3.64	7	Massachusetts	3.78
12	Delaware	3.19	8	New Jersey	3.67
17	Florida	2.87	9	Connecticut	3.64
30	Georgia	1.81	10	Hawaii	3.28
10	Hawaii	3.28	11	Rhode Island	3.20
18	Idaho	2.69	12	Delaware	3.19
16	Illinois	2.99	13	New York	3.12
34	Indiana	1.72	14	Colorado	3.09
47	Iowa	0.95	15	Alaska	3.06
41	Kansas	1.23	16	Illinois	2.99
48	Kentucky	0.93	17	Florida	2.87
27	Louisiana	1.94	18	Idaho	2.69
20	Maine	2.51	19	Arizona	2.58
21	Maryland	2.41	20	Maine	2.51
7	Massachusetts	3.78	21	Maryland	2.41
29	Michigan	1.82	22	Virginia	2.33
24	Minnesota	2.18	23	Montana	2.23
49	Mississippi	0.81	24	Minnesota	2.18
30	Missouri	1.81	25	New Mexico	2.06
23	Montana	2.23	26	Wisconsin	2.01
35	Nebraska	1.60	27	Louisiana	1.94
1	Nevada	5.09	28	Texas	1.92
2	New Hampshire	4.56	29	Michigan	1.82
8	New Jersey	3.67	30	Georgia	1.81
25	New Mexico	2.06	30	Missouri	1.81
13	New York	3.12	32	Wyoming	1.76
39	North Carolina	1.40	33	South Carolina	1.75
40	North Dakota	1.39	34	Indiana	1.72
38	Ohio	1.41	35	Nebraska	1.60
44	Oklahoma	1.13	36	Alabama	1.49
4	Oregon	3.84	37	Pennsylvania	1.47
37	Pennsylvania	1.47	38	Ohio	1.41
11	Rhode Island	3.20	39	North Carolina	1.40
33	South Carolina	1.75	40	North Dakota	1.39
43	South Dakota	1.14	41	Kansas	1.23
42	Tennessee	1.22	42	Tennessee	1.22
28	Texas	1.92	43	South Dakota	1.14
45	Utah	1.08	44	Oklahoma	1.13
5	Vermont	3.83	45	Utah	1.08
22	Virginia	2.33	46	Arkansas	1.04
5	Washington	3.83	47	Iowa	0.95
50	West Virginia	0.74	48	Kentucky	0.93
26	Wisconsin	2.01	49	Mississippi	0.81
32	Wyoming	1.76	50	West Virginia	0.74

District of Columbia   6.31

Source: Morgan Quitno Press using data from Wine Institute as published by the Distilled Spirits Council of the U.S.
"1993 Statistical Information for the Distilled Spirits Industry" (August 31, 1994) and Census
*Apparent consumption is based on several sources which together approximate sales but do not actually measure consumption. Reported state volumes reflect only in-state purchases. Accordingly, figures for some states may be skewed by purchases by nonresidents.

Apparent Distilled Spirits Consumption in 1993

National Total = 338,680,000 Gallons of Distilled Spirits Consumed*

ALPHA ORDER

RANK	STATE	GALLONS	% of USA
26	Alabama	4,582,000	1.35%
46	Alaska	1,047,000	0.31%
22	Arizona	5,868,000	1.73%
33	Arkansas	2,758,000	0.81%
1	California	40,576,000	11.98%
21	Colorado	6,008,000	1.77%
24	Connecticut	5,301,000	1.57%
43	Delaware	1,295,000	0.38%
2	Florida	25,431,000	7.51%
9	Georgia	10,290,000	3.04%
39	Hawaii	1,468,000	0.43%
45	Idaho	1,150,000	0.34%
5	Illinois	16,331,000	4.82%
18	Indiana	6,642,000	1.96%
35	Iowa	2,472,000	0.73%
34	Kansas	2,542,000	0.75%
29	Kentucky	4,138,000	1.22%
20	Louisiana	6,097,000	1.80%
37	Maine	1,851,000	0.55%
14	Maryland	7,736,000	2.28%
11	Massachusetts	9,561,000	2.82%
6	Michigan	12,835,000	3.79%
15	Minnesota	7,317,000	2.16%
32	Mississippi	3,180,000	0.94%
19	Missouri	6,196,000	1.83%
44	Montana	1,172,000	0.35%
38	Nebraska	1,846,000	0.55%
28	Nevada	4,211,000	1.24%
27	New Hampshire	4,323,000	1.28%
7	New Jersey	12,406,000	3.66%
36	New Mexico	1,953,000	0.58%
3	New York	22,353,000	6.60%
13	North Carolina	7,788,000	2.30%
47	North Dakota	1,032,000	0.30%
10	Ohio	10,116,000	2.99%
31	Oklahoma	3,354,000	0.99%
30	Oregon	3,828,000	1.13%
8	Pennsylvania	11,485,000	3.39%
41	Rhode Island	1,377,000	0.41%
25	South Carolina	5,297,000	1.56%
48	South Dakota	993,000	0.29%
23	Tennessee	5,417,000	1.60%
4	Texas	18,089,000	5.34%
42	Utah	1,326,000	0.39%
49	Vermont	830,000	0.25%
17	Virginia	6,898,000	2.04%
16	Washington	7,049,000	2.08%
40	West Virginia	1,462,000	0.43%
12	Wisconsin	8,774,000	2.59%
50	Wyoming	768,000	0.23%

RANK ORDER

RANK	STATE	GALLONS	% of USA
1	California	40,576,000	11.98%
2	Florida	25,431,000	7.51%
3	New York	22,353,000	6.60%
4	Texas	18,089,000	5.34%
5	Illinois	16,331,000	4.82%
6	Michigan	12,835,000	3.79%
7	New Jersey	12,406,000	3.66%
8	Pennsylvania	11,485,000	3.39%
9	Georgia	10,290,000	3.04%
10	Ohio	10,116,000	2.99%
11	Massachusetts	9,561,000	2.82%
12	Wisconsin	8,774,000	2.59%
13	North Carolina	7,788,000	2.30%
14	Maryland	7,736,000	2.28%
15	Minnesota	7,317,000	2.16%
16	Washington	7,049,000	2.08%
17	Virginia	6,898,000	2.04%
18	Indiana	6,642,000	1.96%
19	Missouri	6,196,000	1.83%
20	Louisiana	6,097,000	1.80%
21	Colorado	6,008,000	1.77%
22	Arizona	5,868,000	1.73%
23	Tennessee	5,417,000	1.60%
24	Connecticut	5,301,000	1.57%
25	South Carolina	5,297,000	1.56%
26	Alabama	4,582,000	1.35%
27	New Hampshire	4,323,000	1.28%
28	Nevada	4,211,000	1.24%
29	Kentucky	4,138,000	1.22%
30	Oregon	3,828,000	1.13%
31	Oklahoma	3,354,000	0.99%
32	Mississippi	3,180,000	0.94%
33	Arkansas	2,758,000	0.81%
34	Kansas	2,542,000	0.75%
35	Iowa	2,472,000	0.73%
36	New Mexico	1,953,000	0.58%
37	Maine	1,851,000	0.55%
38	Nebraska	1,846,000	0.55%
39	Hawaii	1,468,000	0.43%
40	West Virginia	1,462,000	0.43%
41	Rhode Island	1,377,000	0.41%
42	Utah	1,326,000	0.39%
43	Delaware	1,295,000	0.38%
44	Montana	1,172,000	0.35%
45	Idaho	1,150,000	0.34%
46	Alaska	1,047,000	0.31%
47	North Dakota	1,032,000	0.30%
48	South Dakota	993,000	0.29%
49	Vermont	830,000	0.25%
50	Wyoming	768,000	0.23%
	District of Columbia	1,861,000	0.55%

Source: Distilled Spirits Council of the United States, Inc.
"1993 Statistical Information for the Distilled Spirits Industry" (August 31, 1994)
Apparent consumption is based on several sources which together approximate sales but do not actually measure consumption. Reported state volumes reflect only in-state purchases. Accordingly, figures for some states may be skewed by purchases by nonresidents.

Adult Per Capita Apparent Distilled Spirits Consumption in 1993

National Per Capita = 1.88 Gallons Consumed per Adult Age 21 Years and Older*

ALPHA ORDER				RANK ORDER		
RANK	STATE	PER CAPITA		RANK	STATE	PER CAPITA
38	Alabama	1.57		1	New Hampshire	5.41
3	Alaska	2.73		2	Nevada	4.26
14	Arizona	2.17		3	Alaska	2.73
36	Arkansas	1.64		4	Delaware	2.60
26	California	1.90		5	Florida	2.53
8	Colorado	2.42		6	Wisconsin	2.51
11	Connecticut	2.22		7	Wyoming	2.48
4	Delaware	2.60		8	Colorado	2.42
5	Florida	2.53		9	North Dakota	2.37
16	Georgia	2.16		10	Minnesota	2.35
30	Hawaii	1.79		11	Connecticut	2.22
37	Idaho	1.61		12	Maryland	2.18
23	Illinois	2.00		12	New Jersey	2.18
35	Indiana	1.66		14	Arizona	2.17
48	Iowa	1.26		14	Massachusetts	2.17
45	Kansas	1.46		16	Georgia	2.16
40	Kentucky	1.56		17	Louisiana	2.13
17	Louisiana	2.13		18	Maine	2.10
18	Maine	2.10		18	South Carolina	2.10
12	Maryland	2.18		20	South Dakota	2.08
14	Massachusetts	2.17		21	Montana	2.05
24	Michigan	1.95		22	Vermont	2.03
10	Minnesota	2.35		23	Illinois	2.00
29	Mississippi	1.81		24	Michigan	1.95
33	Missouri	1.69		25	Washington	1.93
21	Montana	2.05		26	California	1.90
34	Nebraska	1.68		27	Rhode Island	1.89
2	Nevada	4.26		28	New Mexico	1.83
1	New Hampshire	5.41		29	Mississippi	1.81
12	New Jersey	2.18		30	Hawaii	1.79
28	New Mexico	1.83		30	Oregon	1.79
32	New York	1.71		32	New York	1.71
38	North Carolina	1.57		33	Missouri	1.69
9	North Dakota	2.37		34	Nebraska	1.68
47	Ohio	1.30		35	Indiana	1.66
41	Oklahoma	1.51		36	Arkansas	1.64
30	Oregon	1.79		37	Idaho	1.61
46	Pennsylvania	1.32		38	Alabama	1.57
27	Rhode Island	1.89		38	North Carolina	1.57
18	South Carolina	2.10		40	Kentucky	1.56
20	South Dakota	2.08		41	Oklahoma	1.51
42	Tennessee	1.50		42	Tennessee	1.50
42	Texas	1.50		42	Texas	1.50
49	Utah	1.21		44	Virginia	1.49
22	Vermont	2.03		45	Kansas	1.46
44	Virginia	1.49		46	Pennsylvania	1.32
25	Washington	1.93		47	Ohio	1.30
50	West Virginia	1.12		48	Iowa	1.26
6	Wisconsin	2.51		49	Utah	1.21
7	Wyoming	2.48		50	West Virginia	1.12
					District of Columbia	4.19

Source: Morgan Quitno Press using data from Distilled Spirits Council of the United States, Inc.
"1993 Statistical Information for the Distilled Spirits Industry" (August 31, 1994) and Census
*Apparent consumption is based on several sources which together approximate sales but do not actually measure consumption. Reported state volumes reflect only in-state purchases. Accordingly, figures for some states may be skewed by purchases by nonresidents.

Percent of Adults Who Are Binge Drinkers in 1993

National Median = 14.20% of Adults Are Binge Drinkers*

ALPHA ORDER

RANK	STATE	PERCENT
45	Alabama	8.24
4	Alaska	19.25
40	Arizona	10.17
39	Arkansas	10.46
15	California	15.62
14	Colorado	16.65
25	Connecticut	14.24
26	Delaware	14.17
23	Florida	14.29
38	Georgia	10.62
20	Hawaii	15.11
29	Idaho	13.78
30	Illinois	13.74
24	Indiana	14.25
34	Iowa	12.49
37	Kansas	10.74
43	Kentucky	9.15
16	Louisiana	15.27
36	Maine	11.48
42	Maryland	9.49
3	Massachusetts	19.79
8	Michigan	18.45
5	Minnesota	19.18
44	Mississippi	8.51
22	Missouri	14.30
18	Montana	15.13
12	Nebraska	17.18
6	Nevada	18.67
2	New Hampshire	20.42
27	New Jersey	14.00
33	New Mexico	13.00
21	New York	15.09
46	North Carolina	8.13
10	North Dakota	17.52
32	Ohio	13.05
47	Oklahoma	7.29
19	Oregon	15.12
9	Pennsylvania	17.75
7	Rhode Island	18.60
41	South Carolina	9.69
31	South Dakota	13.42
49	Tennessee	4.20
11	Texas	17.26
35	Utah	11.89
13	Vermont	16.70
28	Virginia	13.87
17	Washington	15.20
48	West Virginia	7.12
1	Wisconsin	22.83
NA	Wyoming**	NA

RANK ORDER

RANK	STATE	PERCENT
1	Wisconsin	22.83
2	New Hampshire	20.42
3	Massachusetts	19.79
4	Alaska	19.25
5	Minnesota	19.18
6	Nevada	18.67
7	Rhode Island	18.60
8	Michigan	18.45
9	Pennsylvania	17.75
10	North Dakota	17.52
11	Texas	17.26
12	Nebraska	17.18
13	Vermont	16.70
14	Colorado	16.65
15	California	15.62
16	Louisiana	15.27
17	Washington	15.20
18	Montana	15.13
19	Oregon	15.12
20	Hawaii	15.11
21	New York	15.09
22	Missouri	14.30
23	Florida	14.29
24	Indiana	14.25
25	Connecticut	14.24
26	Delaware	14.17
27	New Jersey	14.00
28	Virginia	13.87
29	Idaho	13.78
30	Illinois	13.74
31	South Dakota	13.42
32	Ohio	13.05
33	New Mexico	13.00
34	Iowa	12.49
35	Utah	11.89
36	Maine	11.48
37	Kansas	10.74
38	Georgia	10.62
39	Arkansas	10.46
40	Arizona	10.17
41	South Carolina	9.69
42	Maryland	9.49
43	Kentucky	9.15
44	Mississippi	8.51
45	Alabama	8.24
46	North Carolina	8.13
47	Oklahoma	7.29
48	West Virginia	7.12
49	Tennessee	4.20
NA	Wyoming**	NA
	District of Columbia	7.98

Source: U.S. Department of Health and Human Services, Centers for Disease Control and Prevention
    "1993 Behavioral Risk Factor Surveillance Summary Prevalence Report" (October 1, 1994)
*Persons 18 and older reporting consumption of five or more alcoholic drinks on one or more occasions during the previous month.
**Not available.

Percent of Adults Who Drink and Drive in 1993

National Median = 2.42% of Adults Drink and Drive*

ALPHA ORDER			RANK ORDER		
RANK	STATE	PERCENT	RANK	STATE	PERCENT
35	Alabama	1.82	1	Wisconsin	5.30
21	Alaska	2.49	2	Michigan	4.63
35	Arizona	1.82	3	Nevada	4.47
40	Arkansas	1.59	4	New Hampshire	4.36
24	California	2.45	5	North Dakota	4.29
20	Colorado	2.50	6	Nebraska	3.80
13	Connecticut	3.00	7	Texas	3.63
27	Delaware	2.33	8	Kansas	3.28
11	Florida	3.16	9	Minnesota	3.21
43	Georgia	1.46	10	Rhode Island	3.19
33	Hawaii	1.96	11	Florida	3.16
29	Idaho	2.18	12	South Dakota	3.04
30	Illinois	2.17	13	Connecticut	3.00
23	Indiana	2.46	14	Iowa	2.88
14	Iowa	2.88	15	Massachusetts	2.76
8	Kansas	3.28	16	New Mexico	2.73
45	Kentucky	0.97	17	Pennsylvania	2.72
26	Louisiana	2.40	18	Missouri	2.71
45	Maine	0.97	19	Vermont	2.67
48	Maryland	0.82	20	Colorado	2.50
15	Massachusetts	2.76	21	Alaska	2.49
2	Michigan	4.63	22	Montana	2.47
9	Minnesota	3.21	23	Indiana	2.46
37	Mississippi	1.78	24	California	2.45
18	Missouri	2.71	25	New Jersey	2.44
22	Montana	2.47	26	Louisiana	2.40
6	Nebraska	3.80	27	Delaware	2.33
3	Nevada	4.47	28	Virginia	2.28
4	New Hampshire	4.36	29	Idaho	2.18
25	New Jersey	2.44	30	Illinois	2.17
16	New Mexico	2.73	31	New York	2.13
31	New York	2.13	32	Washington	1.97
42	North Carolina	1.48	33	Hawaii	1.96
5	North Dakota	4.29	34	Ohio	1.83
34	Ohio	1.83	35	Alabama	1.82
47	Oklahoma	0.86	35	Arizona	1.82
39	Oregon	1.68	37	Mississippi	1.78
17	Pennsylvania	2.72	38	South Carolina	1.71
10	Rhode Island	3.19	39	Oregon	1.68
38	South Carolina	1.71	40	Arkansas	1.59
12	South Dakota	3.04	41	Utah	1.53
48	Tennessee	0.82	42	North Carolina	1.48
7	Texas	3.63	43	Georgia	1.46
41	Utah	1.53	44	West Virginia	1.41
19	Vermont	2.67	45	Kentucky	0.97
28	Virginia	2.28	45	Maine	0.97
32	Washington	1.97	47	Oklahoma	0.86
44	West Virginia	1.41	48	Maryland	0.82
1	Wisconsin	5.30	48	Tennessee	0.82
NA	Wyoming**	NA	NA	Wyoming**	NA
			District of Columbia		1.13

Source: U.S. Department of Health and Human Services, Centers for Disease Control and Prevention
"1993 Behavioral Risk Factor Surveillance Summary Prevalence Report" (October 1, 1994)
*Persons 18 and older who report driving after drinking too much alcohol at least once in the previous month.
**Not available.

Percent of Adults Who Smoke in 1993

National Median = 22.53% of Adults Smoke*

ALPHA ORDER				RANK ORDER		
RANK	STATE	PERCENT		RANK	STATE	PERCENT
47	Alabama	18.53		1	Kentucky	30.05
4	Alaska	26.64		2	Nevada	29.95
37	Arizona	20.74		3	West Virginia	26.83
7	Arkansas	26.42		4	Alaska	26.64
48	California	18.44		5	Missouri	26.61
19	Colorado	23.80		6	Oklahoma	26.60
38	Connecticut	20.64		7	Arkansas	26.42
10	Delaware	26.00		8	Indiana	26.40
29	Florida	21.99		9	Tennessee	26.28
17	Georgia	23.89		10	Delaware	26.00
46	Hawaii	18.86		11	North Carolina	25.80
42	Idaho	20.15		12	Ohio	25.33
23	Illinois	23.16		13	Michigan	25.06
8	Indiana	26.40		14	Maine	24.69
30	Iowa	21.98		15	South Carolina	24.21
41	Kansas	20.21		16	Mississippi	24.06
1	Kentucky	30.05		17	Georgia	23.89
27	Louisiana	22.42		18	Texas	23.82
14	Maine	24.69		19	Colorado	23.80
43	Maryland	19.73		20	New York	23.49
35	Massachusetts	21.17		21	Rhode Island	23.30
13	Michigan	25.06		21	Virginia	23.30
28	Minnesota	22.41		23	Illinois	23.16
16	Mississippi	24.06		24	Wisconsin	22.91
5	Missouri	26.61		25	Pennsylvania	22.60
40	Montana	20.41		26	Washington	22.47
31	Nebraska	21.97		27	Louisiana	22.42
2	Nevada	29.95		28	Minnesota	22.41
39	New Hampshire	20.59		29	Florida	21.99
45	New Jersey	18.92		30	Iowa	21.98
32	New Mexico	21.78		31	Nebraska	21.97
20	New York	23.49		32	New Mexico	21.78
11	North Carolina	25.80		33	Oregon	21.55
44	North Dakota	19.64		34	Vermont	21.29
12	Ohio	25.33		35	Massachusetts	21.17
6	Oklahoma	26.60		36	South Dakota	21.10
33	Oregon	21.55		37	Arizona	20.74
25	Pennsylvania	22.60		38	Connecticut	20.64
21	Rhode Island	23.30		39	New Hampshire	20.59
15	South Carolina	24.21		40	Montana	20.41
36	South Dakota	21.10		41	Kansas	20.21
9	Tennessee	26.28		42	Idaho	20.15
18	Texas	23.82		43	Maryland	19.73
49	Utah	14.45		44	North Dakota	19.64
34	Vermont	21.29		45	New Jersey	18.92
21	Virginia	23.30		46	Hawaii	18.86
26	Washington	22.47		47	Alabama	18.53
3	West Virginia	26.83		48	California	18.44
24	Wisconsin	22.91		49	Utah	14.45
NA	Wyoming**	NA		NA	Wyoming**	NA
					District of Columbia	16.36

Source: U.S. Department of Health and Human Services, Centers for Disease Control and Prevention
"1993 Behavioral Risk Factor Surveillance Summary Prevalence Report" (October 1, 1994)
*Persons 18 and older who have ever smoked 100 cigarettes and currently smoke.
**Not available.

Percent of Adult Smokers Who Would Like to Stop Smoking: 1993

National Median = 72.51% of Current Smokers*

ALPHA ORDER

RANK	STATE	PERCENT
24	Alabama	72.91
15	Alaska	74.01
49	Arizona	58.15
31	Arkansas	71.89
9	California	75.10
45	Colorado	67.06
32	Connecticut	71.49
35	Delaware	70.92
34	Florida	71.12
18	Georgia	73.89
41	Hawaii	68.87
21	Idaho	73.69
30	Illinois	72.01
43	Indiana	68.32
39	Iowa	69.80
46	Kansas	66.65
38	Kentucky	70.02
17	Louisiana	73.98
11	Maine	74.96
33	Maryland	71.23
1	Massachusetts	80.29
3	Michigan	78.90
22	Minnesota	73.68
6	Mississippi	76.21
2	Missouri	79.77
4	Montana	78.84
44	Nebraska	67.44
40	Nevada	69.07
5	New Hampshire	77.48
48	New Jersey	60.14
15	New Mexico	74.01
7	New York	75.92
42	North Carolina	68.60
28	North Dakota	72.28
20	Ohio	73.79
47	Oklahoma	62.12
27	Oregon	72.30
10	Pennsylvania	74.97
13	Rhode Island	74.41
23	South Carolina	72.98
36	South Dakota	70.50
25	Tennessee	72.61
37	Texas	70.14
12	Utah	74.62
26	Vermont	72.41
19	Virginia	73.87
14	Washington	74.35
29	West Virginia	72.17
8	Wisconsin	75.62
NA	Wyoming**	NA

RANK ORDER

RANK	STATE	PERCENT
1	Massachusetts	80.29
2	Missouri	79.77
3	Michigan	78.90
4	Montana	78.84
5	New Hampshire	77.48
6	Mississippi	76.21
7	New York	75.92
8	Wisconsin	75.62
9	California	75.10
10	Pennsylvania	74.97
11	Maine	74.96
12	Utah	74.62
13	Rhode Island	74.41
14	Washington	74.35
15	Alaska	74.01
15	New Mexico	74.01
17	Louisiana	73.98
18	Georgia	73.89
19	Virginia	73.87
20	Ohio	73.79
21	Idaho	73.69
22	Minnesota	73.68
23	South Carolina	72.98
24	Alabama	72.91
25	Tennessee	72.61
26	Vermont	72.41
27	Oregon	72.30
28	North Dakota	72.28
29	West Virginia	72.17
30	Illinois	72.01
31	Arkansas	71.89
32	Connecticut	71.49
33	Maryland	71.23
34	Florida	71.12
35	Delaware	70.92
36	South Dakota	70.50
37	Texas	70.14
38	Kentucky	70.02
39	Iowa	69.80
40	Nevada	69.07
41	Hawaii	68.87
42	North Carolina	68.60
43	Indiana	68.32
44	Nebraska	67.44
45	Colorado	67.06
46	Kansas	66.65
47	Oklahoma	62.12
48	New Jersey	60.14
49	Arizona	58.15
NA	Wyoming**	NA
	District of Columbia	68.65

*Source: U.S. Department of Health and Human Services, Centers for Disease Control and Prevention
"1993 Behavioral Risk Factor Surveillance Summary Prevalence Report" (October 1, 1994)*
*Persons 18 years and older.
**Not available.

Percent of Adults Overweight in 1993

National Median = 25.52 of Adults Are Overweight*

ALPHA ORDER				RANK ORDER		
RANK	**STATE**	**PERCENT**		**RANK**	**STATE**	**PERCENT**
32	Alabama	24.47		1	Mississippi	31.66
35	Alaska	23.70		2	West Virginia	31.10
48	Arizona	20.20		3	Indiana	30.30
4	Arkansas	30.14		4	Arkansas	30.14
31	California	24.53		5	Pennsylvania	28.80
47	Colorado	20.92		6	Michigan	28.72
46	Connecticut	21.79		7	Louisiana	28.50
20	Delaware	26.59		8	South Carolina	28.18
22	Florida	26.21		9	Kentucky	28.09
33	Georgia	24.14		10	Iowa	28.03
48	Hawaii	20.20		11	South Dakota	27.87
30	Idaho	24.63		12	Tennessee	27.33
25	Illinois	25.59		13	Wisconsin	27.32
3	Indiana	30.30		14	North Dakota	27.22
10	Iowa	28.03		15	Minnesota	27.02
34	Kansas	23.94		16	Oklahoma	26.99
9	Kentucky	28.09		17	North Carolina	26.81
7	Louisiana	28.50		18	Nebraska	26.68
19	Maine	26.65		19	Maine	26.65
28	Maryland	24.89		20	Delaware	26.59
41	Massachusetts	22.94		21	Missouri	26.29
6	Michigan	28.72		22	Florida	26.21
15	Minnesota	27.02		23	Texas	26.12
1	Mississippi	31.66		24	Washington	26.01
21	Missouri	26.29		25	Illinois	25.59
37	Montana	23.57		26	Virginia	25.46
18	Nebraska	26.68		27	New York	25.33
40	Nevada	23.34		28	Maryland	24.89
38	New Hampshire	23.40		29	Ohio	24.75
45	New Jersey	21.92		30	Idaho	24.63
42	New Mexico	22.84		31	California	24.53
27	New York	25.33		32	Alabama	24.47
17	North Carolina	26.81		33	Georgia	24.14
14	North Dakota	27.22		34	Kansas	23.94
29	Ohio	24.75		35	Alaska	23.70
16	Oklahoma	26.99		36	Oregon	23.64
36	Oregon	23.64		37	Montana	23.57
5	Pennsylvania	28.80		38	New Hampshire	23.40
39	Rhode Island	23.36		39	Rhode Island	23.36
8	South Carolina	28.18		40	Nevada	23.34
11	South Dakota	27.87		41	Massachusetts	22.94
12	Tennessee	27.33		42	New Mexico	22.84
23	Texas	26.12		43	Vermont	22.75
44	Utah	22.47		44	Utah	22.47
43	Vermont	22.75		45	New Jersey	21.92
26	Virginia	25.46		46	Connecticut	21.79
24	Washington	26.01		47	Colorado	20.92
2	West Virginia	31.10		48	Arizona	20.20
13	Wisconsin	27.32		48	Hawaii	20.20
NA	Wyoming**	NA		NA	Wyoming**	NA
					District of Columbia	20.87

Source: U.S. Department of Health and Human Services, Centers for Disease Control and Prevention
"1993 Behavioral Risk Factor Surveillance Summary Prevalence Report" (October 1, 1994)
*Persons 18 and older. Overweight is defined as men with a body mass index of 27.8 or greater and women with an index of 27.3 or greater.
**Not available.

Number of Days in Past Month When Physical Health was "Not Good": 1993

National Median = 2.94 Days*

ALPHA ORDER

RANK ORDER

RANK	STATE	DAYS
43	Alabama	2.57
46	Alaska	2.29
28	Arizona	2.86
6	Arkansas	3.46
13	California	3.17
23	Colorado	3.00
47	Connecticut	2.27
10	Delaware	3.27
13	Florida	3.17
42	Georgia	2.58
49	Hawaii	2.17
9	Idaho	3.30
36	Illinois	2.68
3	Indiana	3.55
45	Iowa	2.38
48	Kansas	2.20
2	Kentucky	3.80
32	Louisiana	2.80
38	Maine	2.62
37	Maryland	2.67
16	Massachusetts	3.09
26	Michigan	2.92
27	Minnesota	2.87
8	Mississippi	3.33
11	Missouri	3.19
4	Montana	3.48
34	Nebraska	2.75
6	Nevada	3.46
40	New Hampshire	2.61
38	New Jersey	2.62
35	New Mexico	2.70
16	New York	3.09
11	North Carolina	3.19
22	North Dakota	3.01
24	Ohio	2.97
18	Oklahoma	3.07
20	Oregon	3.04
19	Pennsylvania	3.05
5	Rhode Island	3.47
29	South Carolina	2.85
44	South Dakota	2.54
15	Tennessee	3.10
31	Texas	2.82
25	Utah	2.96
33	Vermont	2.77
41	Virginia	2.60
29	Washington	2.85
1	West Virginia	4.10
20	Wisconsin	3.04
NA	Wyoming**	NA

RANK	STATE	DAYS
1	West Virginia	4.10
2	Kentucky	3.80
3	Indiana	3.55
4	Montana	3.48
5	Rhode Island	3.47
6	Arkansas	3.46
6	Nevada	3.46
8	Mississippi	3.33
9	Idaho	3.30
10	Delaware	3.27
11	Missouri	3.19
11	North Carolina	3.19
13	California	3.17
13	Florida	3.17
15	Tennessee	3.10
16	Massachusetts	3.09
16	New York	3.09
18	Oklahoma	3.07
19	Pennsylvania	3.05
20	Oregon	3.04
20	Wisconsin	3.04
22	North Dakota	3.01
23	Colorado	3.00
24	Ohio	2.97
25	Utah	2.96
26	Michigan	2.92
27	Minnesota	2.87
28	Arizona	2.86
29	South Carolina	2.85
29	Washington	2.85
31	Texas	2.82
32	Louisiana	2.80
33	Vermont	2.77
34	Nebraska	2.75
35	New Mexico	2.70
36	Illinois	2.68
37	Maryland	2.67
38	Maine	2.62
38	New Jersey	2.62
40	New Hampshire	2.61
41	Virginia	2.60
42	Georgia	2.58
43	Alabama	2.57
44	South Dakota	2.54
45	Iowa	2.38
46	Alaska	2.29
47	Connecticut	2.27
48	Kansas	2.20
49	Hawaii	2.17
NA	Wyoming**	NA

| | District of Columbia | 1.58 |

Source: U.S. Department of Health and Human Services, Centers for Disease Control and Prevention
"1993 Behavioral Risk Factor Surveillance Summary Prevalence Report" (October 1, 1994)
*Reported by persons 18 years and older.
**Not available.

Percent of Adults Who Have Had Blood Pressure Checked Within the Past 2 Years: 1993

National Median = 93.52% of Adults*

<table>
<tr><th colspan="3">ALPHA ORDER</th><th colspan="3">RANK ORDER</th></tr>
<tr><th>RANK</th><th>STATE</th><th>PERCENT</th><th>RANK</th><th>STATE</th><th>PERCENT</th></tr>
<tr><td>1</td><td>Alabama</td><td>95.95</td><td>1</td><td>Alabama</td><td>95.95</td></tr>
<tr><td>36</td><td>Alaska</td><td>92.48</td><td>2</td><td>Maryland</td><td>95.39</td></tr>
<tr><td>16</td><td>Arizona</td><td>94.23</td><td>3</td><td>Georgia</td><td>95.25</td></tr>
<tr><td>34</td><td>Arkansas</td><td>92.56</td><td>4</td><td>North Carolina</td><td>94.93</td></tr>
<tr><td>42</td><td>California</td><td>91.82</td><td>5</td><td>Hawaii</td><td>94.83</td></tr>
<tr><td>40</td><td>Colorado</td><td>92.11</td><td>5</td><td>Missouri</td><td>94.83</td></tr>
<tr><td>16</td><td>Connecticut</td><td>94.23</td><td>7</td><td>Virginia</td><td>94.79</td></tr>
<tr><td>11</td><td>Delaware</td><td>94.46</td><td>8</td><td>Tennessee</td><td>94.56</td></tr>
<tr><td>31</td><td>Florida</td><td>92.90</td><td>9</td><td>Massachusetts</td><td>94.50</td></tr>
<tr><td>3</td><td>Georgia</td><td>95.25</td><td>9</td><td>Ohio</td><td>94.50</td></tr>
<tr><td>5</td><td>Hawaii</td><td>94.83</td><td>11</td><td>Delaware</td><td>94.46</td></tr>
<tr><td>46</td><td>Idaho</td><td>91.27</td><td>12</td><td>Rhode Island</td><td>94.37</td></tr>
<tr><td>14</td><td>Illinois</td><td>94.33</td><td>13</td><td>West Virginia</td><td>94.36</td></tr>
<tr><td>33</td><td>Indiana</td><td>92.61</td><td>14</td><td>Illinois</td><td>94.33</td></tr>
<tr><td>30</td><td>Iowa</td><td>93.04</td><td>15</td><td>South Carolina</td><td>94.27</td></tr>
<tr><td>24</td><td>Kansas</td><td>93.55</td><td>16</td><td>Arizona</td><td>94.23</td></tr>
<tr><td>26</td><td>Kentucky</td><td>93.22</td><td>16</td><td>Connecticut</td><td>94.23</td></tr>
<tr><td>23</td><td>Louisiana</td><td>93.63</td><td>18</td><td>New Jersey</td><td>94.18</td></tr>
<tr><td>38</td><td>Maine</td><td>92.38</td><td>19</td><td>Pennsylvania</td><td>94.00</td></tr>
<tr><td>2</td><td>Maryland</td><td>95.39</td><td>20</td><td>New York</td><td>93.96</td></tr>
<tr><td>9</td><td>Massachusetts</td><td>94.50</td><td>21</td><td>North Dakota</td><td>93.90</td></tr>
<tr><td>22</td><td>Michigan</td><td>93.80</td><td>22</td><td>Michigan</td><td>93.80</td></tr>
<tr><td>41</td><td>Minnesota</td><td>92.02</td><td>23</td><td>Louisiana</td><td>93.63</td></tr>
<tr><td>25</td><td>Mississippi</td><td>93.49</td><td>24</td><td>Kansas</td><td>93.55</td></tr>
<tr><td>5</td><td>Missouri</td><td>94.83</td><td>25</td><td>Mississippi</td><td>93.49</td></tr>
<tr><td>32</td><td>Montana</td><td>92.83</td><td>26</td><td>Kentucky</td><td>93.22</td></tr>
<tr><td>29</td><td>Nebraska</td><td>93.09</td><td>27</td><td>Wisconsin</td><td>93.20</td></tr>
<tr><td>48</td><td>Nevada</td><td>90.31</td><td>28</td><td>South Dakota</td><td>93.17</td></tr>
<tr><td>44</td><td>New Hampshire</td><td>91.36</td><td>29</td><td>Nebraska</td><td>93.09</td></tr>
<tr><td>18</td><td>New Jersey</td><td>94.18</td><td>30</td><td>Iowa</td><td>93.04</td></tr>
<tr><td>49</td><td>New Mexico</td><td>90.25</td><td>31</td><td>Florida</td><td>92.90</td></tr>
<tr><td>20</td><td>New York</td><td>93.96</td><td>32</td><td>Montana</td><td>92.83</td></tr>
<tr><td>4</td><td>North Carolina</td><td>94.93</td><td>33</td><td>Indiana</td><td>92.61</td></tr>
<tr><td>21</td><td>North Dakota</td><td>93.90</td><td>34</td><td>Arkansas</td><td>92.56</td></tr>
<tr><td>9</td><td>Ohio</td><td>94.50</td><td>35</td><td>Texas</td><td>92.53</td></tr>
<tr><td>37</td><td>Oklahoma</td><td>92.45</td><td>36</td><td>Alaska</td><td>92.48</td></tr>
<tr><td>47</td><td>Oregon</td><td>90.71</td><td>37</td><td>Oklahoma</td><td>92.45</td></tr>
<tr><td>19</td><td>Pennsylvania</td><td>94.00</td><td>38</td><td>Maine</td><td>92.38</td></tr>
<tr><td>12</td><td>Rhode Island</td><td>94.37</td><td>39</td><td>Washington</td><td>92.12</td></tr>
<tr><td>15</td><td>South Carolina</td><td>94.27</td><td>40</td><td>Colorado</td><td>92.11</td></tr>
<tr><td>28</td><td>South Dakota</td><td>93.17</td><td>41</td><td>Minnesota</td><td>92.02</td></tr>
<tr><td>8</td><td>Tennessee</td><td>94.56</td><td>42</td><td>California</td><td>91.82</td></tr>
<tr><td>35</td><td>Texas</td><td>92.53</td><td>43</td><td>Vermont</td><td>91.79</td></tr>
<tr><td>45</td><td>Utah</td><td>91.35</td><td>44</td><td>New Hampshire</td><td>91.36</td></tr>
<tr><td>43</td><td>Vermont</td><td>91.79</td><td>45</td><td>Utah</td><td>91.35</td></tr>
<tr><td>7</td><td>Virginia</td><td>94.79</td><td>46</td><td>Idaho</td><td>91.27</td></tr>
<tr><td>39</td><td>Washington</td><td>92.12</td><td>47</td><td>Oregon</td><td>90.71</td></tr>
<tr><td>13</td><td>West Virginia</td><td>94.36</td><td>48</td><td>Nevada</td><td>90.31</td></tr>
<tr><td>27</td><td>Wisconsin</td><td>93.20</td><td>49</td><td>New Mexico</td><td>90.25</td></tr>
<tr><td>NA</td><td>Wyoming**</td><td>NA</td><td>NA</td><td>Wyoming**</td><td>NA</td></tr>
<tr><td></td><td></td><td></td><td></td><td>District of Columbia</td><td>96.54</td></tr>
</table>

Source: U.S. Department of Health and Human Services, Centers for Disease Control and Prevention
"1993 Behavioral Risk Factor Surveillance Summary Prevalence Report" (October 1, 1994)

*Persons 18 years and older.

**Not available.

Percent of Adult Men Ever Told That Their Blood Pressure is High: 1993

National Median = 20.66% of Adult Men Have Been Told Blood Pressure is High*

ALPHA ORDER

RANK ORDER

RANK	STATE	PERCENT
39	Alabama	18.60
49	Alaska	14.65
48	Arizona	15.74
20	Arkansas	21.42
30	California	20.23
36	Colorado	19.55
11	Connecticut	22.78
19	Delaware	21.68
5	Florida	24.04
43	Georgia	17.98
3	Hawaii	24.69
31	Idaho	20.13
16	Illinois	21.95
7	Indiana	23.40
44	Iowa	17.86
21	Kansas	21.40
22	Kentucky	21.33
35	Louisiana	19.84
10	Maine	22.82
29	Maryland	20.41
27	Massachusetts	20.43
28	Michigan	20.42
15	Minnesota	22.15
1	Mississippi	27.60
23	Missouri	21.20
32	Montana	20.03
13	Nebraska	22.49
14	Nevada	22.29
6	New Hampshire	23.76
2	New Jersey	25.39
47	New Mexico	16.60
24	New York	20.80
46	North Carolina	16.76
9	North Dakota	22.95
45	Ohio	17.38
38	Oklahoma	18.96
34	Oregon	19.90
12	Pennsylvania	22.60
18	Rhode Island	21.89
4	South Carolina	24.38
41	South Dakota	18.16
26	Tennessee	20.62
40	Texas	18.44
42	Utah	18.07
16	Vermont	21.95
33	Virginia	19.97
25	Washington	20.70
8	West Virginia	23.08
37	Wisconsin	19.35
NA	Wyoming**	NA

RANK	STATE	PERCENT
1	Mississippi	27.60
2	New Jersey	25.39
3	Hawaii	24.69
4	South Carolina	24.38
5	Florida	24.04
6	New Hampshire	23.76
7	Indiana	23.40
8	West Virginia	23.08
9	North Dakota	22.95
10	Maine	22.82
11	Connecticut	22.78
12	Pennsylvania	22.60
13	Nebraska	22.49
14	Nevada	22.29
15	Minnesota	22.15
16	Illinois	21.95
16	Vermont	21.95
18	Rhode Island	21.89
19	Delaware	21.68
20	Arkansas	21.42
21	Kansas	21.40
22	Kentucky	21.33
23	Missouri	21.20
24	New York	20.80
25	Washington	20.70
26	Tennessee	20.62
27	Massachusetts	20.43
28	Michigan	20.42
29	Maryland	20.41
30	California	20.23
31	Idaho	20.13
32	Montana	20.03
33	Virginia	19.97
34	Oregon	19.90
35	Louisiana	19.84
36	Colorado	19.55
37	Wisconsin	19.35
38	Oklahoma	18.96
39	Alabama	18.60
40	Texas	18.44
41	South Dakota	18.16
42	Utah	18.07
43	Georgia	17.98
44	Iowa	17.86
45	Ohio	17.38
46	North Carolina	16.76
47	New Mexico	16.60
48	Arizona	15.74
49	Alaska	14.65
NA	Wyoming**	NA
	District of Columbia	15.49

Source: U.S. Department of Health and Human Services, Centers for Disease Control and Prevention
"1993 Behavioral Risk Factor Surveillance Summary Prevalence Report" (October 1, 1994)
*Men 18 years and older ever told that their blood pressure is high.
**Not available.

Percent of Adult Women Ever Told That Their Blood Pressure is High: 1993

National Median = 22.54% of Adult Women Have Been Told Blood Pressure is High*

ALPHA ORDER			RANK ORDER		
RANK	STATE	PERCENT	RANK	STATE	PERCENT
28	Alabama	22.23	1	Mississippi	31.79
41	Alaska	20.13	2	Missouri	27.77
37	Arizona	20.52	3	Tennessee	27.67
9	Arkansas	25.10	4	Indiana	27.04
32	California	21.79	5	South Carolina	25.98
25	Colorado	22.55	6	Idaho	25.82
27	Connecticut	22.42	7	West Virginia	25.70
24	Delaware	22.60	8	Kansas	25.66
12	Florida	24.32	9	Arkansas	25.10
11	Georgia	24.45	10	Louisiana	25.00
46	Hawaii	18.81	11	Georgia	24.45
6	Idaho	25.82	12	Florida	24.32
30	Illinois	21.84	13	Kentucky	23.80
4	Indiana	27.04	14	Rhode Island	23.65
23	Iowa	22.62	15	Nebraska	23.28
8	Kansas	25.66	16	Michigan	23.15
13	Kentucky	23.80	17	Pennsylvania	23.09
10	Louisiana	25.00	18	Oregon	23.08
36	Maine	20.75	19	Wisconsin	22.96
34	Maryland	21.61	20	Oklahoma	22.93
38	Massachusetts	20.46	21	Washington	22.90
16	Michigan	23.15	22	New York	22.68
26	Minnesota	22.54	23	Iowa	22.62
1	Mississippi	31.79	24	Delaware	22.60
2	Missouri	27.77	25	Colorado	22.55
33	Montana	21.70	26	Minnesota	22.54
15	Nebraska	23.28	27	Connecticut	22.42
29	Nevada	22.17	28	Alabama	22.23
42	New Hampshire	19.75	29	Nevada	22.17
48	New Jersey	17.15	30	Illinois	21.84
45	New Mexico	19.40	31	North Dakota	21.83
22	New York	22.68	32	California	21.79
49	North Carolina	17.06	33	Montana	21.70
31	North Dakota	21.83	34	Maryland	21.61
43	Ohio	19.58	35	Virginia	20.78
20	Oklahoma	22.93	36	Maine	20.75
18	Oregon	23.08	37	Arizona	20.52
17	Pennsylvania	23.09	38	Massachusetts	20.46
14	Rhode Island	23.65	39	South Dakota	20.40
5	South Carolina	25.98	40	Vermont	20.16
39	South Dakota	20.40	41	Alaska	20.13
3	Tennessee	27.67	42	New Hampshire	19.75
44	Texas	19.56	43	Ohio	19.58
47	Utah	18.13	44	Texas	19.56
40	Vermont	20.16	45	New Mexico	19.40
35	Virginia	20.78	46	Hawaii	18.81
21	Washington	22.90	47	Utah	18.13
7	West Virginia	25.70	48	New Jersey	17.15
19	Wisconsin	22.96	49	North Carolina	17.06
NA	Wyoming**	NA	NA	Wyoming**	NA
			District of Columbia		17.85

Source: U.S. Department of Health and Human Services, Centers for Disease Control and Prevention
   "1993 Behavioral Risk Factor Surveillance Summary Prevalence Report" (October 1, 1994)
*Women 18 years and older ever told that their blood pressure is high.
**Not available.

Percent of Adults Who Had a Blood Cholesterol Check Within Previous 5 Years: 1993

National Median = 65.02% of Adults Age 18 and Older

ALPHA ORDER

RANK	STATE	PERCENT
37	Alabama	62.21
38	Alaska	62.10
26	Arizona	64.88
46	Arkansas	60.52
15	California	67.10
27	Colorado	64.85
3	Connecticut	70.33
23	Delaware	65.46
4	Florida	69.75
31	Georgia	64.27
11	Hawaii	68.20
34	Idaho	63.19
36	Illinois	62.32
44	Indiana	60.87
13	Iowa	67.77
32	Kansas	63.93
41	Kentucky	61.60
33	Louisiana	63.49
18	Maine	66.72
7	Maryland	69.57
1	Massachusetts	73.43
8	Michigan	69.24
14	Minnesota	67.48
49	Mississippi	57.04
29	Missouri	64.39
28	Montana	64.47
39	Nebraska	62.00
45	Nevada	60.68
10	New Hampshire	68.33
5	New Jersey	69.72
48	New Mexico	59.17
17	New York	66.74
19	North Carolina	66.48
25	North Dakota	65.17
43	Ohio	61.25
35	Oklahoma	62.78
21	Oregon	66.30
20	Pennsylvania	66.42
2	Rhode Island	71.07
16	South Carolina	66.96
42	South Dakota	61.52
24	Tennessee	65.43
22	Texas	65.91
47	Utah	60.07
6	Vermont	69.65
9	Virginia	68.73
12	Washington	67.96
40	West Virginia	61.93
30	Wisconsin	64.37
NA	Wyoming*	NA

RANK ORDER

RANK	STATE	PERCENT
1	Massachusetts	73.43
2	Rhode Island	71.07
3	Connecticut	70.33
4	Florida	69.75
5	New Jersey	69.72
6	Vermont	69.65
7	Maryland	69.57
8	Michigan	69.24
9	Virginia	68.73
10	New Hampshire	68.33
11	Hawaii	68.20
12	Washington	67.96
13	Iowa	67.77
14	Minnesota	67.48
15	California	67.10
16	South Carolina	66.96
17	New York	66.74
18	Maine	66.72
19	North Carolina	66.48
20	Pennsylvania	66.42
21	Oregon	66.30
22	Texas	65.91
23	Delaware	65.46
24	Tennessee	65.43
25	North Dakota	65.17
26	Arizona	64.88
27	Colorado	64.85
28	Montana	64.47
29	Missouri	64.39
30	Wisconsin	64.37
31	Georgia	64.27
32	Kansas	63.93
33	Louisiana	63.49
34	Idaho	63.19
35	Oklahoma	62.78
36	Illinois	62.32
37	Alabama	62.21
38	Alaska	62.10
39	Nebraska	62.00
40	West Virginia	61.93
41	Kentucky	61.60
42	South Dakota	61.52
43	Ohio	61.25
44	Indiana	60.87
45	Nevada	60.68
46	Arkansas	60.52
47	Utah	60.07
48	New Mexico	59.17
49	Mississippi	57.04
NA	Wyoming*	NA

District of Columbia 63.72

Source: U.S. Department of Health and Human Services, Centers for Disease Control and Prevention
"1993 Behavioral Risk Factor Surveillance Summary Prevalence Report" (October 1, 1994)
*Not available.

Percent of Adults Who Have Ever Been Tested for AIDS: 1993

National Median = 24.99% of Adults*

ALPHA ORDER

RANK ORDER

RANK	STATE	PERCENT	RANK	STATE	PERCENT
43	Alabama	19.47	1	Nevada	39.50
2	Alaska	38.60	2	Alaska	38.60
26	Arizona	24.91	3	Florida	35.56
27	Arkansas	24.85	4	Virginia	34.36
6	California	33.59	5	Texas	33.77
8	Colorado	31.78	6	California	33.59
37	Connecticut	21.47	7	Rhode Island	32.21
12	Delaware	30.67	8	Colorado	31.78
3	Florida	35.56	9	Hawaii	31.75
21	Georgia	25.23	10	New Mexico	31.07
9	Hawaii	31.75	11	Maryland	30.87
22	Idaho	25.21	12	Delaware	30.67
25	Illinois	24.98	13	South Carolina	30.00
38	Indiana	21.40	14	Washington	29.59
49	Iowa	15.12	15	Michigan	29.02
46	Kansas	18.24	16	Mississippi	28.94
35	Kentucky	22.70	17	Louisiana	28.71
17	Louisiana	28.71	18	Oregon	27.77
48	Maine	16.00	19	New York	27.02
11	Maryland	30.87	20	New Jersey	25.76
24	Massachusetts	25.00	21	Georgia	25.23
15	Michigan	29.02	22	Idaho	25.21
32	Minnesota	23.19	23	New Hampshire	25.15
16	Mississippi	28.94	24	Massachusetts	25.00
30	Missouri	23.97	25	Illinois	24.98
28	Montana	24.68	26	Arizona	24.91
44	Nebraska	18.81	27	Arkansas	24.85
1	Nevada	39.50	28	Montana	24.68
23	New Hampshire	25.15	29	North Carolina	24.51
20	New Jersey	25.76	30	Missouri	23.97
10	New Mexico	31.07	31	Pennsylvania	23.37
19	New York	27.02	32	Minnesota	23.19
29	North Carolina	24.51	33	Wisconsin	22.96
45	North Dakota	18.69	34	Ohio	22.80
34	Ohio	22.80	35	Kentucky	22.70
39	Oklahoma	21.11	36	Tennessee	22.09
18	Oregon	27.77	37	Connecticut	21.47
31	Pennsylvania	23.37	38	Indiana	21.40
7	Rhode Island	32.21	39	Oklahoma	21.11
13	South Carolina	30.00	40	Vermont	19.87
47	South Dakota	16.62	41	West Virginia	19.68
36	Tennessee	22.09	42	Utah	19.54
5	Texas	33.77	43	Alabama	19.47
42	Utah	19.54	44	Nebraska	18.81
40	Vermont	19.87	45	North Dakota	18.69
4	Virginia	34.36	46	Kansas	18.24
14	Washington	29.59	47	South Dakota	16.62
41	West Virginia	19.68	48	Maine	16.00
33	Wisconsin	22.96	49	Iowa	15.12
NA	Wyoming**	NA	NA	Wyoming**	NA
				District of Columbia	26.98

Source: U.S. Department of Health and Human Services, Centers for Disease Control and Prevention
  "1993 Behavioral Risk Factor Surveillance Summary Prevalence Report" (October 1, 1994)
*Persons 18 to 64 years old.
**Not available.

Percent of Adults Who Believe They Have a High Chance of Getting AIDS: 1993

National Median = 2.09% of Adults*

<u>ALPHA ORDER</u>

RANK	STATE	PERCENT
5	Alabama	2.78
35	Alaska	1.64
31	Arizona	1.72
8	Arkansas	2.75
1	California	3.82
28	Colorado	1.83
25	Connecticut	2.08
6	Delaware	2.76
4	Florida	3.11
36	Georgia	1.62
34	Hawaii	1.66
27	Idaho	1.84
22	Illinois	2.16
41	Indiana	1.44
39	Iowa	1.54
19	Kansas	2.25
13	Kentucky	2.59
14	Louisiana	2.55
2	Maine	3.54
37	Maryland	1.57
45	Massachusetts	1.28
18	Michigan	2.29
42	Minnesota	1.40
9	Mississippi	2.74
33	Missouri	1.69
49	Montana	0.76
38	Nebraska	1.56
16	Nevada	2.39
26	New Hampshire	1.85
24	New Jersey	2.10
9	New Mexico	2.74
17	New York	2.30
20	North Carolina	2.23
44	North Dakota	1.37
29	Ohio	1.75
21	Oklahoma	2.20
31	Oregon	1.72
30	Pennsylvania	1.73
40	Rhode Island	1.50
6	South Carolina	2.76
46	South Dakota	1.27
11	Tennessee	2.71
3	Texas	3.18
47	Utah	1.23
48	Vermont	0.89
15	Virginia	2.40
43	Washington	1.38
12	West Virginia	2.65
22	Wisconsin	2.16
NA	Wyoming**	NA

<u>RANK ORDER</u>

RANK	STATE	PERCENT
1	California	3.82
2	Maine	3.54
3	Texas	3.18
4	Florida	3.11
5	Alabama	2.78
6	Delaware	2.76
6	South Carolina	2.76
8	Arkansas	2.75
9	Mississippi	2.74
9	New Mexico	2.74
11	Tennessee	2.71
12	West Virginia	2.65
13	Kentucky	2.59
14	Louisiana	2.55
15	Virginia	2.40
16	Nevada	2.39
17	New York	2.30
18	Michigan	2.29
19	Kansas	2.25
20	North Carolina	2.23
21	Oklahoma	2.20
22	Illinois	2.16
22	Wisconsin	2.16
24	New Jersey	2.10
25	Connecticut	2.08
26	New Hampshire	1.85
27	Idaho	1.84
28	Colorado	1.83
29	Ohio	1.75
30	Pennsylvania	1.73
31	Arizona	1.72
31	Oregon	1.72
33	Missouri	1.69
34	Hawaii	1.66
35	Alaska	1.64
36	Georgia	1.62
37	Maryland	1.57
38	Nebraska	1.56
39	Iowa	1.54
40	Rhode Island	1.50
41	Indiana	1.44
42	Minnesota	1.40
43	Washington	1.38
44	North Dakota	1.37
45	Massachusetts	1.28
46	South Dakota	1.27
47	Utah	1.23
48	Vermont	0.89
49	Montana	0.76
NA	Wyoming**	NA
	District of Columbia	2.20

Source: U.S. Department of Health and Human Services, Centers for Disease Control and Prevention
"1993 Behavioral Risk Factor Surveillance Summary Prevalence Report" (October 1, 1994)
*Persons 18 to 64 years old.
**Not available.

Percent of Adults Who Would Not Let Child
Attend School with AIDS Infected Classmate: 1993
National Median = 12.16% of Adults*

ALPHA ORDER   RANK ORDER

RANK	STATE	PERCENT		RANK	STATE	PERCENT
4	Alabama	18.75		1	Mississippi	22.60
18	Alaska	13.80		2	Kentucky	19.61
32	Arizona	11.19		3	Florida	18.85
8	Arkansas	17.29		4	Alabama	18.75
9	California	17.06		5	Louisiana	18.58
26	Colorado	11.92		6	Tennessee	18.42
29	Connecticut	11.36		7	Michigan	17.50
22	Delaware	13.34		8	Arkansas	17.29
3	Florida	18.85		9	California	17.06
11	Georgia	16.26		10	South Carolina	16.96
19	Hawaii	13.73		11	Georgia	16.26
24	Idaho	12.20		12	West Virginia	15.20
27	Illinois	11.66		13	Virginia	14.96
31	Indiana	11.29		14	New York	14.95
45	Iowa	7.25		15	New Jersey	14.88
49	Kansas	4.50		16	North Carolina	14.78
2	Kentucky	19.61		17	Texas	14.24
5	Louisiana	18.58		18	Alaska	13.80
47	Maine	6.85		19	Hawaii	13.73
37	Maryland	9.72		20	Missouri	13.72
40	Massachusetts	9.24		20	Pennsylvania	13.72
7	Michigan	17.50		22	Delaware	13.34
44	Minnesota	7.98		23	Montana	12.97
1	Mississippi	22.60		24	Idaho	12.20
20	Missouri	13.72		25	Ohio	12.13
23	Montana	12.97		26	Colorado	11.92
41	Nebraska	9.03		27	Illinois	11.66
28	Nevada	11.43		28	Nevada	11.43
46	New Hampshire	7.22		29	Connecticut	11.36
15	New Jersey	14.88		30	Oklahoma	11.32
33	New Mexico	11.13		31	Indiana	11.29
14	New York	14.95		32	Arizona	11.19
16	North Carolina	14.78		33	New Mexico	11.13
35	North Dakota	10.47		34	Rhode Island	10.81
25	Ohio	12.13		35	North Dakota	10.47
30	Oklahoma	11.32		36	Oregon	10.29
36	Oregon	10.29		37	Maryland	9.72
20	Pennsylvania	13.72		38	Wisconsin	9.42
34	Rhode Island	10.81		39	Washington	9.27
10	South Carolina	16.96		40	Massachusetts	9.24
43	South Dakota	8.00		41	Nebraska	9.03
6	Tennessee	18.42		42	Utah	8.53
17	Texas	14.24		43	South Dakota	8.00
42	Utah	8.53		44	Minnesota	7.98
48	Vermont	5.58		45	Iowa	7.25
13	Virginia	14.96		46	New Hampshire	7.22
39	Washington	9.27		47	Maine	6.85
12	West Virginia	15.20		48	Vermont	5.58
38	Wisconsin	9.42		49	Kansas	4.50
NA	Wyoming**	NA		NA	Wyoming**	NA
					District of Columbia	14.98

Source: U.S. Department of Health and Human Services, Centers for Disease Control and Prevention
"1993 Behavioral Risk Factor Surveillance Summary Prevalence Report" (October 1, 1994)
*Persons 18 to 64 years old with children.
**Not available.

Safety Belt Usage Rate in 1994

National Percent = 66% Use Safety Belts*

ALPHA ORDER			RANK ORDER		
RANK	STATE	PERCENT	RANK	STATE	PERCENT
37	Alabama	55	1	Hawaii	84
16	Alaska	69	2	California	83
7	Arizona	73	3	North Carolina	81
40	Arkansas	51	3	Washington	81
2	California	83	5	New Mexico	79
38	Colorado	54	6	Oregon	77
9	Connecticut	72	7	Arizona	73
26	Delaware	63	7	Iowa	73
29	Florida	61	9	Connecticut	72
34	Georgia	57	9	New York	72
1	Hawaii	84	9	Pennsylvania	72
29	Idaho	61	9	Virginia	72
19	Illinois	68	13	Nevada	71
36	Indiana	56	13	Texas	71
7	Iowa	73	15	Kansas	70
15	Kansas	70	16	Alaska	69
32	Kentucky	58	16	Maryland	69
41	Louisiana	50	16	Montana	69
NA	Maine**	NA	19	Illinois	68
16	Maryland	69	19	Missouri	68
42	Massachusetts	47	19	Vermont	68
22	Michigan	66	22	Michigan	66
34	Minnesota	57	23	New Jersey	64
44	Mississippi	43	23	South Carolina	64
19	Missouri	68	23	Wisconsin	64
16	Montana	69	26	Delaware	63
26	Nebraska	63	26	Nebraska	63
13	Nevada	71	28	Ohio	62
NA	New Hampshire**	NA	29	Florida	61
23	New Jersey	64	29	Idaho	61
5	New Mexico	79	31	Tennessee	60
9	New York	72	32	Kentucky	58
3	North Carolina	81	32	West Virginia	58
46	North Dakota	32	34	Georgia	57
28	Ohio	62	34	Minnesota	57
43	Oklahoma	45	36	Indiana	56
6	Oregon	77	37	Alabama	55
9	Pennsylvania	72	38	Colorado	54
46	Rhode Island	32	39	Utah	53
23	South Carolina	64	40	Arkansas	51
45	South Dakota	40	41	Louisiana	50
31	Tennessee	60	42	Massachusetts	47
13	Texas	71	43	Oklahoma	45
39	Utah	53	44	Mississippi	43
19	Vermont	68	45	South Dakota	40
9	Virginia	72	46	North Dakota	32
3	Washington	81	46	Rhode Island	32
32	West Virginia	58	NA	Maine**	NA
23	Wisconsin	64	NA	New Hampshire**	NA
NA	Wyoming**	NA	NA	Wyoming**	NA
				District of Columbia	62

Source: U.S. Department of Transportation, National Highway Safety Traffic Safety Administration
"Legislative Fact Sheet" (January 1995)
*As of December 1994 except national percent is as of December 1993.
**Not reported.

Percent of Adults Requiring Their Children to Wear Safety Belts: 1993

National Median = 32.77% of Adults*

ALPHA ORDER				RANK ORDER		
RANK	STATE	PERCENT		RANK	STATE	PERCENT
45	Alabama	28.28		1	Utah	42.00
2	Alaska	41.36		2	Alaska	41.36
29	Arizona	32.27		3	California	39.10
33	Arkansas	31.20		4	New Mexico	38.18
3	California	39.10		5	Hawaii	37.78
15	Colorado	34.02		6	Texas	36.81
34	Connecticut	30.70		7	Idaho	36.56
19	Delaware	33.29		8	Oregon	35.07
41	Florida	29.66		9	Maryland	35.00
16	Georgia	33.85		10	South Carolina	34.96
5	Hawaii	37.78		11	Michigan	34.93
7	Idaho	36.56		12	Nevada	34.81
21	Illinois	33.14		13	Washington	34.61
27	Indiana	32.58		14	Virginia	34.31
32	Iowa	31.35		15	Colorado	34.02
40	Kansas	29.72		16	Georgia	33.85
35	Kentucky	30.49		17	Maine	33.66
20	Louisiana	33.28		18	New Jersey	33.52
17	Maine	33.66		19	Delaware	33.29
9	Maryland	35.00		20	Louisiana	33.28
42	Massachusetts	29.38		21	Illinois	33.14
11	Michigan	34.93		22	Minnesota	33.11
22	Minnesota	33.11		22	Montana	33.11
28	Mississippi	32.36		22	North Carolina	33.11
30	Missouri	31.79		25	Tennessee	32.78
22	Montana	33.11		26	New Hampshire	32.77
39	Nebraska	29.81		27	Indiana	32.58
12	Nevada	34.81		28	Mississippi	32.36
26	New Hampshire	32.77		29	Arizona	32.27
18	New Jersey	33.52		30	Missouri	31.79
4	New Mexico	38.18		31	Vermont	31.65
44	New York	28.84		32	Iowa	31.35
22	North Carolina	33.11		33	Arkansas	31.20
46	North Dakota	28.15		34	Connecticut	30.70
37	Ohio	30.09		35	Kentucky	30.49
38	Oklahoma	30.04		36	Wisconsin	30.19
8	Oregon	35.07		37	Ohio	30.09
43	Pennsylvania	28.94		38	Oklahoma	30.04
48	Rhode Island	26.97		39	Nebraska	29.81
10	South Carolina	34.96		40	Kansas	29.72
49	South Dakota	24.09		41	Florida	29.66
25	Tennessee	32.78		42	Massachusetts	29.38
6	Texas	36.81		43	Pennsylvania	28.94
1	Utah	42.00		44	New York	28.84
31	Vermont	31.65		45	Alabama	28.28
14	Virginia	34.31		46	North Dakota	28.15
13	Washington	34.61		47	West Virginia	28.14
47	West Virginia	28.14		48	Rhode Island	26.97
36	Wisconsin	30.19		49	South Dakota	24.09
NA	Wyoming**	NA		NA	Wyoming**	NA
					District of Columbia	16.22

Source: U.S. Department of Health and Human Services, Centers for Disease Control and Prevention
"1993 Behavioral Risk Factor Surveillance Summary Prevalence Report" (October 1, 1994)
*Persons 18 and older with children under 15 years old who always or nearly always require their children to use safety belts.
**Not available.

VIII. APPENDIX

Population Charts

Population in 1994

National Total = 260,341,000*

ALPHA ORDER					RANK ORDER			
RANK	STATE	POPULATION	% of USA		RANK	STATE	POPULATION	% of USA
22	Alabama	4,219,000	1.62%		1	California	31,431,000	12.07%
48	Alaska	606,000	0.23%		2	Texas	18,378,000	7.06%
23	Arizona	4,075,000	1.57%		3	New York	18,169,000	6.98%
33	Arkansas	2,453,000	0.94%		4	Florida	13,953,000	5.36%
1	California	31,431,000	12.07%		5	Pennsylvania	12,052,000	4.63%
26	Colorado	3,656,000	1.40%		6	Illinois	11,752,000	4.51%
27	Connecticut	3,275,000	1.26%		7	Ohio	11,102,000	4.26%
46	Delaware	706,000	0.27%		8	Michigan	9,496,000	3.65%
4	Florida	13,953,000	5.36%		9	New Jersey	7,904,000	3.04%
11	Georgia	7,055,000	2.71%		10	North Carolina	7,070,000	2.72%
40	Hawaii	1,179,000	0.45%		11	Georgia	7,055,000	2.71%
42	Idaho	1,133,000	0.44%		12	Virginia	6,552,000	2.52%
6	Illinois	11,752,000	4.51%		13	Massachusetts	6,041,000	2.32%
14	Indiana	5,752,000	2.21%		14	Indiana	5,752,000	2.21%
30	Iowa	2,829,000	1.09%		15	Washington	5,343,000	2.05%
32	Kansas	2,554,000	0.98%		16	Missouri	5,278,000	2.03%
24	Kentucky	3,827,000	1.47%		17	Tennessee	5,175,000	1.99%
21	Louisiana	4,315,000	1.66%		18	Wisconsin	5,082,000	1.95%
39	Maine	1,240,000	0.48%		19	Maryland	5,006,000	1.92%
19	Maryland	5,006,000	1.92%		20	Minnesota	4,567,000	1.75%
13	Massachusetts	6,041,000	2.32%		21	Louisiana	4,315,000	1.66%
8	Michigan	9,496,000	3.65%		22	Alabama	4,219,000	1.62%
20	Minnesota	4,567,000	1.75%		23	Arizona	4,075,000	1.57%
31	Mississippi	2,669,000	1.03%		24	Kentucky	3,827,000	1.47%
16	Missouri	5,278,000	2.03%		25	South Carolina	3,664,000	1.41%
44	Montana	856,000	0.33%		26	Colorado	3,656,000	1.40%
37	Nebraska	1,623,000	0.62%		27	Connecticut	3,275,000	1.26%
38	Nevada	1,457,000	0.56%		28	Oklahoma	3,258,000	1.25%
41	New Hampshire	1,137,000	0.44%		29	Oregon	3,086,000	1.19%
9	New Jersey	7,904,000	3.04%		30	Iowa	2,829,000	1.09%
36	New Mexico	1,654,000	0.64%		31	Mississippi	2,669,000	1.03%
3	New York	18,169,000	6.98%		32	Kansas	2,554,000	0.98%
10	North Carolina	7,070,000	2.72%		33	Arkansas	2,453,000	0.94%
47	North Dakota	638,000	0.25%		34	Utah	1,908,000	0.73%
7	Ohio	11,102,000	4.26%		35	West Virginia	1,822,000	0.70%
28	Oklahoma	3,258,000	1.25%		36	New Mexico	1,654,000	0.64%
29	Oregon	3,086,000	1.19%		37	Nebraska	1,623,000	0.62%
5	Pennsylvania	12,052,000	4.63%		38	Nevada	1,457,000	0.56%
43	Rhode Island	997,000	0.38%		39	Maine	1,240,000	0.48%
25	South Carolina	3,664,000	1.41%		40	Hawaii	1,179,000	0.45%
45	South Dakota	721,000	0.28%		41	New Hampshire	1,137,000	0.44%
17	Tennessee	5,175,000	1.99%		42	Idaho	1,133,000	0.44%
2	Texas	18,378,000	7.06%		43	Rhode Island	997,000	0.38%
34	Utah	1,908,000	0.73%		44	Montana	856,000	0.33%
49	Vermont	580,000	0.22%		45	South Dakota	721,000	0.28%
12	Virginia	6,552,000	2.52%		46	Delaware	706,000	0.27%
15	Washington	5,343,000	2.05%		47	North Dakota	638,000	0.25%
35	West Virginia	1,822,000	0.70%		48	Alaska	606,000	0.23%
18	Wisconsin	5,082,000	1.95%		49	Vermont	580,000	0.22%
50	Wyoming	476,000	0.18%		50	Wyoming	476,000	0.18%
						District of Columbia	570,000	0.22%

Source: U.S. Bureau of the Census
  Press Release (CB94-204, December 28, 1994)
*Includes armed forces residing in each state.

Male Population in 1994

National Total = 127,076,429

ALPHA ORDER					RANK ORDER			
RANK	STATE	MALES	% of USA		RANK	STATE	MALES	% of USA
22	Alabama	2,023,403	1.59%		1	California	15,720,782	12.37%
47	Alaska	319,598	0.25%		2	Texas	9,060,469	7.13%
23	Arizona	2,013,824	1.58%		3	New York	8,734,152	6.87%
33	Arkansas	1,183,096	0.93%		4	Florida	6,758,180	5.32%
1	California	15,720,782	12.37%		5	Pennsylvania	5,787,005	4.55%
25	Colorado	1,811,503	1.43%		6	Illinois	5,716,632	4.50%
28	Connecticut	1,587,176	1.25%		7	Ohio	5,358,944	4.22%
46	Delaware	343,531	0.27%		8	Michigan	4,616,830	3.63%
4	Florida	6,758,180	5.32%		9	New Jersey	3,823,815	3.01%
11	Georgia	3,429,343	2.70%		10	North Carolina	3,429,722	2.70%
40	Hawaii	596,811	0.47%		11	Georgia	3,429,343	2.70%
41	Idaho	564,945	0.44%		12	Virginia	3,207,571	2.52%
6	Illinois	5,716,632	4.50%		13	Massachusetts	2,907,484	2.29%
14	Indiana	2,793,573	2.20%		14	Indiana	2,793,573	2.20%
30	Iowa	1,374,784	1.08%		15	Washington	2,651,976	2.09%
32	Kansas	1,255,555	0.99%		16	Missouri	2,548,682	2.01%
24	Kentucky	1,854,625	1.46%		17	Tennessee	2,494,696	1.96%
21	Louisiana	2,075,925	1.63%		18	Wisconsin	2,492,094	1.96%
39	Maine	603,754	0.48%		19	Maryland	2,431,171	1.91%
19	Maryland	2,431,171	1.91%		20	Minnesota	2,245,829	1.77%
13	Massachusetts	2,907,484	2.29%		21	Louisiana	2,075,925	1.63%
8	Michigan	4,616,830	3.63%		22	Alabama	2,023,403	1.59%
20	Minnesota	2,245,829	1.77%		23	Arizona	2,013,824	1.58%
31	Mississippi	1,278,831	1.01%		24	Kentucky	1,854,625	1.46%
16	Missouri	2,548,682	2.01%		25	Colorado	1,811,503	1.43%
44	Montana	425,505	0.33%		26	South Carolina	1,770,092	1.39%
37	Nebraska	792,590	0.62%		27	Oklahoma	1,589,126	1.25%
38	Nevada	741,607	0.58%		28	Connecticut	1,587,176	1.25%
42	New Hampshire	557,587	0.44%		29	Oregon	1,520,980	1.20%
9	New Jersey	3,823,815	3.01%		30	Iowa	1,374,784	1.08%
36	New Mexico	814,515	0.64%		31	Mississippi	1,278,831	1.01%
3	New York	8,734,152	6.87%		32	Kansas	1,255,555	0.99%
10	North Carolina	3,429,722	2.70%		33	Arkansas	1,183,096	0.93%
48	North Dakota	317,899	0.25%		34	Utah	948,807	0.75%
7	Ohio	5,358,944	4.22%		35	West Virginia	877,090	0.69%
27	Oklahoma	1,589,126	1.25%		36	New Mexico	814,515	0.64%
29	Oregon	1,520,980	1.20%		37	Nebraska	792,590	0.62%
5	Pennsylvania	5,787,005	4.55%		38	Nevada	741,607	0.58%
43	Rhode Island	478,926	0.38%		39	Maine	603,754	0.48%
26	South Carolina	1,770,092	1.39%		40	Hawaii	596,811	0.47%
45	South Dakota	355,197	0.28%		41	Idaho	564,945	0.44%
17	Tennessee	2,494,696	1.96%		42	New Hampshire	557,587	0.44%
2	Texas	9,060,469	7.13%		43	Rhode Island	478,926	0.38%
34	Utah	948,807	0.75%		44	Montana	425,505	0.33%
49	Vermont	284,935	0.22%		45	South Dakota	355,197	0.28%
12	Virginia	3,207,571	2.52%		46	Delaware	343,531	0.27%
15	Washington	2,651,976	2.09%		47	Alaska	319,598	0.25%
35	West Virginia	877,090	0.69%		48	North Dakota	317,899	0.25%
18	Wisconsin	2,492,094	1.96%		49	Vermont	284,935	0.22%
50	Wyoming	239,218	0.19%		50	Wyoming	239,218	0.19%
						District of Columbia	266,044	0.21%

Source: U.S. Bureau of the Census
Census Advisory (CB95-39, March 1, 1995)

Female Population in 1994

National Total = 133,264,561

ALPHA ORDER					RANK ORDER			
RANK	STATE	FEMALES	% of USA		RANK	STATE	FEMALES	% of USA
22	Alabama	2,195,389	1.65%		1	California	15,709,915	11.79%
49	Alaska	286,678	0.22%		2	New York	9,434,899	7.08%
23	Arizona	2,061,228	1.55%		3	Texas	9,317,716	6.99%
33	Arkansas	1,269,575	0.95%		4	Florida	7,194,534	5.40%
1	California	15,709,915	11.79%		5	Pennsylvania	6,265,362	4.70%
26	Colorado	1,844,144	1.38%		6	Illinois	6,035,142	4.53%
27	Connecticut	1,688,075	1.27%		7	Ohio	5,743,254	4.31%
46	Delaware	362,820	0.27%		8	Michigan	4,879,317	3.66%
4	Florida	7,194,534	5.40%		9	New Jersey	4,080,110	3.06%
11	Georgia	3,625,993	2.72%		10	North Carolina	3,640,114	2.73%
40	Hawaii	581,753	0.44%		11	Georgia	3,625,993	2.72%
42	Idaho	568,089	0.43%		12	Virginia	3,343,951	2.51%
6	Illinois	6,035,142	4.53%		13	Massachusetts	3,133,639	2.35%
14	Indiana	2,958,500	2.22%		14	Indiana	2,958,500	2.22%
30	Iowa	1,454,468	1.09%		15	Missouri	2,728,958	2.05%
32	Kansas	1,298,492	0.97%		16	Washington	2,691,114	2.02%
24	Kentucky	1,972,169	1.48%		17	Tennessee	2,680,544	2.01%
21	Louisiana	2,239,160	1.68%		18	Wisconsin	2,589,564	1.94%
39	Maine	636,455	0.48%		19	Maryland	2,575,094	1.93%
19	Maryland	2,575,094	1.93%		20	Minnesota	2,321,438	1.74%
13	Massachusetts	3,133,639	2.35%		21	Louisiana	2,239,160	1.68%
8	Michigan	4,879,317	3.66%		22	Alabama	2,195,389	1.65%
20	Minnesota	2,321,438	1.74%		23	Arizona	2,061,228	1.55%
31	Mississippi	1,390,280	1.04%		24	Kentucky	1,972,169	1.48%
15	Missouri	2,728,958	2.05%		25	South Carolina	1,893,892	1.42%
44	Montana	430,542	0.32%		26	Colorado	1,844,144	1.38%
37	Nebraska	830,268	0.62%		27	Connecticut	1,688,075	1.27%
38	Nevada	715,421	0.54%		28	Oklahoma	1,668,943	1.25%
41	New Hampshire	579,233	0.43%		29	Oregon	1,565,208	1.17%
9	New Jersey	4,080,110	3.06%		30	Iowa	1,454,468	1.09%
36	New Mexico	839,006	0.63%		31	Mississippi	1,390,280	1.04%
2	New York	9,434,899	7.08%		32	Kansas	1,298,492	0.97%
10	North Carolina	3,640,114	2.73%		33	Arkansas	1,269,575	0.95%
47	North Dakota	320,089	0.24%		34	Utah	959,129	0.72%
7	Ohio	5,743,254	4.31%		35	West Virginia	944,931	0.71%
28	Oklahoma	1,668,943	1.25%		36	New Mexico	839,006	0.63%
29	Oregon	1,565,208	1.17%		37	Nebraska	830,268	0.62%
5	Pennsylvania	6,265,362	4.70%		38	Nevada	715,421	0.54%
43	Rhode Island	517,831	0.39%		39	Maine	636,455	0.48%
25	South Carolina	1,893,892	1.42%		40	Hawaii	581,753	0.44%
45	South Dakota	365,967	0.27%		41	New Hampshire	579,233	0.43%
17	Tennessee	2,680,544	2.01%		42	Idaho	568,089	0.43%
3	Texas	9,317,716	6.99%		43	Rhode Island	517,831	0.39%
34	Utah	959,129	0.72%		44	Montana	430,542	0.32%
48	Vermont	295,274	0.22%		45	South Dakota	365,967	0.27%
12	Virginia	3,343,951	2.51%		46	Delaware	362,820	0.27%
16	Washington	2,691,114	2.02%		47	North Dakota	320,089	0.24%
35	West Virginia	944,931	0.71%		48	Vermont	295,274	0.22%
18	Wisconsin	2,589,564	1.94%		49	Alaska	286,678	0.22%
50	Wyoming	236,763	0.18%		50	Wyoming	236,763	0.18%
					District of Columbia		304,131	0.23%

Source: U.S. Bureau of the Census
  Census Advisory (CB95-39, March 1, 1995)

Population in 1993

National Total = 255,723,000*

ALPHA ORDER					RANK ORDER			
RANK	STATE	POPULATION	% of USA		RANK	STATE	POPULATION	% of USA
22	Alabama	4,181,000	1.63%		1	California	31,217,000	12.20%
48	Alaska	598,000	0.23%		2	New York	18,153,000	7.10%
23	Arizona	3,945,000	1.54%		3	Texas	18,022,000	7.05%
33	Arkansas	2,426,000	0.95%		4	Florida	13,726,000	5.37%
1	California	31,217,000	12.20%		5	Pennsylvania	12,030,000	4.70%
26	Colorado	3,564,000	1.39%		6	Illinois	11,686,000	4.57%
27	Connecticut	3,278,000	1.28%		7	Ohio	11,061,000	4.32%
46	Delaware	698,000	0.27%		8	Michigan	9,460,000	3.70%
4	Florida	13,726,000	5.37%		9	New Jersey	7,859,000	3.07%
11	Georgia	6,902,000	2.70%		10	North Carolina	6,952,000	2.72%
40	Hawaii	1,166,000	0.46%		11	Georgia	6,902,000	2.70%
42	Idaho	1,100,000	0.43%		12	Virginia	6,473,000	2.53%
6	Illinois	11,686,000	4.57%		13	Massachusetts	6,018,000	2.35%
14	Indiana	5,706,000	2.23%		14	Indiana	5,706,000	2.23%
30	Iowa	2,821,000	1.10%		15	Washington	5,259,000	2.06%
32	Kansas	2,535,000	0.99%		16	Missouri	5,235,000	2.05%
24	Kentucky	3,794,000	1.48%		17	Tennessee	5,094,000	1.99%
21	Louisiana	4,290,000	1.68%		18	Wisconsin	5,044,000	1.97%
39	Maine	1,240,000	0.48%		19	Maryland	4,958,000	1.94%
19	Maryland	4,958,000	1.94%		20	Minnesota	4,524,000	1.77%
13	Massachusetts	6,018,000	2.35%		21	Louisiana	4,290,000	1.68%
8	Michigan	9,460,000	3.70%		22	Alabama	4,181,000	1.63%
20	Minnesota	4,524,000	1.77%		23	Arizona	3,945,000	1.54%
31	Mississippi	2,640,000	1.03%		24	Kentucky	3,794,000	1.48%
16	Missouri	5,235,000	2.05%		25	South Carolina	3,630,000	1.42%
44	Montana	841,000	0.33%		26	Colorado	3,564,000	1.39%
37	Nebraska	1,613,000	0.63%		27	Connecticut	3,278,000	1.28%
38	Nevada	1,382,000	0.54%		28	Oklahoma	3,233,000	1.26%
41	New Hampshire	1,124,000	0.44%		29	Oregon	3,035,000	1.19%
9	New Jersey	7,859,000	3.07%		30	Iowa	2,821,000	1.10%
36	New Mexico	1,616,000	0.63%		31	Mississippi	2,640,000	1.03%
2	New York	18,153,000	7.10%		32	Kansas	2,535,000	0.99%
10	North Carolina	6,952,000	2.72%		33	Arkansas	2,426,000	0.95%
47	North Dakota	637,000	0.25%		34	Utah	1,860,000	0.73%
7	Ohio	11,061,000	4.32%		35	West Virginia	1,818,000	0.71%
28	Oklahoma	3,233,000	1.26%		36	New Mexico	1,616,000	0.63%
29	Oregon	3,035,000	1.19%		37	Nebraska	1,613,000	0.63%
5	Pennsylvania	12,030,000	4.70%		38	Nevada	1,382,000	0.54%
43	Rhode Island	1,000,000	0.39%		39	Maine	1,240,000	0.48%
25	South Carolina	3,630,000	1.42%		40	Hawaii	1,166,000	0.46%
45	South Dakota	716,000	0.28%		41	New Hampshire	1,124,000	0.44%
17	Tennessee	5,094,000	1.99%		42	Idaho	1,100,000	0.43%
3	Texas	18,022,000	7.05%		43	Rhode Island	1,000,000	0.39%
34	Utah	1,860,000	0.73%		44	Montana	841,000	0.33%
49	Vermont	576,000	0.23%		45	South Dakota	716,000	0.28%
12	Virginia	6,473,000	2.53%		46	Delaware	698,000	0.27%
15	Washington	5,259,000	2.06%		47	North Dakota	637,000	0.25%
35	West Virginia	1,818,000	0.71%		48	Alaska	598,000	0.23%
18	Wisconsin	5,044,000	1.97%		49	Vermont	576,000	0.23%
50	Wyoming	470,000	0.18%		50	Wyoming	470,000	0.18%
						District of Columbia	579,000	0.23%

Source: U.S. Bureau of the Census
Press Release (CB94-204, December 28, 1994)
Includes armed forces residing in each state. This updates earlier 1993 population estimates.

Population in 1992

National Total = 255,028,000*

ALPHA ORDER

RANK	STATE	POPULATION	% of USA
22	Alabama	4,131,000	1.62%
48	Alaska	587,000	0.23%
23	Arizona	3,835,000	1.50%
33	Arkansas	2,395,000	0.94%
1	California	30,909,000	12.12%
26	Colorado	3,463,000	1.36%
27	Connecticut	3,279,000	1.29%
46	Delaware	690,000	0.27%
4	Florida	13,510,000	5.30%
11	Georgia	6,765,000	2.65%
40	Hawaii	1,153,000	0.45%
42	Idaho	1,066,000	0.42%
6	Illinois	11,610,000	4.55%
14	Indiana	5,652,000	2.22%
30	Iowa	2,808,000	1.10%
32	Kansas	2,518,000	0.99%
24	Kentucky	3,753,000	1.47%
21	Louisiana	4,273,000	1.68%
39	Maine	1,237,000	0.49%
19	Maryland	4,914,000	1.93%
13	Massachusetts	5,999,000	2.35%
8	Michigan	9,423,000	3.69%
20	Minnesota	4,474,000	1.75%
31	Mississippi	2,613,000	1.02%
15	Missouri	5,193,000	2.04%
44	Montana	823,000	0.32%
36	Nebraska	1,604,000	0.63%
38	Nevada	1,331,000	0.52%
41	New Hampshire	1,114,000	0.44%
9	New Jersey	7,813,000	3.06%
37	New Mexico	1,581,000	0.62%
2	New York	18,095,000	7.10%
10	North Carolina	6,838,000	2.68%
47	North Dakota	635,000	0.25%
7	Ohio	11,005,000	4.32%
28	Oklahoma	3,206,000	1.26%
29	Oregon	2,975,000	1.17%
5	Pennsylvania	11,990,000	4.70%
43	Rhode Island	1,002,000	0.39%
25	South Carolina	3,595,000	1.41%
45	South Dakota	709,000	0.28%
17	Tennessee	5,021,000	1.97%
3	Texas	17,667,000	6.93%
34	Utah	1,811,000	0.71%
49	Vermont	571,000	0.22%
12	Virginia	6,389,000	2.51%
16	Washington	5,146,000	2.02%
35	West Virginia	1,807,000	0.71%
18	Wisconsin	4,997,000	1.96%
50	Wyoming	464,000	0.18%

RANK ORDER

RANK	STATE	POPULATION	% of USA
1	California	30,909,000	12.12%
2	New York	18,095,000	7.10%
3	Texas	17,667,000	6.93%
4	Florida	13,510,000	5.30%
5	Pennsylvania	11,990,000	4.70%
6	Illinois	11,610,000	4.55%
7	Ohio	11,005,000	4.32%
8	Michigan	9,423,000	3.69%
9	New Jersey	7,813,000	3.06%
10	North Carolina	6,838,000	2.68%
11	Georgia	6,765,000	2.65%
12	Virginia	6,389,000	2.51%
13	Massachusetts	5,999,000	2.35%
14	Indiana	5,652,000	2.22%
15	Missouri	5,193,000	2.04%
16	Washington	5,146,000	2.02%
17	Tennessee	5,021,000	1.97%
18	Wisconsin	4,997,000	1.96%
19	Maryland	4,914,000	1.93%
20	Minnesota	4,474,000	1.75%
21	Louisiana	4,273,000	1.68%
22	Alabama	4,131,000	1.62%
23	Arizona	3,835,000	1.50%
24	Kentucky	3,753,000	1.47%
25	South Carolina	3,595,000	1.41%
26	Colorado	3,463,000	1.36%
27	Connecticut	3,279,000	1.29%
28	Oklahoma	3,206,000	1.26%
29	Oregon	2,975,000	1.17%
30	Iowa	2,808,000	1.10%
31	Mississippi	2,613,000	1.02%
32	Kansas	2,518,000	0.99%
33	Arkansas	2,395,000	0.94%
34	Utah	1,811,000	0.71%
35	West Virginia	1,807,000	0.71%
36	Nebraska	1,604,000	0.63%
37	New Mexico	1,581,000	0.62%
38	Nevada	1,331,000	0.52%
39	Maine	1,237,000	0.49%
40	Hawaii	1,153,000	0.45%
41	New Hampshire	1,114,000	0.44%
42	Idaho	1,066,000	0.42%
43	Rhode Island	1,002,000	0.39%
44	Montana	823,000	0.32%
45	South Dakota	709,000	0.28%
46	Delaware	690,000	0.27%
47	North Dakota	635,000	0.25%
48	Alaska	587,000	0.23%
49	Vermont	571,000	0.22%
50	Wyoming	464,000	0.18%
	District of Columbia	586,000	0.23%

Source: U.S. Bureau of the Census
Press Release (CB94-204, December 28, 1994)
*Includes armed forces residing in each state. This updates earlier 1992 population estimates.

IX. SOURCES

American Cancer Society, Inc.
1599 Clifton Road, NE
Atlanta, GA   30329-4251
800-227-2345

American Hospital Association
One North Franklin
Chicago, IL   60606-3401
312-422-3501

American Managed Care & Review Assn.
1200 19th Street, NW, Suite 200
Washington, DC   20036-1156
202-728-0506

American Medical Association
P.O. Box 10623
Chicago, IL   60610
312-464-5000

American Osteopathic Association
142 East Ontario Street
Chicago, IL   60611
312-280-5800

American Podiatric Medical Association
9312 Old Georgetown Road
Bethesda, MD   20814
301-571-9200

Bureau of the Census
3 Silver Hill and Suitland Roads
Suitland, MD   20746
301-457-2794

Bureau of Health Professions
U.S. Department of Health and Human Services
5600 Fishers Lane
Rockville, MD   20857
800-767-6732 (Nat'l Practitioners Data Bank)

Centers for Disease Control and Prevention
1600 Clifton Road, NE.
Atlanta, GA   30333
404-639-3286 (Public Affairs)

Distilled Spirits Council of the U.S., Inc.
1250 Eye Street, NW., Ste. 900
Washington, DC   20005
202-628-3544

Families USA Foundation
1334 G Street, NW
Washington, DC   20005
202-628-3030

Federation of Chiropractic Licensing Boards
901 54th Ave., Ste. 101
Greeley, CO   80634
303-356-3500

Group Health Association of America
1129 20th Street, NW Suite 600
Washington, DC   20036-3403
202-778-3200

Health Care Financing Administration
U.S. Department of Health and Human Services
6325 Security Boulevard
Baltimore, MD   21207
410-966-7843 (publications)
202-690-6113 (public affairs)

Health Insurance Association of America
1025 Connecticut Avenue, NW
Washington, DC   20036-3998
202-223-7780

Lewin-VHI, Inc.
9302 Lee Highway, Ste. 500
Fairfax, VA   22031
703-218-5500

National Center for Health Statistics
U.S. Department of Health and Human Services
6525 Belcrest Road
Hyattsville, MD   20782
301-436-8951 (vital statistics division)

National Sporting Goods Assn.
1699 Wall Street
Mt. Prospect, IL   60056
708-439-4000

Public Health Service
U.S. Department of Health and Human Services
200 Independence Avenue, SW
Washington, DC   20201
202-690-6867 (Public Information)

X. INDEX

X. INDEX (continued)

X. INDEX (continued)

CHAPTER INDEX

HOW TO USE THIS INDEX

Place left thumb on the outer edge of this page. To locate the desired entry, fold back the remaining page edges and align the index edge mark with the appropriate page edge mark.